# A Clinician's Guide to Food Allergies

# A Clinician's Guide to Food Allergies

Edited by Kevin Parker

SYRAWOOD
PUBLISHING HOUSE
New York

Published by Syrawood Publishing House,
750 Third Avenue, 9th Floor,
New York, NY 10017, USA
www.syrawoodpublishinghouse.com

**A Clinician's Guide to Food Allergies**
Edited by Kevin Parker



International Standard Book Number: 978-1-68286-451-7 (Hardback)



**Cataloging-in-publication Data**

A clinician's guide to food allergies / edited by Kevin Parker.
p. cm.
Includes bibliographical references and index.
ISBN 978-1-68286-451-7
1. Food allergy. 2. Food allergy--Diagnosis. 3. Clinical immunology. 4. Food allergy--Diet therapy. I. Parker, Kevin.
RC596 .C55 2017
616.975--dc23

Printed in the United States of America.

# TABLE OF CONTENTS

# PREFACE

This book provides comprehensive insights into the field of food allergies. It discusses in detail about the various food allergies and their symptoms and treatment. Food allergies are caused by the abnormal immune response to food. The symptoms include vomiting, hives, itchiness, diarrhea, tongue swelling, etc. The most common allergies are caused by fish, eggs, peanuts, soya, wheat, nuts, milk, etc. The topics included in this book on food allergies are of utmost significance and bound to provide incredible insights to readers. It includes some of the vital pieces of work conducted across the world, on various topics related to food allergies in order to help develop a comprehensive understanding of the discipline. Scientists and students actively engaged in this field will find this text full of crucial and unexplored concepts. It will serve as a valuable source of reference for professionals and students alike.

This book aims to highlight the current researches and provides a platform to further the scope of innovations in this area. This book is a product of the combined efforts of many researchers and scientists from different parts of the world. The objective of this book is to provide the readers with the latest information in the field.

I would like to express my sincere thanks to the authors for their dedicated efforts in the completion of this book. I acknowledge the efforts of the publisher for providing constant support. Lastly, I would like to thank my family for their support in all academic endeavors.

**Editor**

# 1

# Reduction of Cross-Reactive Carbohydrate Determinants in Plant Foodstuff: Elucidation of Clinical Relevance and Implications for Allergy Diagnosis

**Heidi Kaulfürst-Soboll[1]**[☯], **Melanie Mertens[2]**[☯], **Randolf Brehler[2]**, **Antje von Schaewen[1]***

1 Institute of Plant Biology and Biotechnology, University of Münster, Münster, Germany, 2 Department of Dermatology, University of Münster, Münster, Germany

## Abstract

***Background:*** A longstanding debate in allergy is whether or not specific immunoglobulin-E antibodies (sIgE), recognizing cross-reactive carbohydrate determinants (CCD), are able to elicit clinical symptoms. In pollen and food allergy, ≥20% of patients display *in-vitro* CCD reactivity based on presence of α1,3-fucose and/or β1,2-xylose residues on *N*-glycans of plant (xylose/fucose) and insect (fucose) glycoproteins. Because the allergenicity of tomato glycoallergen Lyc e 2 was ascribed to *N*-glycan chains alone, this study aimed at evaluating clinical relevance of CCD-reduced foodstuff in patients with carbohydrate-specific IgE (CCD-sIgE).

***Methodology/Principal Findings:*** Tomato and/or potato plants with stable reduction of Lyc e 2 (tomato) or CCD formation in general were obtained via RNA interference, and gene-silencing was confirmed by immunoblot analyses. Two different CCD-positive patient groups were compared: one with tomato and/or potato food allergy and another with hymenoptera-venom allergy (the latter to distinguish between CCD- and peptide-specific reactions in the food-allergic group). Non-allergic and CCD-negative food-allergic patients served as controls for immunoblot, basophil activation, and ImmunoCAP analyses. Basophil activation tests (BAT) revealed that Lyc e 2 is no key player among other tomato (glyco)allergens. CCD-positive patients showed decreased (re)activity with CCD-reduced foodstuff, most obvious in the hymenoptera venom-allergic but less in the food-allergic group, suggesting that *in-vivo* reactivity is primarily based on peptide- and not CCD-sIgE. Peptide epitopes remained unaffected in CCD-reduced plants, because CCD-negative patient sera showed reactivity similar to wild-type. In-house-made ImmunoCAPs, applied to investigate feasibility in routine diagnosis, confirmed BAT results at the sIgE level.

***Conclusions/Significance:*** CCD-positive hymenoptera venom-allergic patients (control group) showed basophil activation despite no allergic symptoms towards tomato and potato. Therefore, this proof-of-principle study demonstrates feasibility of CCD-reduced foodstuff to minimize 'false-positive results' in routine serum tests. Despite confirming low clinical relevance of CCD antibodies, we identified one patient with ambiguous *in-vitro* results, indicating need for further component-resolved diagnosis.

**Editor:** Lucienne Chatenoud, Université Paris Descartes, France

**Funding:** This work was supported by the Deutsche Forschungsgemeinschaft (DFG-SCHA 541/9) to AvS. The funder had no role in study design, data collection and analysis, decision to publish, or preparation of the manuscript.

**Competing Interests:** The authors have declared that no competing interests exist.

* E-mail: schaewen@uni-muenster.de

☯ These authors contributed equally to this work.

## Introduction

Specific immunoglobulin-E antibodies (sIgE) directed against plant-derived carbohydrate epitopes (cross-reactive carbohydrate determinants, CCD [1]) are ubiquitous among patients with confirmed pollen or food allergy (reviewed by Altmann) [2]. At least 20% of patients with tomato, carrot or celery allergy exhibit CCD-sIgE in their sera [3–6]. The main motifs of these carbohydrate epitopes are asparagine (*N*)-linked glycan chains carrying *core* α1,3-fucose and β1,2-xylose residues [7]. They form essential parts of two independent complex *N*-glycan epitopes found on glycoproteins of plants and lower animals, and occur in pollen, natural rubber latex, vegetables and fruits, hymenoptera venoms (only α1,3-fucose), and in some pathogenic worms but not in mammals (see Altmann) [2]. Therefore, patients with CCD-sIgE display a broad range of cross-reactions when subjected to serum investigations. In non-allergic persons, CCD-sIgE levels are usually below detection limits [8,9].

During the past decades, several investigations have been conducted on carbohydrate-sIgE antibodies concerning their ability to elicit allergic symptoms. Because sufficient evidence for their clinical relevance in pollen, food or hymenoptera-venom allergy is still lacking, CCD epitopes are mainly regarded to obscure *in-vitro* detection of true allergens [2,8,10–13]. On the other hand, some authors have concluded from their studies that in pollen- or plant food-allergic patients (e.g. with symptoms to cypress pollen, tomato, or celery) carbohydrate-specific IgE antibodies may be responsible for the allergic reactions: first, because basophil activation - a crucial type I-allergic event - was observed with native, glycosylated but not with recombinant, non-glycosylated allergens expressed in *Escherichia coli* (*E. coli*), and second, because patient sera predominantly contained CCD-sIgE [7,14–16].

In potato and tomato food allergy, several glycosylated allergens are known [16–20]. Among them are in potato (*Solanum tuberosum*), Sola t 1 (patatin, the main storage protein of tubers) decorated with up to three heterogeneous complex *N*-glycans [21–25], and Sola t 2 (a glycoprotein belonging to the family of soybean trypsin inhibitors [17]). Interestingly in tomato (*Lycopersicon esculentum* alias *Solanum lycopersicum*), only Lyc e 2 (vacuolar β-fructofuranosidase or invertase, a sucrose splitting enzyme appearing during fruit ripening [16,18,19,26,27]), is listed as glycoallergen in the official World Health Organization/ International Union of Immunological Societies (WHO/IUIS) allergen data base, although more glycoproteins of tomato are known to bind specific IgE (e.g. polygalacturonase 2A [18,19], peroxidase I [28], and pectin(-methyl)esterase [18,19]). Importantly, allergenic reactivity of Lyc e 2 (with four potential *N*-glycosylation sites) seems to depend on CCD epitopes alone [7,16].

To challenge the role of CCD-sIgE in plant food allergy, we chose two different RNA interference (RNAi) approaches to minimize CCD epitopes in plant-derived foodstuff: i) reduction of single glycoallergen Lyc e 2 in tomato, and ii) reduction of all CCD epitopes in tomato and potato (Figure 1A). The second approach employed silencing of N-acetylglucosaminyltransferase I (GNTI), an enzyme that catalyses the initial step of complex-type *N*-glycan formation in the Golgi apparatus and thus finally allows addition of *core* α1,3-fucose and β1,2-xylose in plants [29,30], referred to as CCD epitopes (Figure 1B). Both RNAi approaches (Figure 1C, general construct design) intended to maintain in other respects natural allergen composition and offer the opportunity to minimize post-harvest treatment that may influence reactivity of peptide epitopes. Lack of α1,3-fucose and β1,2-xylose residues is tolerated well under standard growth conditions by both, Arabidopsis *complex glycan less1* (*cgl1*, At4g38240) null mutants [29,31] and transgenic plants [30].

Importantly, by the chosen approach only *in-planta* synthesis of CCD epitopes was suppressed and not *N*-glycosylation *per se*, which is indispensable for correct protein folding [32] and plant vitality [33]. Therefore, RNAi-silenced tomato fruits and potato tubers could be compared to the wild-type situation with respect to sIgE and $sIgG_4$ binding as well as basophil reactivity. Two independent patient groups with carbohydrate-specific IgE antibodies were investigated: one with confirmed potato and/or tomato allergy, and another with hymenoptera-venom allergy reporting no symptoms to the plant foods. The latter served as control for solely CCD-based reactions. To investigate possible benefits of CCD-reduced material for routine allergy testing, finally, plant extracts were biotinylated and coupled to streptavidin-ImmunoCAPs.

## Results

### Lyc e 2- and CCD-reduced plant lines are viable and gene-silencing is stable for several generations

For RNAi-mediated gene silencing of glycoallergen Lyc e 2 (β-fructofuranosidase or invertase, vacuolar isoform), initially a constitutive (35S) and a tuber/fruit-specific (B33) promoter were used (Figure 1C). Both promoters proved to be equally efficient in about 30% of the tomato transformants. As revealed by immunoblot analyses with rabbit antisera specific for either Lyc e 2 (α-Le2) or CCD (α-CCD), a glycoprotein of about 52 kDa is

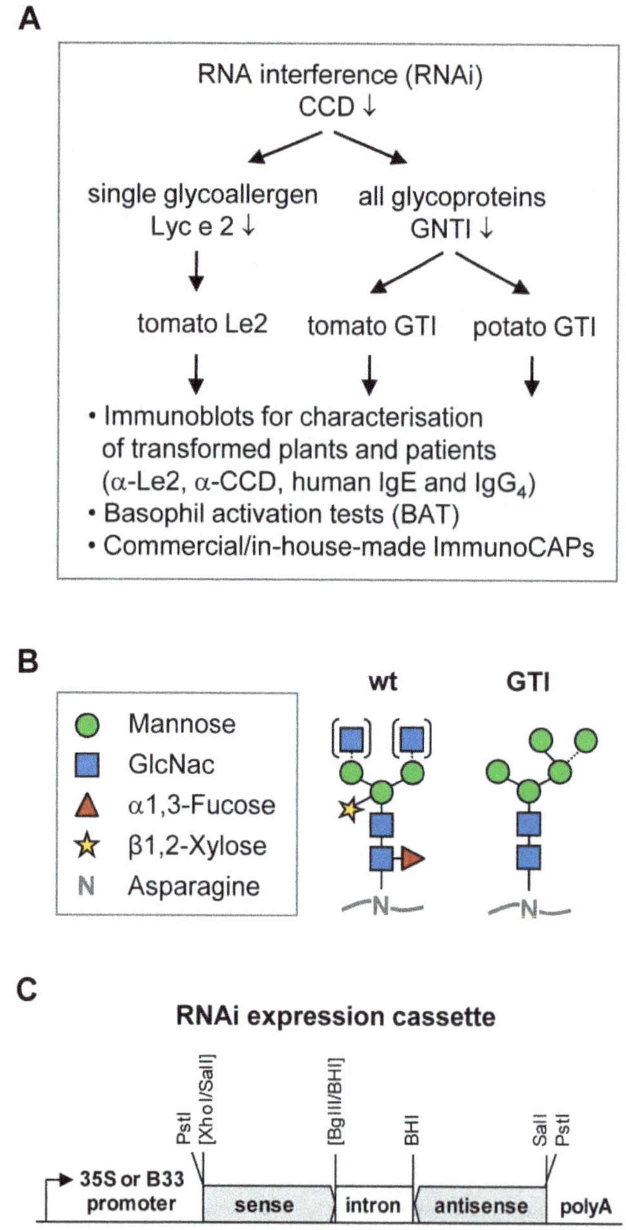


**Figure 1. Schematic of this studies' approach. A:** Flow chart of conducted experimental analyses. The impact of single glycoallergen Lyc e 2 in tomato allergy was studied by establishing Lyc e 2-reduced tomato fruits (plants further referred to as Le2). To evaluate contribution of carbohydrate- *versus* peptide-specific determinants in reactivity to foodstuff, CCD-reduced tomato and potato plants were created by silencing N-acetylglucosaminyltransferase-I (GNTI, plants further also referred to as GTI), catalyzing the crucial step leading to CCD formation in the Golgi apparatus. **B:** Predominant protein-bound *N*-glycan structures prevailing in wild-type (wt) and in GTI transformants (no CCD epitopes). *N*-glycan structures are depicted according to the proglycan system (www.proglycan.com). Note that terminal GlcNac (N-acetylglucosamine) residues are not present on fully trimmed wild-type *N*-glycans (dotted lines and brackets). **C:** RNAi-expression cassette used for Lyc e 2- or GNTI-silencing; restriction sites are indicated (destroyed ones in brackets). (BHI: BamHI; B33: tuber/fruit-specific promoter; CCD: cross-reactive carbohydrate determinants; polyA: polyadenylation signal; 35S: constitutive promoter of Cauliflower Mosaic Virus).

missing from tomato pulp tissue of Lyc e 2-silenced plants (further referred to as Le2, Figure 2A). However, since more than one band was recognized by α-Le2 in wild-type fruit extracts, proper designation of the missing band required additional analyses using peptide: N-glycosidase F (PNGase F) treatment (compare wt and Le2 *versus* a crossed Le2xGTI line, Figure S1 and Text S1). Notably, Le2 plants showed no striking phenotype in the greenhouse (Figure 2B), despite missing vacuolar β-fructofuranosidase activity (not shown).

In tomato, efficient general CCD reduction via GNTI-silencing was only achieved with the constitutive (35S) promoter. Out of 91 regenerated plants 6 (7%) displayed reduced CCD patterns. The two best lines carried CCD reduction beyond transformant generation T6. Immunoblot analyses conducted with α-CCD

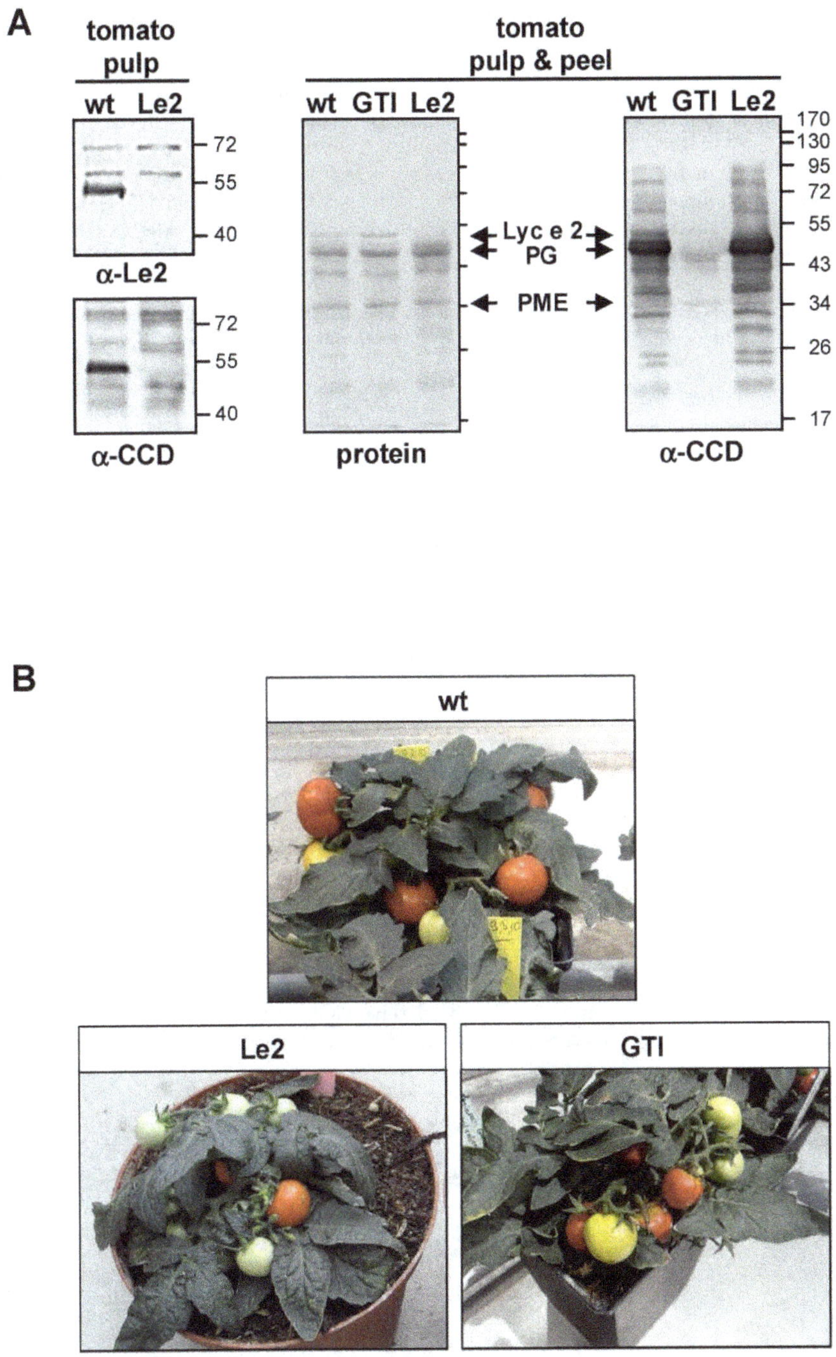


**Figure 2. Verification of successful Lyc e 2- and GNTI-silencing in tomato. A**: Immunoblots prepared with tomato fruit extracts of wild-type (wt), Lyc e 2-silenced (Le2), or GNTI-silenced (GTI) lines were developed either with α-Le2 or α-CCD polyclonal rabbit antiserum. Protein staining is shown as loading control for the blot developed with α-CCD. Note that the CCD pattern of Le2 is similar to wt, except for a faint band corresponding to Lyc e 2. Consistently with the immunoblots, enzymatic activity of vacuolar β-fructofuranosidase (invertase) was undetectable in Le2-fruit extracts (data not shown). Sizes of glycoprotein allergens are indicated: Lyc e 2 (~52 kDa), PG (polygalacturonase 2A, 46 kDa), and PME (pectin(methyl)esterase, ~35 kDa). **B**: Le2 and GTI tomato plants compared to wt. Note that both transformants are viable and form mature fruits.

showed that whole fruit extracts of selected GNTI-silenced plants (further referred to as GTI) have clearly reduced CCD patterns (Figure 2A). Compared to wild-type, only faint recognition of most abundant glycoproteins remained, namely a double band around 45 kDa and a second glycoprotein of about 35 kDa (possibly pectin(methyl)esterase, PME). In the greenhouse, GTI plants were more susceptible to stray pathogen attack compared to tomato wild-type and Le2 plants, as already observed for corresponding Arabidopsis GNTI null-mutant *cgl1* [29]. Furthermore, directly stem-associated fruit parts turned necrotic during ripening (Figure 2B and Figure S1C), and especially fruits of older plants showed a patchy, yellow-red coloration.

In potato, transformation was successful with both promoter constructs resulting in efficiently reduced CCD patterns. With the constitutive promoter, 28 out of 187 (15%) original transformants were strongly silenced, whereas with the tuber-specific promoter this was only the case for 5 out of 167 (3%) generated plants. Selected lines maintained low CCD levels during several vegetative reproduction cycles and showed no phenotype under greenhouse conditions, i.e. were indistinguishable from potato wild-type (not shown). Similarly to tomato, in CCD-reduced potato tubers only residual detection of abundant glycoproteins remained, most likely Sola t 1 (patatin of about 43 kDa) and Sola t 2 (cathepsin D-protease inhibitor of about 21 kDa) (Figure 3 and Figure S2B). From each tomato and potato set, best suppressed plants were chosen for further breeding and analyses.

## Le2 tomato fruit extracts activate basophils comparable to wild-type

Since Lyc e 2-reactivity was ascribed to CCD epitopes alone [7,16] and 32 individuals with sIgE to tomato gave no signals with recombinant, unglycosylated Lyc e 2 on immunoblots (not shown), one aim of the present study was to investigate in CCD-positive patients what impact Lyc e 2 has among all tomato allergens. When blotted Le2 extracts of whole fruits (pulp with peel) were challenged with sera of CCD-positive patients (labeled (+), Table 1), Lyc e 2 reduction was detectable but less obvious, due to many other prominent glycoproteins of similar size (exemplarily shown for PT-02(+) and PT-06(+), Figure 4A, arrows). Interestingly, in CCD-positive food-allergic patients, basophil activation

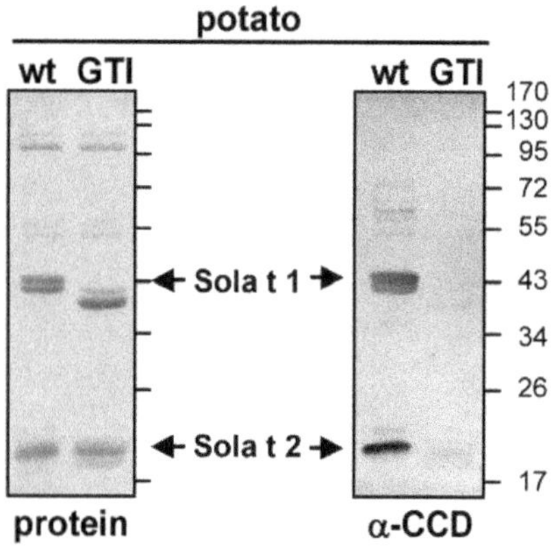


**Figure 3. Verification of successful GNTI-silencing in potato.** The immunoblot was prepared with extracts of wild-type (wt) and GNTI-silenced (GTI) tubers and developed with the CCD-specific rabbit antiserum (α-CCD). Sizes of known glycoprotein allergens Sola t 1 and Sola t 2 are indicated. The protein-stained blot confirms equal loading and reveals band shifts around 40–43 kDa in GTI extracts, likely due to different Sola t 1 (patatin) isoforms.

with Le2 extracts was comparable to wild-type (exemplarily shown for PT-02(+), Figure 4B).

## Selective loss of CCD epitopes in GTI plants

As initially observed with the CCD-specific rabbit antiserum (Figure 2A and Figure 3), all patient sera with confirmed CCD-sIgE showed strongly reduced binding to GTI samples upon immunoblot analyses with wild-type and GNTI-silenced plant extracts (Figure 5A). However, there were no obvious differences between food- and hymenoptera venom-allergic patients. As expected, sera of non-allergic subjects (NA) did not show specific IgE binding and CCD-sIgE negative sera of potato/tomato-allergic control patients did not discriminate between wild-type and GTI (Figure 5A). Furthermore, blots of additionally investigated patient sera imply that known tomato and potato allergens are detectable in both, wild-type and GTI extracts to similar extent (independent of CCD epitopes, Figure S2).

Additional analyses of CCD-sIgG$_4$ abundance also revealed clear discrimination between wild-type and CCD-reduced food-stuff for some patients (Figure 5B, marked pink), and moreover, unchanged peptide-specific binding. However, not all patients with CCD-sIgE also displayed CCD-sIgG$_4$ and *vice versa* (Figure 5, compare panels A and B), particularly obvious for PT-03(−) (CCD-sIgE negative but CCD-sIgG$_4$ positive), and PT-06(+) or BW-39(+) (CCD-sIgE positive but CCD-sIgG$_4$ negative).

## Reduced basophil activation by GTI extracts in CCD-positive patients

To investigate the capability of CCD-sIgE to trigger effector-cell activation, and to elucidate whether presence of CCD-sIgG$_4$ might have an influence, basophil-activation tests (BAT) with native plant food extracts or single plant glycoprotein horseradish peroxidase (HRP, routinely used to assess activation via CCD epitopes) were performed in a total of eight patients. Initially, three healthy non-allergic subjects were analyzed, and showed basophil activation with the positive control (α-IgE, ~20%) but not with plant food extracts or HRP (data not shown).

Interestingly, basophils of all patients with confirmed sIgE to tomato or potato (Table 1) could be activated with wild-type plant food extracts, regardless whether symptoms were reported (potato/tomato-allergic group) or not (hymenoptera venom-allergic group) (Figure 6 and Figure S3). Activation by HRP was only observed for clear-cut CCD-positive patients (Figure 6B and C, dotted line), whereas patients without CCD-sIgE (PT-03(−), Figure 6A), or borderline CCD-positive potato/tomato-allergic patients (PT-01(+) and PT-09(+), Figure S3) revealed no activation upon HRP stimulation.

For patients without HRP response, stimulation with either wild-type or GTI extracts activated basophils similarly (Figure 6A and Figure S3). In contrast, basophils of HRP-responsive patients showed clearly reduced activation by GTI extracts. For PT-38(+), BAT results differed by up to one order of magnitude between wild-type and GTI extracts, whereas PT-02(+) showed weaker but detectable CCD discrimination (Figure 6B). Best discrimination was obtained with basophils of hymenoptera venom-allergic blood donors. In this CCD-positive patient group, stimulation differed by up to two orders of magnitude between wild-type and GTI extracts (Figure 6C). CCD-sIgG$_4$ clearly present in some sera of the two CCD-positive patient groups (Figure 5B, marked pink), however, had no influence on the outcome of the BAT. For example, stimulation with potato and tomato wild-type extracts resulted in similarly strong basophil activation of BW-39(+) without CCD-sIgG$_4$ and BW-42(+) with CCD-sIgG$_4$ (compare Figure 6B and C).

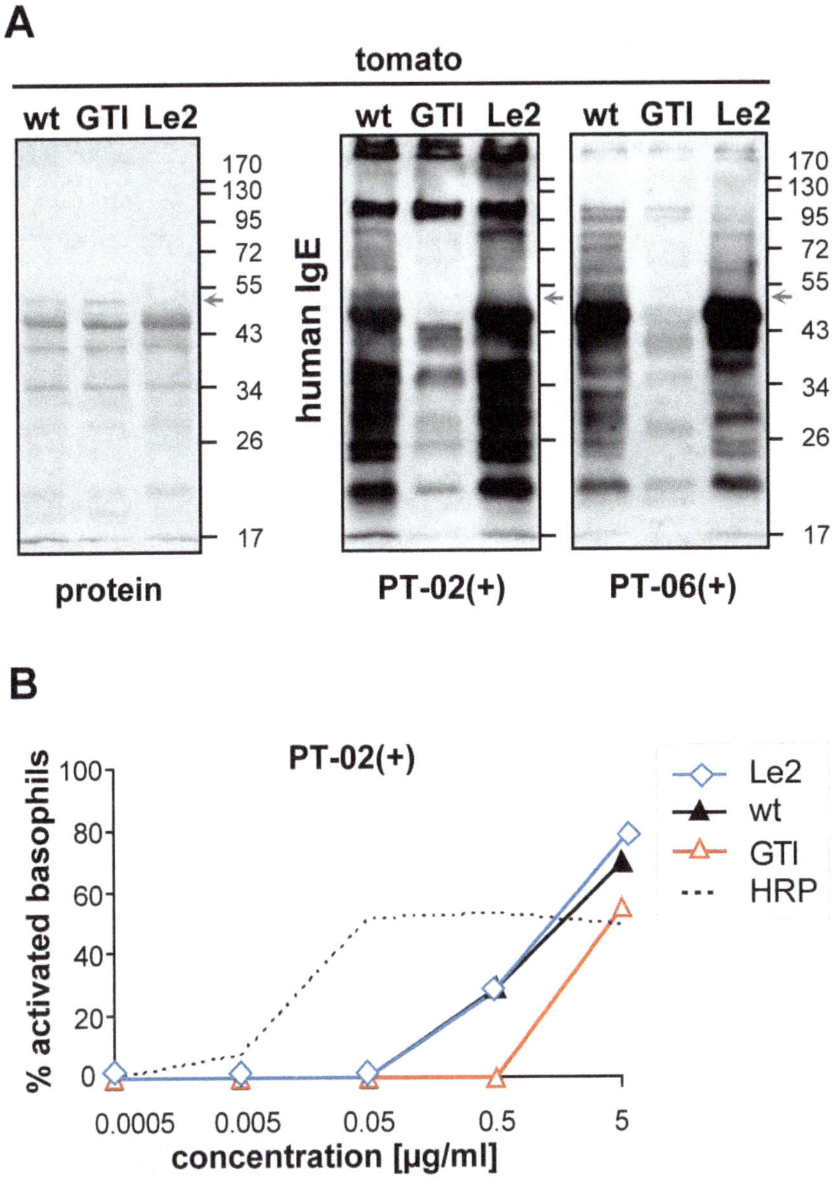


**Figure 4. Lyc e 2 seems to be no key player among other CCD-bearing glycoproteins of tomato. A**: Immunoblots prepared with whole fruit extracts (pulp with peel) of wild-type (wt), Le2, and GTI plants were developed with CCD-positive potato/tomato-allergic patient sera (PT-02(+) and PT-06(+)). Arrows point to a faint band around 52 kDa missing in Le2 (for Lyc e 2 size, compare Figure 2 and Figure S1). Protein staining is shown for equal loading. **B**: Basophil activation test of PT-02(+) with indicated tomato fruit extracts. Horseradish peroxidase (HRP), a vacuolar glycoprotein with plant-specific CCD epitopes, was used as control for CCD-dependent stimulation (dotted line).

## ImmunoCAP analyses reveal benefits of GTI extracts for allergy testing

To investigate feasibility of CCD-reduced foodstuff for allergy diagnosis, biotinylated wild-type and GTI extracts were coupled to streptavidin-ImmunoCAPs. For better comparison, sIgE values (Table 1) were plotted against each other or those obtained with commercial ImmunoCAPs (Figure 7), and additionally also against those obtained with HRP ImmunoCAP o400 (Figure S4 and Text S1). Specific IgE results determined with wild-type extracts were similar to those determined with commercial tomato (f25) and potato (f35) ImmunoCAPs (Table 1, Figure 7A and B). Furthermore, when analyzing sIgE results of wild-type and GTI ImmunoCAPs, sera of CCD-negative food-allergic patients (black circles) revealed no differences for potato and only slight differences for tomato (Figure 7C and D). By contrast, sIgE values of CCD-positive potato/tomato (PT, red squares) food-allergic and especially bee/wasp (BW, yellow triangles) hymenoptera venom-allergic patients were much lower with coupled GTI extracts as compared to wild-type (Figure 7C and D, more evident for tomato than potato), however not in all cases below the 0.35 kU/l (kilounits per liter) threshold.

## CCD inhibition reduces potato-specific IgE levels of one potato-allergic patient below threshold

To determine whether remaining sIgE recognition of GTI extracts by CCD-positive patient sera is due to residual CCD or to protein epitopes, we conducted inhibition experiments with HRP as CCD-competing glycoprotein. Initial dose-response tests

**Table 1.** Allergic symptoms (patient history), specific and total IgE (ImmunoCAP analyses) of all patients investigated.

| | | Allergic symptoms to | | | Specific IgE (kU/l) | | | | | | | | | | |
|---|---|---|---|---|---|---|---|---|---|---|---|---|---|---|---|
| | | | | | MUXF | HRP | YJV | HBV | Potato | | | Tomato | | | |
| | **Patient** | **Potato** | **Tomato** | **HV** | **o214** | **o400** | **i3** | **i1** | **f35** | **wt** | **GTI** | **f25** | **wt** | **GTI** | **Total IgE (kU/l)** |
| **CCD-negative** | **PT-03(−)** | CU (3) | OAS | – | 0.11 | 0.18 | 0.66 | 1.12 | 0.29 | 0.58 | 0.52 | 1.21 | 1.05 | 0.73 | 541 |
| | **PT-16(−)** | CU (1) | – | – | 0 | 0 | 0.01 | 0.03 | 5.02 | 3.28 | 4.08 | 0.03 | 0.02 | 0.06 | 166 |
| | **PT-20(−)** | – | OAS | – | 0 | 0 | 0 | 0 | 0.16 | 0.04 | 0.04 | 2.20 | 0.35 | 0.35 | 162 |
| | **PT-21(−)** | CU (3) | – | – | 0.03 | 0.06 | 0.02 | 0.07 | 1.44 | 1.07 | 1.21 | 0.28 | 0.13 | 0.2 | 221 |
| | **PT-23(−)** | CU (3) | OAS, dyspnoea | – | 0 | 0 | 0 | 0 | 1.42‡ | 4.15‡ | 3.85‡ | 1.92‡ | 1.71‡ | 3.24‡ | 35.9 |
| | **PT-26(−)** | – | OAS | – | 0.19 | 0.24 | 0.11 | 0.20 | 0.57 | 0.39 | 0.34 | 2.08 | 0.80 | 0.56 | 77.4 |
| | **PT-27(−)** | CU (1) | CU (1) | – | 0.08 | 0.11 | 0.05 | 0.11 | 1.88 | 0.90 | 1.05 | 0.36 | 0.29 | 0.19 | 557 |
| **CCD-positive** | **PT-01(+)*** | RC | CU (1) | – | 0.20 | 0.62 | 0.66 | 1.90 | 3.93 | 1.20 | 1.06 | 3.76 | 0.29 | 0.91 | 552 |
| | **PT-02(+)** | CU (1) | OAS | – | 22.3 | 27.4 | 24.7 | 33.3 | 34.9‡ | 36.4‡ | 32.6‡ | 38.9‡ | 31.4‡ | 17.2‡ | 6840 |
| | **PT-06(+)** | CU (1) | – | – | 0.11 | 1.72 | 0.28 | 0.23 | 2.43 | 2.17 | 0.80 | 2.20 | 1.97 | 0.16 | 393 |
| | **PT-09(+)*** | OAS; CU (1) | OAS | – | 0.10 | 0.56 | 1.06 | 1.67 | 0.64 | 0.80 | 0.55 | 0.66 | 0.63 | 0.17 | 200 |
| | **PT-22(+)** | – | GI | – | 2.68 | 2.65 | 2.76 | 2.86 | 3.65 | 2.92 | 1.27 | 3.96 | 3.88 | 0.83 | 352 |
| | **PT-34(+)** | – | OAS | – | 2.44 | 0.49 | 0.11 | 0.45 | 4.17 | 1.43 | 0.84 | 3.55 | 4.23 | 0.35 | 332 |
| | **PT-38(+)** | CU (1) | – | – | 28.8 | 24.8 | 21.1 | 51.9# | 35.8‡ | 34.5‡ | 18.0‡ | 25.4‡ | 27.6‡ | 3.74‡ | 1122 |
| | **BW-28(+)** | – | – | systemic (YJV) | 1.12 | 1.26 | 27.6 | 9.16 | 1.32 | 0.79 | 0.30 | 1.48 | 0.92 | 0.09 | 796 |
| | **BW-32(+)** | – | – | systemic (YJV) | 6.70 | 9.33 | 9.92 | 15.8 | 11.7 | 20.1 | 7.47 | 9.83 | 16.8 | 1.19 | 1000 |
| | **BW-39(+)** | – | – | systemic (YJV) | 1.07 | 2.28 | 14.8 | 3.13 | 1.74 | 1.02 | 0.83 | 1.79 | 0.9 | 0.29 | 68.5 |
| | **BW-40(+)** | – | – | systemic (YJV) | 7.51 | 4.55 | 63.3 | 11.3 | 5.34‡ | 6.52‡ | 3.72‡ | 4.40‡ | 5.51‡ | 0.98‡ | 737 |
| | **BW-42(+)** | – | – | systemic (HBV) | 1.40 | 3.05 | 2.18 | 9.52 | 2.19‡ | 2.71‡ | 1.94‡ | 2.21‡ | 2.35‡ | 0.69‡ | 41.6 |
| | **BW-43(+)** | – | – | systemic (YJV) | 2.77 | 1.61 | >100 | 3.65 | 2.98 | 2.49 | 2.04 | 3.51 | 3.40 | 1.14 | 1610 |
| **control** | **NA-05** | – | – | – | 0 | 0 | 0 | 0 | 0.01 | 0.002 | 0 | 0.01 | 0.01 | 0.03 | 56.1 |
| | **NA-16** | – | – | – | 0 | 0 | 0.03 | 0.04 | 0.02 | 0.001 | 0.004 | 0.01 | 0.01 | 0.03 | 30.8 |
| | **NA-18** | – | – | – | 0 | 0 | 0.02 | 0.03 | 0 | 0 | 0 | 0 | 0.004 | 0.03 | 10.7 |

Allergic symptoms after contact with potato, tomato or hymenoptera venoms are listed according to patient history. Contact urticaria (CU, after direct contact with raw potato or tomato) was classified from 1 to 4 according to von Krogh and Maibach [51]. Total and specific IgE levels were measured with the UniCAP100 instrument (Phadia) using either commercial ImmunoCAPs for tomato (f25), potato (f35), HBV (i1), YJV (i3), HRP (o400), and MUXF (o214), or in-house-made ImmunoCAPs (wt and GTI). Specific IgE values ≥0.35 kU/l were considered positive.

*Borderline patients due to negative MUXF-sIgE and borderline positive HRP-sIgE levels.

#Recently stung by a honeybee but without allergic symptoms.

‡For CCD inhibition with HRP, see Table 2. (BW: bee/wasp hymenoptera venom-allergic; CU: contact urticaria; GI: gastro-intestinal symptoms; GTI: GNTI-silenced; HBV: honeybee venom; HRP: horseradish peroxidase; HV: hymenoptera venom; MUXF: *N*-glycan structure according to the proglycan system (www.proglycan.com); NA: non-allergic control; OAS: oral allergy syndrome; PT: potato/tomato-allergic; RC: rhinoconjunctivitis; systemic: systemic reaction; wt: wild-type; YJV: yellow jacket venom).

identified 10 mg/ml HRP as sufficient for inhibiting CCD-sIgE (Figure S5A), and showed that in CCD-negative patient PT-23(−) sIgE recognition of tomato and potato is not affected (Table 2, Figure S5B). Five patient sera were investigated in detail, comprising two CCD-positive plant food-allergic and two hymenoptera venom-allergic patients (PT-02(+), PT-38(+), BW-40(+), BW-42(+); Table 2). HRP pre-incubation revealed that sIgE binding of CCD-positive sera to plant proteins can be inhibited to almost equal levels when comparing commercial, wild-type, and CCD-reduced ImmunoCAPs. This suggested that tomato and potato GTI extracts still contain residual CCD epitopes (compare immunoblot and BAT analyses), especially obvious for the two potato/tomato allergic patients with high CCD-sIgE levels (PT-02(+) and PT-38(+), Table 1). Sera of hymenoptera venom-allergic patients displayed inhibition below the 0.35 kU/l threshold, confirming that no peptide-sIgE antibodies to the plant food extracts are present. Surprisingly, the same was true for potato-allergic patient PT-38(+) using in-house-made potato wild-type and also commercial ImmunoCAP f35, albeit only at elevated inhibitor concentration (compare Table 2, Figure S5B), whereas potato/tomato-allergic patient PT-02(+) still displayed high sIgE levels after CCD inhibition for both plant foods.

As independent control, similar experiments were conducted with in-house-made ImmunoCAPs of Arabidopsis wild-type and GNTI-null mutant *cgl1*. All CCD-specific patient sera clearly discriminated between the two, but sIgE values of the two plant

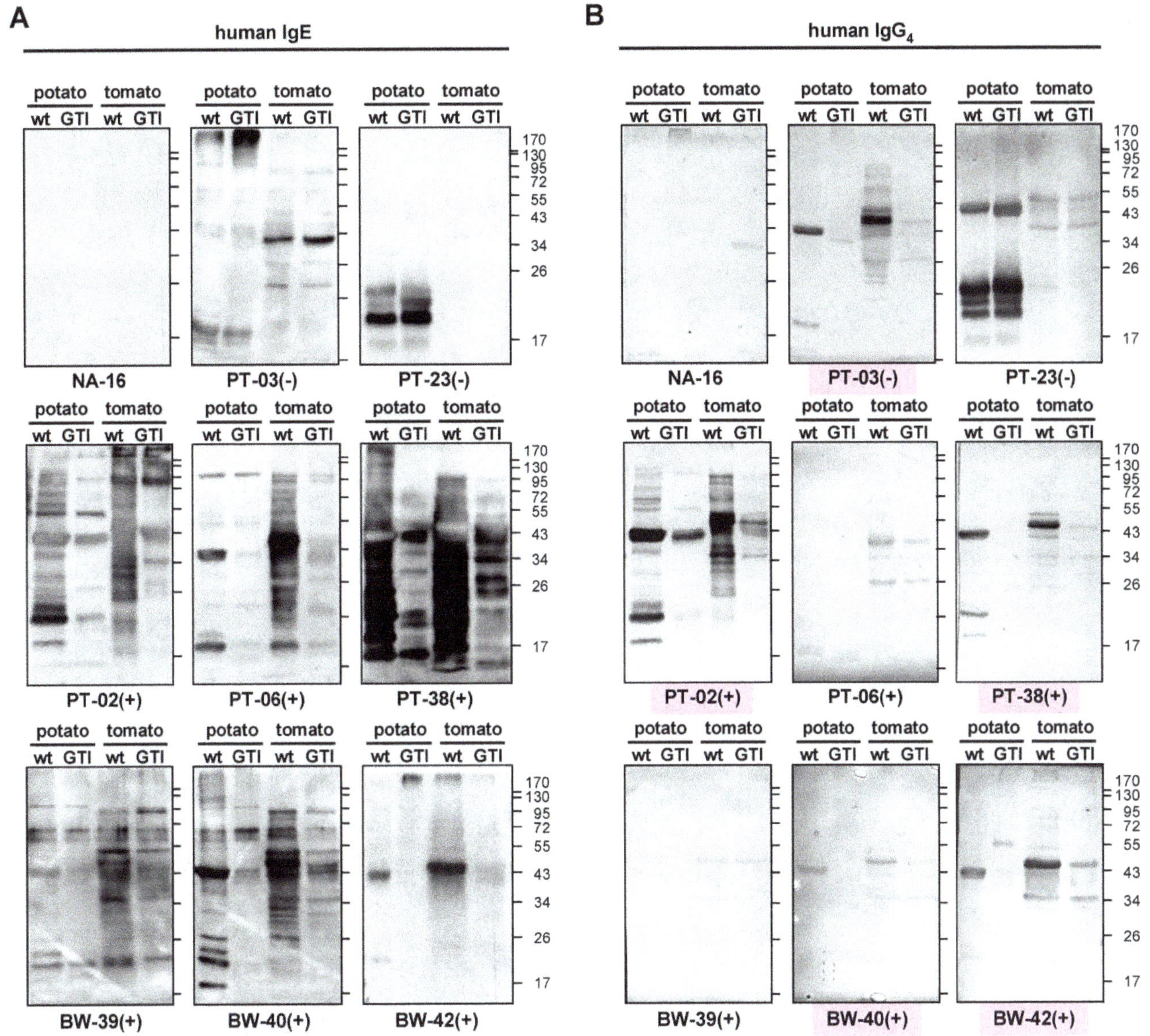


**Figure 5. Blotted GTI extracts show reduced binding of CCD-positive patient sera and reveal differences in specific IgE and $IgG_4$ patterns. A**: Immunoblots of potato tuber and tomato fruit extracts (pulp with peel) were incubated with selected patient sera (NA: non-allergic control; PT: potato/tomato food-allergic; BW: bee/wasp hymenoptera venom-allergic) and developed for detection of human IgE. CCD-sIgE negative patients are labeled (−) and CCD-sIgE positive patients (+) (compare Table 1). **B**: After sensitive ECL detection of IgE binding, blots were additionally subjected to colorimetric development for visualizing bound $IgG_4$. Sera that differentiate between wild-type (wt) and CCD-reduced (GTI) plant extracts at the $IgG_4$ level are labeled pink.

food-allergic patients did not lie below threshold with *cgl1*. Upon HRP inhibition, *cgl1*-sIgE values decreased below threshold only for PT-38(+) but lay clearly above threshold (2.73 kU/l) for PT-02(+).

## Discussion

Since protein- and carbohydrate-based allergic immune reactions are difficult to distinguish, this proof-of-principle study intended to explore the usefulness of selectively Lyc e 2- and CCD-reduced foodstuff. Importantly, our RNAi-based approaches represent more or less the physiological situation after contact with or ingestion of plant foods (i.e. challenge with an allergen mixture), in contrast to previous studies that reported histamine release assays conducted with only a single native, glycosylated allergen *versus* the recombinant, non-glycosylated allergen form [7,14–16].

In this context it is noteworthy that tomato glycoallergen Lyc e 2, whose effector-cell triggering depends on CCD epitopes alone [7,16], was no key player for reducing the allergenic potential of tomato fruits. An explanation for this finding is given by the recent study of Mertens and coworkers, revealing that CCD may induce basophil activation without clinical relevance in hymenoptera venom allergy [34]. We therefore doubt that Lyc e 2 is a true allergen, albeit inducing histamine release [7,16] that appears to result from application of a single plant glycoprotein in high concentration, similar to HRP used as control in our BAT assays.

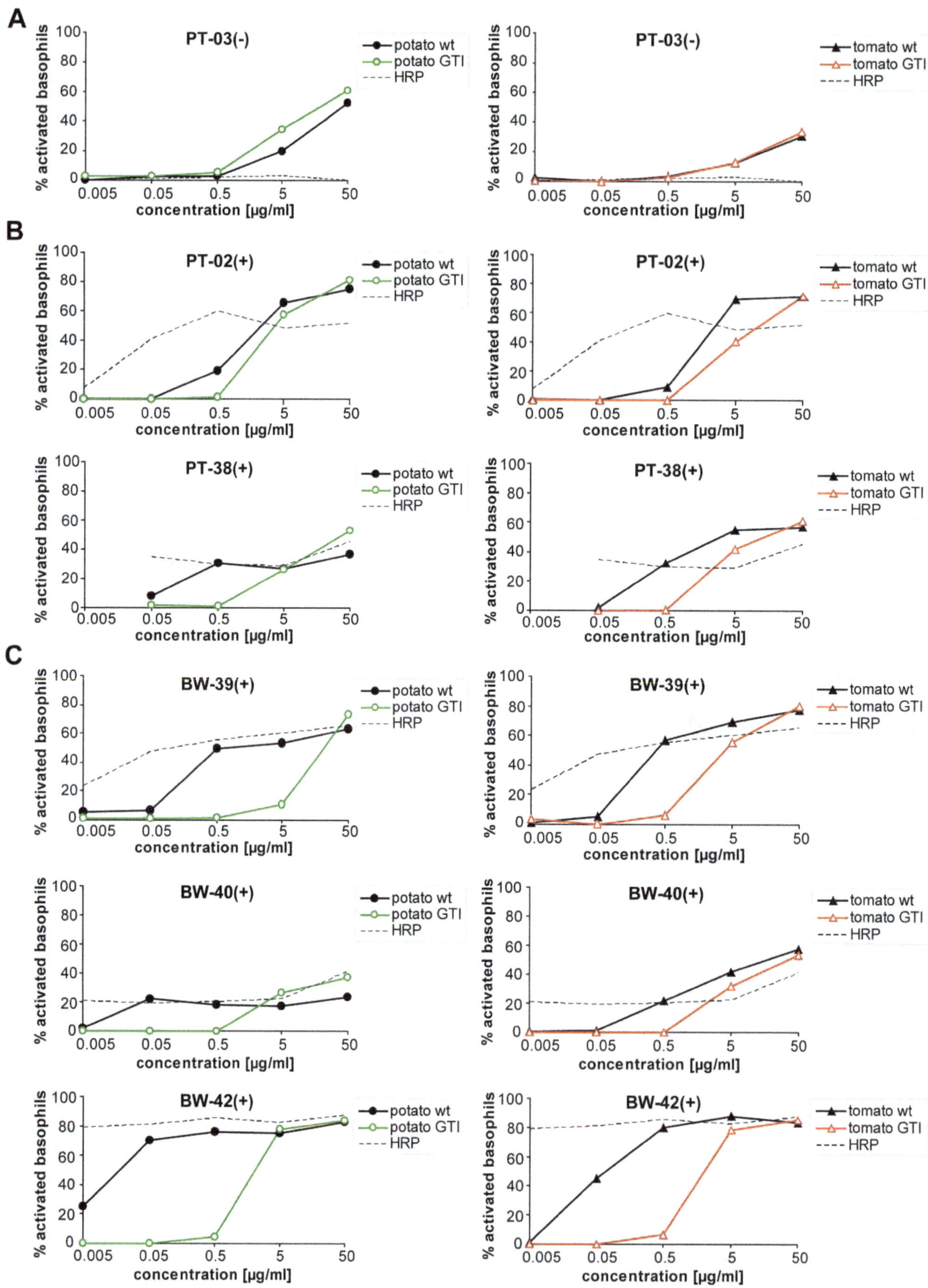
A
B
C
PT-03(-)
PT-02(+)
PT-38(+)
BW-39(+)
BW-40(+)
BW-42(+)
potato wt
potato GTI
tomato wt
tomato GTI
HRP
% activated basophils
concentration [μg/ml]
0.005
0.05
0.5
5
50

**Figure 6. CCD-positive patients show decreased basophil activation with GTI extracts.** Comparison of basophils stimulated with potato tuber (left panels) or tomato fruit extracts (right panels) of either wild-type (wt) or GTI plants. In all tests, horseradish peroxidase (HRP, dotted line) served as control for CCD-dependent stimulation. The percentage of activated basophils was calculated by subtracting values of spontaneous CD203c expression (negative control, PBS) from the values obtained with the particular allergen challenge. **A**: Potato/tomato-allergic patient without CCD-sIgE; **B**: Potato/tomato-allergic patients with CCD-sIgE; **C**: Hymenoptera venom-allergic patients with CCD-sIgE but no allergic symptoms to potato or tomato (for patient details, see Table 1).

Compared to silencing only one CCD-bearing glycoprotein (Lyc e 2), GNTI silencing offered the possibility to remove essentially all CCD epitopes from the plant extracts investigated, without additional chemical treatment. In all clear-cut CCD-positive patients tested, BAT analyses conducted with CCD-reduced GTI foodstuff revealed diminished effector-cell triggering to various extents. This was especially obvious in the hymenoptera venom-allergic group reporting no symptoms to potato and/or tomato. Since analyses with CCD-negative patients verified that peptide epitopes are unaffected, biological activity of CCD-sIgE without obvious link to clinical symptoms was confirmed (compare [34]). Notably, decreased effector-cell stimulation detected with CCD-reduced GTI plant extracts lay in the same range as previously reported for basophil histamine-release assays obtained with extracts of either LTP-silenced (Lyc e 3, a true allergen) [35,36] or profilin-silenced (Lyc e 1, a debated allergen [10]) [37] tomato plants, demonstrating equal relevance of CCD-sIgE and peptide-sIgE at this level.

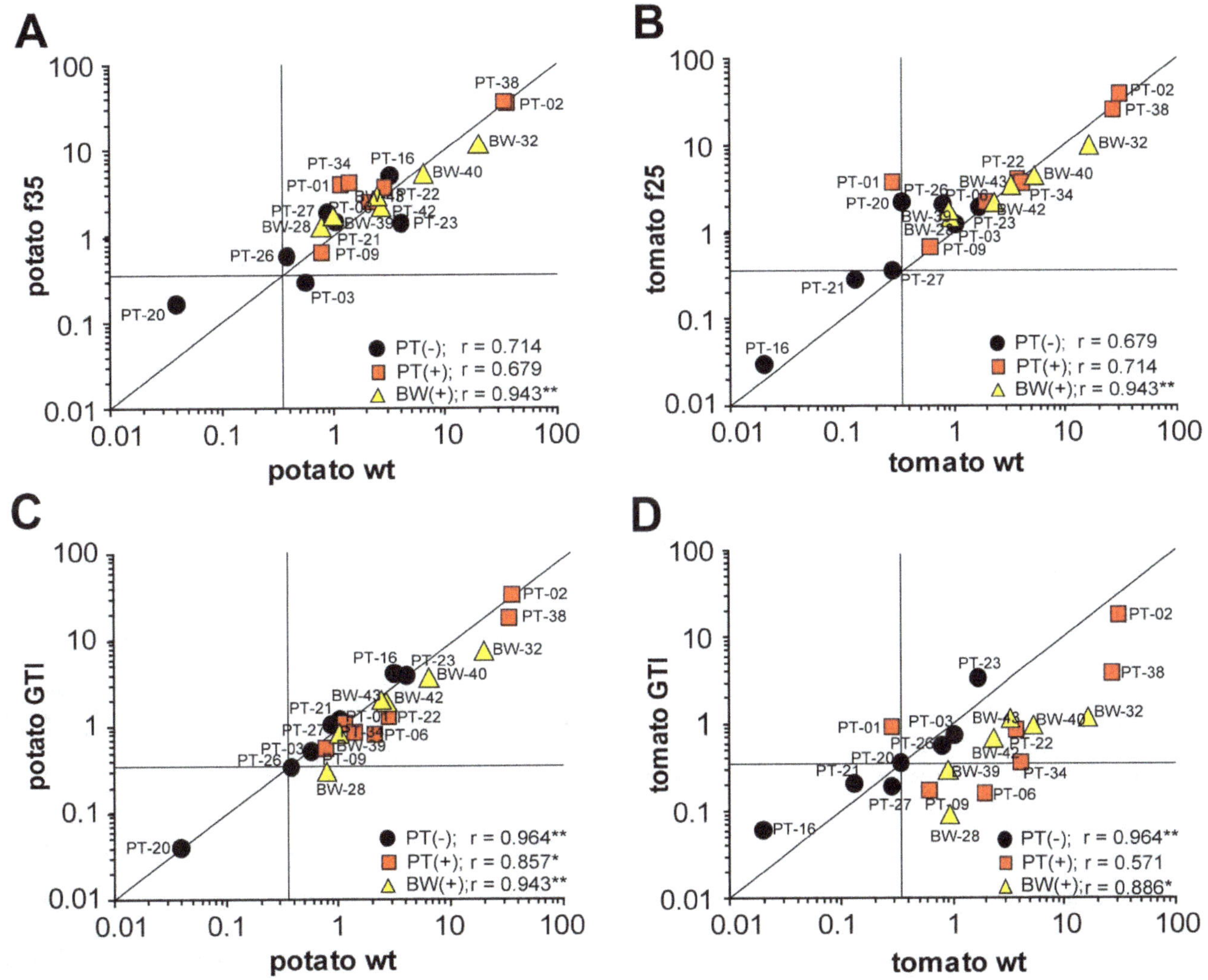


**Figure 7. Correlation plots of specific IgE values determined with commercial and in-house-made ImmunoCAPs.** Comparison of sIgE values in three different patient groups. **A**: Potato, commercial (f35) *versus* in-house-made wild-type (wt). **B**: Tomato, commercial (f25) *versus* in-house-made wt. **C**: Potato, in-house-made wt *versus* GTI. **D**: Tomato, in-house-made wt *versus* GTI. (Black circles: CCD-negative potato/tomato-allergic patients, red squares: CCD-positive potato/tomato-allergic patients, yellow triangles: CCD-positive hymenoptera venom-allergic patients). For sIgE values compare Table 1. Note that sIgE values of CCD-negative food-allergic patients (black circles) match more or less the bisecting line and those of CCD-positive patients (red squares and yellow triangles) shift downwards with GTI extracts (especially obvious for tomato). For better illustration, zero values were set to 0.01. Horizontal and vertical lines indicate the 0.35 kU/l threshold for sIgE positivity, bisecting lines congruency. Correlation coefficient r was calculated by the Spearman's rank correlation test, r = +1/−1 would be ideal (*: $p<0.05$; **: $p<0.01$).

**Table 2.** Specific IgE values of commercial and in-house-made ImmunoCAPs including HRP-mediated CCD inhibition for selected patients.

| Patient | Potato | | | | | | Tomato | | | | | | Arabidopsis | | | |
|---|---|---|---|---|---|---|---|---|---|---|---|---|---|---|---|---|
| | f35 | | wt | | GTI | | f25 | | wt | | GTI | | wt | | *cgl1* | |
| | − | + | − | + | − | + | − | + | − | + | − | + | − | + | − | + |
| **PT-23(−)** | 1.37 | 1.40 | 1.41 | 1.24 | 1.18 | 1.07 | 2.23 | 2.11 | 0.84 | 0.86 | 2.36 | 2.42 | 0.10 | 0.10 | 0.06 | 0.06 |
| **PT-02(+)** | 41.2 | 2.37 | 31.5 | 3.98 | 21.4 | 2.67 | 47.2 | 4.13 | 30.6 | 3.11 | 14.6 | 3.53 | 28.6 | 3.31 | 4.83 | 2.73 |
| **PT-38(+)** | 34.8 | 0.42[‡] | 31.8 | 0.26 | 7.88 | 0.09 | 30.8 | 0.21 | 23.3 | 0.17 | 3.71 | 0.09 | 18.9 | 0.28 | 0.67 | 0.20 |
| **BW-40(+)** | 5.90 | 0.10 | 5.31 | 0.05 | 1.71 | 0.02 | 5.05 | 0.05 | 4.01 | 0.11 | 1.05 | 0.05 | 3.55 | 0.13 | 0.26 | 0.09 |
| **BW-42(+)** | 2.61 | 0.04 | 2.09 | 0.01 | 1.06 | 0.01 | 2.54 | 0.03 | 1.75 | 0.08 | 0.66 | 0.07 | 1.74 | 0.09 | 0.11 | 0.08 |

CCD inhibition was done by incubating the respective patient sera over night at 4°C with HRP (10 mg/ml final concentration). Arabidopsis was included as control.
[‡]When conducted with a final inhibitor concentration of 33.3 mg/ml HRP, the sIgE value decreased to 0.22 kU/l (below the 0.35 kU/l threshold, compare Figure S5B). (BW: bee/wasp hymenoptera venom-allergic; *cgl1*: *complex glycan-less* GNTI-null mutant; f25: commercial tomato ImmunoCAP; f35: commercial potato ImmunoCAP; GTI: GNTI-silenced; PT: potato/tomato-allergic; wt: wild-type).

Nevertheless, reasons for the apparent clinical insignificance of CCD-sIgE are not obvious and have been extensively discussed [reviewed in 2]. Low binding affinity of carbohydrate-specific IgE antibodies was previously ruled out [9]. Instead, to explain tolerance in allergy, it was hypothesized that some IgG fraction might function as CCD-blocking antibody [9,38,39]. If this assumption was correct, an influence on our BAT analyses would be expected, because whole blood was used that retains the individual balance between sIgE and $sIgG_4$. However, results obtained with CCD-$sIgG_4$ positive and negative patients revealed no effect of CCD-$sIgG_4$ upon basophil activation with native potato or tomato wild-type extracts. Furthermore, despite clear IgE binding to wild-type plant food extracts, lack of clinical symptoms in the hymenoptera venom-allergic group was not accompanied by high $sIgG_4$ levels. Therefore, blocking of CCD epitopes by CCD-$sIgG_4$ antibodies can be probably ruled out.

The overall opinion that CCD-sIgE is irrelevant for triggering allergic symptoms and causes only 'false-positive results' in serum tests [2,10] recently received support by a study in which plant-derived, CCD-decorated human lactoferrin did not elicit allergic symptoms among a limited number of patients (n = 3) upon double-blind placebo-controlled food challenge [12]. But remarkably our study identified one patient with symptoms to potato (PT-38(+)) as potential candidate for clinical relevance of CCD-sIgE, because after serum inhibition with HRP, potato-sIgE values lay below threshold. This finding is especially striking, since plant food-allergic patient PT-02(+) still displayed high sIgE levels after HRP inhibition (for both, tomato and potato), indicating presence of peptide-sIgE that would also explain the minimal differences observed in the BAT.

To assure that CCD epitopes may be needed occasionally to trigger allergic symptoms, identification of more patients like PT-38(+) is required to perform double-blind placebo-controlled challenges with cognate, essentially CCD-free plant material. However, as unsolved issue remains that stability and composition of plant-derived extracts is a general problem for routine *in-vitro* diagnosis [40,41]. Thus, it is also possible that the causative potato allergen for PT-38(+) was missing from both, in-house-made and commercial ImmunoCAPs.

In order to improve routine testing for the majority of CCD-positive patients (i.e. those with clinically irrelevant CCD sensitization), GTI potato and tomato extracts were coupled to streptavidin-ImmunoCAPs. These in-house-made ImmunoCAPs resulted in clearly reduced sIgE values compared to the corresponding wild-types and commercial references, thus confirming the outcome of our initial immunoblot and BAT analyses. As an aside, commercial and streptavidin-ImmunoCAPs coupled with wild-type food extracts amounted to similar sIgE values, implying high quality of our in-house-made ImmunoCAPs. For selected patients with very high CCD-sIgE titers, HRP-inhibition experiments suggested that CCD reduction of the GNTI-silenced foodstuff might not be complete, especially in potato. However, HRP inhibition also reduced sIgE binding to Arabidopsis GNTI-null mutant *cgl1* (definitely lacking CCD [42]), indicating that some IgE antibodies also bound to the HRP backbone. This alternatively might explain the under-threshold potato-sIgE values of PT-38(+) observed upon HRP inhibition. By contrast, PT-02(+) still showed strong residual sIgE binding to *cgl1* after HRP inhibition, pointing to recognition of additional peptide epitope(s) in leaf extracts. Since PT-02(+) displays symptoms to diverse pollens and other plant sources, this finding is interesting but not that surprising.

As inferred from another study on tobacco GTI-antisense plants lacking measurable GNTI activity despite almost wild-type-like CCD patterns on immunoblots [43], GNTI is likely suppressed below detection limits in our potato and tomato GTI-RNAi lines. CCD-reduced foodstuff therefore provides the possibility to improve allergy testing with whole extracts. Furthermore, such CCD-reduced plants also offer the opportunity of heterologous protein expression, especially when post-translational modification without perturbation by CCD epitopes is required. Despite availability of GNTI-null mutant *cgl1*, Arabidopsis - as a small weed - is not suitable for high yield applications. Also, the protein pattern of leaves is much more complex (than e.g. of seeds, fruits, or tubers), which could interfere with protein purification.

In summary, the GNTI-silenced tomato and potato lines described in this study proved to be a valuable tool for evaluating contribution of CCD- *versus* peptide-specific determinants to food-allergic reactions. We confirmed that for most patients investigated (except PT-38(+)) presence of CCD-sIgE is clinically irrelevant. Hence, the described approach bears the potential to improve existing diagnostic tools (BAT and sIgE determination). Since phenotypic deviations are negligible, CCD-reduced plants likely constitute an ideal expression system for glycosylated allergens. Thus, they should be perfectly suited for state-of-the-art component-resolved allergy diagnosis in the near future.

## Materials and Methods

### Ethics Statement

The study protocol was approved by the ethics committee of the Institutional Review Board of Münster University, School of Medicine (Permit no. 2007-451-f-S, 'Investigations concerning CCD epitopes of allergenic glycoproteins'). Blood samples (50 ml per donor) were obtained under written informed consent and used for immunoblot development, basophil-activation tests, and ImmunoCAP analyses.

### Tomato and potato RNAi transformants, Arabidopsis *cgl1* mutant

For creation of tomato and potato RNAi transformants, total RNA was purified from tomato (*Lycopersicon esculentum* cv. Moneymaker 'Micro-Tom') or potato (*Solanum tuberosum* cv. Désirée) leaf tissue. GNTI-specific cDNA sequences were amplified for each cultivar using oligo-dT-primed reverse transcription with primers 5′-N$_6$-GTCGAC CAA TTA AGG GCT CTT GTT C-3′ and 5′-N$_6$-GGATCCGG CCA CTT TGG AG- 3′. Similarly, Lyc e 2-specific cDNA was obtained from tomato-fruit RNA using primers 5′-N$_3$-GTCGACA CGA AGA GTA CTG TGG GGA TG-3′ and 5′-N$_3$-GGATCCCT AGT TTG ATC AGC ACA GAA GTG AGT CTC-3′ (SalI and BamHI sites underlined). The resulting fragments were cloned in vector pUC-RNAi [44], and introduced into binary plant-expression vectors, driven either by a constitutive (35S) [45] or a tuber/fruit-specific (B33) [44] promoter (Figure 1C). Binary constructs were introduced into Agrobacteria and used to transform the corresponding plant cultivars [46,47]. Arabidopsis GTI-null mutant *cgl1-3* (described in Frank et al.) [42] served as control for ImmunoCAP analyses.

### Preparation of protein extracts

Fresh tomato fruits without seeds or potato tubers were cut into small pieces and ground in liquid nitrogen to yield fine powder. For SDS-PAGE and immunoblot analyses, frozen powder was extracted with ice-cold buffer (50 mM of HEPES-NaOH pH 8, 250 mM NaCl, 2 mM $Na_2S_2O_5$, 1 mM EDTA), 1 mM Pefabloc SC (Serva, Heidelberg, Germany), and Polyvinylpolypyrrolidone (0.1 mg/ml, Sigma-Aldrich, Taufkirchen, Germany) to prevent protein oxidation. For basophil activation tests (BAT), frozen powder was extracted with phosphate-buffered saline (PBS; pH 8 for tomato and pH 7.4 for potato), supplemented with 1 mM Pefabloc SC and processed as above. For preparation of in-house-made ImmunoCAPs, extraction of potato tubers was done as described for BAT. Due to low pH and protein contents, tomato fruit extracts were prepared with 'high' PBS (200 mM $Na_2HPO_4$ pH 9, 250 mM NaCl, 2 mM $Na_2S_2O_5$, 1 mM EDTA, and 0.05% (v/v) Triton-X100) and supplements as above. Extraction of Arabidopsis leaves was done with last mentioned buffer. Protein contents were determined with Bradford reagent (Bio-Rad, Munich, Germany) and bovine serum albumin (BSA) as standard protein. Aliquots were stored at −80°C until use.

### Preparation of recombinant Lyc e 2 antigen for rabbit immunization

The coding sequence of mature vacuolar β-fructofuranosidase (Lyc e 2) [48] was used for *E. coli*-based expression and purification of recombinant protein. RT-PCR was conducted with tomato (*Lycopersicon esculentum* cv. Moneymaker "Micro-Tom") fruit RNA using primers 5′-N$_3$-CATATG TAT GCG TGG TCC AAT GCT ATG CTT AG-3′ and 5′-N$_3$-GGATCCTT ACA AGT CTT GCA AAG GAA GGA TTG-3′ (NdeI and BamHI sites underlined). Amplified cDNA fragments were inserted into vector pET16b, allowing for overexpression in *E. coli* BL21(DE3):pLysS cells (Novagen/Merck, Darmstadt, Germany). Recombinant Lyc e 2 protein with His-tag was isolated with Ni-NTA agarose (Qiagen, Hilden, Germany) under denaturing conditions. This fraction was used in a pre-study with sera of subjects showing reactivity to tomato extracts, and for production of a polypeptide-specific polyclonal rabbit antiserum (α-Le2; Eurogentec, Seraing, Belgium).

### Immunoblot analyses

Prior to blot development, protein extracts (20 μg for tomato, 12 μg for potato) were separated by SDS-PAGE, blotted to nitrocellulose and stained with Ponceau S (Serva) as described previously [42]. For Lyc e 2 detection, the polypeptide-specific α-Le2 antiserum (described above) served as first antibody (1:5,000 in 2% skimmed milk/2× Tris-buffered saline (TBS) with 0.1% [v/v] Tween-20 (TBST) for 2 hours) and HRP-labeled goat anti-rabbit IgG conjugate (Bio-Rad) as second antibody (1:10,000 in 2% skimmed milk/TBST for 1 hour). For detection of CCD epitopes, a polyclonal rabbit anti-HRP serum (α-CCD, Sigma-Aldrich, Taufkirchen, Germany) was used as first antibody (1:10,000 in 2% skimmed milk/2× TBST for 2 hours) followed by the second antibody (as above). For detection of sIgE, blots were first incubated with patient sera (1:10 in 2% skimmed milk/TBST for 3 hours) followed by HRP-labeled affinity-purified goat antibodies to human IgE (KPL, Gaithersburg, Maryland, USA; 1:10,000 in TBST for 1 hour). Signals were visualized with the ECL-Advance Western-Blot Detection Kit (Amersham/GE Healthcare, Freiburg, Germany). After chemiluminescent IgE detection, bound $IgG_4$ was visualized via alkaline phosphatase (AP)-conjugated mouse anti-human $IgG_4$ monoclonal antibodies (BD Biosciences; Heidelberg, Germany; 1:500 in TBST for 1 hour) using colorimetric AP substrates (Promega, Mannheim, Germany).

### Patient selection and sera characterization

Two patient groups were recruited separately according to patient history and specific IgE levels determined by ImmunoCAP analyses (a routine *in-vitro* method used for allergy diagnosis): the potato and/or tomato allergic group comprised initially 26 patients with reported symptoms. Due to negative potato- and tomato-sIgE 12 patients were subsequently excluded. Of the remaining 14 patients seven displayed CCD-sIgE to HRP and MUXF (isolated *N*-glycan chains of bromelain). The others served as CCD-negative control. The second group comprised hymenoptera venom-allergic patients with confirmed sIgE towards CCD, but without reported symptoms to potato and tomato. CCD-sIgE negative patients are labeled (−) and CCD-sIgE positive patients (+) (compare Table 1). Additionally, three healthy subjects without history of allergic reactions and confirmed absence of sIgE to potato, tomato, hymenoptera venoms, HRP, and MUXF served as non-allergic controls (for an overview of investigated patients, see Table 1).

### Basophil-activation test (BAT)

BAT was performed as described earlier by Mertens et al. [34]. In brief, heparinized whole blood was incubated for 15 min at 37°C with 10-fold serial dilutions of the allergen extracts in PBS ranging from 50 to 0.005 or 5 to 0.0005 μg/ml. To determine reactivity towards plant-derived CCD, HRP was included in the same concentration range. To confirm cell responsiveness, 0.2 μg of a monoclonal anti-IgE antibody (clone BE5; EurobioSciences,

Friesoythe, Germany) served as CCD-independent positive control. After stimulation, the reaction was stopped by addition of 20 mM EDTA in PBS and centrifugation at 400×g. Basophils were stained with 10 µl anti-CD203c-PE (Beckman-Coulter, Krefeld, Germany) for 45 min at room temperature in the dark. Erythrocytes were destroyed using 'whole blood lysing reagent' (Beckman-Coulter). After washing and resuspending the cells in PBS with 1% BSA, a total of 60,000 cells were measured using the FACSCalibur flow cytometer equipped with CellQuestPro software (BD Biosciences) and subsequently the percentage of activated cells was determined.

### Preparation of in-house-made ImmunoCAPs

In-house-made ImmunoCAPs were prepared by coupling biotinylated plant extracts to streptavidin-ImmunoCAPs (o212, Phadia, Freiburg, Germany). Coupling followed basically previous protocols [49,50]. In brief, biotinylation was performed using the EZ-Link® Sulfo-NHS-Biotinylation Kit (PIERCE, Rockford, IL, USA) at pH 9 for 30 min at room temperature in 2.5-fold molar excess based on major proteins. To remove excess biotin, desalting spin columns were used, equilibrated with PBS (pH 8) and 0.05% Triton-X100. For coupling, 50 µl of each biotinylated extract were added to a streptavidin-CAP and incubated for 30 min in the UniCAP100 instrument (Phadia) before performing specific IgE assays (described below).

### ImmunoCAP analyses

Total and specific IgE levels were measured with UniCAP100 and corresponding kits (Phadia) using either commercial ImmunoCAPs for tomato (f25), potato (f35), hymenoptera venoms (i1 and i3), HRP (o400), and MUXF (o214), or the in-house-made ImmunoCAPs. Specific IgE values ≥0.35 kU/l were considered positive. Correlations between commercial and in-house-made ImmunoCAPs were statistically analyzed using the Spearman's rank correlation test and SPSS version 15.0 (SPSS Inc., Chicago, IL, USA). For CCD inhibition, the optimal HRP concentration was determined in a pre-study using 0.67 to 33.3 mg/ml HRP (final concentration) and over-night incubation with patient sera at 4°C prior to sIgE determination with commercial HRP ImmunoCAP o400. A final concentration of 10 mg/ml was found to be sufficient and used for further analyses.

## Supporting Information

**Text S1** Supporting Methods, Results & Discussion, References, and Figure Legends.
(DOC)

**Figure S1** PNGase-F treatment of tomato fruit extracts verifies efficient Lyc e 2-silencing.
(TIFF)

**Figure S2** GNTI-silenced plants maintain CCD-independent specific IgE and $IgG_4$ binding.
(TIFF)

**Figure S3** Basophil activation in borderline CCD-positive potato/tomato-allergic patients.
(TIFF)

**Figure S4** Correlation plots of specific IgE values determined with commercial and in-house-made ImmunoCAPs.
(TIFF)

**Figure S5** Inhibition of CCD-specific IgE binding by horseradish peroxidase (HRP).
(TIFF)

## Acknowledgments

The authors thank K. Fischer, J. Hausfeld, and D. Schubert for taking care of plants in tissue culture and the greenhouse. Vector pUC-RNAi, tomato seeds, and the tomato transformation protocol were provided by the group of U. Sonnewald (University of Erlangen-Nuremberg, Germany). Tobacco suspension-culture cells for tomato feeder-layers were a kind gift of B. Kost (University of Agricultural Sciences, Uppsala, Sweden).

## Author Contributions

Conceived and designed the experiments: HK-S MM RB AvS. Performed the experiments: HK-S MM. Analyzed the data: HK-S MM RB AvS. Contributed reagents/materials/analysis tools: RB AvS. Wrote the paper: HK-S MM AvS. Final approval of the version to be published: RB.

## References

1. Aalberse RC, Koshte V, Clemens JG (1981) Immunoglobulin E antibodies that crossreact with vegetable foods, pollen, and Hymenoptera venom. J Allergy Clin Immunol 68: 356–364.
2. Altmann F (2007) The role of protein glycosylation in allergy. Int Arch Allergy Immunol 142: 99–115.
3. Fötisch K, Altmann F, Haustein D, Vieths S (1999) Involvement of carbohydrate epitopes in the IgE response of celery-allergic patients. Int Arch Allergy Immunol 120: 30–42.
4. Lüttkopf D, Ballmer-Weber BK, Wüthrich B, Vieths S (2000) Celery allergens in patients with positive double-blind placebo-controlled food challenge. J Allergy Clin Immunol 106: 390–399.
5. Ballmer-Weber BK, Wüthrich B, Wangorsch A, Fötisch K, Altmann F, et al. (2001) Carrot allergy: double-blinded, placebo-controlled food challenge and identification of allergens. J Allergy Clin Immunol 108: 301–307.
6. Fötisch K, Westphal S, Lauer I, Retzek M, Altmann F, et al. (2003) Biological activity of IgE specific for cross-reactive carbohydrate determinants. J Allergy Clin Immunol 111: 889–896.
7. van Ree R, Cabanes-Macheteau M, Akkerdaas J, Milazzo JP, Loutelier-Bourhis C, et al. (2000) Beta(1,2)-xylose and alpha(1,3)-fucose residues have a strong contribution in IgE binding to plant glycoallergens. J Biol Chem 275: 11451–11458.
8. Mari A (2002) IgE to cross-reactive carbohydrate determinants: analysis of the distribution and appraisal of the in vivo and in vitro reactivity. Int Arch Allergy Immunol 129: 286–295.
9. Jin C, Hantusch B, Hemmer W, Stadlmann J, Altmann F (2008) Affinity of IgE and IgG against cross-reactive carbohydrate determinants on plant and insect glycoproteins. J Allergy Clin Immunol 121: 185–190.
10. Ebo DG, Hagendorens MM, Bridts CH, De Clerck LS, Stevens WJ (2004) Sensitization to cross-reactive carbohydrate determinants and the ubiquitous protein profilin: mimickers of allergy. Clin Exp Allergy 34: 137–144.
11. Mari A, Iacovacci P, Afferni C, Barletta B, Tinghino R, et al. (1999) Specific IgE to cross-reactive carbohydrate determinants strongly affect the in vitro diagnosis of allergic diseases. J Allergy Clin Immunol 103: 1005–1011.
12. Mari A, Ooievaar-de Heer P, Scala E, Giani M, Pirrotta L, et al. (2008) Evaluation by double-blind placebo-controlled oral challenge of the clinical relevance of IgE antibodies against plant glycans. Allergy 63: 891–896.
13. van der Veen MJ, van Ree R, Aalberse RC, Akkerdaas J, Koppelman SJ, et al. (1997) Poor biologic activity of cross-reactive IgE directed to carbohydrate determinants of glycoproteins. J Allergy Clin Immunol 100: 327–334.
14. Iacovacci P, Afferni C, Butteroni C, Pironi L, Puggioni EMR, et al. (2002) Comparison between the native glycosylated and the recombinant Cup a1 allergen: role of carbohydrates in the histamine release from basophils. Clin Exp Allergy 32: 1620–1627.
15. Bublin M, Radauer C, Wilson IBH, Kraft D, Scheiner O, et al. (2003) Cross-reactive N-glycans of Api g 5, a high molecular weight glycoprotein allergen from celery, are required for immunoglobulin E binding and activation of effector cells from allergic patients. FASEB J 17: 1697–1699.
16. Westphal S, Kolarich D, Foetisch K, Lauer I, Altmann F, et al. (2003) Molecular characterization and allergenic activity of Lyc e 2 (beta-fructofuranosidase), a glycosylated allergen of tomato. Eur J Biochem 270: 1327–1337.
17. Seppälä U, Majamaa H, Turjanmaa K, Helin J, Reunala T, et al. (2001) Identification of four novel potato (*Solanum tuberosum*) allergens belonging to the family of soybean trypsin inhibitors. Allergy 56: 619–626.

18. Fötisch K, Son DY, Altmann F, Aulepp H, Conti A, et al. (2001) Tomato (*Lycopersicon esculentum*) allergens in pollen-allergic patients. Eur Food Res Technol 213: 259–266.
19. Kondo Y, Urisu A, Tokuda R (2001) Identification and characterization of the allergens in the tomato fruit by immunoblotting. Int Arch Allergy Immunol 126: 294–299.
20. Bässler OY, Weiss J, Wienkoop S, Lehmann K, Scheler C, et al. (2009) Evidence for novel tomato seed allergens: IgE-reactive legumin and vicilin proteins identified by multidimensional protein fractionation-mass spectrometry and in silico epitope modeling. J Proteome Res 8: 1111–1122.
21. Park WD, Blackwood C, Mignery GA, Hermodson MA, Lister RM (1983) Analysis of the Heterogeneity of the 40,000 Molecular Weight Tuber Glycoprotein of Potatoes by Immunological Methods and by NH(2)-Terminal Sequence Analysis. Plant Physiol 71: 156–160.
22. Sonnewald U, Sturm A, Chrispeels MJ, Willmitzer L (1989) Targeting and glycosylation of patatin, the major tuber protein in leaves of transgenic tobacco. Planta 179: 171–180.
23. Pots AM, Gruppen H, Hessing M, van Boekel MA, Voragen AG (1999) Isolation and characterization of patatin isoforms. J Agric Food Chem 47: 4587–4592.
24. Seppälä U, Alenius H, Turjanmaa K, Reunala T, Palosuo T, et al. (1999) Identification of patatin as a novel allergen for children with positive skin prick test responses to raw potato. J Allergy Clin Immunol 103: 165–171.
25. Majamaa H, Seppälä U, Palosuo T, Turjanmaa K, Kalkkinen N, et al. (2001) Positive skin and oral challenge responses to potato and occurrence of immunoglobulin E antibodies to patatin (Sol t 1) in infants with atopic dermatitis. Pediatr Allergy Immunol 12: 283–288.
26. Ohyama A, Hirai M, Nishimura S (1992) A novel cDNA clone for acid invertase in tomato fruit. Jpn J Genet 67: 491–492.
27. Petersen A, Vieths S, Aulepp H, Schlaak M, Becker WM (1996) Ubiquitous structures responsible for IgE cross-reactivity between tomato fruit and grass pollen allergens. J Allergy Clin Immunol 98: 805–815.
28. Weangsripanaval T, Nomura N, Moriyama T, Ohta N, Ogawa T (2003) Identification of suberization-associated anionic peroxidase as a possible allergenic protein from tomato. Biosci Biotechnol Biochem 67: 1299–1304.
29. von Schaewen A, Sturm A, O'Neill J, Chrispeels MJ (1993) Isolation of a mutant Arabidopsis plant that lacks N-acetyl glucosaminyl transferase I and is unable to synthesize Golgi-modified complex N-linked glycans. Plant Physiol 102: 1109–1118.
30. Wenderoth I, von Schaewen A (2000) Isolation and characterization of plant *N*-acetyl glucosaminyltransferase I (*GntI*) cDNA sequences. Functional analyses in the Arabidopsis *cgl* mutant and in antisense plants. Plant Physiol 123: 1097–1108.
31. Kang JS, Frank J, Kang CH, Kajiura H, Vikram M, et al. (2008) Salt tolerance of *Arabidopsis thaliana* requires maturation of *N*-glycosylated proteins in the Golgi apparatus. Proc Natl Acad Sci U S A 105: 5933–5938.
32. Bosques CJ, Tschampel SM, Woods RJ, Imperiali B (2004) Effects of glycosylation on peptide conformation: a synergistic experimental and computational study. J Am Chem Soc 126: 8421–8425.
33. Lerouge P, Cabanes-Macheteau M, Rayon C, Fischette-Lainé AC, Gomord V, et al. (1998) N-glycoprotein biosynthesis in plants: recent developments and future trends. Plant Mol Biol 38: 31–48.
34. Mertens M, Amler S, Moerschbacher BM, Brehler R (2010) Cross-reactive carbohydrate determinants strongly affect the results of the basophil activation test in hymenoptera-venom allergy. Clin Exp Allergy 40: 1333–1345.
35. Lorenz Y, Enrique E, Le QL, Fötisch K, Retzek M, et al. (2006) Skin prick tests reveal stable and heritable reduction of allergenic potency of gene-silenced tomato fruits. J Allergy Clin Immunol 118: 711–718.
36. Le LQ, Lorenz Y, Scheurer S, Fötisch K, Enrique E, et al. (2006) Design of tomato fruits with reduced allergenicity by dsRNAi-mediated inhibition of ns-LTP (Lyc e 3) expression. Plant Biotechnol J 4: 231–242.
37. Le LQ, Mahler V, Lorenz Y, Scheurer S, Biemelt S, et al. (2006) Reduced allergenicity of tomato fruits harvested from Lyc e 1-silenced transgenic tomato plants. J Allergy Clin Immunol 118: 1176–1183.
38. Nouri-Aria KT, Wachholz PA, Francis JN, Jacobson MR, Walker SM, et al. (2004) Grass pollen immunotherapy induces mucosal and peripheral IL-10 responses and blocking IgG activity. J Immunol 172: 3252–3259.
39. Turner JD, Faulkner H, Kamgno J, Kennedy MW, Behnke J, et al. (2005) Allergen-specific IgE and IgG4 are markers of resistance and susceptibility in a human intestinal nematode infection. Microbes Infect 7: 990–996.
40. Ortolani C, Ispano M, Pastorello EA, Ansaloni R, Magri GC (1989) Comparison of results of skin prick tests (with fresh foods and commercial food extracts) and RAST in 100 patients with oral allergy syndrome. J Allergy Clin Immunol 83: 683–690.
41. Rudeschko O, Fahlbusch B, Henzgen M, Schlenvoigt G, Herrmann D, et al. (1995) Optimization of apple allergen preparation for in vivo and in vitro diagnostics. Allergy 50: 262–268.
42. Frank J, Kaulfürst-Soboll H, Rips S, Koiwa H, von Schaewen A (2008) Comparative analyses of Arabidopsis *complex glycan1* mutants and genetic interaction with *staurosporin and temperature sensitive3a*. Plant Physiol 148: 1354–1367.
43. Strasser R, Altmann F, Glössl J, Steinkellner H (2004) Unaltered complex N-glycan profiles in *Nicotiana benthamiana* despite drastic reduction of beta1,2-N-acetylglucosaminyltransferase I activity. Glycoconj J 21: 275–282.
44. Chen S, Hofius D, Sonnewald U, Börnke F (2003) Temporal and spatial control of gene silencing in transgenic plants by inducible expression of double-stranded RNA. Plant J 36: 731–740.
45. Höfgen R, Willmitzer L (1990) Biochemical and genetic analysis of different patatin isoforms expressed in various organs of potato (*Solanum tuberosum*). Plant Sci 66: 221–230.
46. Rocha-Sosa M, Sonnewald U, Frommer W, Stratmann M, Schell J, et al. (1989) Both developmental and metabolic signals activate the promoter of a class I patatin gene. EMBO J 8: 23–29.
47. Ling H-Q, Kriseleit D, Ganal MW (1998) Effect of ticarcillin/potassium clavulanate on callus growth and shoot regeneration in Agrobacterium-mediated transformation of tomato (*Lycopersicon esculentum* Mill.). Plant Cell Reports 17: 843–847.
48. Klann E, Yelle S, Bennett AB (1992) Tomato fruit Acid Invertase Complementary DNA – Nucleotide and deduced amino acid sequences. Plant Physiol 99: 351–353.
49. Sander I, Kespohl S, Merget R, Goldscheid N, Degens PO, et al. (2005) A new method to bind allergens for the measurement of specific IgE antibodies. Int Arch Allergy Immunol 136: 39–44.
50. Erwin EA, Custis NJ, Satinover SM, Perzanowski MS, Woodfolk JA, et al. (2005) Quantitative measurement of IgE antibodies to purified allergens using streptavidin linked to a high-capacity solid phase. J Allergy Clin Immunol 115: 1029–1035.
51. von Krogh G, Maibach HI (1981) The contact urticaria syndrome: an updated review. J Am Acad Dermatol 5: 328–342.

2

# Tolerability of a Fully Maturated Cheese in Cow's Milk Allergic Children: Biochemical, Immunochemical, and Clinical Aspects

**Claudia Alessandri[1], Stefano Sforza[2], Paola Palazzo[1], Francesca Lambertini[2], Sara Paolella[2], Danila Zennaro[1], Chiara Rafaiani[1], Rosetta Ferrara[1], Maria Livia Bernardi[1], Mario Santoro[1], Sara Zuzzi[1], Ivana Giangrieco[1], Arnaldo Dossena[2], Adriano Mari[1]***

**1** Center for Molecular Allergology, IDI-IRCCS, Rome, Italy, **2** Department of Organic and Industrial Chemistry, University of Parma, Parma, Italy

## Abstract

***Background:*** From patients' reports and our preliminary observations, a fully maturated cheese (*Parmigiano-Reggiano;* PR) seems to be well tolerated by a subset of cow's milk (CM) allergic patients.

***Objective and Methods:*** To biochemically and immunologically characterize PR samples at different maturation stage and to verify PR tolerability in CM allergic children. Seventy patients, with suspected CM allergy, were enrolled. IgE to CM, α-lactalbumin (ALA), β-lactoglobulin (BLG) and caseins (CAS) were tested using ImmunoCAP, ISAC103 and skin prick test. Patients underwent a double-blind, placebo-controlled food challenge with CM, and an open food challenge with 36 months-maturated PR. Extracts obtained from PR samples were biochemically analyzed in order to determine protein and peptide contents. Pepsin and trypsin-chymotrypsin-pepsin simulated digestions were applied to PR extracts. Each PR extract was investigated by IgE Single Point Highest Inhibition Achievable assay (SPHIAa). The efficiency analysis was carried out using CM and PR oral challenges as gold standards.

***Results:*** The IgE binding to milk allergens was 100% inhibited by almost all PR preparations; the only difference was for CAS, mainly $\alpha_{S1}$-CAS. Sixteen patients sensitized to CM tolerated both CM and PR; 29 patients tolerated PR only; 21 patients, reacted to both CM and PR, whereas 4 patients reactive to CM refused to ingest PR. ROC analysis showed that the absence of IgE to BLG measured by ISAC could be a good marker of PR tolerance. The SPHIAa using digested PR preparations showed a marked effect on IgE binding to CAS and almost none on ALA and BLG.

***Conclusions:*** 58% of patients clinically reactive to CM tolerated fully maturated PR. The preliminary digestion of CAS induced by PR maturation process, facilitating a further loss of allergenic reactivity during gut digestion, might explain the tolerance. This hypothesis seems to work when no IgE sensitization to ISAC BLG is detected.

**Editor:** Christian Taube, Leiden University Medical Center, The Netherlands

**Funding:** This study has been funded by Centro Ricerche Produzioni Animali S.p.a. (www.crpa.it) and by the Italian Ministry of Health, Current Research Program 2008–2010. The funders had no role in the study design, data collection and analysis, decision to publish, or preparation of the manuscript.

**Competing Interests:** The authors have declared that no competing interests exist.

* E-mail: adriano.mari@idi.it

## Introduction

Cow's milk allergy (CM) is the most common food allergy during early infancy. CM contains allergenic proteins, caseins (CAS) and whey proteins, being the former a fraction accounting for 80% of total CM proteins, and including four different proteins: $\alpha_{S1}$-, $\alpha_{S2}$-, β- and κ-CAS [1–3]. β-lactoglobulin (BLG), whose homolog is not present in human milk, represents 50% of the CM whey proteins. The first line treatment for CM allergy is CM and dairy products avoidance [4,5], sometime leading to growth impairment [4]. Hydrolyzed formulas are good alternatives in CM allergic children though not always well accepted because of their not excellent taste [6]. They are produced by combined enzymatic and heat treatments and ultra-filtration of cow's milk proteins. According to the degree of protein modifications, hydrolyzed CM formulas are differentiated in partially and extensively hydrolyzed whey or CAS hydrolysates. Studies have supported the safety of including extensively heated products containing milk into the diet for those patients who are non-reactive [7].

Beside the clinical history and the oral food challenge, the diagnostic workup to correctly identify CM protein allergic patients is based on the use of *in vivo* or *in vitro* approaches, skin test and IgE detection respectively. Both approaches can be based on a fresh milk preparation (prick-prick test) and CM extracts [5], or discrete CM allergenic molecules [3]. The *in vitro* testing using allergenic molecules can be performed either in a singleplex way, like most of the currently used laboratory systems (*e.g.* ImmunoCAP, Immulite) or by multiplex testing using the allergenic molecule-based microarray technology (*e.g.* ISAC system) [8,9].

The latter laboratory approach allows IgE detection for a panel of CM-related and non-related allergenic molecules in a single run giving a broader view on patients' sensitization profiles [8,10].

*Parmigiano-Reggiano* (PR) is an Italian CM-based cheese with a variable but long and natural maturation process (12–36 months), produced in the place of origin and appointed for that with the "Protected Designation of Origin - PDO". Production is carried out under rigid specifications (http://www.parmigianoreggiano.com/consortium/rules_regulation_2/specification_single_document.aspx). The milk used in the process, obtained by cows fed with locally grown forage, is monitored to ensure the high quality and the presence of special characteristics. One kg of PR is made using 16 litres of CM. The partially skimmed milk is poured into copper cauldrons where calf rennet and fermented whey, rich in natural lactic ferments obtained from the processing of the day before, are added. The milk coagulates and the curd is then broken down into minuscule granules. After a cooking process, at 55°C, the cheesy granules form a single mass that will be placed in a mould which will give PR its final shape. After a few days the process of salting closes the production cycle and opens the maturation cycle. During maturation rennet's and lactic acid bacteria's proteases digest milk proteins. The full production cycle releases a cheese having a content of 30% water and 70% nutrients [11], mainly constituted by highly hydrolyzed proteins [12]. Different production procedures and maturation length adopted by other Italian and non-Italian parmesan producers give raise to different biochemical products as showed by Sforza et al. [12].

During the maturation, CAS are gradually and constantly broken down by the proteolytic enzymes of milk, rennet and lactic acid bacteria, yielding a nitrogen fraction which is continuously changing during the cheese maturation, gradually shifting from full proteins to longer peptides, then to shorter peptides and free amino acids. The peptide fraction of aged cheese is thus extremely complex, being formed by proteins, hundreds of different peptides, mostly deriving from $\alpha_{S1}$- and β-CAS, the two most abundant proteins in the CAS fraction, and free amino acids. The composition of this fraction is related to the month of maturation, and also, to a lesser extent, to the single producer [12,13].

Up to now allergenicity of PR proteins has never been studied. From patients' and caregivers' reports and from our preliminary observations, original PR cheese seemed to be well tolerated by a subset of CM allergic patients unless having generalized reactions on CM protein exposure.

In the present study, we sought to define the clinical tolerability of PR in CM allergic patients, characterizing the biochemical, immunochemical, and clinical aspects of the condition, trying to understand the underlying mechanisms and searching for a possible marker of PR reactivity/tolerability.

## Methods

### Patients' Selection and Allergy Testing

The study was carried out at the Center of Molecular Allergology, IDI-IRCCS, Rome, Italy, during the period December 2009–June 2011. Seventy-five patients referred to our center by the family pediatricians for suspected CM allergy have been enrolled. Seventy patients (47 male), age ranging from 6 months to 16 years (3 years old median age), agreed to participate. The suspicious of CM allergy was based on history of reactions after ingestion or contact with CM, or positive SPT or IgE to CM extracts. At the time of consultation, all patients were following a CM elimination diet set before by other physicians. All *in vivo* and *in vitro* tests performed in the present study are part of the routine diagnostic workup for CM allergic patients. Institutional Ethics Committee approval was obtained for using data, biological material, and performs PR challenge (29/CE/2009). Informed signed consent to perform food challenges was obtained from caregivers. *In vivo* tests have been performed in a highly protected environment in the day care centre.

Demographics, clinical data, namely respiratory and ingestion-related symptoms on CM exposure, and *in vivo* and *in vitro* test results, were recorded for all patients by an allergy specialist using the InterAll software, a customized allergy electronic record for diagnostic and clinical data storing (version 3.0, Allergy Data Laboratories, Latina, Italy).

Specifications on allergenic proteins used in the present study are given in Table 1. SPT were performed and measured as previously reported [10] using fresh skimmed CM, α-lactalbumin (ALA), BLG, CAS, and milk extract commercial preparations (Lofarma, Milan, Italy). A wheal area greater than 7 $mm^2$ was scored positive. Specific IgE towards CM, ALA, BLG and CAS were measured using the ImmunoCAP system (Phadia, Sweden); positive values were deemed when >0.35 kUa/l. Specific IgE for the same three allergen preparations *plus* bovine serum albumin (BSA) were measured using the ISAC 103 (Phadia Multiplexing Diagnostics, PMD, Vienna, Austria) as previously reported [14]; positive threshold value was set at 0.01 kUa/l.

### Food Challenges and Tolerance Follow Up

In order to verify the consistency of CM allergy diagnosis, a double blind placebo controlled CM challenge (DBPCFC) has been carried out in patients without recent CM anaphylaxis using fresh pasteurized skimmed milk (3.5% fat, 3.2 gr proteins/100 ml) following current international recommendations [15,16]. A preparation of 150 ml of skimmed milk and two spoons of white sugar were used as *verum*. The same preparation without CM but with soy or rice milk, depending on patient's use, was served as placebo. To mask smell, taste, and consistency differences, three teaspoons of sugarless cocoa (Cacao Amaro, Perugina, Italy), free of any nut contamination, were used for all preparations. In order to verify PR tolerability within the subset of CM allergic children, patients underwent challenge with 36 months matured PR preparation provided as a single lot from a single dairy by the PR consortium, and kept frozen at −20°C until used. An open food challenge procedure (OFC) has been adopted as it was impossible to adequately mask by any mean the strong PR taste to perform a DBPCFC. Patients were admitted to our centre in the morning, in a fasting state; administration of antihistamines, if any, was stopped at least one week prior to skin test and oral challenge, in order to avoid any effect on test outcomes. None of the patients was under steroid treatment. Blinded active and placebo meals were randomly administered in identical doses on separate days, prepared immediately before challenge [15,16]. CM challenge was performed as shown in Table 2, administering increasing doses every 20 minutes. PR challenge was performed taking into account the estimated CM proteins equivalent of 200 ml CM = 13.3 gr PR, as shown in Table 2. Only symptoms appearing soon after the challenge have been considered, whereas eczema flare up appearing the following days to the oral challenge was not considered as any objective evaluation was possible.

PR tolerant subjects were invited to continue consuming the 36 months maturated PR by using commercially available preparations as certified by the PR consortium. Symptoms recording in the follow up phase was made possible by using scheduled control visit attendance, or, if the visit was delayed for any reason, by email contacts or telephone calls.

**Table 1.** Cow's milk allergenic protein nomenclature and short names as adopted within the present study.

| Milk Allergen Nomenclature | | | | | Used for Diagnosis and Experiments# | | | |
|---|---|---|---|---|---|---|---|---|
| **Common Name** | **Short Name°** | **WHO-IUIS Nomenclature*** | **Allergome Name§** | **Allergome Code§** | **Skin Prick Test** | **CAP** | **ISAC 103** | **ISAC 89** |
| Cow's Milk | CM | N.A. | Bos d [Milk] | 1747 | Tested | Tested | N.T. | N.T. |
| α-Lactalbumin | ALA | Bos d 4 | Bos d 4 | 163 | Tested | Tested | Tested | Tested |
| β-lactoglobulin | BLG | Bos d 5 | Bos d 5 | 164 | Tested | Tested | Tested | N.T. |
| β-lactoglobulin A | BLG-A | N.A. | Bos d 5.0102 | 2738 | N.T. | N.T. | N.T. | Tested |
| β-lactoglobulin B | BLG-B | Bos d 5.0101 | Bos d 5.0101 | 2739 | N.T. | N.T. | N.T. | Tested |
| Serum Albumin | BSA | Bos d 6 | Bos d 6 | 165 | N.T. | N.T. | Tested | Tested |
| Lactoferrin | LCF | N.A. | Bos d Lactoferrin | 1065 | N.T. | N.T. | Tested | Tested |
| Caseins | CAS | Bos d 8 | Bos d 8 | 167 | Tested | Tested | Tested | Tested |
| $\alpha_{s1}$-Casein | $\alpha_{s1}$-CAS | N.A. | Bos d 8 alphaS1 | 2734 | N.T. | N.T. | N.T. | Tested |
| $\alpha_{s2}$-Casein | | N.A. | Bos d 8 alphaS2 | 2735 | N.T. | N.T. | N.T. | N.T. |
| β-Casein | β-CAS | N.A. | Bos d 8 beta | 2736 | N.T. | N.T. | N.T. | Tested |
| κ-Casein | κ-CAS | N.A. | Bos d 8 kappa | 2737 | N.T. | N.T. | N.T. | Tested |

Allergen specifications for each diagnostic or experimental testing are included.
°As used in the present paper;
*www.allergen.org.
§www.allergome.org.
#The test for diagnosis and experiments were provided as follows: Skin prick test by Lofarma, excepting cow's milk which was also used as fresh skimmed preparation by prick-prick testing; CAP by Phadia; ISAC 103 by PMD; ISAC 89 by VBC-Genomics;
N.A.: Not available, N.T.: not tested in the present study.

## Preparation of Water Soluble Extracts of PR Cheese

Forty six PR samples (1.5 kg each), at maturation ages between 6 and 41 months, were received from six producers as detailed in Table 3. Ninety two water soluble extracts (WSE) were obtained from the 46 PR samples and were prepared by homogenizing 20 gr of finely grated cheese by Ultra Turrax T50 Basic (IKA-Werke, Staufen, Germany) for 1.5 minutes at 4000 rpm in 90 ml of deionised water. The mixture was then filtered through filter paper to obtain a limpid extract.

**Table 2.** Oral Challenge schedules in patients with reported cow's milk sensitization.

| | Cow's Milk* | | *Parmigiano-Reggiano*° | | |
|---|---|---|---|---|---|
| **Dose** | **ml** | **Amount** | **Gr** | **Amount** | |
| 1 | 0.05 | 1 drop | 0.003 | 1 drop | PR (1 gr) *plus* water (14 ml) |
| 2 | 0.15 | 3 drops | 0.01 | 3 drops | |
| 3 | 0.3 | 6 drops | 0.02 | 6 drops | |
| 4 | 1 | 1 ml | 0.07 | 1 ml | |
| 5 | 3 | 3 ml | 0.2 | 3 ml | |
| 6 | 10 | 10 ml | 0.7 | 10 ml | |
| 7 | 30 | 30 ml | 2.00 | 2 gr | PR as is |
| 8 | 50 | 50 ml | 3.03 | 3 gr | |
| 9 | 100 | 100 ml | 6.07 | 7 gr | |
| Cumulative | 195 | | 13.0 | | |

*Cow's Milk: Double Blind Placebo Controlled Food Challenge;
°*Parmigiano-Reggiano*: Open Food Challenge;
PR: *Parmigiano-Reggiano* cheese;
Protein equivalence (aprox): 200 ml Cow's Milk = 13.3 gr PR.

## SDS-PAGE of PR Water Soluble Extracts

SDS-PAGE was performed on CriterionTM XT Precast gels 12% Bis-Tris (Bio Rad) according to the standard procedures indicated by the manufacturer (Bio-Rad). 100 µl of WSE were dried by nitrogen flow, re-dissolved in 25 µl of reducing sample buffer, and incubated at 95°C for 5 minutes. About 1 mg of ALA, BLG, α-CAS, β-CAS and κ-CAS were dissolved in 1 ml of deionised water and the volume corresponding to 5 µg of each protein was dried under nitrogen flow. Solid residue was dissolved in 25 µl of reducing sample buffer and incubated at 95°C for 5 minutes. The run was performed at 150 V and lasted about 55 minutes, using 1% of Coomassie blue in the sample buffer as indicator. The gel was transferred into a vessel with the staining solution covering it and placed in swelling for at least 1 hour. After that, the gel was rinsed with de-staining solution in order to achieve the desired contrast. Gel was acquired by GS-800 Calibrated Densitometer with Quantity One software (Bio Rad).

## Peptide and Whey Protein Determination by UHPLC/ESI-MS Analysis

For UHPLC analysis, 900 µl of WSE were transferred into a vial and dried under nitrogen flow, then dissolved in 150 µl, of 0.1% formic acid solution. UHPLC/ESI-MS analysis was performed by using an Acquity UPLC separation system (Waters, Milford, Ma, USA) with an Acquity BEH C18 2.1×150 mm column (Waters), 1.7 µm particle size, according to a previous published methodology [Sforza S, Cavatorta V, Lambertini F, Galaverna G, Dossena A et al. J Dairy Sci 2012; accepted for publication]. Each UHPLC/ESI-MS chromatogram was analyzed in order to determine the molecular weight and the characteristic ions of the main peaks. In the case of molecular weights higher than 1 kDa, reconstructed mass peaks were obtained by MaxEnt 1, application of Masslynx 4.0 software (Waters, Milford, Ma, USA). Peptides were mostly identified according to their MW and

**Table 3.** Ninety two *PR* water soluble extracts from 46 samples as provided by six producers at different maturation ages.

| Sample | Protein (mg/ml) | Sample | Protein (mg/ml) | Sample | Protein (mg/ml) | Sample | Protein (mg/ml) | Sample | Protein (mg/ml) |
|---|---|---|---|---|---|---|---|---|---|
| **A-6-1-a** | 2,19 | A-6-2-a | 1,71 | **C-6-1-a** | 1,43 | C-6-2-a | 0,89 | E-6-1-a | 0,82 |
| A-12-1-a | 2,18 | A-12-2-a | 1,21 | C-14-1-a | 0,93 | C-13-2-a | 0,97 | E-12-1-a | 1,26 |
| **A-16-1-a** | 1,88 | A-16-2-a | 1,05 | **C-18-1-a** | 1,14 | C-18-2-a | 1,14 | E-24-1-a | 0,98 |
| A-24-1-a | 1,17 | A-24-2-a | 2,00 | C-24-1-a | 0,91 | C-23-2-a | 1,12 | E-37-1-a | 0,73 |
| **A-36-1-a** | 1,55 | A-36-2-a | 2,17 | **C-38-1-a** | 1,06 | | | E-41-1-a | 0,72 |
| A-6-1-b | 1,27 | A-6-2-b | 2,35 | C-6-1-b | 1,42 | C-6-2-b | 1,02 | E-6-1-b | 0,85 |
| A-12-1-b | 1,76 | A-12-2-b | 1,97 | C-14-1-b | 2,03 | C-13-2-b | 1,21 | E-12-1-b | 1,18 |
| A-16-1-b | 1,05 | A-16-2-b | 2,44 | C-18-1-b | 1,26 | C-18-2-b | 1,10 | E-24-1-b | 0,98 |
| A-24-1-b | 1,36 | A-24-2-b | 1,88 | C-24-1-b | 1,85 | C-24-2-b | 1,41 | E-37-1-b | 0,80 |
| A-36-1-b | 1,38 | A-36-2-b | 2,01 | C-38-1-b | 1,15 | | | E-41-1-b | 0,80 |
| **B-6-1-a** | 1,37 | B-6-2-a | 1,20 | **D-7-1-a** | 1,37 | D-6-2-a | 1,43 | | |
| B-12-1-a | 2,60 | B-12-2-a | 1,29 | D-12-1-a | 1,37 | D-12-2-a | 1,20 | F-11-1-a | 1,43 |
| **B-18-1-a** | 2,10 | B-18-2-a | 1,14 | **D-20-1-a** | 1,67 | D-24-2-a | 1,21 | F-24-1-a | 1,66 |
| B-25-1-a | 2,00 | B-24-2-a | 1,25 | D-26-1-a | 1,07 | D-36-2-a | 1,37 | F-33-1-a | 1,75 |
| **B-36-1-a** | 2,39 | B-36-2-a | | **D-41-1-a** | 1,12 | | | | |
| B-6-1-b | 1,37 | B-6-2-b | 1,17 | D-7-1-b | 1,35 | D-6-2-b | 1,15 | | |
| B-12-1-b | 1,75 | B-12-2-b | 1,06 | D-12-1-b | 1,64 | D-12-2-b | 0,99 | F-11-1-b | 2,10 |
| B-18-1-b | 1,09 | B-18-2-b | 1,49 | D-20-1-b | 1,54 | D-24-2-b | 1,11 | F-24-1-b | 1,61 |
| B-25-1-b | 1,33 | B-24-2-b | 1,21 | D-26-1-b | 1,13 | D-36-2-b | 1,35 | F-33-1-b | 1,94 |
| B-36-1-b | 1,40 | B-36-2-b | 1,46 | D-41-1-b | 1,11 | | | | |

One or two samples were provided, and one or two water soluble extracts were prepared.
Footnote: Each water soluble extract has been identified using an uppercase letter for the producer, a number indicating the maturation age in months, a second number indicating the first or second sample when available, and a lowercase letter indicating the performed extractions. Protein yield in mg/ml are given for each extract. Extracts marked in bold have been used for the simulated gastrointestinal digestion experiments.

to fragments present in the mass spectra, according to a methodology previously developed [12,13], also using a suitably developed software for assisting the identification, by narrowing the possibilities according to the proteins generating the proteolytic peptides (Pep Sirio software, Biodigital Valley, Italy).

The quantification of ALA and BLG in the extracts was performed by UHPLC/ESI-MS applying the same method as above, with the external standard method for quantification. Calibration curves were obtained by injecting in the UHPLC/ESI-MS systems standard solutions of ALA and BLG at different concentrations. All standards and samples were analyzed by extracting from the full scan chromatograms the selected ion chromatograms for the two proteins, by using the following ions: m/z 1418.3, 1575.8 for ALA; m/z 1143.0, 1219.1 for BLG-B, and 1148.3, 1224.9 for BLG-A. The chromatographic peaks were integrated in all the extracted chromatograms, and the standard solutions were used as reference for the quantification of the same proteins in the samples.

## In vitro Simulated Gastrointestinal Digestion of PR Water Soluble Extracts

Two different digestion models were applied: the first simulating the gastric transit, using pepsin, and a second one using all three major digestive enzymes, namely trypsin and chymotripsin after pepsin treatment (TCP), in order to simulate the digestion in the gastric and the intestinal tracts. The 12 WSE marked in Table 3 were used in the digestion experiments. For preparing standard solutions, 10 mg of pepsin were dissolved in 10 ml of hydrochloric acid solution at pH 4.4 and stored at $-20°C$, 10 mg of trypsin were dissolved in 10 ml of hydrochloric acid solution 1 mM at pH 3.0 and stored at $-20°C$, 10 mg of chymotrypsin were dissolved in 10 ml of hydrochloric acid solution 1 mM containing $CaCl_2$ 2 mM and stored at $-20°C$. 5 ml of WSE were acidified to pH 2.2 by the addition of hydrochloric acid 1 mM and 50 μl of pepsin stock solution were added (enzyme:protein ratio 1:100). The mixture was incubated in horizontal swelling for 3 hours at 37°C in order to simulate the gastric transit. The solution was then neutralized by the addition of $NH_4HCO_3$ to pH 7.5 and 50 μl of trypsin and 50 μl of chymotrypsin stock solutions (enzyme:protein ratio 1:100) were then added. The mixture was incubated in horizontal swelling for 4 hours at 37°C in order to simulate intestinal transit. In order to stop the digestion at the end of the simulation, 1 ml of acetonitrile was mixed with the solution. Finally, 1 ml of digested WSE was centrifuged at 16000 *g* for 15 minutes. The supernatant was stored at $-20°C$.

## Immunochemical Characterization of PR Water Soluble Extracts

The qualitative allergen composition of each PR WSE was investigated by the Single Point Highest Inhibition Achievable assay (SPHIAa) [17] performed by detecting IgE on the ISAC 89 microarray (VBC-Genomics, Vienna, Austria), where purified natural milk allergens are immobilized. The ISAC 89 microarray was used as, along with other milk allergens, it bears purified CAS, $\alpha_{S1}$-CAS, β-CAS, κ-CAS as well as the two BLG natural variants (Table 1). A pool of sera of allergic subjects known having IgE for

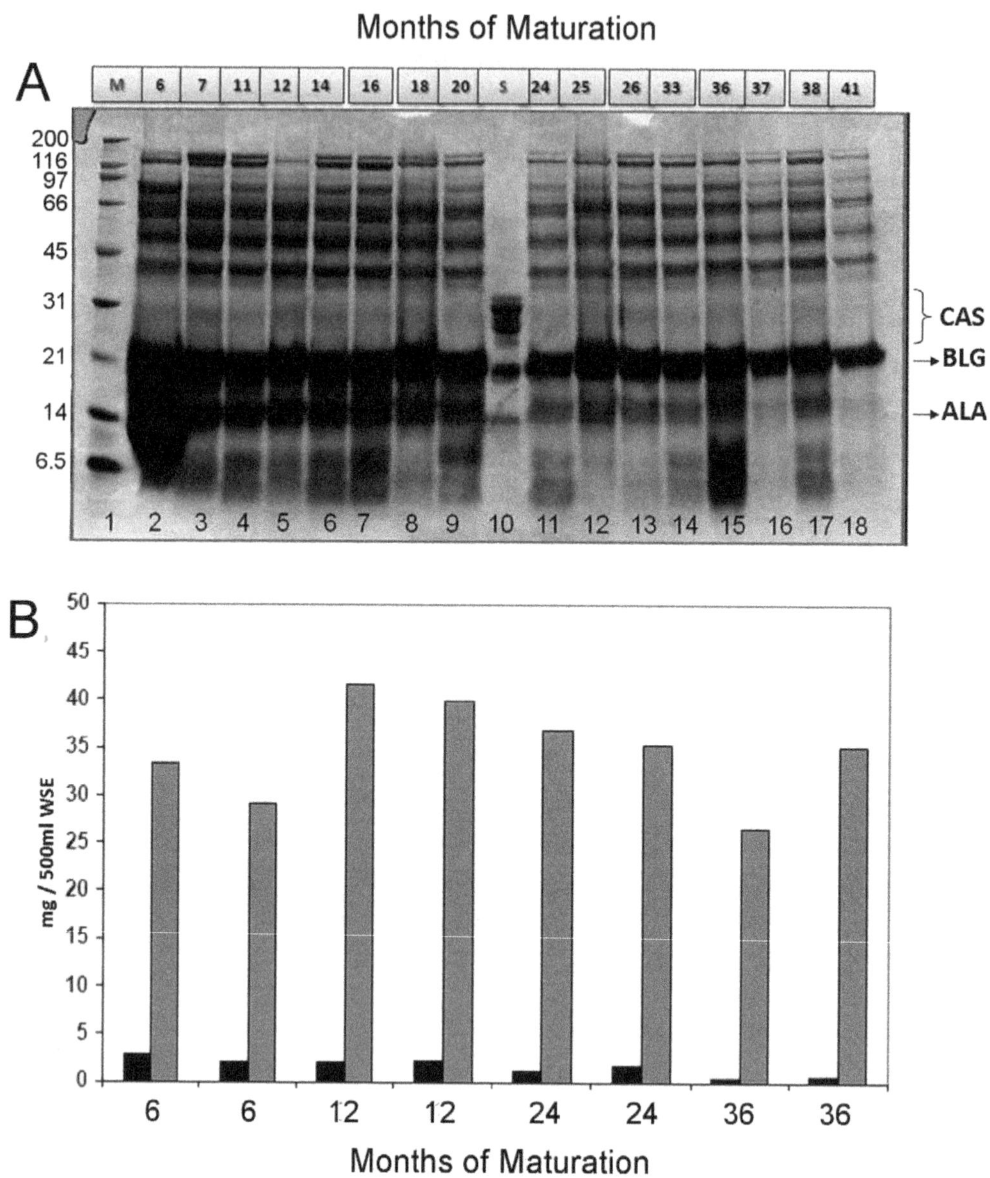


**Figure 1. Biochemical evaluation of cow's milk proteins in *Parmigiano-Reggiano* preparations at different maturation stages.** Panel A: SDS-PAGE of *Parmigiano-Reggiano* (PR) water soluble extracts at different maturation time (6–41 months). Extracts from different producers, as detailed in Table 3, are shown to give a comprehensive description of maturation effect on (PR); Lane 2: A-6-1-a; Lane 3: D-7-1-a; Lane 4: F-11-1-b; Lane 5: B-12-1-a; Lane 6: C-14-1-a; Lane 7: A-16-1-a; Lane 8: B-18-1-a; Lane 9: B-20-1-a; Lane11: E-24-1-a; Lane 12: B-25-1-a; Lane 13: D-26-1-a; Lane 14: F-33-1-a; Lane 15: A-36-1-a; Lane 16: E-37-1-a; Lane 17: C-38-1-a; Lane 18: E-41-1-b. The molecular weight marker (M, lane 1) and a standard solution (S, lane 10) containing α-lactalbumin, β-lactoglobulin, α-caseins, β-casein, κ-casein are also included. ALA: α-lactalbumin; BLG: β-lactoglobulin; CAS: casein fraction. Numbers above lanes indicate the month of maturation (lanes 2–9 and 11–18); numbers below indicate lanes. Panel B: Amounts of α-lactalbumin and β-lactoglobulin in the PR aqueous extracts having different maturation ages, as measured by UHPLC/ESI-MS. Some of the analyzed samples from different producers are shown. Preparations shown in the graph can be identified in Table 3 as follows, from left to right: 6 months: A-6-1-a; 7 months: B-6-1-a; 12 months: B-12-1-a; 12 months: D-12-1-a; 24 months: A-24-1-a; 24 months: C-24-1-a; 36 months: A-36-1-a; 36 months: B-36-1-a. Values are expressed as mg/100 gr Water Soluble Extract, and reported as average of two independent analyses (standard deviations aprox 10%). Black bars: α-lactalbumin (ALA); Grey bars: β-lactoglobulin (BLG).

all the above allergen specificities was used. Serum donors were not the same patients enrolled in the study because to perform all inhibitions a quite large amount of serum had to be used, thus requiring a higher number of donors. As far as the pooled sera were used as probes for allergen detection in extract by the SPHIAa, sera selection did not influence the experimental outcome. The same pool was used throughout the study for all IgE inhibition experiments. Fifteen μl of the serum pool were incubated overnight with the PR WSE both in the first set of experiments comparing the 92 different PR preparations and in the experiments using digested PR WSE as detailed in Table 3. As non-inhibited control the same serum pool was incubated with D-PBS (Euroclone, Milan, Italy). For the SPHIAa experiments as reported above, using digested PR, preparations from four producers at three maturation stages, young, medium and aged, respectively, were used, as shown in Table 3. ISAC 89 testing for IgE was performed as previously reported [14].

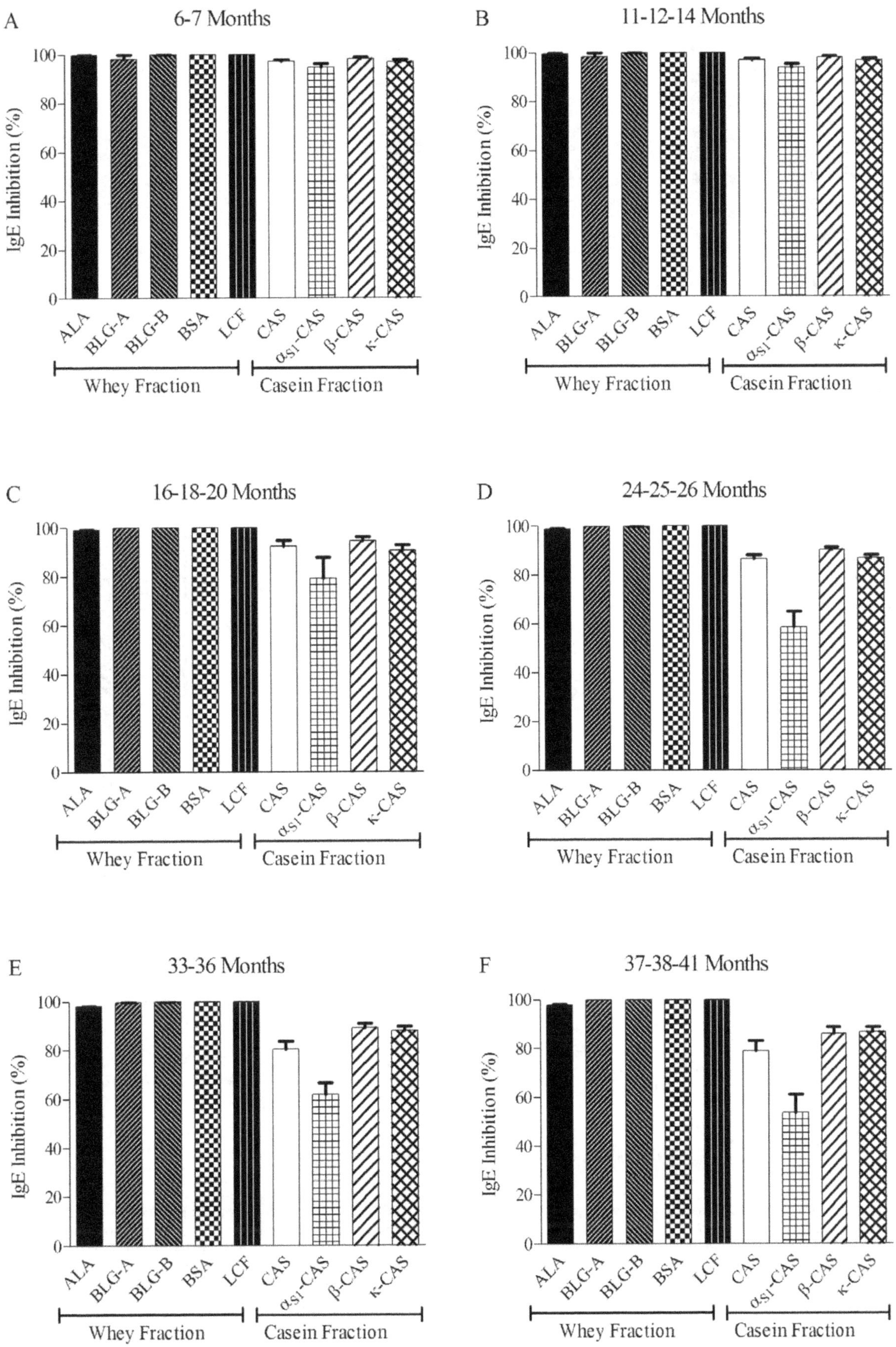
A
6-7 Months
IgE Inhibition (%)
0
20
40
60
80
100
ALA
BLG-A
BLG-B
BSA
LCF
CAS
αS1-CAS
β-CAS
κ-CAS
Whey Fraction
Casein Fraction
B
11-12-14 Months
IgE Inhibition (%)
0
20
40
60
80
100
ALA
BLG-A
BLG-B
BSA
LCF
CAS
αS1-CAS
β-CAS
κ-CAS
Whey Fraction
Casein Fraction
C
16-18-20 Months
IgE Inhibition (%)
0
20
40
60
80
100
ALA
BLG-A
BLG-B
BSA
LCF
CAS
αS1-CAS
β-CAS
κ-CAS
Whey Fraction
Casein Fraction
D
24-25-26 Months
IgE Inhibition (%)
0
20
40
60
80
100
ALA
BLG-A
BLG-B
BSA
LCF
CAS
αS1-CAS
β-CAS
κ-CAS
Whey Fraction
Casein Fraction
E
33-36 Months
IgE Inhibition (%)
0
20
40
60
80
100
ALA
BLG-A
BLG-B
BSA
LCF
CAS
αS1-CAS
β-CAS
κ-CAS
Whey Fraction
Casein Fraction
F
37-38-41 Months
IgE Inhibition (%)
0
20
40
60
80
100
ALA
BLG-A
BLG-B
BSA
LCF
CAS
αS1-CAS
β-CAS
κ-CAS
Whey Fraction
Casein Fraction

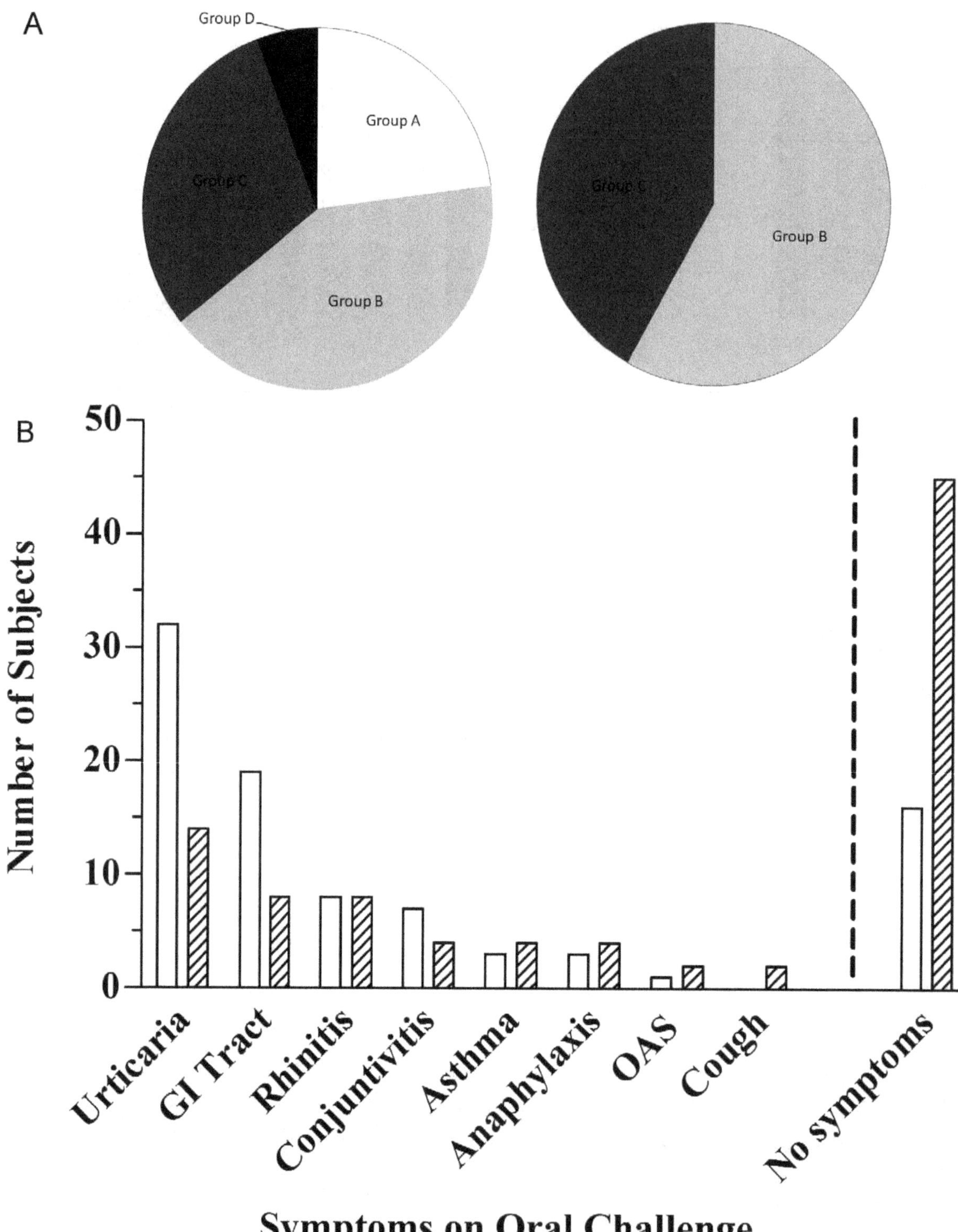


**Figure 3.** ***In vivo*** **test reactivity distribution and symptoms recorded on DBPCFC with fresh cow's milk and OFC with 36 months maturated *Parmigiano-Reggiano.*** Panel A, left graph, includes all 70 patients either tested or not for both milk and PR preparations. Group A includes Cow's Milk (CM) and *Parmigiano-Reggiano* (PR) Tolerant subjects: 16 (22.86%); Group B includes CM Reactive PR Tolerant subjects: 29 (41.43%); Group C includes CM and PR Reactive subjects: 21 (30%); Group D includes CM Reactive PR not tested subjects: 4 (5.71%). Panel A, right graph, includes the 50 patients who reacted to CM DBPCFC and differently to PR OFC. Group B includes CM Reactive PR Tolerant subjects: 29 (58%); Group C includes CM and PR Reactive subjects: 21 (42%). Panel B includes the 66 patients tested by both CM DBPCFC and PR OFC; White bars: symptoms recorded after CM DBPCFC in 50 reactive subjects; Hatched bars: symptoms recorded after PR OFC in 21 reactive subjects; The four subjects not tested with PR OFC are not included in the graph. GI Tract: symptoms related to the gastrointestinal tract including vomiting and diarrhea, excluding oral allergy syndrome (OAS). Urticaria, GI tract symptoms and no symptom prevalence differed by the Fisher's exact test in a

statistically significant way for p<0.0017, 0.0297, 0.0001, respectively.

## Statistics

Descriptive statistics included relative frequencies for qualitative and quantitative variables. Specific IgE and SPT results were expressed using median values. Graphpad Prism version 5.02 has been used for advanced statistics and graphs (Graphpad Software Inc., La Jolla, CA, USA). Fisher's exact test has been used to compare prevalence. To assess test performances, receiver operating characteristic (ROC) analyses were performed using MedCalc (MedCalc SW, Mariakerke, Belgium) on SPT, ImmunoCAP and ISAC specific IgE data, using both CM DBPCFC and PR OFC as gold standard. Sensitivity and specificity, proving the diagnostic performance of each test, were estimated at the optimal cut-off level. Statistically significance level was set at a p value <0.05.

# Results

## Casein and Whey Protein Content of PR Water Soluble Extracts

SDS-PAGE of PR WSE samples was obtained. Sixteen samples, received from different producers and having different maturation times, are reported as an example in Figure 1, panel A, to provide an overall picture of the maturation effect on PR. All other samples were consistent with those in the figure (data not shown). The most abundant proteins of the extracts were found to be whey proteins, ALA and BLG, whereas CAS where nearly absent in all the samples (Figure 1, panel A). The most intense protein band, corresponding to the BLG MW, seems to be resistant to PR proteolytic degradation, giving intense bands also in very aged samples, whereas the protein having a MW of about 14 kDa, deemed to be ALA, seems to be partly degraded along the maturation. Quantification of the two whey proteins, performed by UHPLC/ESI-MS on several samples, confirmed what described above from SDS-PAGE results, indicating for intact BLG a content ranging from 30 to 40 mg/500 ml of PR WSE, which was found to be independent from the maturation time, whereas a much lower content of ALA was detected, of about 3–5 mg/500 ml of WSE in the younger samples, which reduced to 1 mg or less in the most aged samples. Figure 1, panel B shows some examples among the 92 analyzed; all other samples were consistent with those in the figure (data not shown).

## Peptide Content of PR Water Soluble Extracts

The WSE were also analyzed by UHPLC-ESI/MS in order to determine the main composition of the peptide fraction. Focusing only on the most abundant peptides, the compounds giving a signal intensity equivalent to at least 30% of the signal of the most abundant compounds were considered. Several peptides were traced and identified in all compounds. Peptides could be divided in two groups: proteolytic compounds, derived from CAS breakdown, where only $\alpha_{S1}$-CAS and β-CAS fragments were identified, being these proteins the most abundant in the CM CAS fraction, and non-proteolytic aminoacyl derivatives, derived from the recombination of the free amino acids in unusual dipeptide like structures (γ-glutamyl-amino acids, lactoyl-amino acids, pyroglutamyl-amino acids) [18].

The quantitative trends observed were quite clear: proteolytic compounds deriving from CAS fragmentation were found to be the most abundant in the less aged samples (6 months) and then continuously decreasing with the increasing of the maturation time, whereas non-proteolytic compounds always increased or

**Table 4.** Demographics and *in vivo* and *in vitro* diagnostic test results in patients referring to our allergy Centre with a previous diagnosis of cow's milk allergy.

| | DBPCFC | OFC | Subjects | Demographics | | Total IgE |
|---|---|---|---|---|---|---|
| Groups | CM | PR | N | Age° | F/M | IU/ml° |
| A | Neg | Neg | 16 | 5 | 6/10 | 632 |
| B | Pos | Neg | 29 | 3.9 | 17/12 | 1257 |
| C | Pos | Pos | 21 | 3.6 | 5/16 | 424 |
| D | Pos | N.T. | 4 | 2.3 | 4/0 | 393 |

| | DBPCFC | OFC | P-P* | Skin Prick Test* | | | | IgE ImmunoCAP* | | | | IgE ISAC* | | |
|---|---|---|---|---|---|---|---|---|---|---|---|---|---|---|
| Groups | CM | PR | CM | CM | ALA | BLG | CAS | CM | ALA | BLG | CAS | ALA | BLG | CAS |
| A | Neg | Neg | 75 | 56 | 44 | 56 | 31 | 75 | 50 | 38 | 44 | 13 | 6 | 19 |
| B | Pos | Neg | 90 | 69 | 54 | 65 | 29 | 93 | 62 | 66 | 76 | 48 | 17 | 41 |
| C | Pos | Pos | 95 | 80 | 85 | 100 | 62 | 100 | 86 | 90 | 90 | 67 | 76 | 71 |
| D | Pos | N.T. | 100 | 50 | 100 | 75 | 50 | 100 | 100 | 75 | 75 | 75 | 25 | 25 |

CM: Cow's milk; PR: *Parmigiano-Reggiano* cheese;
Group A: CM and PR tolerant; Group B: Allergic to CM, PR tolerant; Group C: Allergic to CM and PR; Group D: Allergic to CM, but not tested for PR OFC.
Allergen short names are as in Table 1. P-P: prick-prick technique with fresh CM.
*Values are expressed as percentage of all test results in the group, considering positive values above each specific test cut-off (P-P and skin prick test >7 mm$^2$, IgE ImmunoCAP>0.35 kUa/l, IgE ISAC 0.01 kUa/l).
°Age and total IgE are expressed as medians in years and IU/l, respectively.

**Table 5.** ROC analyses of performed tests using cow's milk DBPCFC and PR OFC as gold standards.

| **Cow's Milk DBPCFC** | | **Criterion**[§] | **Sensitivity** | **Specificity** | **+LR** | **−LR** | **PPV** | **NPV** |
|---|---|---|---|---|---|---|---|---|
| | Total IgE | >101 | 66.0 | 56.2 | 1.51 | 0.60 | 82.5 | 34.6 |
| Prick-Prick test | CM* | >56.3 | 64.0 | 68.7 | 2.05 | 0.52 | 86.5 | 37.9 |
| Skin prick test | CM° | >2.8 | 86.0 | 43.7 | 1.53 | 0.32 | 82.7 | 50.0 |
| | ALA | >16 | 64.0 | 75.0 | 2.56 | 0.48 | 88.9 | 40.0 |
| | BLG | >13.5 | 72.0 | 62.5 | 1.92 | 0.45 | 85.7 | 41.7 |
| | CAS | >17.7 | 32.0 | 93.7 | 5.12 | 0.73 | 94.1 | 30.6 |
| ImmunoCAP | CM | >0.52 | 94.0 | 50.0 | 1.88 | 0.12 | 85.5 | 72.7 |
| | ALA | >1.02 | 58.0 | 81.2 | 3.09 | 0.52 | 90.6 | 38.2 |
| | BLG | >0 | 90.0 | 50.0 | 1.80 | 0.20 | 84.9 | 61.5 |
| | CAS | >0.44 | 82.0 | 62.5 | 2.19 | 0.29 | 87.2 | 52.6 |
| ISAC | ALA | >0 | 56.0 | 87.5 | 4.48 | 0.50 | 93.3 | 38.9 |
| | BLG | >0 | 40.0 | 93.7 | 6.40 | 0.64 | 95.2 | 33.3 |
| | CAS | >0 | 54.0 | 81.2 | 2.88 | 0.57 | 90.0 | 36.1 |
| ***Parmigiano-Reggiano* OFC** | | **Criterion**[§] | **Sensitivity** | **Specificity** | **+LR** | **−LR** | **PPV** | **NPV** |
| | Total IgE | ≤628 | 85.7 | 33.3 | 1.29 | 0.43 | 37.5 | 83.3 |
| Prick-Prick test | CM* | >59,3 | 90.5 | 62.2 | 2.39 | 0.15 | 52.8 | 93.3 |
| Skin prick test | CM° | >26 | 76.2 | 66.7 | 2.29 | 0.36 | 51.6 | 85.7 |
| | ALA | >16 | 80.9 | 57. 8 | 1.92 | 0.33 | 47.2 | 86.7 |
| | BLG | >28.26 | 80.9 | 73.3 | 3.04 | 0.26 | 58.6 | 89.2 |
| | CAS | >17.7 | 57.1 | 88.9 | 5.14 | 0.48 | 70.6 | 81.6 |
| ImmunoCAP | CM | >3.99 | 85.7 | 71.1 | 2.97 | 0.20 | 58.1 | 91.4 |
| | ALA | >1.93 | 76.2 | 80.0 | 3.81 | 0.30 | 64.0 | 87.8 |
| | BLG | >2.54 | 66.7 | 84.4 | 4.29 | 0.39 | 66.7 | 84.4 |
| | CAS | >5.25 | 76.2 | 82.2 | 4.29 | 0.29 | 66.7 | 88.1 |
| ISAC | ALA | >0.14 | 66.7 | 73.3 | 2.50 | 0.45 | 53.8 | 82.5 |
| | BLG | >0.15 | 71.4 | 91.1 | 8.04 | 0.31 | 78.9 | 87.2 |
| | CAS | >0.43 | 66.7 | 75.6 | 2.73 | 0.44 | 56.0 | 82.9 |

Allergen short names are as in Table 1.
DBPCFC: Double blind placebo controlled food challenge;
OFC: Open food challenge;
PR: *Parmigiano-Reggiano;*
*Fresh cow's milk tested by skin prick-prick technique;
°Cow's milk extract tested by skin prick test;
§Criteria for applied tests are reported depending on specific test units: Total IgE = IU/l; Skin prick test = $mm^2$; IgE by ImmunoCAP and ISAC = kUa/l;
+LR: Positive likelihood ratio; −LR: Negative likelihood ratio; NPV: Negative predictive value;
PPV: Positive predictive value.

maintained a constant amount by increasing the maturation time (data not shown).

These results on the composition of peptide fraction were in perfect agreement with previous works on PR WSE [12,13] and on recent report detailing the evolution along time of the peptide fraction [Sforza S, Cavatorta V, Lambertini F, Galaverna G, Dossena A et al. J Dairy Sci 2012; accepted for publication].

## Immunochemical Features of PR Water Soluble Extracts

In agreement with the molecular composition reported above, the main results of SPHIAa experiments performed on the 92 PR WSE are shown in Figure 2 and can be summarized as follows: the tested PR WSE samples showed to contain all proteins known as allergens, including milk whey proteins, as all preparation were equally able to exert IgE inhibition on allergens immobilized on the ISAC microarray (Figure 2). No major differences were observed depending on the producer. Extracts of PR matured up to 20 months have an almost intact ability to inhibit specific IgE binding on all ISAC allergens. This result implies that all CM IgE-binding epitopes recognized on ISAC allergens by the serum pool are preserved intact in "young" PR preparations. This applies to all CAS and whey proteins (Figure 2, panel A to C). PR extracts older than 20 months behaved on whey proteins similarly to those of 20 months or younger, whilst for CAS a decreasing IgE inhibition ability was found as a function of PR maturation (Figure 2, panels D to F). This behaviour is more pronounced for $\alpha_{S1}$-CAS, whose IgE binding inhibition gradually decreases to 45% with PR samples of 37–41 months maturation, whilst the IgE binding on β-CAS and κ-CAS slightly decreased reaching an 83–85% inhibition value.

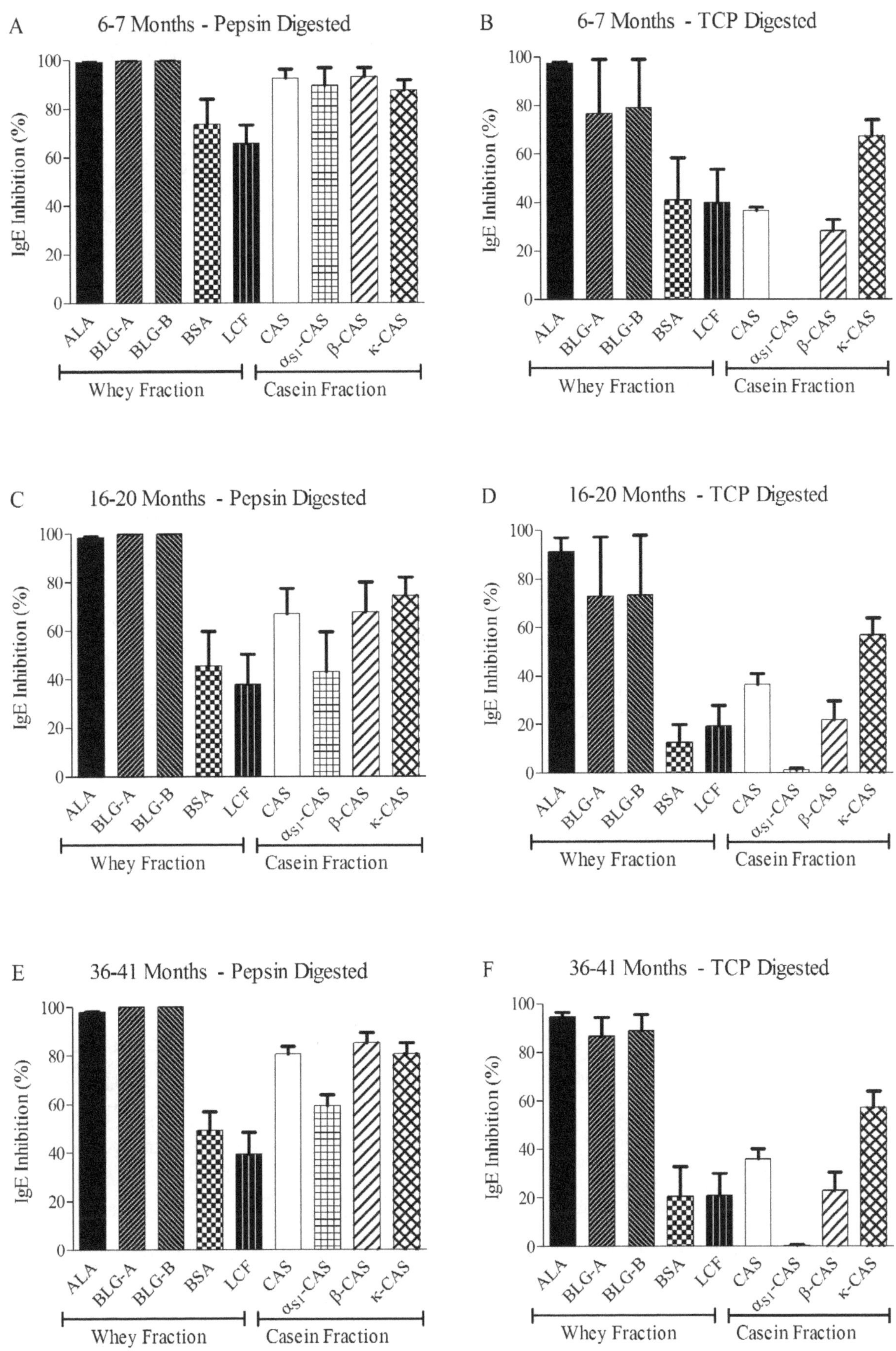
A
6-7 Months - Pepsin Digested
B
6-7 Months - TCP Digested
C
16-20 Months - Pepsin Digested
D
16-20 Months - TCP Digested
E
36-41 Months - Pepsin Digested
F
36-41 Months - TCP Digested
IgE Inhibition (%)
0
20
40
60
80
100
ALA
BLG-A
BLG-B
BSA
LCF
CAS
αS1-CAS
β-CAS
κ-CAS
Whey Fraction
Casein Fraction

**Figure 4. Single Point Highest Inhibition Achievable assay (SPHIAa) IgE experiments with simulated digestions of *Parmigiano-Reggiano* water soluble extracts at three different maturation stages.** Results are the average of water soluble extracts obtained from four producers. Error bars, indicating variability among four assays, are reported above each allergen result. TCP: Trypsin, Chimotrypsin, Pepsin.

## Oral Challenge with PR

Considering SPT, CM and CM allergen ImmunoCAP IgE and ISAC IgE performed tests, all 70 patients reacted to at least one allergen of at least one of the performed test. As shown in Figure 3, panel A left part, the analysis of the CM DBPCFC and PR OFC allowed us dividing the 70 CM sensitized patients in four groups: group A, 16 patients, tolerated both CM and PR; group B, 29 patients, tolerated PR only; group C, 21 patients, reacted to both CM and PR, while 4 patients in group D, reacted to CM but refused to undergo PR OFC thus dropped off the study. Overall, 29 of 50 patients allergic to CM (58%) tolerated 36 months maturated PR (Figure 3, panel A right part). Symptoms of the patients reacting on DBPCFC to CM and OFC to PR are shown in Figure 3, panel B. Statistical analysis is reported in the Figure 3 legend.

For all performed tests (SPT, ImmunoCAP, ISAC) a common trend was found: percentages of test results above their cut-off gradually increased shifting from group A to B to C (Table 4), with the only exception of CAS SPT. The best marker of PR tolerance seems to be the absence of IgE to BLG on ISAC testing, providing specificity greater than 91.1% at the optimum cut-off of 0.15 kUa/l against PR OFC as gold standard (Table 5).

## IgE Inhibition Using SPHIAa and Digested PR Water Soluble Extracts

Simulated gastrointestinal digestion effects applied to PR WSE at different maturation stages were studied by SPHIAa on IgE. Enzymes without any PR preparation and PR WSE at the same maturation stages without enzyme preparations acted as negative and positive controls, respectively. Recorded results of no IgE inhibition for the former and full IgE binding inhibitions, in an almost overlapping way as in Figure 2, for the latter were obtained (data not shown). SPHIAa for IgE were then carried out on three different maturation ages of PR WSE samples coming from four different dairies, as marked in Table 3. Aggregated data are reported in Figure 4. Whey-derived proteins were differently affected by the two simulated digestions, having no effect at all for ALA, little or even doubtful effect for both BLG variants, and a progressive additive effect on BSA and LCF by both pepsin and TCP digestions, reaching an almost total loss of the IgE binding inhibition capacity for the average and the most aged PR WSE preparations under TCP digestion (Figure 4). Almost the same effect as described for BSA and LCF was recorded for CAS, with a different behaviour of the three purified CAS. $\alpha_{S1}$-CAS, already having its IgE binding inhibition capacity partially reduced by PR maturation (Figure 2), totally lost its IgE inhibitory capability in a progressive and increasing manner with increasing PR maturation age, mainly under TCP digestion (Figure 4). A very partial effect was also recorded during pepsin digestion. ß-CAS and κ-CAS, whose IgE binding inhibition capability was almost not affected by PR maturation (Figure 2), were not influenced by the pepsin digestion, whereas had their IgE inhibition activity reduced by TCP digestion, more pronounced though not total for ß-CAS (Figure 4).

## PR Medium-long Term "Real Life" Tolerance

All PR tolerant subjects were in the follow up phase. Parents were instructed to continue using the 36 months maturated PR at home by using the commercially available preparations as certified by the producer on the marketed packages. No specific weekly schedule of PR intake was given assuming its use as normal in Italians daily life. Overall follow up period lasted from December 2009 up to December 2011, with the shortest observation time of six months just for one child. None of the PR tolerant subjects reported any minor or major complaint in the follow up phase, all using PR as in the usual family habit.

## IgE Detection Toward Additional Non-CM Food and Inhalant Allergens

Testing 103 allergenic molecules for IgE using the microarray approach allowed us to detect sensitizations also to other important allergens from other sources as shown in Figure 5. Allergenic molecules were considered either as markers of allergen group sensitization (Figure 5, Panel A) or as markers of sensitization to a given allergenic source (Figure 5, Panel B–C; *i.e.* Gal d 1, 2, 3, and 5 for hen's egg allergy, Phl p 1, 2, 4, 5, 6, and 11 for grass pollen allergy). Additional details on allergens are given in Figure 5 legend. Eleven patients had no additional IgE detectable sensitizations on the ISAC103; 5 were in the group A, 5 in the group B, and 1 in the group C. Evaluating the 55 subjects being positive for at least one non-CM allergen, a general trend was recorded for having higher sensitization prevalence, mainly in group C, to some of the other food allergens, namely the markers for hen's egg, seeds excluding peanuts, soy, and kiwifruit, or to food panallergens like lipid transfer proteins from plant-derived foods and parvalbumins from fishes. Such trend was not recorded for allergens causing sensitization by inhalation like those from pollen, mites, mammal epithelia, and moulds.

## Discussion

Although other authors already reported tolerance to baked CM proteins in CM allergic children [7,19,20], we herein prove for the first time how CM allergic children can tolerate a dairy product as PR cheese, lacking CM high temperature processing. Although all CM allergenic proteins extracted from PR in its various maturation stages largely retained their ability to bind IgE, the clinical findings prompted us to investigate the clinical tolerance mechanism of this non-baked product. Among the CM proteins, CAS seems to behave differently from the others, as the proteolytic enzymes activity during the maturation process reduces, at least partially, their IgE binding capability. The presence of CAS derived peptides indicate that an intense proteolytic process on the CAS fraction is continuously acting, degrading the full proteins and the peptides derived from them, making aged PR very poor in CAS in their native structure. The absence of CAS in the extracts might thus be due in part to the poor CAS solubility in water, but mostly to their proteolytic degradation which takes place during PR manufacturing and maturation; actually, older samples were accordingly poorer in CAS than younger ones.

Conversely, no peptides derived from whey proteins were observed, indicating that the proteolysis does not affect these proteins, and actually whey protein content seems not to be affected by the maturation time. As for CAS, whey proteins retain an almost intact ability to bind IgE also in very aged PR preparations.

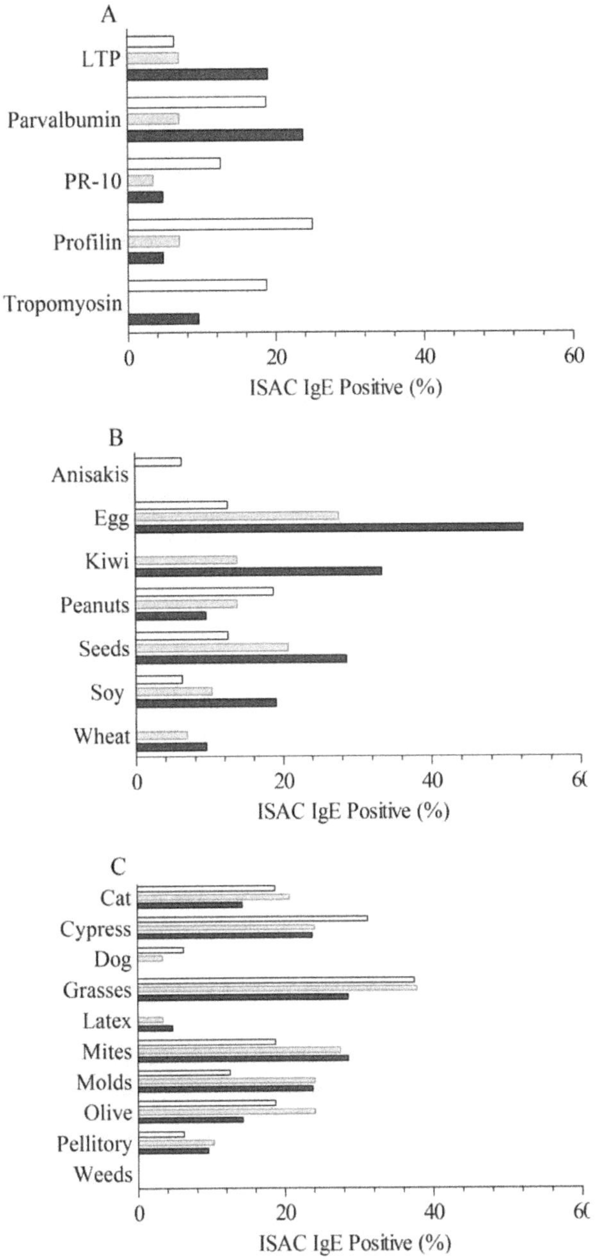


**Figure 5. Additional allergen sensitizations detecting IgE using the ISAC103 microarray system in the three CM sensitised subsets depending on their response to CM and PR oral challenges: A (CM- PR-: white bar); B (CM+ PR−: light grey bar); Group C (CM+ PR+: dark grey bar).** At least one positive IgE result for one of the following allergens has been evaluated for grouping by allergenic molecule groups and allergenic sources: Panel A - LTP: Cor a 8, Pru p 3; Parvalbumin: Cyp c 1, Gad c 1; PR-10: Act d 11, Api g 1, Ara h 8, Bet v 1, Cor a 1.0101, Cora 1.0401, Dau c 1, Mal d 1, Pru p 1, Gly m 4; Profilin: Bet v 2, Hev b 8, Mer a 1, Ole e 2, Phl p 12; Tropomyosin: Der p 10, Ani s 3, Pen a 1, Pen i 1, Pen m 1; Panel B - Anisakis: Ani s 1; Hen's egg: Gal d 1, Gal d 2, Gal d 3, Gal d 5; Kiwi: Act d 1, Act d 2, Act d 5; Peanuts: Ara h 1, Ara h 2, Ara h 3; Seeds: Ana o 2, Ber e 1, Cor a 9, Ses i 1; Soy: Gly m 5, Gly m 6; Wheat: Tri a 18, Tri a 19, Tri a Gliadin; Panel C - Cat: Fel d 1, Cypress: Cry j 1, Cup a 1; Dog: Can f 1, Can f 3; Grasses: Phl p 1, Phl p 2, Phl p 4, Phl p 5, Phl p 6, Phl p 11; Latex: Hev b 1, Hev b 3,, Hev b 5, Hev b 6; Mites: Der p 1, Der p 2, Der f 1, Der f 2, Eur m 2; Moulds: Alt a 1, Alt a 6, Asp f 1, Asp f 2, Asp f 3, Asp f 4, Asp f 6; Olive: Ole e 1; Pellitory: Par j 2; Weeds: Art v 1, Art v 3, Amb a 1, Sal k 1. Detailed information about the nature of additional IgE positive allergens detected by ISAC microarray system can be obtained from www.allergome.org.

Whey proteins were unexpectedly present in all WSE, albeit the fact that during cheese making only CAS precipitate in the curd and become part of the cheese, whereas most of the whey proteins should remain in solution and used for other diary production purposes. Anyway, since some whey is always included in the curd, it is quite obvious to presume that part of the whey proteins become trapped in the PR.

As shown in the first part of simulated digestion, pepsin treatment of WSE further reduces the IgE binding inhibition to CAS, and start decreasing the one to BSA, and to LCF. The effect of pepsin was better seen when it acted on aged PR WSE. Digestion with TCP, however, can greatly reduce the IgE binding to CAS, almost abolishing the one to $\alpha_{S1}$-CAS, markedly reducing the one to β-CAS, BSA, LCF, and reducing by a 50% the one to κ-CAS. Overall, PR maturation combined with gastro-duodenal digestion brought to a marked decrease of the IgE binding inhibition capability of WSE. Opposite to CAS and other whey proteins, ALA and BLG IgE binding inhibition were almost not affected by the combined PR and simulated digestions. ALA, BLG and CAS resistance/sensitivity to digestion has been already reported by many authors in the past and recently [2,21,22], and it seems to largely depend on the kind of enzymatic treatment used and additional experimental conditions (*e.g.* heating) [2,23,24]. Reduction in the antigenicity of CM proteins can be also achieved using fermentation with lactic acid bacteria [25], the same microorganisms added to produce PR, though in experimental models BLG seems to be fully degraded [26,27]. The clinical outcome of our study clearly shows the beneficial effect of the PR production procedures, though the clinical tolerance seems to be achieved combining the partial proteolysis degrading some CM proteins in highly aged PR, the gut digestion and a specific IgE reactivity to allergenic molecule defined by diagnostic profiling with the ISAC microarray. BLG IgE reactivity seems to play a critical role at this regard as shown by their presence in sera of PR-reactive patients. These findings are in line with those previously reported of preserved IgE binding by BLG peptides [28].

IgE detection by SPHIAa is a simple method to identify allergenic molecules in foods [17]. It provides a preliminary estimate of allergen presence in the source, though the result largely depends on concentration, affinity, and avidity of the allergenic molecules under study. Inhibition can be achieved by a molecular structure with preserved IgE epitopes as shown for BLG and CAS by Cerecedo et al. [29], not necessarily still biologically active. Hence, as in the present study, SPHIAa results suggest the presence of peptides and other structures still able to bind CM allergic patients' IgE. These IgE binding structures might not trigger mast cell activation. Nevertheless, the usefulness of a multiplexed IgE inhibition retains its validity as it gives the full profile of proteins present or not in a preparation. Notably, in our experiments the availability of fractionated CAS on ISAC 89 lead to differentiate the sensitivity to digestion of each of them. As reported by Bernard et al. [30], IgE reactivity to different CAS is part of the personal profile of each CM allergic patient, and CAS should be not considered as unique entity. The biochemical and immunochemical experiments run in the present study show an unexpected presence of seemingly intact whey proteins in matured PR. Whey, a by-product from cheese or CAS manufacture, contains less than 1% proteins: ALA, BLG, immunoglobulins and protease peptones, as well as several minor proteins including lactoferrin, glycoproteins, lactoperoxidase and transferrin [1]. Recognition of still present whey proteins could thus explain PR allergy. Although CM allergy is often due to more than one epitope present on different CM proteins, up to now no specific CM protein has ever been identified as 'major and unique milk allergen' [31,32]. In terms of PR tolerance, a good marker has been identified in BLG negative IgE results obtained by ISAC, with specificity greater than 91% on ISAC test. At the moment we are not aware of the reasons behind a better performance of IgE detection made by ISAC rather than by ImmunoCAP, though we might speculate that a different antigen/antibody interaction kinetic could exist in the micro *versus* the macro system. Even in those favourable cases, where a large rate of success is expected when giving patients with fully matured PR, oral food challenge in a supervised setting to assess PR tolerability in CM allergic children is strongly suggested. PR allergic reaction, though rarer, could be very severe, as shown in the present study, being PR a CM protein concentrates. Conversely, specific markers of PR clinical reactivity are still to be identified.

The tested PR tolerant children are going ahead consuming PR without any problem. The clinical follow up study is thus supporting that unless the PR product is not a truly industrial one, it achieves "reproducibility" in production as documented by our biochemical and immunochemical evaluations. Further studies are required to verify if regular PR ingestion might anticipate CM tolerance as reported in studies using baked CM products [7]. Published studies on children outgrowing CM allergy have shown levels of CM specific IgE antibodies lower than those of persistent allergic patients [9,33], therefore a low IgE response to all CM proteins on microarray testing, as reported in the present study, could be a good marker of PR tolerability toward the following CM reintroduction.

As for our previous study on hen's egg allergic children [10], some differences in the overall allergenic molecule-based diagnostic profile were found when comparing the three groups of children. Beside the problematic CM allergy and not being tolerant to PR ingestion, group C had also a higher number of additional food sensitization, which, with a timely diagnosis, could prevent major allergic reactions to food sources other than CM.

In conclusion, even if SPHIAa results on PR analysis show the presence of either proteins, or peptides or other compounds at different molecular weight still able to bind IgE, a significant proportion (58%) of patients reacting to CM tolerate PR. A possible explanation is the CAS partial hydrolysis induced by the 36 months PR maturation process, additionally digested in the gastro-intestinal tract. Although the best marker of PR tolerance seems to be an IgE BLG negative result on ISAC testing, a fully reliable model to identify patients tolerating PR without a risky oral challenge is still to be finalized. Our combined biochemical, immunological, and diagnostic methods should be encouraged in study protocols exploring CM protein clinical tolerance to allow comparability among different approaches. Reintroduction of a tasty food as PR was highly appreciated by tolerant children and their relatives leading to an improvement of the overall family quality of life. Hence, PR could be added to baked products for CM allergic children management.

## Acknowledgments

We thank Silvia Monti and Giorgio Perotti for their timely support in patient data management.

The use of the Allergome-InterAll software was generously made available for free by Allergy Data Laboratories s.c., Italy.

## Author Contributions

Conceived and designed the experiments: AM CA SS AD. Performed the experiments: CA SS PP FL SP DZ CR RF MLB IG. Analyzed the data: MS SZ CA. Contributed reagents/materials/analysis tools: AM SF AD. Wrote the paper: AM CA SF.

## References

1. Wal JM (2001) Structure and function of milk allergens. Allergy 56: 35–8.
2. Wal JM (2004) Bovine milk allergenicity. Ann Allergy Asthma Immunol 93: S2–S11.
3. Fiocchi A, Bouygue GR, Albarini M, Restani P (2011) Molecular diagnosis of cow's milk allergy. Curr Opin Allergy Clin Immunol 11: 216–21.
4. Sampson HA (1999) Food allergy. Part 2: diagnosis and management. J Allergy Clin Immunol 103: 981–9.
5. Fiocchi A, Schunemann HJ, Brozek J, Restani P, Beyer K, et al. (2010) Diagnosis and Rationale for Action against Cow's Milk Allergy (DRACMA): A summary report. J Allergy Clin Immunol 126: 1119–28.
6. Allen KJ, Davidson GP, Day AS, Hill DJ, Kemp AS, et al. (2009) Management of cow's milk protein allergy in infants and young children: an expert panel perspective. J Paediatr Child Health 45: 481–6.
7. Konstantinou GN, Kim JS (2012) Paradigm shift in the management of milk and egg allergy: baked milk and egg diet. Immunol Allergy Clin North Am 32: 151–64.
8. Mari A, Alessandri C, Bernardi ML, Ferrara R, Scala E, et al. (2010) Microarrayed Allergen Molecules for the Diagnosis of Allergic Diseases. Curr Allergy Asthma Rep 10: 357–64.
9. Hochwallner H, Schulmeister U, Swoboda I, Balic N, Geller B, et al. (2010) Microarray and allergenic activity assessment of milk allergens. Clin Exp Allergy 40: 1809–18.
10. Alessandri C, Zennaro D, Scala E, Ferrara R, Bernardi ML, et al. (2012) Ovomucoid (Gal d 1) specific IgE detected by microarray system predict tolerability to boiled hen's egg and an increased risk to progress to multiple environmental allergen sensitisation. Clin Exp Allergy 42: 441–50.
11. Malacarne M, Summer A, Fossa E, Formaggioni P, Franceschi P, et al. (2006) Composition, coagulation properties and Parmigiano-Reggiano cheese yield of Italian Brown and Italian Friesian herd milks. J Dairy Res 73: 171–7.
12. Sforza S, Galaverna G, Dossena A, Marchelli R, Neviani E, et al. (2004) Study of the oligopeptide fraction in Grana Padano and Parmigiano-Reggiano cheeses by liquid chromatography electrospray ionization mass spectrometry. Eur J Mass Spectrom (Chichester, Eng) 10: 421–7.
13. Sforza S, Ferroni L, Galaverna G, Dossena A, Marchelli R (2003) Extraction, semi-quantification, and fast on-line identification of oligopeptides in Grana Padano cheese by HPLC-MS. J Agric Food Chem 51: 2130–5.
14. Scala E, Alessandri C, Bernardi ML, Ferrara R, Palazzo P, et al. (2010) Cross-sectional survey on immunoglobulin E reactivity in 23 077 subjects using an allergenic molecule-based microarray detection system. Clin Exp Allergy 40: 911–21.
15. Bindslev-Jensen C, Ballmer-Weber BK, Bengtsson U, Blanco C, Ebner C, et al. (2004) Standardization of food challenges in patients with immediate reactions to foods - position paper from the European Academy of Allergology and Clinical Immunology. Allergy 59: 690–7.
16. Nowak-Wegrzyn A, Assa'ad AH, Bahna SL, Bock SA, Sicherer SH, et al. (2009) Work Group report: Oral food challenge testing. J Allergy Clin Immunol 123: S365–S383.
17. Bernardi ML, Giangrieco I, Camardella L, Ferrara R, Palazzo P, et al. (2011) Allergenic Lipid Transfer Proteins from Plant-Derived Foods Do Not Immunologically and Clinically Behave Homogeneously: The Kiwifruit LTP as a Model. PLoS ONE 6: e27856.
18. Sforza S, Cavatorta V, Galaverna G, Dossena A, Marchelli R (2009) Accumulation of non-proteolytic aminoacyl derivatives in Parmigiano-Reggiano cheese during ripening. Int Dairy J 19: 582–7.
19. Nowak-Wegrzyn A, Bloom KA, Sicherer S, Shreffler WG, Noone S, et al. (2008) Tolerance to extensively heated milk in children with cow's milk allergy. J Allergy Clin Immunol 122: 342–7.
20. Kim JS, Nowak-Wegrzyn A, Sicherer SH, Noone S, Moshier EL, et al. (2011) Dietary baked milk accelerates the resolution of cow's milk allergy in children. J Allergy Clin Immunol 128: 125–31.e2.
21. Maier I, Okun VM, Pittner F, Lindner W (2006) Changes in peptic digestibility of bovine beta-lactoglobulin as a result of food processing studied by capillary electrophoresis and immunochemical methods. J Chromatogr B Analyt Technol Biomed Life Sci 841: 160–7.
22. Bossios A, Theodoropoulou M, Mondoulet L, Rigby N, Papadopoulos N, et al. (2011) Effect of simulated gastro-duodenal digestion on the allergenic reactivity of beta-lactoglobulin. Clin Transl Allergy 1: 6.

23. Bonomi F, Fiocchi A, Frokiaer H, Gaiaschi A, Iametti S, et al. (2003) Reduction of immunoreactivity of bovine beta-lactoglobulin upon combined physical and proteolytic treatment. J Dairy Res 70: 51–9.
24. Chiancone E, Gattoni M, Giampietro PG, Ragno V, Businco L (1995) Detection of undegraded beta-lactoglobulins and evaluation of the molecular weight of peptides in hydrolysate cow's milk formulae. J Investig Allergol Clin Immunol 5: 228–31.
25. Bu G, Luo Y, Zhang Y, Chen F (2010) Effects of fermentation by lactic acid bacteria on the antigenicity of bovine whey proteins. J Sci Food Agric 90: 2015–20.
26. Pescuma M, Hebert EM, Dalgalarrondo M, Haertle T, Mozzi F, et al. (2009) Effect of Exopolysaccharides on the Hydrolysis of beta-Lactoglobulin by Lactobacillus acidophilus CRL 636 in an in Vitro Gastric/Pancreatic System. J Agric Food Chem 57: 5571–7.
27. Ehn BM, Allmere T, Telemo E, Bengtsson U, Ekstrand B (2005) Modification of IgE Binding to beta-Lactoglobulin by Fermentation and Proteolysis of Cow's Milk. J Agric Food Chem 53: 3743–8.
28. Selo I, Clement G, Bernard H, Chatel J, Creminon C, et al. (1999) Allergy to bovine beta-lactoglobulin: specificity of human IgE to tryptic peptides. Clin Exp Allergy 29: 1055–63.
29. Cerecedo I, Zamora J, Shreffler WG, Lin J, Bardina L, et al. (2008) Mapping of the IgE and IgG4 sequential epitopes of milk allergens with a peptide microarray-based immunoassay. J Allergy Clin Immunol 122: 589–94.
30. Bernard H, Creminon C, Yvon M, Wal JM (1998) Specificity of the human IgE response to the different purified caseins in allergy to cow's milk proteins. Int Arch Allergy Immunol 115: 235–44.
31. Savilahti E, Kuitunen M (1992) Allergenicity of cow milk proteins. J Pediatr 121: S12–S20.
32. Schulmeister U, Hochwallner H, Swoboda I, Focke-Tejkl M, Geller B, et al. (2009) Cloning, expression, and mapping of allergenic determinants of alphaS1-casein, a major cow's milk allergen. J Immunol 182: 7019–29.
33. Hill DJ, Firer MA, Ball G, Hosking CS (1993) Natural history of cows' milk allergy in children: immunological outcome over 2 years. Clin Exp Allergy 23: 124–31.

3

# Graph Based Study of Allergen Cross-Reactivity of Plant Lipid Transfer Proteins (LTPs) Using Microarray in a Multicenter Study

**Arantxa Palacín[1], Cristina Gómez-Casado[1], Luis A. Rivas[2], Jacobo Aguirre[2], Leticia Tordesillas[1], Joan Bartra[3], Carlos Blanco[4], Teresa Carrillo[5], Javier Cuesta-Herranz[6], Consolación de Frutos[4], Genoveva García Álvarez-Eire[8], Francisco J. Fernández[7], Pedro Gamboa[10], Rosa Muñoz[3], Rosa Sánchez-Monge[1], Sofía Sirvent[11], María J. Torres[9], Susana Varela-Losada[8], Rosalía Rodríguez[11], Victor Parro[2], Miguel Blanca[9], Gabriel Salcedo[12], Araceli Díaz-Perales[1]***

**1** Centro de Biotecnología y Genómica de Plantas (UPM-INIA), Campus de Montegancedo, Pozuelo de Alarcón, Madrid, Spain, **2** Departamento de Evolución Molecular, Centro de Astrobiología (INTA-CSIC), Torrejón de Ardoz, Madrid, Spain, **3** Unitat d'Alèrgia Servei Pneumologia i Alèrgia Respiratòria Universitat de Barcelona, Institut d'Investigacions Biomèdiques August Pi i Sunyer (IDIBAPS), Centro de Investigaciones Biomédicas en Red de Enfermedades Respiratorias (CIBERES), Barcelona, Spain, **4** Servicio de Alergia, Hospital Universitario de la Princesa, Instituto de Investigación Sanitaria Princesa (IP), Madrid, Spain, **5** Servicio de Alergología, Hospital Universitario de Gran Canaria Dr. Negrín, Las Palmas de Gran Canaria, Spain, **6** Unidad Servicio de Alergia, Fundación Jiménez Díaz, Madrid, Spain, **7** Allergy Section, General University Hospital, Miguel Hernández University, Elche, Spain, **8** Unidad de Alergología, Complexo Hospitalario, Ourense, Spain, **9** Research Laboratory, Fundación IMABIS-Carlos Haya Hospital; Hospital Civil, Málaga, Spain, **10** Servicio de Alergia, Hospital de Basurto, Bilbao, Spain, **11** Departamento de Bioquímica y Biología Molecular I, Facultad de Químicas, Universidad Complutense, Madrid, Spain, **12** Departamento de Biotecnología, ETSI Agrónomos, Universidad Politécnica, Madrid, Spain

## Abstract

The study of cross-reactivity in allergy is key to both understanding. the allergic response of many patients and providing them with a rational treatment In the present study, protein microarrays and a co-sensitization graph approach were used in conjunction with an allergen microarray immunoassay. This enabled us to include a wide number of proteins and a large number of patients, and to study sensitization profiles among members of the LTP family. Fourteen LTPs from the most frequent plant food-induced allergies in the geographical area studied were printed into a microarray specifically designed for this research. 212 patients with fruit allergy and 117 food-tolerant pollen allergic subjects were recruited from seven regions of Spain with different pollen profiles, and their sera were tested with allergen microarray. This approach has proven itself to be a good tool to study cross-reactivity between members of LTP family, and could become a useful strategy to analyze other families of allergens.

**Editor:** Phillip A. Stumbles, Murdoch University, Australia

**Funding:** Ministerio de Ciencia e Innovación (projects BIO2009-07050 and SAF2008-04053) and FIS-Thematic Networks, and Co-operative Research Centers: RIRAAF (RD07/0064). C Gómez Casado and L Tordesillas have been supported by training grants from the Spanish Government (FPI and FPU programmes, MEC, respectively). J Aguirre has been supported by the Ministerio de Ciencia e Innovación (project FIS2011-27569) and Comunidad de Madrid, R&D Program of Activities, grant MODELICO-CM S2009ESP-1691. The funders had no role in the study design, data collection and analysis, decision to publish, or preparation of the manuscript.

**Competing Interests:** None of the authors has any conflict of interest, or has received any money from biotechnology and/or pharmaceutical manufacturers for the present study.

* E-mail: araceli.diaz@upm.es

## Introduction

The fact that allergic patients sensitized to a particular allergen can exhibit an allergic response to other agents shows that the same IgE antibodies are able to recognize homologous allergens from different species that share the same epitopes. This phenomenon is known as cross-reactivity [1] and is a major concern in allergy. The cross-reactivity allergens share the same epitopes but can differ mainly in the identity of their primary sequences and often in their three-dimensional structure. Understanding the factors and identifying the number of allergenic sources that are involved in cross-reactivity are essential for improving the diagnosis and treatment of allergic diseases [2,3]. To address these issues, a large number of allergens of the same family and sera from a large number of patients are needed because of the heterogeneity of patients' responses. These requirements make the study of cross-reactivity using classical approaches difficult [4,5] and require the use of higher capacity technologies.

The introduction of microarray techniques featuring a large panel of purified allergens has been a major advance in the diagnosis of allergic diseases [6,7,8]. Simultaneous measurements of IgEs specific to many proteins from the same family using minimal quantity of allergen and sera are now possible, allowing many samples to be screened at reasonable cost. The huge amount of information generated by these microarrays also demands more powerful analytical strategies to identify associations within the obtained data [5,6,7,8,9,10].

In the context of graph theory, graphs, also known as networks [7,10], represent relationships between objects and have been used to obtain reliable information from many different biological systems [11–16], including a network that has been established for human diseases [17]. In particular, the graph theory has recently been used to describe cross-reactions between antibodies in a sandwich microarray immunoassay [17], and we use it in a similar way here to study allergen cross-reactivity.

The family of plant lipid transfer proteins (LTPs) has been widely studied with respect to plant food allergenic reactions and their role in food and/or pollen cross-reactivities. Allergens from this family have been found in most vegetable sources. Pru p 3, the peach LTP, is the model member of this family. It is recognized by 75% of patients who suffer from peach allergy, the most frequent plant food allergy in Spain [18,19]. Pru p 3 has been implicated in food cross-reactivities, especially those involving fruits and nuts, and pollens such as those of mugwort and plane [20,21].

The principal aim of this study was to study cross-reactivity in plant foods using as models the LTP family and their recognition by fruit-allergic patients from several regions of Spain, taking into account the different pollen profiles in these areas. For this purpose we used competitive cross-inhibition immunoassay and the analytical potential of the theory of graphs.

## Results

### Cross-reactivity between LTPs

Considering the allergies most frequently associated with peach sensitization in Spain [19,22,23], 14 LTPs from those foods and pollens relevant to the study population (Table 1; see Materials and Methods for details) were selected to construct a homemade microarray (LTP microarray). All of the allergens were tested by Western-blot with a polyclonal antibody against Pru p 3 (peach LTP; 20) (Figure 1) as well as by N-terminal amino acid-sequencing and mass spectrometry (Table 1). A comparison of the group of fruit allergic patients with food-tolerant pollen allergic subjects (Table 2) confirmed an association between LTP sensitization and fruit allergy (Figure 2A). By contrast, LTP frequencies were very similar in the group of fruit allergic patients, regardless of their inhalant sensitization profiles.

As expected, the most prevalent LTP was Pru p 3, which was slightly more frequently recognized by fruit-allergic patients without pollen allergy than by those who also had respiratory diseases, although these differences (74% versus 67%; Figure 2A) were not statistically significant. This tendency was observed for other allergens such as Sin a 3 (58% versus 47%) and Jug r 3 (53% versus 43%).

Cross-reactivity between LTPs was demonstrated by inhibition assays, selecting three allergens as models: Pru p 3 (from fruit), Art v 3 (from pollen) and Cas s 8 (from nuts) (Figure 2B). The peach LTP, Pru p 3, was able to completely inhibit the IgE binding of printed LTPs, with the exception of Sin a 3. Cas s 8 and Art v 3 were more specific in their inhibition, although both were also able to inhibit the IgE binding of the other. These data suggest that Pru p 3 acts as the principal primary sensitizer of these types of allergies and as the main gateway to patients' poly-sensitization to LTPs.

### Graph-based analysis of the LTP microarray immunoassay

In this study, graph theory has been used not only as a way to represent LTP-microarray immunoassay data, but also to gain insight into co-sensitization patterns of the LTP allergens in the selected allergic population. The construction of the co-sensitization graph associated to our LTP microarray immunoassay, shown in Figure 3, is explained in detail in *Materials and methods*. In summary, two allergens are connected by a link of the graph if at least one serum gave a positive reaction to both allergens. The weight of such a link is a measure of the degree of similarity between the sera that reacted positively to each of the allergens; the maximum weight of 1 is obtained when both allergens were recognized by exactly the same group of reacting sera (irrespective of the size of the group).

In this way, we were able to confirm that our co-sensitization graph was totally connected (i.e., all allergens were interconnected). This means that at least one serum reacted positively to any given pair of allergens, that is, there were no incompatible pairs of co-sensitizations. Therefore, there are $(20\times19)/2 = 190$ links in the graph, although in order to clarify the interpretation of results only the 35 with a weight greater than 0.55 are plotted in Figure 3. The allergens connected with the highest weights, i.e., those undergo-

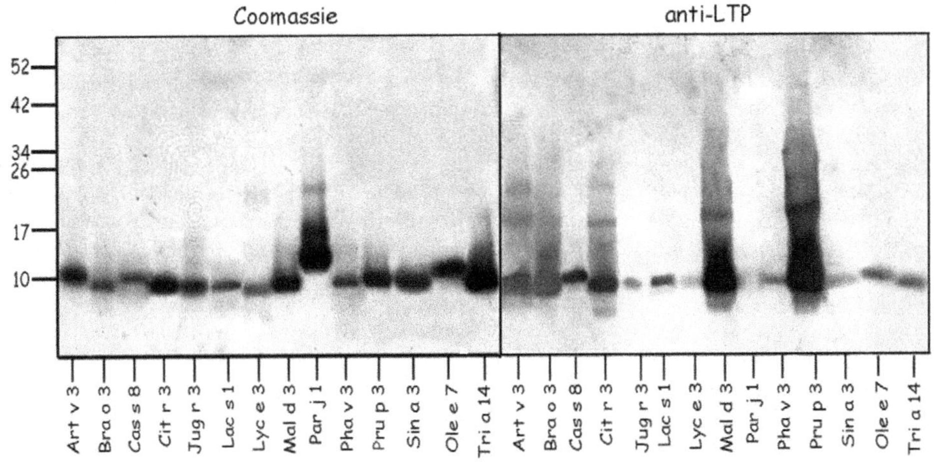


**Figure 1. Lipid transfer proteins (LTP) included in the homemade array were separated by SDS-PAGE and stained with Coomassie Blue.** Replicas were electrotransferred and incubated with polyclonal antibodies produced against peach LTP (dilution 1:500). The name of the proteins corresponds to Table I.

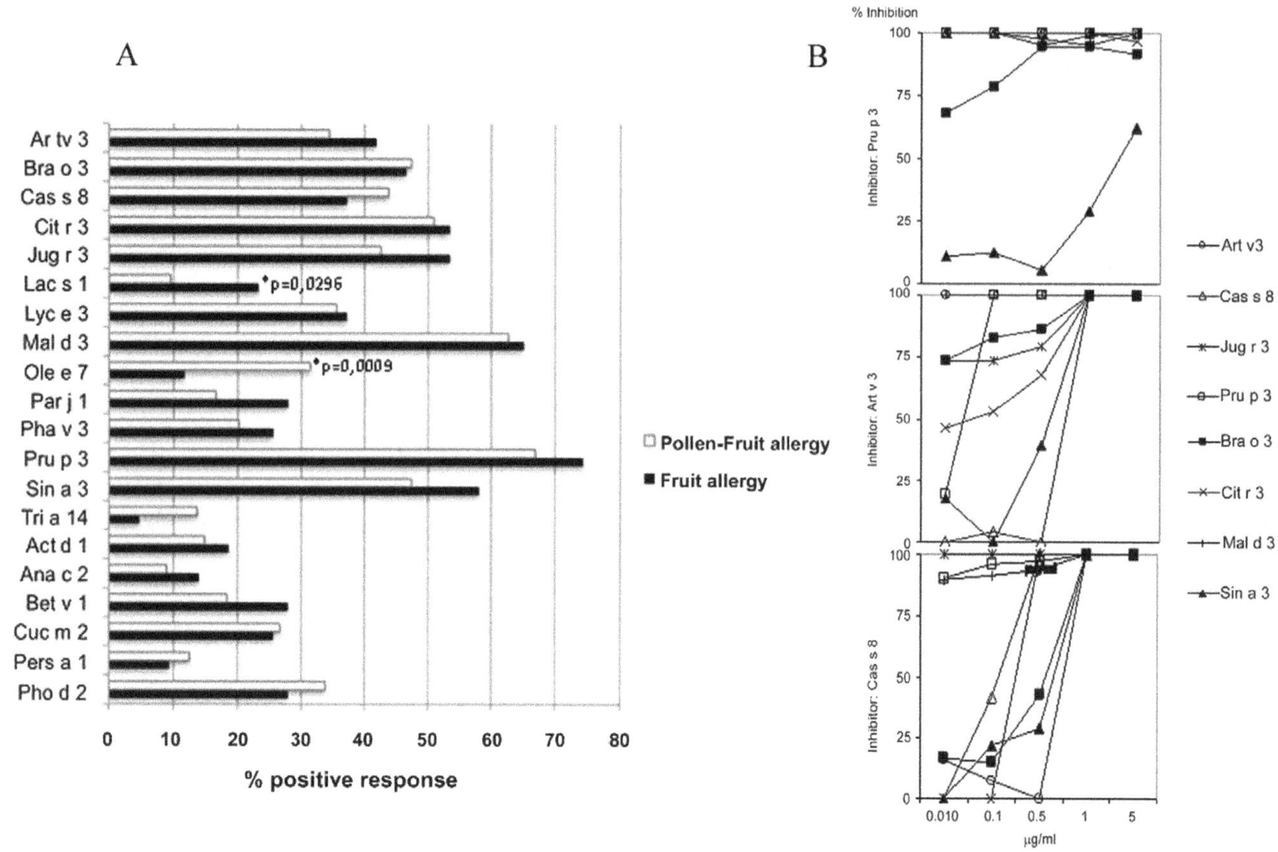


**Figure 2. Frequency of LTP sensitization. A**. Recognition frequencies of food and pollen LTPs comparing fruit allergic patients with and without pollen sensitization (Pollen Fruit Allergy and Fruit Allergy, respectively). The recognition frequencies, shown as percentage of positive response (%), were obtained incubating the LTP microarray with single sera from allergic patients. **B**. Analysis of LTP crossreactivities by inhibition assays using the LTP microarray as solid phase and Pru p 3, Art v 3 and Cas s 8 (5, 1, 0.1, 0.01 µg/mL) as inhibitors. The inhibition percentage of the IgE binding capacity is indicated. Means (n = 3) and SDs (bars) are represented. All tests were performed in triplicate.

ing the strongest co-sensitization, were Pru p 3 and Mal d 3 (0.89), Mal d 3 and Cit r 3 (0.82) and the non-LTP allergens Cuc m 2 and Pho d 2 (0.80). As expected, the lowest co-sensitizations were found between LTP allergens and non-LTP allergens: Pers a 1 and Tri a 14 (0.19) and Ana c 2 and Ole e 7 (0.19). The lowest co-sensitizations between two LTP allergens were found in Par j 1 and Lyc e 3 (0.29) and Par j 1 and Sin a 3 (0.31).

The average weights shown in Table 3 and mathematically defined in *Materials and methods* are a measure of the average degree of co-sensitization that an allergen showed with the other allergens in the graph. As expected, Pru p 3 had a very high average weight of 0.49, meaning that it is one of the most robustly connected nodes of the network. Bra o 3, Cit r 3 and Mal d 3 had the highest average weights and were all above 0.5, while the non-LTP allergens had very low average weights (all less than 0.37). The case of the non-LTP allergens Cuc m 2 and Pho d 2 is amazing, since these allergens are very highly co-sensitized because they belong to the same protein family (the profilins), but their average weight was extremely low because, as non-LTP allergens, their co-sensitizations with the rest of the nodes were very low. Finally, it is useful to highlight attention the case of Par j 1 and Tri a 14, the LTP-allergens with the lowest average weight (0.36 and 0.34, respectively).

## Pattern of responses by geographical area

Subjects with fruit allergy and without any inhalant symptoms tended to recognize more LTPs ($\tilde{\alpha} = 6$) than those who were sensitized to fruit and pollen ($\tilde{\alpha} = 5$), although the difference was not significant (Mann-Whitney U test: $p = 0.0561$). Curiously, individuals from Barcelona and the Canary Islands showed a high degree of polysensitization ($\tilde{\alpha} = 9$ and $\tilde{\alpha} = 7$ LTPs, respectively; Mann-Whitney test: $p = 0.0010$). This was markedly higher than those from Ourense ($\tilde{\alpha} = 3$), who exhibited the lowest frequencies for most of the LTPs analyzed.

The frequencies of recognition in most areas for Pru p 3 were very similar, except in Ourense, where fewer than 40% of patients recognized Pru p 3 (Figure 4). In this area, Cas s 8, the chestnut LTP, was the most prevalent LTP with recognition of more than 80%. Considerable consumption of chestnut is typical in this area, where patients suffer from pollen and nut allergy. With respect to the other nut LTP, Jug r 3, people from the Canary Islands, Barcelona and Málaga, but not subjects from Madrid, Bilbao or Alicante, exhibited the highest recognition frequencies (Figure 4).

Of the pollen LTPs included in this study, only Art v 3 was clearly associated with fruit sensitization (Figure 3; $\chi^2 = 0.001$). Areas such as Barcelona, the Canary Islands and Bilbao had the highest frequencies of this allergen (>50%). The high frequency in the Canary Islands could be due to the presence of this pollen, but cross-reactivity may explain the high degree of recognition of this pollen allergen (40%) by patients from Barcelona and Bilbao.

**Table 1.** Purified proteins included in the LTP microarray.

| Protein | Family | Species/Tissue | N-terminal or internal peptide sequence | Accession number | Reference |
|---|---|---|---|---|---|
| **Art v 3** | LTP | *Artemisia vulgaris*/pollen | ALTXSDV | P0C088 | [20] |
| **Bra o 3** | LTP | *Brassica oleracea*/leaf | AISXGTVTSNLAPXAVYLMK | Q9ZSL7 | [31] |
| **Cas s 8** | LTP | *Castanea sativa*/fruit | SITXTQVSKLMPXL | Q42952 | [20] |
| **Cit r 3** | LTP | *Citrus reticulata*/fruit | ITXGQVTGSLAPCIAFRLTG | P84161 | [32] |
| **Jug r 3** | LTP | *Juglans regia*/fruit | VITXGQVASS | C5H617 | [33] |
| **Lac s 1** | LTP | *Lactuca sativa*/leaf | AISXGQVTANLAGXL | A1E2H5 | [34] |
| **Lyc e 3** | LTP | *Lycopersicon esculentum*/fruit | AITXGQVDAN | P27056 | [35] |
| **rMal d 3** | LTP | *Malus domestica*/fruit | EITCGTV | Q9M5X7 | [36] |
| **Ole e 7** | LTP | *Olea europaea*/pollen | APSQSTVTALLTSCVSYIDDQ | P81430 | [29] |
| **rPar j 1** | LTP | *Parietaria judaica*/pollen | AGLAWTSLASVAP | P43217 | Commercial |
| **Pha v 3** | LTP | *Phaseolus vulgaris*/fruit | K.QLSASVPGVNANNAAALPGK.C K.CGVNVPYK.IKQLSASVPGVNANNAAALPGKC KCGVNVPYKI | Q9M5X8 (O24440) | [37] |
| **rPru p 3** | LTP | *Prunus persica*/fruit | ITCGQE | Q9LED1 | [36] |
| **rSin a 3** | LTP | *Sinapis alba*/seed | ALSXG | EF626938 | [38] |
| **rTri a 14** | LTP | *Triticum aestivum*/wheat | IDCGHVD | AJ852536 | [28] |
| ***Act d 1** | Cysteine protease | *Actinidia deliciosa*/fruit | LPSYV | P00785 | [39] |
| ***Ana c 2** | Cysteine protease | *Ananas comosus/pineapple* commercial | MAEYGRVYKDNDE | BAA21929 | Commercial |
| ***Bet v 1** | PR10 | *Betula verrucosa*/pollen | ARLFKAFILDGDNL | P15494 | Commercial |
| ***Cuc m 2** | Profilin | *Cucumis melon*/fruit | MSWGAYVDDHLMC | AJ565931 | [40] |
| ***Pers a 1** | Class I chitinase | *Persea americana*/fruit | EQHGR | P93680 | [41] |
| ***Pho d 2** | Profilin | *Phoenix dactylifera*/pollen | MSWGAYVDEHLMC | AJ417566 | Commercial |

r recombinant protein;
*non-LTPs or control proteins included in the array are marked with an asterisk.

**Table 2.** Clinical data of patients included in this study.

| | Fruit allergic patients | Pollen-food tolerant allergic patients |
|---|---|---|
| Number of patients | 212 | 117 |
| **Allergy Symptoms (%)** | | |
| Rhinitis | 76 | 87 |
| Asthma | 27 | 43 |
| Oral allergy syndrome | 42 | 0 |
| Anaphylactic reaction | 14 | 0 |
| Urticaria | 50 | 2 |
| Angio-edema | 13 | 0 |
| Gastrointestinal | 7 | 0 |
| Others | 3 | 0 |
| **SPT (%)**[3] | | |
| Mugwort | 40 | 45 |
| Cypress | 22 | 31 |
| Grass | 40 | 88 |
| Plane | 42 | 31 |
| Olive | 43 | 39 |
| Pellitory | 4 | 13 |

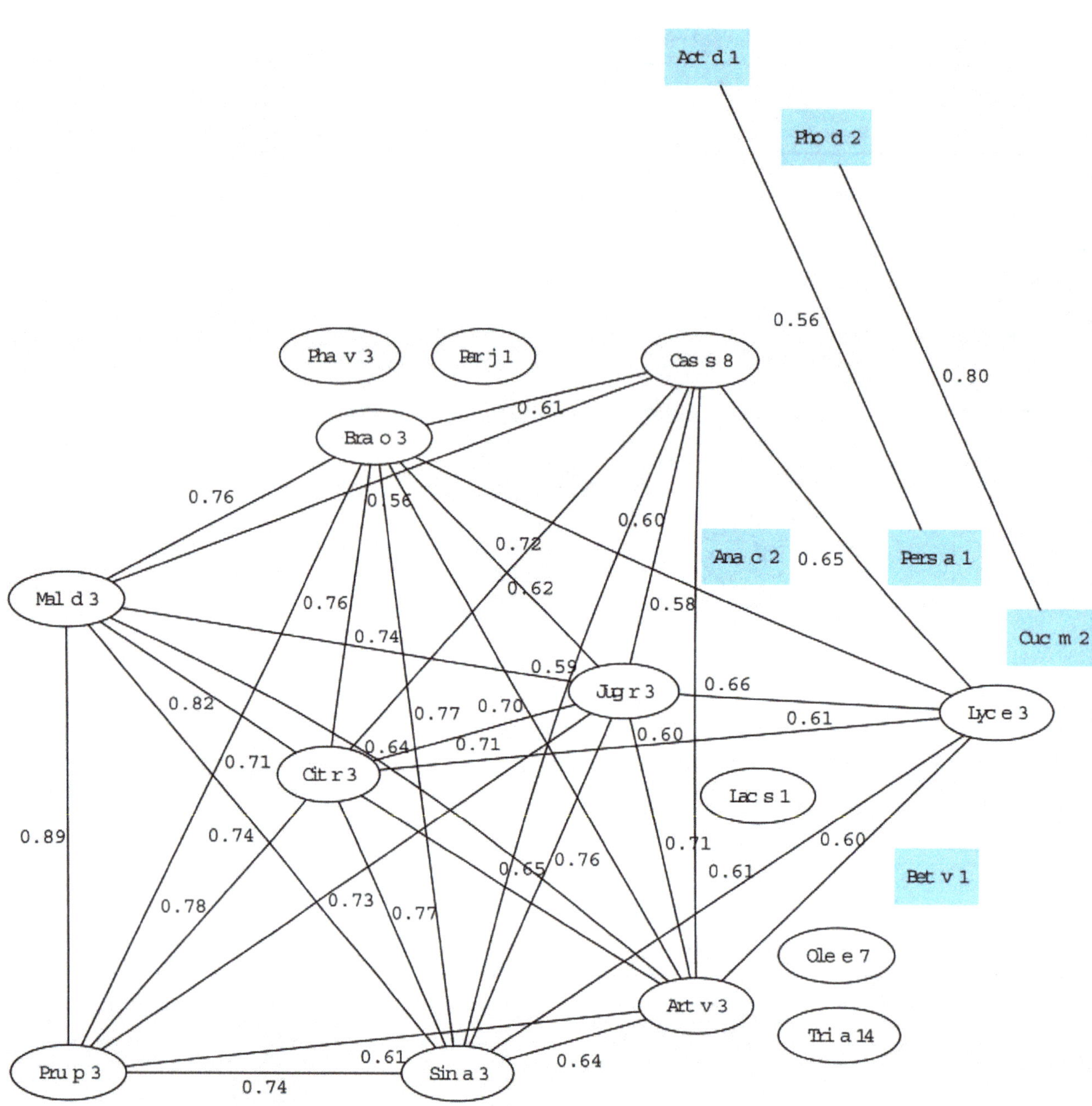


**Figure 3. Co-sensitization graph of LTP allergens.** Each node represents one allergen (LTP, white ovals non-LTP allergens, blue squares) and the links represent co-sensitization of one or more sera for the linked allergens. The weight of each link, between 0 and 1, measures the degree of co-sensitization. For the sake of clarity, only the 35 links of weights greater than 0.55 of the total 190 existing links are plotted.

## Discussion

The analysis of the IgE binding of members of the same allergenic family using data from large numbers of patients could clarify recognition patterns and help us to predict cross-reactivity in food allergy. In order to study plant food cross-reactivity, a representative panel of LTP allergens was produced, based on the most frequent sensitizations associated with plant food allergy in our area [19,22,23]. The quantity of proteins required and the number of patients led us to adopt the microarray approach to ensure the accuracy of our study. Analysis of sensitization profiles for allergies using microarray strategies is a powerful method, and several research groups have obtained relevant results with this technique [7,8,9,24–26] for a variety of pathologies. It can help us to improve the diagnosis and treatment of allergy because many allergens can be tested in a large number of patients in the same assay. The lower cost and the more rapid processing of samples are also advantages [5,7].

Lipid transfer proteins have been classified as important food allergens and are often involved in many plant food and food/pollen cross-reactivities [27]. In our study, Pru p 3 yielded the highest recognition frequencies, followed by Mal d 3, Cit r 3, Bra o 3 and Sin a 3 LTP (all of them around 50%). The nut LTPs, Jug r 3 and Cas s 8, also had a very high prevalence (>40%). These values were consistent with previously published results concerning one of the most frequent cross-reactivities with peach observed in

**Table 3.** Average weight of allergens included in the co-sensitization graph.

| Protein | Family | Average weight |
|---|---|---|
| Bra o 3 | LTP | 0.52 |
| Cit r 3 | LTP | 0.51 |
| Mal d 3 | LTP | 0.50 |
| Jug r 3 | LTP | 0.50 |
| Art v 3 | LTP | 0.50 |
| Sin a 3 | LTP | 0.49 |
| Pru p 3 | LTP | 0.49 |
| Cas s 8 | LTP | 0.48 |
| Lyc e 3 | LTP | 0.46 |
| Lac s 1 | LTP | 0.40 |
| Pha v 3 | LTP | 0.40 |
| Pho d 2 | Profilin | 0.38 |
| Ole e 7 | LTP | 0.37 |
| Cuc m 2 | Profilin | 0.37 |
| Par j 1 | LTP | 0.36 |
| Act d 1 | Cysteine protease | 0.35 |
| Tri a 14 | LTP | 0.34 |
| Bet v 1 | PR10 | 0.32 |
| Ana c 2 | Cysteine protease | 0.31 |
| Pers a 1 | Class I chitinase | 0.30 |

the routine clinical milieu [19,22,23]. By contrast, Tri a 14, the wheat LTP responsible for baker's asthma [28] was seldom recognized in the population that we studied. The low response to Tri a 14 suggests that this LTP is of no relevance in fruit allergy.

With respect to inhaled LTPs, Art v 3 was the only one clearly associated with fruit allergy, in accordance with previously described results [20]. However, the other pollen allergens, Ole e 7 and Par j 1, gave very different recognition patterns from that of Pru p 3. The lack of any relation between Ole e 7/Par j 1 sensitization and peach allergy has recently been described [29].

The study of LTP cross-reactivity by IgE binding inhibition suggested that Pru p 3 was the primary sensitizing in the majority of reactions, but not the only one. Pru p 3 was not able to fully inhibit IgE binding of Sin a 3, or mustard LTP. This peculiarity implies that the mustard LTP includes specific epitopes, being other gateway into the syndrome of LTPs.

The fruit-allergic patients recognizing the largest number of LTPs came from Barcelona and the Canary Islands. The presence of cross-reactive pollen LTPs such as Pla a 3, from plane pollen, and Art v 3, from mugwort pollen [20,21], may increase the polysensitization to this allergenic family. The pollen season is annual and may favour constant LTP sensitizations and, unlike food, it is unavoidable.

The graph analysis also revealed strong associations between allergens. Pru p 3 presented very high co-sensitizations with many other allergens, suggesting that a fruit-allergic patient has a high probability of being sensitive in turn to apple, cabbage, nut, mustard and tangerine. However, it seems that subjects do not easily develop allergy against green beans or lettuce in the first stage of polysensitization. All these results are known in routine clinical circumstances but they represent the first experimental evidence of the syndrome of LTPs with a large number of allergens. Therefore, our model is valuable due to its ability to illustrate i) the degree of cross-reactivity between LTP members and ii) the probability that patients allergic to a given LTP will be sensitized to others. These results open up the possibility of analyzing other routes of sensitization obtained from the graph analysis, and therefore represent a promising line of future work.

In summary, the array approach and the application of graph theory have proved to be useful tools in this type of study. Fruit-allergic patients from Spain were usually polysensitized to multiple members of the LTP family, with the sensitizations to peach, apple, tangerine, cabbage, mustard and nuts being the most noteworthy. LTP recognition profiles may be influenced by local pollen patterns, especially by some pollen LTPs such as mugwort and plane allergens.

## Materials and Methods

### Selection and purification of allergens

Thirteen LTPs were purified by Diaz Perales' and Rodriguez's laboratories following a previously published method from natural source or as recombinant protein in the yeast *Pichia pastoris* (rMal d 3, rPru p 3, rSin a 3, rTri a 14), and one, Par j 1, was produced as recombinant in *Escherichia coli* by Bial Aristegui (Bilbao, Spain) [19–21,28]. These proteins were chosen on the basis of their previously described allergenic properties and their relationship with peach allergy. Additional allergens were obtained to complete the allergen array: Pru p 2.0102 (TLP, peach allergen), Act d 1 (cysteine protease, kiwi allergen), Ana c 2 (pineapple allergen), Bet v 1 (PR10 from birch pollen), Cuc m 2 (melon fruit profilin), Pers a 1 (avocado latex-fruit allergen) and Pho d 2 (palm-pollen profilin).

All purified proteins were identified by trypsin peptide- and/or N-terminal amino acid-sequencing and mass spectrometry (MALDI-TOF-TOF Autoflex, Bruker, Bremen, Germany) in the Proteomic Service of CIB, CSIC (Madrid, Spain). In addition, every purified protein (5 µg) was visualized on Coomassie-stained SDS-PAGE and by incubation with rabbit polyclonal antibodies to Pru p 3 (1:500 dilution). Protein preparations were considered to contain homogeneous molecules after adequate verification to rule out the possibility of contamination.

### Characteristics of the allergic population included

Patients from seven different regions of Spain were selected following the same criteria. The regions were chosen based on the regions with the highest pollen counts (Table 4, pollen count average of the last 10 years). Fruit-allergic patients (n = 212) were included in the study, prospectively among the adult population (Table 2). Criteria for inclusion were: i) a consistent history of adverse reaction to fruits, indicative of IgE-mediated allergy and ii) giving positive results to the skin-prick test and open food challenge, following the diagnostic algorithm recommended by official allergy academies [30]. SPT responses were performed following EAACI recommendations [30]. The Ethics Committee of each hospital approved the study: the Ethic Committee of Hospital Clinic de Barcelona; the Ethic Committee of Hospital Universitario de la Princesa; the Ethic Committee of Hospital Universitario de Gran Canaria Dr. Negrín; the Ethic Committee of Fundación Jiménez Díaz; the Hospital General de Alicante; the Ethic Committee of Complexo Hospitalario de Ourense the Ethic Committee of Hospital Civil, Málaga; the Ethic Committee of Hospital de Basurto, Bilbao; the Ethic Committee of Universidad Politécnica de Madrid (Spain). Patients and control volunteers also gave their written informed consent to their participation.

Patients with seasonal rhinitis and food tolerance were included as a control group with the following criteria: a compatible clinical

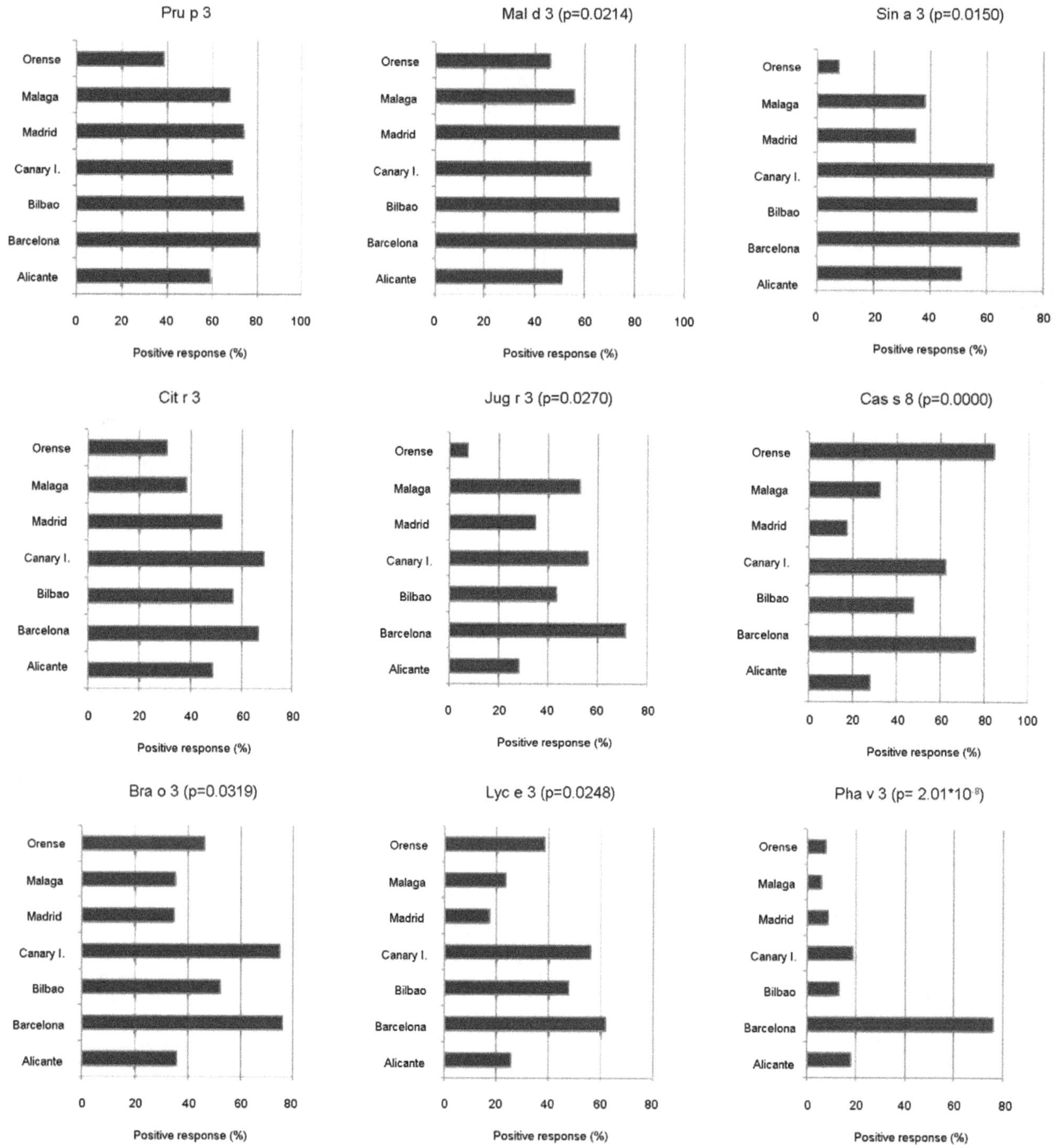


**Figure 4. Recognition frequencies of food and pollen LTPs by geographical area.** The recognition frequencies, shown as percentage of positive response (%), were obtained incubating the LTP microarray with single sera from allergic patients. Only LTPs with a positive response of more than 20% (taking all patients into account) are represented. Percentage positive responses and significant differences ($p<0.05$) are indicated.

history of pollinosis confirmed by positive skin-prick tests to pollen allergens, but without any symptoms of plant food allergy and negative responses to food extracts by SPTs (n = 117). These patients showed mainly positive responses to mugwort, olive and grass pollen (Table 2). An additional group of food-tolerant volunteers without pollinosis (n = 35; 5 per region) was recruited as a negative control. Most of them (n = 27) were atopic suffering from dust mite and animal dander allergies.

## Production of allergen microarray and immunoassay

Purified proteins (0.25 mg/ml and 0.125 mg/ml in 1X Protein Binding Buffer (Whatman, USA) containing 0.02% Tween 20) were applied on epoxy-activated glass slides (TeleChem International, Sunnyvale, CA, USA) with 16 microarrays per slide, using a MicroGrid II TAS arrayer (BioRobotics, Genomic Solutions, Ann Arbor, MI, USA). Several protein concentrations (1, 0.75, 0.5, 0.25 and 0.125 mg/ml) were tested and those that resolved best

**Table 4.** Pollen counts (grains/m$^3$ of air) of the regions included in the study.

| Region Pollen* | Alicante (Elche) (2001–2011) | Barcelona (2001–2011) | Bilbao (2001–2011) | Canary Islands (2008–2011) | Madrid (2001–2011) | Málaga (1995–1999) | Ourense (1996–1999) |
|---|---|---|---|---|---|---|---|
| Grass | - | - | - | - | 200 | - | - |
| Birch | - | - | 100 | - | - | - | 120 |
| Plane | - | 1800 | - | - | 1050 | 225 | - |
| Oak | - | 375 | 330 | - | 520 | - | 100 |
| Pine | 375 | 200 | 620 | 100 | 160 | - | 130 |
| Cypress | 175 | 525 | - | - | 200 | 250 | 470 |
| Mugwort | - | - | - | 150 | - | - | - |
| Pellitory | - | - | - | 110 | - | - | - |
| Olive | 355 | 125 | - | - | 473 | 1250 | - |
| Palm | 220 | - | - | - | - | - | - |

*Average pollen counts (grains/m$^3$). The period is indicated in brackets.
Data were obtained as the average of the previous years (period in parentheses), from the Comité de Aerobiología-SEAIC (http://www.polenes.com/concentraciones.html) and the PIA-Punto de información de Aerobiología-UAB (http://lap.uab.cat/aerobiologia/).

were chosen (data not shown). Labelled pre-immune antibody was spotted as a guide dot to support automatic image analysis. Gaskets (TeleChem International, Sunnyvale, CA, USA) were attached to the slides to create a barrier between the 16 arrays and sealed to prevent evaporation. Each array well was incubated for 1 hour at room temperature with blocking solution (Sigma, St. Louis, CO, USA) and then incubated overnight with 80 ul undiluted serum at 4°C. To detect bound IgE antibodies, the slides were incubated for 1 hour at room temperature with anti-human IgE labelled with PE-DY 647 (Thermo Scientific, Rockford, IL, USA) diluted 1:100. As a blank control, one array well per slide was always incubated with PBS alone (Sigma, St. Louis, CO, USA) instead of serum, and after washing, incubated with the fluorescence secondary antibody. PBS containing 0.1% Tween 20 was used as washing solution. Three spots from the same sample were included in each array, and two replicates of each assay were performed (Pearson correlation = 0.83; $p<0.0001$).

Spots with obvious defects and those replicate spots with a signal-to-noise ratio less than 3, as measured by GenePix$^{TM}$ software (Genomics Solutions, PE, USA), were removed from the analysis. Only those allergen spots with at least two to three replicates fulfilling the analysis criteria were considered for quantification. The IgE binding of each allergen spot was calculated as the final fluorescence intensity, obtained by subtracting the local background $B$ from the observed value, measured by GenePix$^{TM}$ software and then the fluorescence intensity from the blank control by applying the equation: $I = (F_{645} - B)_{sample} - (F_{645} - B)_{blank}$. Fluorescence intensity levels >200 units were considered to be positive (highest value of mean +3× SD of negative control spots, those containing only blocking solution).

## Immunoinhibition assay on the LTP array

The inhibition assays were carried out as explained in the former section for immunoassays, but with the following modifications. A pool of sera (n = 20 fruit allergic patients) was incubated with increasing amounts of LTPs used as inhibitors (0.01, 0.1, 0.5, 1, 5 mg/mL) for 3 hours at room temperature: Pru p 3, as fruit LTP; Cas s 8, as nut LTP; and Art v 3, as pollen LTP. The preincubated pool was then added to the LTP array blocked with blocking solution. All tests were performed in triplicate. The inhibition (%) of IgE binding was determined as:

$$\text{Inhibition}(\%) = 100 \times ([1 - (\text{Fluorescence} - \text{Fluorescence}_{100\%}) / (\text{Fluorescence}_{0\%} - \text{Fluorescence}_{100\%})]).$$

Fluorescence stands for the result of the immuno-inhibition incubating the pool of sera with LTP inhibitor, $\text{Fluorescence}_{0\%}$ stands for the result incubating the pool of sera without LTP inhibitor, and $\text{Fluorescence}_{100\%}$ stands for the result incubating LTP inhibitor in the absence of the pool of sera.

## Construction of the co-sensitization graph associated with an LTP microarray immunoassay

A weighted and undirected co-sensitization graph $G_A$ can be associated with an LTP microarray immunoassay to study the co-sensitization between LTPs as follows. The elements of the matrix of fluorescence intensities $I$ are first defined as the fluorescence $I_{ij}$ obtained when the serum IgE $i$ binds to the allergen $j$. Therefore, each column of $I$ represents the average of two microarray immunoassays in which the same patient serum is incubated on the LTP-microarray and revealed with fluorescently labelled anti-human IgE (see former subsection). We call $B$ the matrix defined by $B_{ij} = 1$ when $A_{ij} > 0$; otherwise, $B_{ij} = 0$.

Graphs are bipartite when they have two or more types of nodes, and links only connect nodes of different type. Graph $\boldsymbol{B}$ associated with matrix $\boldsymbol{B}$ is a bipartite graph. Nodes of type S represent the $N_S = 329$ sera and nodes of type A represent the $N_A = 20$ allergens (14 LTPs and 6 non-LTP allergens). Two nodes, $i$ (serum) and $j$ (allergen), are connected in the bipartite graph $\boldsymbol{B}$ if the value $B_{ij} = 1$, which means that subject $i$ has given a positive allergic reaction to the allergen $j$.

We then project the bipartite graph $\boldsymbol{B}$ onto graph $\boldsymbol{G_A}$, a graph with nodes of only one type (allergens). We call it the co-sensitization graph and visualize it using the open source graph visualization software GRAPHVIZ (tool NEATO). The links in graph $\boldsymbol{G_A}$ connect two allergens $m$ and $n$ if, in the original bipartite graph $\boldsymbol{B}$, these two allergens were connected to one or more common sera. The weight $w_{m,n}$ of such a link between $m$ and $n$ takes values from 0 to 1 and measures the *similarity* between the neighbors of allergens $m$ and $n$ in the bipartite graph. We use the cosine distance between two vectors to calculate $w_{m,n}$:

$$w_{m,n} = \frac{B_m \cdot B_n}{|B_m| \cdot |B_n|} = \frac{\sum_{k=1}^{N_S} B_{k,m} \cdot B_{k,n}}{\sqrt{\sum_{k=1}^{N_S} B_{k,m}^2 \cdot \sum_{k=1}^{N_S} B_{k,n}^2}}$$

where $B_m$ and $B_n$ are the $m$- and $n$- columns of matrix $B$, respectively. Therefore, the weight $w_{m,n}$ is zero, and there is no link between $m$ and $n$, when $B_m$ and $B_n$ have no common elements (that is, when not even one serum has a positive reaction to both allergens $m$ and $n$), while $w_{m,n}$ reaches its maximum value of one when both vectors are identical (that is, when allergens $m$ and $n$ are recognized by the same group of reacting sera).

Finally, the average weight of a node is calculated as:

$$\bar{w}_l = \frac{\sum_{k=1}^{N_A} w_{l,k}}{N_A}.$$

The average weight of an allergen $l$ measures the average value of the co-sensitizations between $l$ and all other allergens represented in the graph.

## Statistical analysis

Fluorescence levels (in arbitrary units) obtained from each patient's serum were analyzed using contingency tests. Differences in the quantitative variables were analyzed by the non-parametric Mann-Whitney U and Kruskal-Wallis tests. Differences among frequencies were analyzed by the Chi-square test. Values of $p<0.05$ were considered significant for all tests.

## Author Contributions

Conceived and designed the experiments: AP CGC LAR JA LT VP RSM GS ADP. Performed the experiments: AP CGC LAR JA LT. Analyzed the data: AP CGC LAR JA LT VP. Contributed reagents/materials/analysis tools: AP CGC LAR JA LT VP RSM GS ADP JB CB TC JCH CF GGAE FJF PG RM SS MJT SVL RR MB. Wrote the paper: LAR JA GS MB ADP.

## References


1. Holgate ST, Church MK, Lichtenstein LM (2006) Allergy. Third Edition, Mosby Elsevier: 458pp.
2. Aalberse RC, Crameri R (2011) IgE-binding epitopes: a reappraisal. Allergy 66: 1261–1274.
3. Crameri R (2007) Allergy vaccines: dreams and reality. Expert Rev Vaccines 6: 991–999.
4. Valenta R, Lidholm J, Niederberger V, Hayek B, Kraft D, et al. (1999) The recombinant allergen-based concept of component-resolved diagnostics and immunotherapy (CRD and CRIT). Clin Exp Allergy 29: 896–904.
5. Salcedo G, Díaz-Perales A (2010) Component-resolved diagnosis of allergy: more is better? Clin Exp Allergy 40: 836–838.
6. Hiller R, Laffer S, Harwanegg C, Huber M, Schmidt WM, et al. (2002) Microarrayed allergen molecules: diagnostic gatekeepers for allergy treatment. FASEB J 16: 414–416.
7. Palacín A, Rivas LA, Gomez-Casado C, Aguirre J, Tordesillas L, et al. (2012) The Involvement of Thaumatin-Like Proteins in Plant Food Cross-Reactivity: A Multicenter Study Using a Specific Protein Microarray. Plos ONE 7: e44088.
8. Scala E, Alessandri C, Bernardi ML, Ferrara R, Palazzo P, et al. (2010) Cross-sectional survey on immunoglobulin E reactivity in 23,077 subjects using an allergenic molecule-based microarray detection system. Clin Exp Allergy 40: 911–921.
9. Bernardi ML, Giangrieco I, Camardella L, Ferrara R, Palazzo P, et al. (2011) Allergenic lipid transfer proteins from plant-derived foods do not immunologically and clinically behave homogeneously: the kiwifruit LTP as a model. PLoS One 6: e27856.
10. Boccaletti S, Latora V, Moreno Y, Chavez M, Hwang DU (2006) Complex networks: structure and dynamics. Phys Rep 424: 175–308.
11. Jeong H, Mason SP, Barabási AL, Oltvai ZN (2001) Lethality and centrality in protein networks. Nature 411: 41–42.
12. Albert R (2005) Scale-free networks in cell biology. J Cell Sci 118: 4947–4957.
13. Huber W, Carey VJ, Long L, Falcon S, Gentleman R (2007) Graphs in molecular biology. BMC Bioinformatics 8 Suppl 6: S8.
14. Arenas A, Díaz-Guilera A, Kurths J, Moreno Y, Zhou C (2008) Synchronization in complex networks. Phys Rep 469: 93–153.
15. Aguirre J, Buldú JM, Stich M, Manrubia SC (2011) Topological structure of the space of phenotypes: the case of RNA neutral networks. PLoS One 6: e26324.
16. Goh KI, Cusick ME, Valle D, Childs B, Vidal M, Barabási AL (2007) The human disease network. PNAS 104: 8685–8690.
17. Rivas LA, Aguirre J, Blanco Y, González-Toril E, Parro V (2011) Graph-based deconvolution analysis of multiplex sandwich microarray immunoassays: applications for environmental monitoring. Environ Microbiol 13: 1421–1432.
18. Salcedo G, Sánchez-Monge R, Díaz-Perales A, García-Casado G, Barber D (2004) Plant non-specific lipid transfer proteins as food and pollen allergens. Clin Exp Allergy 34: 1336–1341.
19. Cuesta-Herranz J, Barber D, Blanco C, Cistero-Bahima A, Crespo JF, et al. (2010) Differences among pollen-allergic patients with and without plant food allergy. Int Arch Allergy Immunol 153: 182–192.
20. Díaz-Perales A, Lombardero M, Sánchez-Monge R, García-Selles FJ, Pernas M, et al. (2000) Lipid-transfer proteins as potential plant panallergens: cross-reactivity among proteins of Artemisia pollen, Castanea nut and Rosaceae fruits, with different IgE-binding capacities. Clin Exp Allergy 30: 1403–1410.
21. Lauer I, Miguel-Moncin MS, Abel T, Foetisch K, Hartz C, et al. (2007) Identification of a plane pollen lipid transfer protein (Pla a 3) and its immunological relation to the peach lipid-transfer protein, Pru p 3. Clin Exp Allergy 37: 261–269.
22. Fernández Rivas M (2009) Food allergy in Alergologica-2005. J Investig Allergol Clin Immunol 19 Suppl 2: 37–44.
23. Barber D, de la Torre F, Lombardero M, Antepara I, Colas C, et al. (2009) Component-resolved diagnosis of pollen allergy based on skin testing with profilin, polcalcin and lipid transfer protein pan-allergens. Clin Exp Allergy 39: 1764–1773.
24. Sanz ML, Blázquez AB, García BE (2011) Microarray of allergenic component-based diagnosis in food allergy. Curr Opin Allergy Clin Immunol 11: 204–209.
25. Shreffler WG (2011) Microarrayed recombinant allergens for diagnostic testing. J Allergy Clin Immunol 127: 843–849.
26. Beyer K, Teuber SS (2005) Food allergy diagnostics: scientific and unproven procedures. Curr Opin Allergy Clin Immunol 5: 261–266.
27. Salcedo G, Sánchez-Monge R, Barber D, Díaz-Perales A (2007) Plant non-specific lipid transfer proteins: an interface between plant defence and human allergy. Biochim Biophys Acta 1771: 781–791.
28. Palacín A, Varela J, Quirce S, del Pozo V, Tordesillas L, et al. (2009) Recombinant lipid transfer protein Tri a 14: a novel heat and proteolytic resistant tool for the diagnosis of baker's asthma. Clin Exp Allergy 39: 1267–1276.
29. Tordesillas L, Sirvent S, Díaz-Perales A, Villalba M, Cuesta-Herranz J, et al. (2011) Plant lipid transfer protein allergens: no cross-reactivity between those from foods and olive and parietaria pollen. Int Arch Allergy Immunol 156: 291–296.
30. EAACI Sostaas (1989) Skin tests for diagnosis of IgE-mediated allergy. Allergy 44: 31–37.
31. Palacín A, Cumplido J, Figueroa J, Ahrazem O, Sánchez-Monge R, et al. (2006) Cabbage lipid transfer protein Bra o 3 is a major allergen responsible for cross-

reactivity between plant foods and pollens. J Allergy Clin Immunol 117: 1423–1429.
32. Ahrazem O, Ibáñez MD, López-Torrejón G, Sánchez-Monge R, Sastre J, et al. (2005) Lipid transfer proteins and allergy to oranges. Int Arch Allergy Immunol. 137:201–10.
33. Pastorello EA, Farioli L, Pravettoni V, Robino AM, Scibilia J, et al. (2004) Lipid transfer protein and vicilin are important walnut allergens in patients not allergic to pollen. J Allergy Clin Immunol 114: 908–914.
34. Hartz C, San Miguel-Moncin M, Cistero-Bahima A, Fotisch K, Metzner KJ, et al. (2007) Molecular characterisation of Lac s 1, the major allergen from lettuce (Lactuca sativa). Mol Immunol 44: 2820–2830.
35. Le LQ, Lorenz Y, Scheurer S, Fotisch K, Enrique E, et al. (2006) Design of tomato fruits with reduced allergenicity by dsRNAi-mediated inhibition of ns-LTP (Lyc e 3) expression. Plant Biotechnol J 4: 231–242.
36. Díaz-Perales A, García-Casado G, Sánchez-Monge R, García-Selles FJ, Barber D, et al. (2002) cDNA cloning and heterologous expression of the major allergens from peach and apple belonging to the lipid-transfer protein family. Clin Exp Allergy 32: 87–92.
37. Pastorello EA, Pravettoni V, Farioli L, Primavesi L, Scibilia J, et al. (2008) Green bean (Phaseolus vulgaris): a new source of IgE-binding lipid transfer protein. J Agric Food Chem 58: 4513–4516.
38. Sirvent S, Palomares O, Vereda A, Villalba M, Cuesta-Herranz J, et al. (2009) nsLTP and profilin are allergens in mustard seeds: cloning, sequencing and recombinant production of Sin a 3 and Sin a 4. Clin Exp Allergy 39: 1929–1936.
39. Palacín A, Rodríguez J, Blanco C, López-Torrejón G, Sánchez-Monge R, et al. (2008) Immunoglobulin E recognition patterns to purified Kiwifruit (Actinidinia deliciosa) allergens in patients sensitized to Kiwi with different clinical symptoms. Clin Exp Allergy 38:1220–1228.
40. López-Torrejón G, Crespo JF, Sánchez-Monge R, Sánchez-Jimenez M, Alvarez J, et al. (2005) Allergenic reactivity of the melon profilin Cuc m 2 and its identification as major allergen. Clin Exp Allergy 35: 1065–1072.
41. Díaz-Perales A, Blanco C, Sánchez-Monge R, Varela J, Carrillo T, et al. (2003) Analysis of avocado allergen (Prs a 1) IgE-binding peptides generated by simulated gastric fluid digestion. J Allergy Clin Immunol 112: 1002–1007.

4

# *Nigella sativa* (Black Cumin) Seed Extract Alleviates Symptoms of Allergic Diarrhea in Mice, Involving Opioid Receptors

**Swantje C. Duncker*, David Philippe, Christine Martin-Paschoud, Mireille Moser, Annick Mercenier, Sophie Nutten**

Nestlé Research Center, Nestec Ltd., Vers-chez-les-Blancs, Lausanne, Switzerland

**Abstract**

The incidence of food hypersensitivity and food allergies is on the rise and new treatment approaches are needed. We investigated whether *N. sativa*, one of its components, thymoquinone, or synthetic opioid receptor (OR)-agonists can alleviate food allergy. Hence, ovalbumin (OVA) -sensitized *BALB/c*-mice were pre-treated either with a hexanic *N. sativa* seed extract, thymoquinone, kappa- (U50'4889) or mu-OR-agonists (DAMGO) and subsequently challenged intra-gastrically with OVA. All 4 treatments significantly decreased clinical scores of OVA-induced diarrhea. *N. sativa* seed extract, thymoquinone, and U50'488 also decreased intestinal mast cell numbers and plasma mouse mast cell protease-1 (MMCP-1). DAMGO, in contrast, had no effect on mast cell parameters but decreased IFNγ, IL-4, IL-5, and IL-10 concentration after *ex vivo* re-stimulation of mesenteric lymphocytes. The effects on allergy symptoms were reversible by OR-antagonist pre-treatment, whereas most of the effects on immunological parameter were not. We demonstrate that *N. sativa* seed extract significantly improves symptoms and immune parameters in murine OVA-induced allergic diarrhea; this effect is at least partially mediated by thymoquinone. ORs may also be involved and could be a new target for intestinal allergy symptom alleviation. *N. sativa* seed extract seems to be a promising candidate for nutritional interventions in humans with food allergy.

**Editor:** Henri Salmon, INRA, UR1282, France

**Funding:** These authors have no support or funding to report.

**Competing Interests:** All authors of the manuscript are employees of Nestec Ltd. A patent was submitted (patent #: EP 2 263 664 A1 "Opioid receptors stimulating compounds (thymoquinone, Nigella sativa) and food allergy") using some of the results that are presented in this paper.

* E-mail: swantje.duncker@rdls.nestle.com

## Introduction

The last few decades have seen a constant increase in allergic manifestations with a striking prevalence in Western Countries [1,2]. In infants and children, food proteins are among the most potent inducers of allergic reactions. Depending on the country, the prevalence of diagnosed food allergies (double-blinded, placebo-controlled, food challenge confirmed) in the general population is between 2.4% and 4% [3–5] and it can increase up to 6% in children under 3 years of age [6–8]. Sensitization to food antigens often results in intestinal symptoms such as oral allergy syndrome, vomiting and diarrhea [9]. However, allergic reactions to food are not limited to symptoms in the gastrointestinal tract but can involve other body sites such as the skin in atopic eczema. Food allergies are often caused by different allergens according to the age of the patient. The most prevalent allergenic foods in infants and children are milk and egg [3]. Most children have outgrown their food allergies when reaching school age [10], but in some of them, symptoms persist and, moreover, they often develop allergic symptoms against other types of food such as peanut, nuts, fish, soybeans or cereals [3]. Food related allergic reactions represent a significant burden for patients and their families and cause considerable health care costs. In most of these patients, avoidance of the allergen is the only efficient treatment. This bares the risk of nutritional deficiencies, especially in children and almost always results in impairment of quality of life for the patients as well as their families. Therefore, alternative treatments are needed. As one way to find solutions research groups have conducted clinical trials with remedies from complementary and alternative medicine [11] like *Tylophora indica* in asthma [12], butterbur in allergic rhinitis [13] and St. John's wort in atopic dermatitis [14]. Another plant that has gained more and more interest for potential medical use in recent years is *Nigella sativa* (*N. sativa*). *N. sativa*, a member of the *Ranonuculaceae* family, also known as black cumin or black caraway has been shown to be rich in polyunsaturated fatty acids [15], phospholipids [16] and contains a number of active ingredients like thymoquinone, hydrothymoquinone and nigellone [17,18]. *N. sativa* is used in the Middle East as remedy for a number of different diseases [19,20]. Various biological effects have been linked to the use of *N. sativa* and some of its active ingredients. In particular thymoquinone has been reported to have anti-inflammatory [21–23] and anti-cancer [24] properties and to alleviate allergic asthma [25–27]. Additionally, *N. sativa* and its component thymoquinone have been linked to anticonvulsive effects and pain protection, possibly through opioid receptor (OR) mediated mechanisms [28–30].

ORs belong to the G protein-coupled receptor superfamily. According to their pharmacological activity they are defined into three classes, mu-OR (MOR), kappa-OR (KOR), and delta-OR (DOR). They have first been described in the central nervous system for their involvement in pain regulation but have now been found to be widely expressed in peripheral tissues including the gastrointestinal tract. Intestinal ORs are involved in regulation of motility [31], intestinal secretion [32] and bowel transit time [33], these are mechanisms also involved in development of intestinal symptoms of food allergy. Recently, molecular and functional investigations have revealed that all three OR-subtypes are also expressed on immune cells, where they have been shown to modulate cytokine and chemokine production as well as the expression of their receptors [34].

In the present study we investigated the effect of oral hexanic *N. sativa* seed extract in ovalbumin (OVA)-induced allergic diarrhea in mice. In this well described food allergy model [35], OVA-sensitized mice develop transient diarrhea with progressively increasing severity following multiple OVA-challenges. Clinical symptoms are accompanied by elevated plasma mouse mast cell protease-1 (MMCP-1, a marker for mast cell degranulation), mastocytosis in the jejunum, elevated plasma IgE, and Th2-type intestinal responses. We demonstrated that *N. sativa* seed extract significantly improves symptoms and immune related markers in murine OVA-induced allergic diarrhea and that the effect is partially mediated by thymoquinone involving ORs.

## Results

### *N. sativa* seed extract alleviates symptoms and modulates immune markers in mice with OVA-induced allergic diarrhea

*N. sativa* seed extract significantly attenuated the diarrhea severity (clinical macroscopic scores) at the final OVA-challenge ($p<0.001$, **Figure 1A+B**) as well as the sum of clinical scores from consecutive challenges ($p<0.001$, data not shown) when compared to non-treated OVA-challenged controls. The decrease in clinical symptoms was accompanied by a decrease in plasma concentration of MMCP-1 ($p=0.006$, **Figure 1C**) and intestinal mast cell numbers ($p=0.005$, **Figure 1D**) in mice supplemented with *N. sativa* seed extract. Total IgE or OVA-specific IgE concentrations were not significantly decreased. *N. sativa* seed extract administration did not cause any change in IL-4, IL-5, IL-10 or IFNγ release from mesenteric lymphocytes following *ex vivo* re-stimulation with OVA (data not shown).

### Thymoquinone, one of the active components of *N. sativa* seeds, alleviates symptoms and decreases immune markers in mice with OVA-induced allergic diarrhea

One of the most potent components of *N. sativa*, shown to modulate immune reactions, is the quinolone, thymoquinone [21,36]. To investigate if thymoquinone was involved in mediating the positive effects of *N. sativa*, mice were treated intragastrically with thymoquinone, in a concentration corresponding to the one that had been given with *N. sativa* seed extract in previous experiments (13 μg/kg BW). Thymoquinone treatment resulted in a decrease of the sum of clinical scores ($p=0.006$, **Figure 2A**, two pooled experiments) and the diarrhea severity at the final challenge ($p=0.001$, data not shown). Treatment with thymoquinone also decreased plasma MMCP-1 concentration ($p=0.01$, **Figure 2B**) and intestinal mast cell numbers ($p<0.001$, **Figure 2C and 2D–F**). Similarly to what was shown with *N. sativa*, no significant changes in total plasma IgE and OVA-specific IgE were observed and intragastric treatment of mice with thymoquinone did not cause any modulation in IL-4, IL-5, IL- 10 or IFNγ secretion by mesenteric lymphocytes after *ex vivo* re-stimulation with OVA.

### Thymoquinone displaces OR-ligands *in vitro*

Thymoquinone has been suggested to activate ORs. To investigate whether ORs play a role mediating the positive effects of thymoquinone and *N. sativa* in OVA-induced allergic diarrhea, we first tested possible interactions of thymoquinone with ORs *in vitro*. At a concentration of 100 μM thymoquinone showed displacement of specific OR-ligands from their receptors in a radio-ligand displacement assay. 45% of [$^3$H]DAMGO were displaced from MOR, 35% of [$^3$H]U-69,593 from KOR, and 48% of [$^3$H]DADLE from DOR, indicating possible binding and subsequent signalling of thymoquinone through OR (**Table 1**).

### ORs are involved in mediating the positive effect of thymoquinone and *N. sativa*

We next investigated the effect of OR-antagonist pre-treatment on thymoquinone induced alleviation of allergic diarrhea in mice. Subcutaneous pre-treatment of mice with the peripheral OR-antagonist, naloxone-methiodide (30 mg/kg BW), strongly reduced the positive effect of thymoquinone on the sum of clinical scores in OVA-allergic mice ($p=0.01$, **Figure 2A**) as well as the thymoquinone-induced decrease in plasma MMCP-1 ($p=0.02$, **Figure 2B**) and intestinal mast cell numbers ($p=0.001$, **Figure 2C and 2G**).

Pre-treatment with 10 mg/kg BW of naloxone-methiodide also reversed the protective effect of *N. sativa* seed extract (**Figure 1A**) whereas, surprisingly, 30 mg/kg did not (**Figure 1B**). Pre-treatment with Naloxone-methiodide did not have any impact on *N. sativa* mediated decrease of MMCP-1 and intestinal mastocytosis (**Figure 1C+D**). Naloxone-methiodide alone showed no effect at 10 mg/kg BW and a mild effect when given at 30 mg/kg BW when compared to positive control groups (**Figures 1A and 1B**).

### MOR- and KOR are involved in allergic diarrhea

Since the role of ORs in OVA-induced allergic diarrhea of mice has not been demonstrated previously, we next assessed the influence of OR activation on clinical symptoms and immune parameters, using known OR-agonists. Involvement of DOR, MOR and KOR was tested using the chemical agonists SNC80 and DPDPE, DAMGO, and U50'488, respectively. No measurable effect was observed using the DOR-agonist but pre-treating mice by subcutaneous injection with the KOR-agonist U50'488 at a concentration of 5 mg/kg BW, resulted in a significant, reproducible decrease of the sum of clinical scores ($p<0.001$), due to continuously lower scores from the 3$^{rd}$ challenge onwards (**Figure 3A**), and a low clinical macroscopic diarrhea scores at the last challenge ($p=0.005$, data not shown). The beneficial effect of U50'488 was strongly reduced in mice pre-treated with the subcutaneous KOR-specific antagonist NorBNI (**Figure 3A**). Administration of NorBNI alone had no effect on diarrhea scores (**Figure 3A**). In order to investigate whether the effect seen with the KOR-agonist U50'488 was purely anti-diarrheic, mice were treated with U50'488 only at the time of diarrhea induction (for two days before the 6$^{th}$ challenge). This short term treatment failed to protect mice from OVA-induced diarrhea.

As with U50'488, subcutaneous injection with the MOR-agonist DAMGO at a concentration of 5 mg/kg BW, resulted in a significant decrease in the sum of clinical scores ($p=0.038$) due to decreased scores from the 3$^{rd}$ challenge onwards (**Figure 3B**). Subcutaneous injection of OR-antagonist naloxone-methiodide at

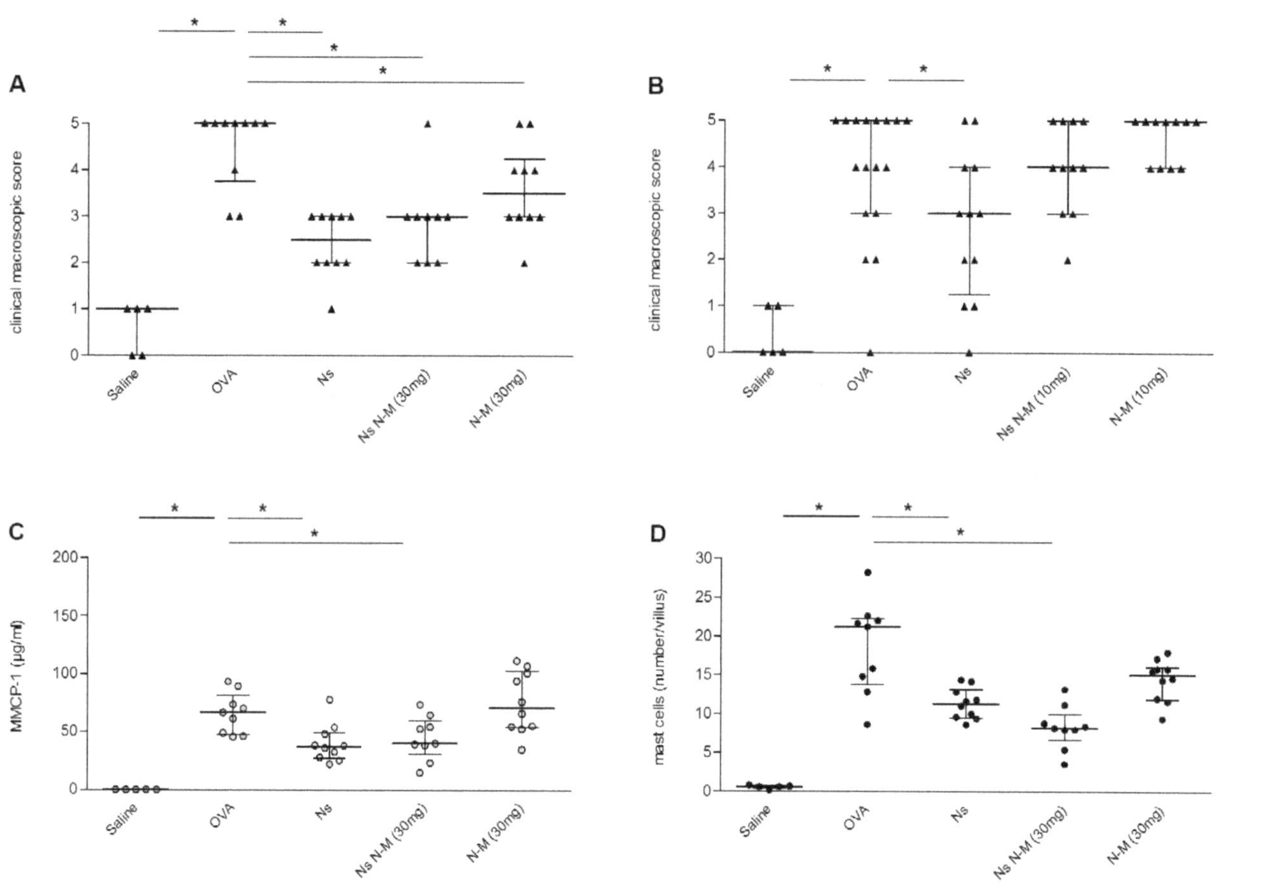


**Figure 1. *N. sativa* seed extract decreases clinical macroscopic scores and immune parameters in OVA-allergic mice.** OVA-sensitized mice were challenged with saline (Saline), OVA (OVA), or with OVA after intragastric administration of *N. sativa* seed extract (Ns) with the OR antagonist naloxone-methiodide pre-treatment at the dose indicated (Ns N-M), or with naloxone-methiodide alone (N-M). Panels **A** and **B** represent the median of clinical macroscopic scores at sacrifice. Panels **C** and **D** show the plasma concentration of MMCP-1 (**C**) and the numbers of mast cells per intestinal villus (**D**) at sacrifice. Each dot represents the corresponding value for one animal and the bars represent the median with interquartile range, * = $p<0.05$; n = 5–19.

a concentration of 1 mg/kg BW (a concentration suggested to preferably inhibit MOR) one hour before the administration of DAMGO further attenuated the diarrhea scores, whereas administration of naloxone-methiodide alone showed no effect (**Figure 3B**).

## MOR- and KOR-agonists differ in their effect on allergy related immune parameters

KOR-agonist U50'488 decreased the plasma level of MMCP-1 ($p = 0.01$, **Figure 4A**) and total plasma IgE ($p = 0.043$, **Figure S1**). Contrary to the results for clinical symptoms NorBNI pre-treatment did not reverse the effect on MMCP-1 (**Figure 4A**) and only partially reversed the effect on plasma IgE (**Figure S1**). U50'488 showed no significant effect on cytokine release from mesenteric lymphocytes after *ex vivo* stimulation with OVA (data not shown). We next investigated the effect of DAMGO on allergy-related immune parameters. DAMGO had no effect on MMCP-1 and total plasma IgE (data not shown) but decreased the concentration of IL-4 ($p = 0.02$, **Figure 4B**), IFNγ ($p = 0.02$, **Figure 4C**), IL-5 ($p = 0.02$, **Figure S2A**), and IL-10 ($p = 0.04$, **Figure S2B**) after *ex vivo* re-stimulation of mesenteric lymphocytes with OVA. The concentrations of these cytokines were further decreased when mice were pre-treated with naloxone-methiodide whereas naloxone-methiodide alone had no significant effect on cytokine release (**Figure 4B–C** and **Figure S2**).

## Discussion

Here we demonstrate that a hexanic extract of *N. sativa* seeds decreases diarrhea scores and allergy related immune markers in mice with OVA-induced allergic diarrhea. Recent results from the literature indicate beneficial effects of *N. sativa* in respiratory allergies [25,26]. Detailed studies conducted in *in vivo* allergy models showed a decrease in blood eosinophils, total IgG1, total IgG2 and lung inflammatory cells in mice with allergic asthma [37]. Consistent with these effects, we show that *N. sativa* seed extract also reliably decreased symptoms of food allergy reducing the overall severity of OVA-induced diarrhea in OVA-allergic mice. This effect of *N. sativa* was confirmed in four independent experiments, using two different batches of hexanic *N. sativa* seed extract. The reduction of symptoms is accompanied by a decreased number of OVA-induced intestinal mucosal mast cells and a reduction of OVA-induced plasma MMCP-1 increase. In this mouse model, mast cells have been described as the main mediators of symptoms, which has led to it being considered as a model of local intestinal anaphylaxis [35]. It has been shown that diarrhea is prevented when mast cells were depleted by

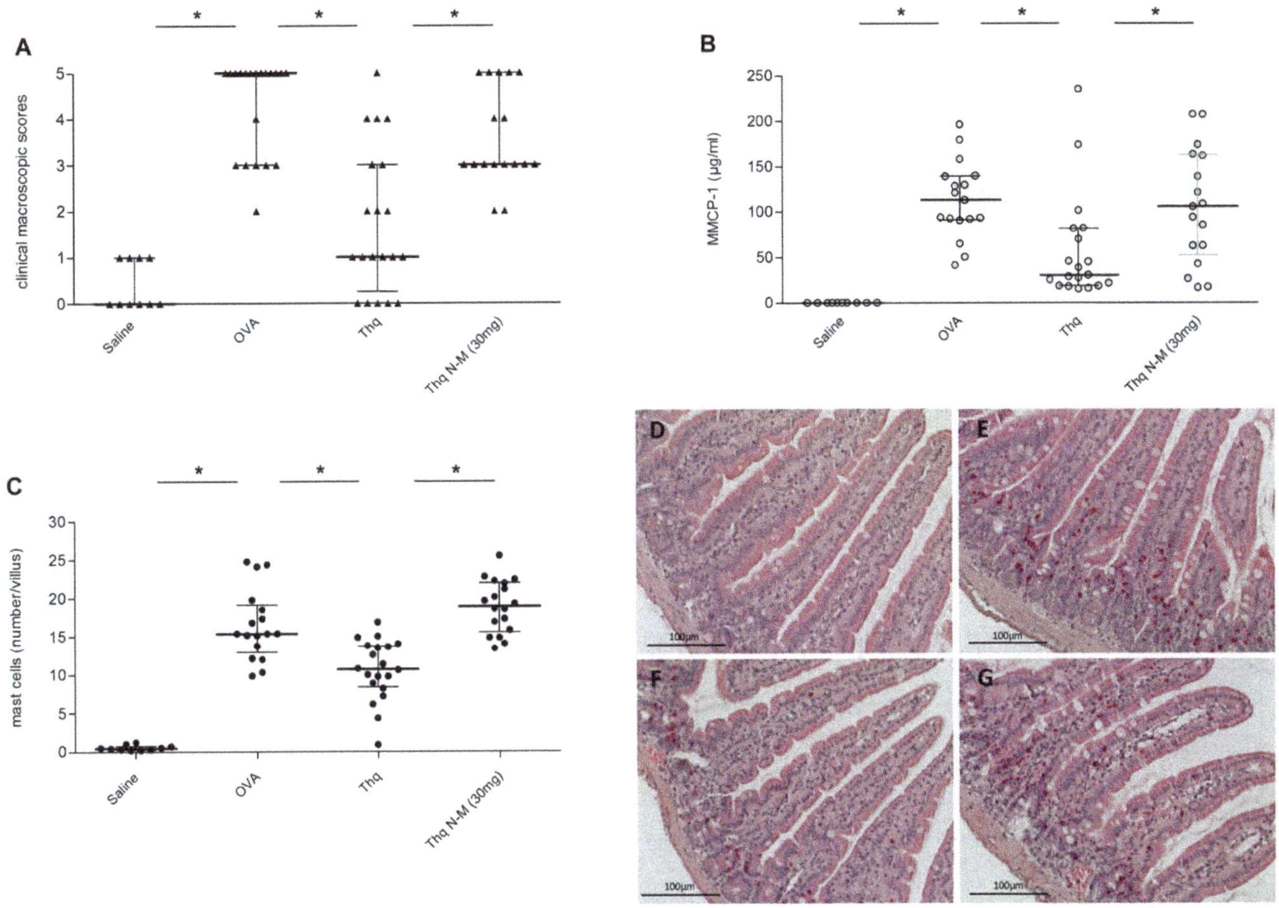


**Figure 2. Thymoquinone decreases clinical symptoms, plasma MMCP-1 levels, and mast cell numbers in OVA-allergic mice.** OVA-sensitized mice were challenged with saline (Saline), OVA (OVA), or with OVA after intragastric treatment with 13 mg/kgBW thymoquinone (Thq) and with thymoquinone after 30 mg/kgBW naloxone-methiodide pre-treatment (Thq N-M). Panel **A** represent the median of clinical macroscopic scores at sacrifice. Panel **B** shows the plasma concentrations of MMCP-1 and Panel **C** the numbers of mast cells per intestinal villus at sacrifice. The dots correspond to results from individual animals and the bars represent the median with interquartile range, * = $p<0.05$, panels show the results from two pooled experiments, n = 10–20. Panel **D–G** are representative histological pictures of mast cells in the jejunum of OVA-sensitized mice challenged with saline (**D**), OVA (**E**), or with OVA after intragastric treatment with 13 mg/kgBW thymoquinone (**F**) and with thymoquinone after 30 mg/kgBW naloxone-methiodide pre-treatment (**G**). Mast cells appear in bright red.

administration of anti-c-kit antibody or when the effect of mast cell mediators (platelet activating factor and serotonin) was inhibited [35]. Mast cell stabilization and/or decrease in mast cell numbers could therefore be involved in mediating the beneficial effect of *N. sativa* seed extract. Previous data from the literature, regarding *N. sativa* effect on mast cells, substantiate this hypothesis. *In vitro* experiments in rat peritoneal mast cells, pre-treated with nigellone, a carbonyl polymer of thymoquinone (one of the active compounds in *N. sativa*) demonstrated an inhibition of histamine release in response to antigen-specific activation [38]. Furthermore, Kanter and colleagues have reported that protection from gastric ulcers with *N. sativa* treatment in rats was mediated by a decrease in gastric mast cell numbers [39].

**Table 1.** *In vitro* ligand displacement by thymoquinone.

| Opioid receptor | % ligand displacement with 100 µM Thymoquinone[a] |
|---|---|
| MOR | 45 |
| KOR | 35 |
| DOR | 48 |

[a]20–50% = moderate displacement (Abbr.: MOR = µ-opioid receptor, KOR = ê-opioid receptor, DOR = δ-opioid receptor).

In the attempt to also test the influence of *N. sativa* on the adaptive immune response, we re-stimulated murine mesenteric lymph node (MLN) lymphocytes *ex vivo* with OVA to measure cytokine release. Consistent with previously published results [40], cells of *N. sativa* treated mice failed to demonstrate changes in cytokine release. Together these changes suggest that local effector mechanisms rather than changes in sensitization mediate the beneficial effect of *N. sativa* in OVA-allergic mice.

The quinolone, thymoquinone, one of the lipophilic compounds in hexanic extract from *N. sativa* seeds, has been shown to mediate anti-cancer [41], anti-inflammatory [22], and anti-allergic [36] benefits of *N. sativa* in animal models. We have demonstrated with oral administration of thymoquinone to OVA-allergic mice that, similar to the results with *N. sativa* seed extract, thymoquinone provokes a decrease in symptoms, plasma MMCP-1 levels and mast cell numbers in OVA-induced diarrhea. Contrary to

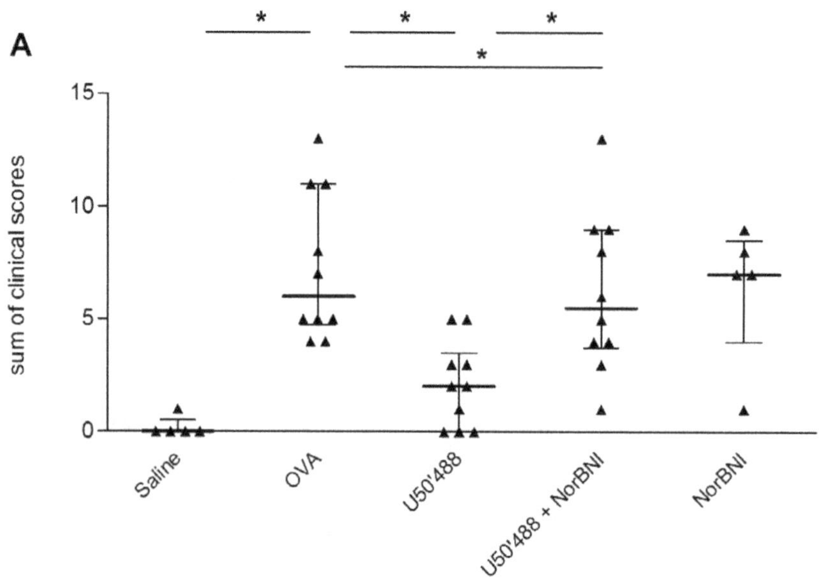


Median clinical score from the 3rd to the 6th challenge

| | 3rd Challenge | 4th challenge | 5th challenge | 6th challenge |
|---|---|---|---|---|
| Saline | 0 | 0 | 0 | 0 |
| OVA | 1 | 1 | 2.5 | 3 |
| U50'488 | 0 | 0 | 0 | 0.5 |
| U50'488 + NorBNI | 0 | 1 | 2 | 3 |
| NorBNI | 0 | 1 | 3 | 3 |

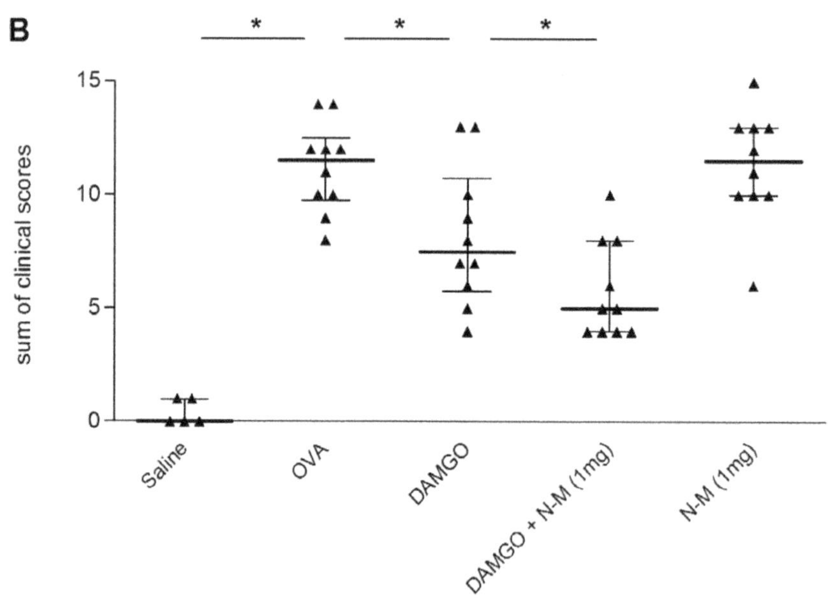


Median clinical score from the 3rd to the 6th challenge

| | 3rd Challenge | 4th challenge | 5th challenge | 6th challenge |
|---|---|---|---|---|
| Saline | 0 | 0 | 0 | 0 |
| OVA | 1.5 | 3 | 4 | 4 |
| DAMGO | 1 | 1 | 3 | 3 |
| DAMGO + N -M (1mg) | 1 | 1 | 2 | 2 |
| N-M (1mg) | 1.5 | 3 | 3 | 4 |

**Figure 3. KOR-agonist (U50'488) and MOR-agonist (DAMGO) decrease symptoms in OVA-allergic mice.** OVA-sensitized mice were challenged with saline (Saline) or OVA (OVA) with or without pre-treatment. Panel **A** shows the sum of clinical symptoms after subcutaneous treatment with 5 mg/kgBW KOR-agonist U50'488 (U50'488) and 20 mg/kgBW NorBNI (U50'488+NorBNI), or with NorBNI alone (NorBNI). Panel **B** shows the sum of clinical symptoms after subcutaneous treatment with 5 mg/kgBW MOR-agonist (DAMGO) and naloxone-methiodide (DAMGO+N-M 1 mg), or naloxone-methiodide alone (N-M 1 mg). Each dot represents the corresponding value for one animal and the bars represent the median with interquartile range, $* = p < 0.05$; n = 5–10. For both panels the table shows the median clinical score for each challenge from the 3$^{rd}$ to 6$^{th}$ challenge.

previous results in the literature, we did not consistently detect changes in total or OVA-specific IgE after thymoquinone treatment. This discrepancy can most likely be linked to the route of administration (intraperitoneal versus oral). Interestingly, a milk-based extraction of *N. sativa* seeds, containing no thymoquinone, had no effect on allergic diarrhea (data not shown). Together these results suggest that thymoquinone could be a major active component mediating the beneficial effect of *N. sativa* seed extract in OVA-induced allergic diarrhea.

Various mechanisms of action have been suggested for thymoquinone such as inhibition of the cyclooxygenase and 5-lipoxidase pathways [42], and regulation of the toll-like receptor 4/NF êB pathway [43]. It has also been reported that oral thymoquinone as well as *N. sativa* have an analgesic effect in protection from peripheral pain in mice through an OR-mediated mechanism [28]. OR-activation has recently also been reported to have anti-inflammatory properties [44]. We were able to show that thymoquinone displaces OR-agonists *in vitro* suggesting a possible implication of OR-pathways in *N. sativa* and thymoquinone effects. To our knowledge the effects of ORs in food allergy have not been investigated *in vivo*. Thus, we first tested the functional effect of OR-agonists in our mouse model. MOR and KOR are the two ORs that are most widely expressed in the gut, whereas DOR is less abundant. Treatment with either DAMGO (MOR-agonist) or U50'488 (KOR-agonist) significantly improved the severity of OVA-induced allergic diarrhea whereas DOR-agonist showed inconclusive results (data not shown). Peripheral OR-agonists have been demonstrated in the past to delay intestinal transit time and decrease intestinal secretion through neurogenic mechanisms resulting in a beneficial effect on diarrhea [32,33]. Interestingly, KOR-agonist treatment did not only decrease diarrhea – OR-agonist have long history as anti-diarrhoeic drugs [45,46] – but also mast cell numbers and plasma MMCP-1 concentration in OVA-allergic mice. This suggests an effect that involves the mucosal immune response. Immune cells, specifically mucosal mast cells have been shown to be in close proximity to neurons [47] in the intestine and they functionally interact [48,49]. OR could be involved in this interaction since *Ussing* chamber experiments with intestine from beta–lactoglobulin sensitized pigs, revealed that beta–lactoglobulin specific, mast cell induced, neurogenic increase of intestinal secretion is alleviated by OR-agonist treatment [48]. However, future experiments are required to determine the mechanism of the KOR effect. It is noteworthy that KOR-agonist did not show an effect on allergic diarrhea in our mouse model when administered for only two days before the final challenge, reinforcing the suggestion that the benefit of KOR activation in allergic diarrhea goes beyond an anti-diarrheic effect and that a more extended agonist treatment is required to show an effect.

Contrary to KOR-agonist treatment, injection with MOR-agonist DAMGO influenced neither serum MMCP-1 concentration nor mast cell numbers. In line with previous work on MORs [50], which revealed an influence on immune mediator release from inflammatory cells, we observed a significant decrease of cytokines secreted from *ex vivo* OVA-stimulated mesenteric lymphocytes in DAMGO-treated mice. The fact that U50'488 and DAMGO show different immune modulating capacities suggests different mechanisms of action in murine allergic diarrhea but may also result from differences in the expression pattern of KOR and MOR on allergy-related immune cells.

In the experiments with DAMGO we used low dose (1 mg/kg BW) naloxone-methiodide as MOR antagonist, according to its high affinity to MOR. Paradoxically, treatment with low dose DAMGO enhanced the beneficial effect on allergic diarrhea. It has been reported in the literature that MOR-expression on the cell surface is highly regulated and influenced by long term agonist treatment, which can lead to OR-tolerance and opioid dependence. For recycling of functionality following activation, MORs need to be internalized, remodelled, and re-expressed on the surface. Thus one of the mechanisms of agonist tolerance is inactivation of cell surface ORs by circumvention of internalization [51]. On the contrary, low dose, long term antagonist treatment (as used in our model) has been shown to enhance internalization of MOR, resulting in recycling and functional re-expression of the receptor on the cell surface [52]. Combination of high dose agonist and low dose antagonist (like done in our study) could hence, paradoxically increase the total DAMGO signalling through increased availability of functional MOR on the cell surface (functional supersensitivity) and consequently result in an increase of the beneficial effect. This has been reported for low dose OR-antagonist treatment by others [52]. It also needs to be considered that endogenous opioid receptor agonists, like beta-endorphin, could be involved in the regulation of MOR expression and might influence the effect of exogenous MOR agonist [53]. Further investigations measuring the expression of MOR and binding studies using selective MOR-antagonists are needed to fully explain these observations.

When testing the involvement of OR in the beneficial effect of thymoquinone and *N. sativa*, antagonist pre-treatment inhibited the effect of thymoquinone and *N. sativa* on diarrhea, mast cell numbers, and plasma MMCP-1 concentration. We hence conclude that the beneficial effect of *N. sativa* seed extract in allergic diarrhea involves OR-signalling, most possibly through thymoquinone. *N. sativa* seed extract, however, contains other active compounds and we can hence not exclude that non-OR-related pathways are involved. Especially, when keeping in mind that the beneficial effect of *N. sativa* was inhibited by antagonist pre-treatment with moderate dose (10 mg/kg BW) but, contrary to thymoquinone, pre-treatment with high dose of 30 mg/kg BW was not effective. Additional work is required to fully understand the underlying mechanisms.

In conclusion, we have shown for the first time, that MOR- and KOR-signalling are involved in murine allergic diarrhea and that treatment with their respective agonists can decrease symptoms by mechanisms that are going beyond a purely anti-diarrheic effect and that involve modulation of immune parameters associated with food allergy. Furthermore, we were able to show that this pathway might have a clinical application by using an extract from *N. sativa* seeds, which alleviates symptoms of allergic diarrhea and modulates immune parameters in mice. The beneficial effect of *N. sativa* extract seems to be at least partially mediated by its active ingredient thymoquinone and involves OR-signalling. *N. sativa*

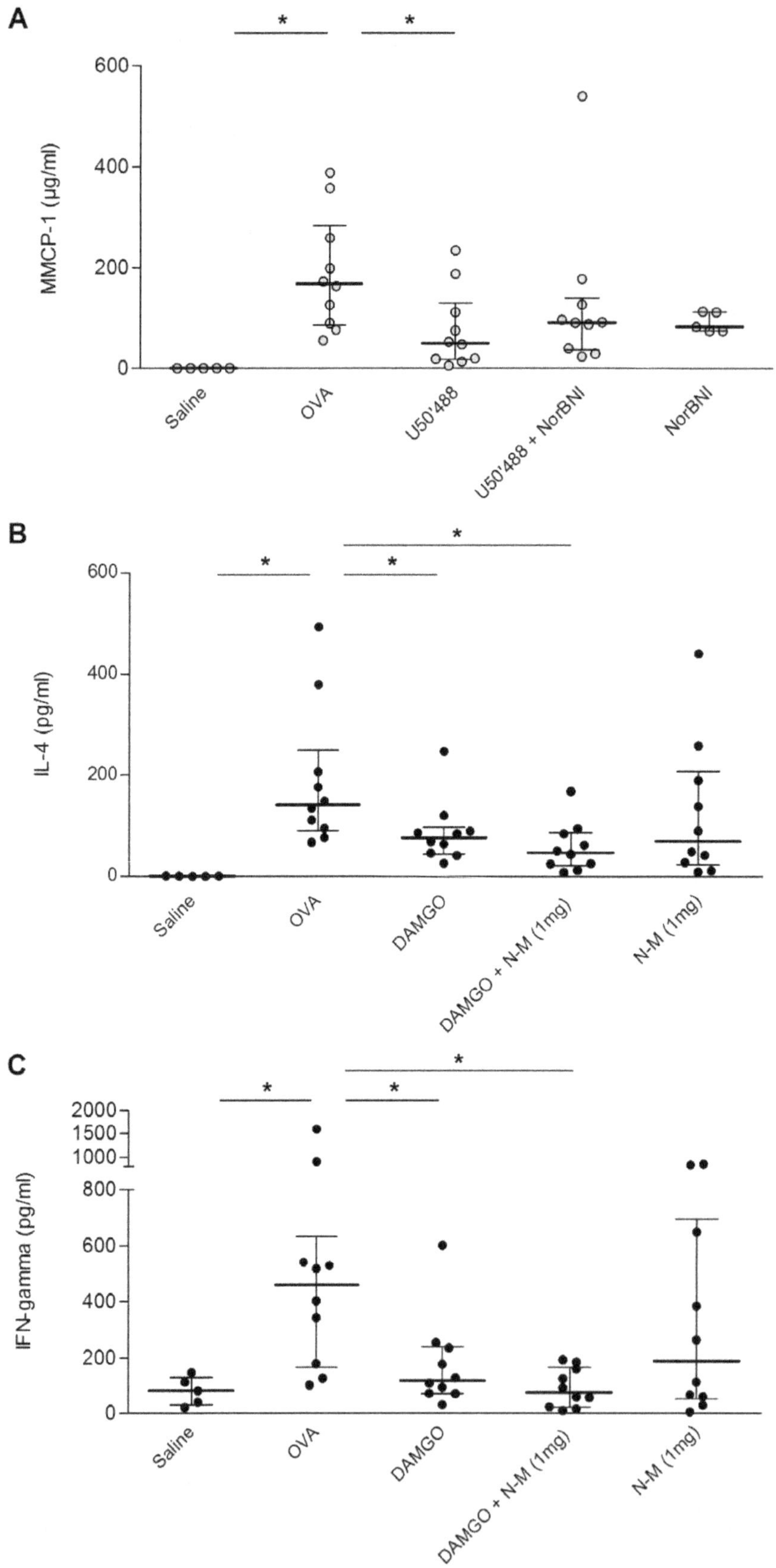


**Figure 4. KOR-agonist (U50'488) and MOR-agonist (DAMGO) alleviate allergy related immune markers in OVA-allergic mice.** OVA-sensitized mice were challenged with saline (Saline) or OVA (OVA) with or without pre-treatment. The graph shows the concentration of total plasma MMCP-1 (**A**) at sacrifice after subcutaneous treatment with 5 mg/kgBW KOR-agonist U50'488 (U50'488), with 20 mg/kgBW NorBNI (U50'488+NorBNI),

or with NorBNI alone (NorBNI), and the concentration of plasma IL-4 (**B**) and IFN-gamma (**C**) after subcutaneous treatment with 5 mg/kgBW MOR-agonist (DAMGO) and naloxone-methiodide (DAMGO+N-M 1 mg), or naloxone-methiodide alone (N-M 1 mg). MMCP-1 levels were unchanged with MOR-agonist and IL-4 and IFN-gamma levels were unchanged with KOR-agonist respectively (data not shown). Each dot represents the corresponding value for one animal and the bars represent the median and interquartile range, * $p<0.05$; n = 5–10.

seed extract might be a promising candidate for nutritional interventions in humans suffering from food allergy.

## Materials and Methods

### Ethics statement

All experiments were approved by the District Veterinary Office of the Canton Vaud, Lausanne, Switzerland and all procedures conducted according to the Swiss Animal Protection Law (Authorization # 1822 VD).

### Animals

Male *BALB/c* mice (Charles River Breeding Laboratories, France) were housed in groups of 5 animals in micro-isolator cages in the Central Animal Facilities at the Nestlé Research Centre, Lausanne, Switzerland. The cages were equipped with filter hoods and kept under controlled temperature (20°C) with a 12:12 h light-dark cycle and free access to food and water. The animals were given one week after arrival at the animal facility to adapt to the new environment and minimize stress. Afterwards they were randomized by weight into the different experimental groups.

### Sensitization and challenges (OVA-induced allergic diarrhea)

Sensitization and challenge procedures were conducted as previously published [35]. Briefly, the mice (6 weeks old) received two intra-peritoneal injections with 50 µg chicken OVA (Sigma-Aldrich, Germany) and 1 mg aluminium potassium sulphate adjuvant (Alum) (Sigma-Aldrich, Germany) at intervals of two weeks (**Figure 5**). Tail vein blood samples were tested for OVA-specific IgE one week after the second i.p. injection to assess sensitization levels. Thirteen days after the second sensitization the mice were challenged with 50 mg OVA by intra-gastric gavage, placed in individual cages and monitored for diarrhea symptoms during one hour. The mice were scored according to feces appearance as follows: score 0 = no changes; score 1 = soft but well formed; score 2 = soft, non-formed; score 3 = one episode of liquid diarrhea; score 4 = at least two episodes of liquid diarrhea; score 5 (only at sacrifice) = score 4 and only clear liquid in the colon at sacrifice. One hour after the 6$^{th}$ challenge mice were sacrificed by exsanguination under inhalation anaesthesia (isoflurane) and blood, MLN, and intestinal tissue were taken for further analysis.

### Hexanic extraction of *N. sativa* seeds

500 g of *N. sativa* seeds (Mehran Spice & Food Industries, Pakistan) were ground using a laboratory mill. The ground seeds were placed in a flask equipped with an overhead stirrer Heidolph 2041 (Heidolph Instruments GmbH & Co KG, Germany). The oil was extracted twice for 1 hour using hexane (2×2500 ml). The mixture was filtered and the solvent was removed using a rotatory evaporator. The oil was recovered and stored at −20°C until use.

### Treatments

*N. sativa* seed hexanic extract and thymoquinone (Sigma-Aldrich, Germany) were given by intra-gastric gavage once a day for 4 days starting 3 days before the two intraperitoneal sensitizations. Treatment was started again 3 days before the first challenge and continued daily until sacrifice (**Figure 5**). The DOR-agonist 4-[(*R*)-[(2*S*,5*R*)-4-allyl-2,5-dimethylpiperazin-1-yl](3-methoxyphenyl)methyl]-*N*, *N*-diethylbenzamide (SNC80) or [D-Pen2,5]-Enkephalin (DPDPE), the MOR-agonist [D-Ala$^2$, N-MePhe$^4$, Gly-ol]-enkephalin (DAMGO), and the KOR-agonist 2-(3,4-dichlorophenyl)-N-methyl-N-[(1R,2R)-2-pyrrolidin-1-ylcyclo-hexyl]acetamide (U50'488) (all agonists from Sigma-Aldrich, Germany) were injected subcutaneously at a concentration of 5 mg/kg BW once a day. When indicated, mice were injected subcutaneously with the peripheral OR-antagonist naloxone–methiodide (N-M) (concentration of 1 mg/kg, 10 mg/kg or 30 mg/kg) or the KOR-antagonist Norbinaltorphimine (NorBNI) (concentration 20 mg/kg) (both Sigma-Aldrich, Germany) 1 h prior to the agonist treatment. All subcutaneous administered substances were dissolved in sterile saline. Due to the long lasting antagonist effect of NorBNI the injection was given every other day.

### *In vitro* OR-binding assay

Interaction of thymoquinone with OR was tested *in vitro* for MOR, KOR and DOR at CEREP (Le Bois l'Evêque, BP 1, 88660 Celle l'Evescault) using previously published radiolabel-binding assays [54–56] with the conditions displayed in **Table 2**. In each

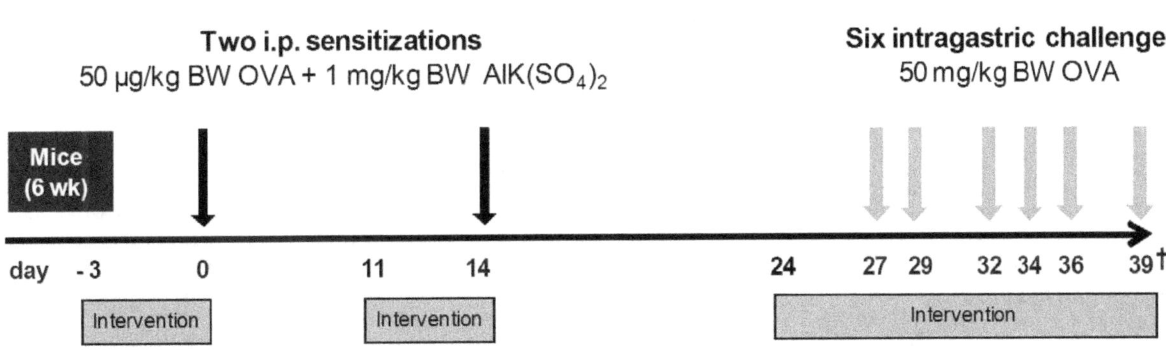


**Figure 5. Experimental set up for OVA-induced allergic diarrhea.** Intervention corresponds to either intragastric *N. sativa* or thymoquinone (with or without sub-cutaneous OR-antagonist pre-treatment) or subcutaneous OR-agonists (with or without sub-cutaneous OR-antagonist pre-treatment). (Abbreviations: i.p. = intraperitoneal, OR = opioid receptor, OVA = ovalbumin, BW = body weight, † = sacrifice).

**Table 2.** *In vitro* opioid receptor-displacement assay.

| Assay used | Receptors/Cells used | Reference compound | Reference of assay | Radio- ligand (concentration) | Incubation |
|---|---|---|---|---|---|
| *δ₂(h)* (DOP) | human recomb./CHO cells | DPDPE | Simonin *et al.* (1994) | [$^3$H]DADLE (0.5 nM) | 120 min/22°C |
| κ (KOP) | rat recomb./CHO cells | U 50'488 | Meng *et al.* (1993) | [$^3$H]U 69'593 (1 nM) | 60 min/22°C |
| *μ(h)* (MOP) | human recomb./HEK-293 cells | DAMGO | Wang *et al.* (1994) | [$^3$H]DAMGO (0.5 nM) | 120 min/22°C |

(Abbr.: CHO = Chinese hamster Ovary, HEK = Human embryonic kidney, DOP = delta opioid; KOP = kappa opioid, MOP = mu opioid, recomb. = recombinant).

of the assays, thymoquinone was tested concurrently with the respective reference compound (MOR-agonist (DAMGO), KOR-agonist (U-50'488) or DOR-agonist (DPDPE)) at several concentrations ($10^{-6}$, $10^{-5}$, $10^{-4}$ M). Displacement of radiolabled ligands was measured by scintillation counts. The specific binding was determined as the difference between total binding of the radiolabeled ligands and nonspecific binding, determined in the presence of an excess of unlabelled ligands. Results were displayed in % dislocation of radiolabeled MOR-agonist ([$^3$H]DAMGO), KOR-agonist ([$^3$H]U-69,593) or DOR-agonist ([$^3$H]DADLE). Displacement of 25–50% was rated as moderate displacement and 51–100% as strong displacement.

## *Ex vivo* re-stimulation of mesenteric lymph node

MLN isolated cells were re-stimulated *ex vivo* with OVA as described previously [57]. Briefly, MLNs were homogenized with a syringe plunger in a cell strainer (BD Falcon, Switzerland). Cells were centrifuged and washed 2× in RPMI medium (Sigma) complemented with 10% fetal bovine serum (FBS; Bioconcept, France), 1% L-glutamine, 1% Penicillin/Streptomycin 0.1% Gentamycin, 50 mM β-mercaptoethanol (all: Sigma-Aldrich, Germany). Cells ($3\times10^5$ cells/well) were cultured in 96 well flat bottom plate (Milian, Switzerland) in the absence or presence of OVA (1 mg/ml). After 72 hrs of culture, plates (including supernatant and cells) were frozen at −20°C.

## Quantification of cytokines in cell culture supernatant

Mouse IL-4, IL-5, IL-10, and IFNγ were measured using the mouse Th-1/Th-2 4-plex multiplex kit (MesoScale Discovery®, USA) according to the manufacturer's instructions.

## Quantification of total plasma IgE and OVA-specific IgE by ELISA

Blood was collected in heparin tubes at sacrifice, centrifuged, aliquoted, and stored at −20°C until use. Total IgE concentration and mouse mast cell protease-1 (MMCP-1) were measured by ELISA Kit (BD Bioscience, USA and Moredune Scientific, UK, respectively) according to the manufacturer's instructions. For detection of OVA-specific IgE [58], 96 well plates were coated with anti-mouse IgE antibody (BD Pharmingen, Switzerland) over night. The next day plates were blocked with 1% bovine serum albumin in phosphate buffered saline plus 0.5% Tween20 (Sigma Aldrich, Germany) (PBSAT) for 1 h at 37°C, washed with PBSAT and samples were added starting with a dilution serum to PBSAT 1:10 diluting sequentially 1:2. Mouse anti-OVA IgE (Serotec, UK) served as standard with a starting concentration of 200 ng/ml. Following incubation at 37°C for 2 h, plates were washed and biotinylated OVA (see below) was added at a concentration of 4 μg/ml with a subsequent incubation for 1 h at 37°C. Before development with 3,3′,5,5′ – tetramethylbenzidine (KPL, US) plates were incubated for 30 min in the dark at 37°C with horse radish peroxidase-conjugated streptavidine (KPL, US). Colorimetric reaction was stopped with 1 N HCl.

The ODs of all ELISAs were read at 450 nm with a Dynex MRX II (Dynex Technologies, Germany). For biotinylation, 2 ml of OVA (10 mg/ml) and 1 mg of sulfo-LC-NHS-biotin (Molecular Biosciences, US) were incubated on a rotating wheel for 1 h at RT. The solution was then loaded on a PD-10 Sephadex G25M column (Amersham Biosciences, Sweden) to remove excess biotin. Protein concentration was determined using standard procedures and biotinylation was verified by Western Blot analysis.

## Mast cell quantification

For mast cell quantification in the small intestinal mucosa 0.5 cm of the proximal jejunum were rinsed with PBS, placed in 10% formalin (Sigma-Aldrich, Germany), and embedded in paraffin using standard histological techniques. Slides (5 μm) were cut and mucosal mast cells stained for chloroacetate esterase activity [35] and tissue counter stained with haematoxylin. Mast cell numbers were determined by counting chloroacetate-positive cells under a light microscope (400× magnification). Mast cells in at least 5 villi (OVA-challenged groups) or 10 villi (saline-challenged groups) were counted and the results were expressed in number of mast cells/villus.

## Statistics

For each experiment a gate keeper strategy was used, that allowed comparisons between treatment groups and OVA-challenged positive controls only if the groups "saline" and "OVA" showed significant differences. Results are expressed as median with interquartile ranges. Clinical macroscopic scores at the 6th challenge comprised clinical and *in situ* observations (scores 1–5). Clinical sum of scores was calculated as sum of the clinical scores (scores 1–4) from all 6 challenges with a score of 0 assigned to the 1st and 2nd challenge according to the progressive nature of the symptoms with multiple challenges. Wilcoxon-Test was used to analyze differences between groups. Tests were performed two-sided. *P*-values of less than 0.05 were considered significant. The software used for the calculations was R 2.6.1 (http://www.r-project.org).

## Supporting Information

**Figure S1 KOR-agonist (U50'488) decreases total plasma IgE in OVA-allergic mice.** OVA-sensitized mice were challenged with saline (Saline) or OVA (OVA) with or without pre-treatment. The graph shows the concentration of plasma IgE at sacrifice after subcutaneous treatment with 5 mg/kgBW KOR-agonist U50'488 (U50'488), with 20 mg/kgBW NorBNI (U50'488+NorBNI), or with NorBNI alone (NorBNI). Each dot represents the corresponding value for one animal and the bars represent the median and interquartile range, * $p<0.05$; n = 5–10. (TIF)

**Figure S2 MOR-agonist (DAMGO) decreases IL-5 and IL-10 in OVA-allergic mice.** OVA-sensitized mice were challenged with saline (Saline) or OVA (OVA) with or without pre-treatment. Panels **A** and **B** show the concentration of IL-5 (**A**) and IL-10 (**B**) in supernatant from *ex vivo* re-stimulated mesenteric lymphocytes of mice subcutaneously treated with 5 mg/kgBW MOR-agonist (DAMGO) and naloxone-methiodide (DAMGO+N-M 1 mg), or naloxone methiodide alone (N-M 1 mg). Each dot represents the corresponding value for one animal and the bars represent the median and interquartile range, * $p<0.05$; n = 5–10.
(TIF)

## Acknowledgments

We warmly thank J. Husson and D. Courtois from the Nestlé Research and Development Centre Tours for providing the hexanic *N. sativa seed* extracts and quantification of thymoquinone. From the Nestlé Research Center, Lausanne we express our gratitude to C. Schwarz for her work with the animals, to A. Demont, S. Holvoet, Tristan Bourdeau, and A. Singh for their help with the laboratory analysis and C. Blanchard for proofreading and constructive discussions.

## Author Contributions

Conceived and designed the experiments: SD AM SN. Performed the experiments: SD SN CMP. Analyzed the data: SD MM. Contributed reagents/materials/analysis tools: DP. Wrote the paper: SD. Developed original hypothesis: DP SN.

## References


1. Gerez IF, Lee BW, van Bever HP, Shek LP (2010) Allergies in Asia: differences in prevalence and management compared with western populations. Expert Rev Clin Immunol 6: 279–289.
2. Zuercher AW, Fritsche R, Corthesy B, Mercenier A (2006) Food products and allergy development, prevention and treatment. Curr Opin Biotechnol 17: 198–203. S0958-1669(06)00024-3 [pii];10.1016/j.copbio.2006.01.010 [doi].
3. Ramesh S (2008) Food allergy overview in children. Clin Rev Allergy Immunol 34: 217–230. 10.1007/s12016-007-8034-1 [doi].
4. Sicherer SH, Sampson HA (2010) Food allergy. J Allergy Clin Immunol 125: S116–S125. S0091-6749(09)01270-6 [pii];10.1016/j.jaci.2009.08.028 [doi].
5. Sicherer SH (2011) Epidemiology of food allergy. J Allergy Clin Immunol. S0091-6749(10)01868-3 [pii];10.1016/j.jaci.2010.11.044 [doi].
6. Bock SA (1987) Prospective appraisal of complaints of adverse reactions to foods in children during the first 3 years of life. Pediatrics 79: 683–688.
7. Luccioli S, Ross M, Labiner-Wolfe J, Fein SB (2008) Maternally reported food allergies and other food-related health problems in infants: characteristics and associated factors. Pediatrics 122 Suppl 2: S105–S112. 122/Supplement_2/S105 [pii];10.1542/peds.2008-1315n [doi].
8. Venter C, Pereira B, Voigt K, Grundy J, Clayton CB, Higgins B, et al. (2008) Prevalence and cumulative incidence of food hypersensitivity in the first 3 years of life. Allergy 63: 354–359. ALL1570 [pii];10.1111/j.1398-9995.2007.01570.x [doi].
9. Garcia-Careaga M Jr, Kerner JA Jr (2005) Gastrointestinal manifestations of food allergies in pediatric patients. Nutr Clin Pract 20: 526–535. 20/5/526 [pii].
10. Prescott S, Allen KJ (2011) Food allergy: Riding the second wave of the allergy epidemic. Pediatr Allergy Immunol 22: 155–160. 10.1111/j.1399-3038.2011.01145.x [doi].
11. Mainardi T, Kapoor S, Bielory L (2009) Complementary and alternative medicine: herbs, phytochemicals and vitamins and their immunologic effects. J Allergy Clin Immunol 123: 283–294. S0091-6749(08)02439-1 [pii];10.1016/j.jaci.2008.12.023 [doi].
12. Gupta S, George P, Gupta V, Tandon VR, Sundaram KR (1979) Tylophora indica in bronchial asthma–a double blind study. Indian J Med Res 69: 981–989.
13. Lee DK, Carstairs IJ, Haggart K, Jackson CM, Currie GP, et al. (2003) Butterbur, a herbal remedy, attenuates adenosine monophosphate induced nasal responsiveness in seasonal allergic rhinitis. Clin Exp Allergy 33: 882–886. 1705 [pii].
14. Schempp CM, Windeck T, Hezel S, Simon JC (2003) Topical treatment of atopic dermatitis with St. John's wort cream–a randomized, placebo controlled, double blind half-side comparison. Phytomedicine 10 Suppl 4: 31–37.
15. Lutterodt H, Luther M, Salvin M, Yin J-J, Perry J, Gao J-M, et al. (2011) Fatty acid profile, thymoquinone content, oxidative stability, and antioxidative properties of cold-pressed black cumin seed oils. LWT-Food Science and Technology 43: 1409–1413.
16. Ramadan MF, Morsel JT (2002) AID-FOOD240>3.0.CO;2-1 [doi].
17. Ghosheh OA, Houdi AA, Crooks PA (1999) High performance liquid chromatographic analysis of the pharmacologically active quinones and related compounds in the oil of the black seed (Nigella sativa L.). J Pharm Biomed Anal 19: 757–762. S0731-7085(98)00300-8 [pii].
18. Tiruppur Venkatachallam SK, Pattekhan H, Divakar S, Kadimi US (2010) Chemical composition of *Nigella sativa* L. seed extracts obtained by supercritical carbon dioxide. J Food Sci Technol 47: 598–605.
19. Padhye S, Banerjee S, Ahmad A, Mohammad R, Sarkar FH (2008) From here to eternity – the secret of Pharaohs: Therapeutic potential of black cumin seeds and beyond. Cancer Ther 6: 495–510.
20. Butt MS, Sultan MT (2010) Nigella sativa: reduces the risk of various maladies. Crit Rev Food Sci Nutr 50: 654–665. 925289763 [pii];10.1080/10408390902768797 [doi].
21. Mansour M, Tornhamre S (2004) Inhibition of 5-lipoxygenase and leukotriene C4 synthase in human blood cells by thymoquinone. J Enzyme Inhib Med Chem 19: 431–436. 10.1080/14756360400002072 [doi].
22. Vaillancourt F, Silva P, Shi Q, Fahmi H, Fernandes JC, et al. (2011) Elucidation of molecular mechanisms underlying the protective effects of thymoquinone against rheumatoid arthritis. J Cell Biochem 112: 107–117. 10.1002/jcb.22884 [doi].
23. Isik F, Tunali AT, Yarat A, Genc Z, Pisiriciler R, et al. (2011) Protective effects of black cumin (Nigella sativa) oil on TNBS-induced experimental colitis in rats. Dig Dis Sci 56: 721–730. 10.1007/s10620-010-1333-z [doi].
24. Banerjee S, Padhye S, Azmi A, Wang Z, Philip PA, et al. (2010) Review on molecular and therapeutic potential of thymoquinone in cancer. Nutr Cancer 62: 938–946. 927591507 [pii];10.1080/01635581.2010.509832 [doi].
25. Nikakhlagh S, Rahim F, Aryani FH, Syahpoush A, Brougerdnya MG, et al. (2010) Herbal treatment of allergic rhinitis: the use of Nigella sativa. Am J Otolaryngol. S0196-0709(10)00140-7 [pii];10.1016/j.amjoto.2010.07.019 [doi].
26. Boskabady MH, Mohsenpoor N, Takaloo L (2010) Antiasthmatic effect of Nigella sativa in airways of asthmatic patients. Phytomedicine 17: 707–713. S0944-7113(10)00018-8 [pii];10.1016/j.phymed.2010.01.002 [doi].
27. El Gazzar M, El Mezayen R, Nicolls MR, Marecki JC, Dreskin SC (2006) Downregulation of leukotriene biosynthesis by thymoquinone attenuates airway inflammation in a mouse model of allergic asthma. Biochim Biophys Acta 1760: 1088–1095. S0304-4165(06)00072-9 [pii];10.1016/j.bbagen.2006.03.006 [doi].
28. Abdel-Fattah AM, Matsumoto K, Watanabe H (2000) Antinociceptive effects of Nigella sativa oil and its major component, thymoquinone, in mice. Eur J Pharmacol 400: 89–97. S001429990000340X [pii].
29. Hosseinzadeh H, Parvardeh S (2004) Anticonvulsant effects of thymoquinone, the major constituent of Nigella sativa seeds, in mice. Phytomedicine 11: 56–64.
30. Hosseinzadeh H, Parvardeh S, Nassiri-Asl M, Mansouri MT (2005) Intracerebroventricular administration of thymoquinone, the major constituent of Nigella sativa seeds, suppresses epileptic seizures in rats. Med Sci Monit 11: BR106-BR110. 5295 [pii].
31. Shahbazian A, Heinemann A, Schmidhammer H, Beubler E, Holzer-Petsche U, et al. (2002) Involvement of mu- and kappa-, but not delta-, opioid receptors in the peristaltic motor depression caused by endogenous and exogenous opioids in the guinea-pig intestine. Br J Pharmacol 135: 741–750. 10.1038/sj.bjp.0704527 [doi].
32. Shook JE, Lemcke PK, Gehrig CA, Hruby VJ, Burks TF (1989) Antidiarrheal properties of supraspinal mu and delta and peripheral mu, delta and kappa opioid receptors: inhibition of diarrhea without constipation. J Pharmacol Exp Ther 249: 83–90.
33. Wood JD, Galligan JJ (2004) Function of opioids in the enteric nervous system. Neurogastroenterol Motil 16 Suppl 2: 17–28. 10.1111/j.1743-3150.2004.00554.x [doi]; NMO554 [pii].
34. Rogers TJ, Peterson PK (2003) Opioid G protein-coupled receptors: signals at the crossroads of inflammation. Trends Immunol 24: 116–121. S1471490603000036 [pii].
35. Brandt EB, Strait RT, Hershko D, Wang Q, Muntel EE, et al. (2003) Mast cells are required for experimental oral allergen-induced diarrhea. J Clin Invest 112: 1666–1677.
36. El Gazzar M, El Mezayen R, Marecki JC, Nicolls MR, Canastar A, et al. (2006) Anti-inflammatory effect of thymoquinone in a mouse model of allergic lung inflammation. Int Immunopharmacol 6: 1135–1142. S1567-5769(06)00060-9 [pii];10.1016/j.intimp.2006.02.004 [doi].
37. Abbas AT, Abdel-Aziz MM, Zalata KR, Tel AA-G (2005) Effect of dexamethasone and Nigella sativa on peripheral blood eosinophil count, IgG1 and IgG2a, cytokine profiles and lung inflammation in murine model of allergic asthma. Egypt J Immunol 12: 95–102.
38. Chakravarty N (1993) Inhibition of histamine release from mast cells by nigellone. Ann Allergy 70: 237–242.
39. Kanter M, Coskun O, Uysal H (2006) The antioxidative and antihistaminic effect of Nigella sativa and its major constituent, thymoquinone on ethanol-induced gastric mucosal damage. Arch Toxicol 80: 217–224. 10.1007/s00204-005-0037-1 [doi].

40. Buyukozturk S, Gelincik A, Ozseker F, Genc S, Savran FO, et al. (2005) Nigella sativa (black seed) oil does not affect the T-helper 1 and T-helper 2 type cytokine production from splenic mononuclear cells in allergen sensitized mice. J Ethnopharmacol 100: 295–298. S0378-8741(05)00214-X [pii];10.1016/j.jep.2005.03.007 [doi].
41. Badary OA, Gamal El-Din AM (2001) Inhibitory effects of thymoquinone against 20-methylcholanthrene-induced fibrosarcoma tumorigenesis. Cancer Detect Prev 25: 362–368.
42. Houghton PJ, Zarka R, de las Heras B, Hoult JR (1995) Fixed oil of Nigella sativa and derived thymoquinone inhibit eicosanoid generation in leukocytes and membrane lipid peroxidation. Planta Med 61: 33–36. 10.1055/s-2006-957994 [doi].
43. Finlay TM, Abdulkhalek S, Gilmour A, Guzzo C, Jayanth P, et al. (2010) Thymoquinone-induced Neu4 sialidase activates NFkappaB in macrophage cells and pro-inflammatory cytokines in vivo. Glycoconj J 27: 583–600. 10.1007/s10719-010-9302-5 [doi].
44. Philippe D, Dubuquoy L, Groux H, Brun V, Chuoi-Mariot MT, et al. (2003) Anti-inflammatory properties of the mu opioid receptor support its use in the treatment of colon inflammation. J Clin Invest 111: 1329–1338.
45. Barbezat GO, Clain JE, Halter F (1979) A double-blind trial of loperamide in the treatment of chronic diarrhoea. S Afr Med J 55: 502–503.
46. Jaffe G (1977) A comparison of lomotil and imodium in acute non-specific diarrhoea. J Int Med Res 5: 195–198.
47. Stead RH, Dixon MF, Bramwell NH, Riddell RH, Bienenstock J (1989) Mast cells are closely apposed to nerves in the human gastrointestinal mucosa. Gastroenterology 97: 575–585. S0016508589002738 [pii].
48. Poonyachoti S, Brown DR (2001) delta-opioid receptors inhibit neurogenic intestinal secretion evoked by mast cell degranulation and type I hypersensitivity. J Neuroimmunol 112: 89–96.
49. Stead RH, Colley EC, Wang B, Partosoedarso E, Lin J, et al. (2006) Vagal influences over mast cells. Auton Neurosci 125: 53–61. S1566-0702(06)00004-X [pii];10.1016/j.autneu.2006.01.002 [doi].
50. Philippe D, Dubuquoy L, Groux H, Brun V, Chuoi-Mariot MT, et al. (2003) Anti-inflammatory properties of the mu opioid receptor support its use in the treatment of colon inflammation. J Clin Invest 111: 1329–1338. 10.1172/JCI16750 [doi].
51. Whistler JL, Chuang HH, Chu P, Jan LY, von Zastrow M (1999) Functional dissociation of mu opioid receptor signaling and endocytosis: implications for the biology of opiate tolerance and addiction. Neuron 23: 737–746. S0896-6273(01)80032-5 [pii].
52. Sirohi S, Kumar P, Yoburn BC (2007) Mu-opioid receptor up-regulation and functional supersensitivity are independent of antagonist efficacy. J Pharmacol Exp Ther 323: 701–707. jpet.107.127019 [pii];10.1124/jpet.107.127019 [doi].
53. Verma-Gandhu M, Verdu EF, Cohen-Lyons D, Collins SM (2007) Lymphocyte-mediated regulation of beta-endorphin in the myenteric plexus. Am J Physiol Gastrointest Liver Physiol 292: G344-G348. 00318.2006 [pii];10.1152/ajpgi.00318.2006 [doi].
54. Meng F, Xie GX, Thompson RC, Mansour A, Goldstein A, et al. (1993) Cloning and pharmacological characterization of a rat kappa opioid receptor. Proc Natl Acad Sci U S A 90: 9954–9958.
55. Simonin F, Befort K, Gaveriaux-Ruff C, Matthes H, Nappey V, et al. (1994) The human delta-opioid receptor: genomic organization, cDNA cloning, functional expression, and distribution in human brain. Mol Pharmacol 46: 1015–1021.
56. Wang JB, Johnson PS, Persico AM, Hawkins AL, Griffin CA, et al. (1994) Human mu opiate receptor. cDNA and genomic clones, pharmacologic characterization and chromosomal assignment. FEBS Lett 338: 217–222. 0014-5793(94)80368-4 [pii].
57. Zuercher AW, Holvoet S, Weiss M, Mercenier A (2010) Polyphenol-enriched apple extract attenuates food allergy in mice. Clin Exp Allergy 40: 942–950. CEA3460 [pii];10.1111/j.1365-2222.2010.03460.x [doi].
58. Perrier C, Thierry AC, Mercenier A, Corthesy B (2010) Allergen-specific antibody and cytokine responses, mast cell reactivity and intestinal permeability upon oral challenge of sensitized and tolerized mice. Clin Exp Allergy 40: 153–162. CEA3329 [pii];10.1111/j.1365-2222.2009.03329.x [doi].

5

# Acid Hydrolysis of Wheat Gluten Induces Formation of New Epitopes but Does Not Enhance Sensitizing Capacity by the Oral Route: A Study in "Gluten Free" Brown Norway Rats

**Stine Kroghsbo[1¤], Nanna B. Andersen[1], Tina F. Rasmussen[1], Susanne Jacobsen[2]†, Charlotte B. Madsen[1*]**

**1** National Food Institute, Technical University of Denmark, Søborg, Denmark, **2** Enzyme and Protein Chemistry, Department of Systems Biology, Technical University of Denmark, Lyngby, Denmark

## Abstract

***Background:*** Acid hydrolyzed wheat proteins (HWPs) are used in the food and cosmetic industry as emulsifiers. Cases of severe food allergic reactions caused by HWPs have been reported. Recent data suggest that these reactions are caused by HWPs produced by acid hydrolysis.

***Objectives:*** To examine the sensitizing capacity of gluten proteins *per se* when altered by acid or enzymatic hydrolysis relative to unmodified gluten in rats naïve to gluten.

***Methods:*** High IgE-responder Brown Norway (BN) rats bred on a gluten-free diet were sensitized without the use of adjuvant to three different gluten products (unmodified, acid hydrolyzed and enzymatic hydrolyzed). Rats were sensitized by intraperitoneal (i.p.) immunization three times with 200 µg gluten protein/rat or by oral dosing for 35 days with 0.2, 2 or 20 mg gluten protein/rat/day. Sera were analyzed for specific IgG and IgE and IgG-binding capacity by ELISA. IgE functionality was measured by rat basophilic leukemia (RBL) assay.

***Results:*** Regardless of the route of dosing, all products had sensitizing capacity. When sensitized i.p., all three gluten products induced a strong IgG1 response in all animals. Acid hydrolyzed gluten induced the highest level of specific IgE but with a low functionality. Orally all three gluten products induced specific IgG1 and IgE but with different dose-response relations. Sensitizing rats i.p. or orally with unmodified or enzymatic hydrolyzed gluten induced specific IgG1 responses with similar binding capacity which was different from that of acid hydrolyzed gluten indicating that acid hydrolysis of gluten proteins induces formation of 'new' epitopes.

***Conclusions:*** In rats not tolerant to gluten acid hydrolysis of gluten enhances the sensitizing capacity by the i.p. but not by the oral route. In addition, acid hydrolysis induces formation of new epitopes. This is in contrast to the enzymatic hydrolyzed gluten having an epitope pattern similar to unmodified gluten.

**Editor:** Nicholas J. Mantis, New York State Dept. Health, United States of America

**Funding:** This work was financially supported by Tereos Syral, Aalst, Belgium who also provided the gluten proteins used, Danish Veterinary and Food Administration, and the Danish Research Council grant 0603-00199B. The funders had no role in study design, data collection and analysis, decision to publish, or preparation of the manuscript.

**Competing Interests:** Tereos Syral, a company producing wheat gluten and proteins under the name Meripro, provided funding towards this study. There are no further patents, products in development or marketed products to declare.

† Deceased.

* Email: charm@food.dtu.dk

¤ Current address: Unisensor A/S, Allerød, Denmark

## Introduction

Gluten proteins are wheat storage proteins, constituting about 10% of wheat, and give wheat dough functional properties such as water absorption capacity, viscosity and elasticity, which contribute to the unique baking properties [1–3]. Gluten proteins are among the most complex proteins in nature containing hundreds of components present as monomers, oligomers and polymers. Oligomers and polymers are linked by disul-phide bonds between the S-containing amino acid cysteine, which make up approximately 2% of gluten. Based on their physical characteristics, gluten proteins can be divided into gliadins and glutenins. Gliadins, also known as wheat prolamins, are soluble in alcohol and are mainly present in gluten as monomers interacting by non-covalent forces.

Glutenins are soluble in dilute acid and are mainly present as aggregated proteins linked by intra- and interchain disulphide bonds. Gliadins and glutenins consist mainly of glutamine, proline and the essential amino acid phenylalanine [3,4]. Another unique feature about gluten proteins is their structures, which are dynamic, comprise interchanging conformations and do not unfold when exposed to heating like most other proteins [5].

Gluten proteins are by definition not soluble in water but enzymatic or acid hydrolysis can alter their structure and size and thereby resulting in soluble protein hydrolysates. Acid hydrolyses also result in partial deamidation of the proteins [6]. Acid hydrolyzed wheat gluten obtain emulsifying properties which make them useful in food products such as coffee creamers and shake-and-bake products but also in cosmetic products for hair and body [6,7].

The digestibility of wheat depends on the degree of processing and grinding [8]. Results from *in vitro* digestion studies of wheat proteins indicate that gluten proteins partially resist digestion in the stomach and intestine and thus may be absorbed as structurally intact proteins [9]. However, when gluten proteins are deamidated, it may result in increased digestibility [10]. In general, hydrolysis can alter the way proteins are broken down, digested and absorbed across the gut mucosal barrier [5]. Hence, there is a possibility that the mucosal immune system is not exposed to hydrolyzed gluten proteins in the same way as gluten proteins [5,11].

The default immunological reaction to ingested food proteins is tolerance. However, in susceptible individuals an otherwise harmless food or food component can induce an IgE-mediated food allergy, which involves an abnormal response of the immune system to specific food proteins. IgE-mediated wheat allergy appears in three different types; wheat food allergy, wheat-dependent exercise-induced anaphylaxis (WDEIA) and baker's asthma, which must be distinguished from each other [12]. Recently allergy to HWPs was recognized as a fourth type of IgE-mediated allergy to wheat. Most interestingly, HWPs have been reported to cause food allergic reactions in patients who are tolerant to wheat [11,13–17]. Allergic skin reactions after application of cosmetic products containing HWPs have also been described [7,14,15,18,19]. However, the type of hydrolysis (enzymatic or acid) in the papers on HWP's is not always clearly defined. In Japan the use of a facial soap containing acid hydrolyzed wheat protein has caused allergic skin symptoms and WDEIA i.e. allergic reactions to wheat products [20,21]. A wide spectrum of wheat proteins belonging to the albumin/globulin fraction (salt-soluble), gliadin fraction (alcohol-soluble) and glutenin fraction (soluble in dilute acid) [9,11,13–15,19,22,23] have been reported to be involved in IgE-mediated allergic reactions to wheat. However, at present no study has clearly demonstrated a correlation between the type of IgE-mediated wheat allergy and pattern of IgE-reactivity to a specific fraction of wheat proteins. In general, food allergens have a high resistance to heat. This is also the case of gluten proteins that contain potentially thermo-stable IgE-epitopes [5,9,25]. The route of sensitization can occur via the gastrointestinal tract, via the respiratory tract (wheat flour) or via the skin [12,25–27].

Solubility increases when gluten is hydrolyzed by enzymes. This type of product is used in food as a protein supplement. When gluten is hydrolyzed by acid, emulsifying properties are created. This type of product is used as emulsifier in food and in cosmetics.

To investigate if hydrolysis alters the immunogenicity of gluten proteins we have studied the sensitization capacity of unmodified, enzymatic hydrolyzed and acid hydrolyzed wheat gluten. To be able to compare the immune response *per se* the influence from gluten tolerance was excluded by performing the studies in Brown Norway rats naïve to gluten (bred for more than three generations on a gluten free diet). Rats were dosed intraperitoneally or orally.

## Material and Methods

### Ethics statement

Animal experiments were carried out at the DTU Food (Mørkhøj, Denmark) facilities. Ethical approval was given by the Danish Animal Experiments Inspectorate. The authorization number given: 2009/561-01710. The experiments were overseen by the National Food Institutes in-house Animal Welfare Committee for animal care and use.

### Wheat gluten products

Wheat gluten (unmodified), enzymatic hydrolyzed wheat gluten and acid hydrolyzed wheat gluten were provided by Tereos Syral, Aalst, Belgium. The enzyme used in the production of enzyme hydrolyzed gluten was an endoprotease with no transglutaminase activity. Compared to the conditions of acid hydrolysis, the enzymatic reaction occurs at more neutral pH and moderate temperature. The acid hydrolyzed gluten is produced at very low pH (below pH 2.5) and at high temperature (above 80°C). For technical information on gluten products see Table 1. It can be seen that acid hydrolysis results in substantial deamidation. The level of endotoxin in gluten proteins were analyzed according to manufacturer's instructions (Pierce LAL Chromogenic Endotoxin Quantitation kit; Fisher Scientific ApS, Slangerup, Denmark). Endotoxin levels were below 50 EU/mg gluten protein for all products.

### Preparation of soluble fractions of wheat gluten products for analysis of antibody response

Gluten products were dissolved by carefully adding 1 mg/mL unmodified gluten or hydrolyzed gluten products to phosphate buffered saline (PBS; 137 mM NaCl, 3 mM KCl, 8 mM $Na_2HPO_4$, 1 mM $KH_2PO_4$; pH 7.2) before magnetic stirring for 2 hours at room temperature (RT) followed by ultrasonication for 3–5 hours. After centrifugation at 2000×*g* for 20 min. at 4°C, supernatants were collected and stored at ÷20°C. Protein concentrations in supernatants were determined by amino acid analysis [28].

As approximately 35% of proteins in unmodified gluten were soluble in PBS, gluten proteins were extracted by ethanol (gliadin fraction) followed by sodium oleate (glutenin fraction) for measurement of the specific antibody response to 'total' gluten proteins. Briefly, unmodified gluten were suspended in 50% ethanol (2 mg gluten protein/mL), mixed carefully for 10 min. before ultrasonication for 2–3 hours. The gliadin fraction was obtained by collecting the supernatant after centrifugation (2000×*g*, RT, 5 min.). The glutenin fraction was obtained by suspending the remaining pellet in 0.1% (w/v) sodium oleate solution before carefully mixing for 10 min. followed by ultrasonication for 2 hours and collection of supernatant after centrifugation (2000×*g*, RT, 15 min.). Gliadin and glutenin fractions were stored at RT.

### Animals

Inbred high IgE-responder Brown Norway (BN) rats were from our in-house colony at the National Food Institute (DTU, Denmark). Rats were bred and kept for at least three generations on a gluten free diet developed and produced at the National Food Institute (DTU, Denmark) [29] to ensure immunologically naïve animals with respect to wheat proteins. The diet was analyzed for

**Table 1.** Technical information on unmodified, enzymatic hydrolyzed and acid hydrolyzed wheat gluten provided by Tereos Syral.

| | Unmodified wheat gluten | Enzymatic hydrolyzed wheat gluten | Acid hydrolyzed wheat gluten |
|---|---|---|---|
| **% relative protein (SDS soluble)*** | | | |
| F1>779.6 kDa | 9.8 | 0.7 | 0.9 |
| 779.6 kDa>F2>96.7 kDa | 26.0 | 4.3 | 13.6 |
| 96.7 kDa>F3>58.1 kDa | 7.7 | 2.8 | 9.5 |
| 58.1 kDa>F4>20.5 kDa | 42.7 | 21.7 | 40.3 |
| 20.5 kDa>F5>6.2 kDa | 12.7 | 60.4 | 34.4 |
| 6.2 kDa>F6>0.47 kDa | 1.1 | 10.2 | 1.3 |
| **Degree of deamidation (%)**¤ | ~3 | ~3 | 60 |
| **Emulsifying capacity**† | - | - | 950 |
| **Solubility in PBS (%)**‡ | 35 | 100 | 98 |

*Weight distribution for SDS soluble protein in gluten products expressed as relative % of different fractions. 15.3% of unmodified gluten was not soluble in SDS whereas enzymatic and acid hydrolyzed gluten products were completely soluble.
¤Degree of deamidation was measured by a titrimetric determination of the free ammonia in native, enzyme hydrolyzed and acid hydrolyzed wheat gluten, expressed as % of the free ammonia after total deamidation of wheat gluten.
†Emulsifying capacity denotes the maximum amount of oil that is emulsified by a standard amount of protein (g oil/g product).
‡Solubility of gluten proteins in phosphate buffered saline (PBS) based on protein concentration measured by amino acid analysis. Determined as % protein extracted from 1 mg/mL solutions of gluten products. Own results.
-: not tested.

wheat proteins using a sensitive commercial kit for detection of gliadin peptide fragments in accordance with manufacturer's instructions (Art.no. R7011, RIDASCREEN Gliadin competitive; Food Diagnostics, Grenaa, Denmark). For sensitization studies, 4–6 weeks old rats, were allocated into groups and housed in macrolon cages (two/cage) at 22±1°C, relative humidity 55±5%, air change 10 times/h, and electric light from 9.00 am – 9.00 pm. Diet and acidified water (pH 3.5) were given *ad libitum*. Animals were inspected twice daily and body weights recorded weekly. At termination of sensitization experiments all animals were anaesthetized by hypnorm-dormicum and killed by exsanguinations. Animal experiments were carried out at the National Food Institute (DTU, Denmark) facilities and performed under conditions approved by the Danish Animal Experiments Inspectorate and by the in-house Animal Welfare Committee for animal care and use.

## Animal sensitization studies

Sensitization capacity of unmodified gluten and hydrolyzed gluten products were studied in two different rat models; an i.p. model based on intraperitoneal immunization with the soluble fraction of gluten products and an oral model based on intragastric dosing of rats with 'whole' gluten products suspended in water.

For each of the gluten products, positive control sera were produced in BN rats by i.p. immunization with 200 µg gluten product adsorbed on Alhydrogel (Brenntag Biosector, Frederikssund, Denmark) at day 0 and with 20 µg gluten product suspended in 0.9% NaCl at day 14, 21 and 28. Rats were immunized with 0.2 mL per rat and blood was collected at sacrifice (day 35).

Sera from all animal experiments were stored at ÷20°C until analysis.

**I.p. study with gluten products.** Groups of 16 BN rats (8 rats per sex) were immunized i.p. on day 0, 14 and 28 with unmodified gluten or hydrolyzed gluten products extracted in PBS (200 µg protein/rat/immunization). Blood was collected on day 35.

**Oral sensitization studies with gluten products.** Only female BN rats (12 per group) were included in these studies as it has previously been shown that significantly more responders are found amongst female BN rats than among males when dosed by gavage [30]. Rats were dosed by gavage each day for 35 days (day 1–35) with 0.2, 2 or 20 mg of unmodified gluten or hydrolyzed gluten products suspended in PBS. Suspensions were carefully mixed between dosing of rats to avoid precipitation. For all feeding studies, the dosing volume was 0.5 mL per rat per day and blood was collected on day 0, 14, 28 and 42 (sacrifice).

## Enzyme-Linked Immuno Sorbent Assay (ELISA)

Sera from sensitization studies were analyzed for specific IgG1 and IgE by ELISA. Positive and negative serum control pools were included on each plate. Antibody titers were expressed as log2 titers and calculated using four-parameter analysis, Gen5 (Bio-Tek Instruments Inc., Winooski, VT, USA). Detection limits were determined as the mean absorbance for the negative control serum+3 standard deviations (SD). For all ELISA experiments washing procedures and development of enzymatic reaction were as described previously [31]. All reagents and incubation periods were at RT for 1 hour unless otherwise noted.

**Detection of specific IgG1 by direct ELISA.** For detection of specific IgG1, plates (96-well, MaxiSorp; Nunc, Roskilde, Denmark) were coated overnight at 4°C with 100 µL/well of 2 µg/mL of the soluble fraction of unmodified gluten or hydrolyzed gluten products, gliadin fraction or glutenin fraction in carbonate buffer (15 mM $Na_2CO_3$, 35 mM $NaHCO_3$; pH 9.6). Plates were incubated with serially two-fold diluted rat sera in PBS containing 0.01% Tween (PBS-T) before incubation with horseradish peroxidase (HRP)-labeled mouse anti-rat IgG1 (1:20,000; SouthernBiotech cat. no. 3060-05, Birmingham, AL, USA) in PBS-T followed by development with TMB-one (Kem-En-Tec, Copenhagen, Denmark) for 10 min in the dark. Absorbance values for detection limits were calculated to 0.1 for all IgG1 assays.

**Inhibition ELISAs for examination of IgG1-binding capacity.** Assay procedures were as described for measurement of specific IgG1 except that sera were preincubated with inhibitor solutions. Sera from individual rats were diluted to reach an OD between 0.8 and 1.0 and preincubated for 1 hour at RT with serial ten-fold dilutions of the soluble fraction of gluten products (50 pg/mL to 50 μg/mL) before triplicates of serum/inhibitor mix (and sera with no inhibitor as a control) were added to the wells. Results were expressed as % $B/B_0$ where $B$ corresponds to the specific IgG1-binding to immobilized gluten protein when a known concentration of inhibitor is present and $B_0$ corresponds to the binding in the absence of inhibitor. For each serum pool, the concentration of inhibitor that inhibits 50% of the binding to the immobilized antigen ($IC_{50}$) was determined, where an increase in $IC_{50}$ value is correlated to a lower IgG1-reactivity of the product used as inhibitor. Inhibition curves were analyzed by GraphPad Prism (GraphPad Software, San Diego, CA, USA) to examine if curves were parallel (no significant difference between slopes) which is important for appropriate comparison of $IC_{50}$ values.

**Detection of specific IgE by antibody-capture ELISAs.** To avoid the interference of the much higher level of IgG than IgE in rat sera, assays based on selective IgE capture were established for detection of specific IgE responses. Plates were coated overnight at 4°C with 0.5 μg/mL of mouse anti-rat IgE (HPMAB-123 HybriDomus, Cytotech, Hellebæk, Denmark) in carbonate buffer. After blocking of remaining active sites for 1 hour at 37°C with PBS-T containing 3% bovine serum albumin (BSA; A2153, Sigma, Copenhagen, Denmark), plates were incubated with serially two-fold diluted rat sera and then with biotin-coupled gluten products or gliadin diluted in PBS-T containing 3% BSA (biotin-gluten 1:200, biotin-enzymatic hydrolyzed gluten 1:1500, biotin-acid hydrolyzed gluten 1:800 and biotin-gliadin 1:250). After washing, plates were incubated with HRP-labeled NeutrAvidin (cat. no. 31030; ThermoScientific, Slangerup, Denmark) diluted in PBS-T containing 3% BSA (diluted 1:4000 for detection of anti-gluten IgE, anti-acid hydrolyzed gluten IgE and anti-gliadin IgE or diluted 1:8000 for detection of anti-enzymatic hydrolyzed gluten IgE). Plates were developed for 10 min in the dark and absorbance values for detection limits were calculated to 0.1 for all IgE assays.

Biotin was coupled to each of the gluten products or gliadin using a biotin protein-labeling kit (Pierce EZ-Link Sulfo-NHS-LC-Biotinylation Kit; ThermoScientific) in accordance with the manufacturer's instructions. For gluten products, proteins soluble in PBS were used for biotinylation whereas the gliadin fraction of unmodified gluten was dissolved in 50% ethanol before biotinylation. The highest stability of biotin-coupled gluten proteins was obtained when biotin-gliadin was stored at ÷20°C and biotinylated gluten products were stored at 4°C.

### Rat Basophilic Leukemia (RBL) Assay

The biological functionality of specific IgE was examined by RBL assay as described previously [29] with minor modifications. Briefly, RBL-2H3 cells (kindly provided by Prof. Stefan Vieths, Paul-Ehrlich Institute, Langen, Germany) were harvested in the stationary phase, after over-confluence had been reached. Cells were re-suspended ($1\times10^6$ cells/mL) in assay medium (Eagle MEM supplemented with 100 U/100 μg/mL penicillin/streptomycin solution, 2.5 μg/mL amphotericin, and 2 mM L-glutamine) and incubated overnight (100 μL/well) in flat-bottomed cell culture microtitre plates (Nunc) for attachment. Attached cells were sensitized passively with 50 μL/well of undiluted rat serum pools for 2 hours (37°C, 5% $CO_2$) and then washed twice before incubation with 100 μL/well of five-fold diluted extracts of gluten products (0.02–350 μg protein/mL) for 60 min for cross-linking. After incubation plates were centrifuged ($200\times g$, 5 min) and 50 μL of supernatant (Specific release) was transferred to a microtitre plate (Nunc) for measurement of $\beta$-hexosaminidase enzymatic activity. Total release from remaining intact cells was measured for each well by addition of detergent (50 μL/well of 0.1% Triton X-100; X100, Sigma), incubated for 30 min before centrifugation and transfer of 50 μL supernatant (Total release) to a second microtitre plate.

For control of IgE-mediated degranulation (total biological release), serum-sensitized cells were stimulated with 1.25 μg/mL of mouse anti-rat IgE (553914, BD Pharmingen, San Diego, CA, USA). Negative controls were included on each plate to measure spontaneous release (equivalent to background reading).

For each serum sample $\beta$-hexosaminidase release was calculated according to the following equation:

$$\%\ \textit{Specific release} = \frac{\text{Specific release (stimulated with extracts of gluten products)}}{\text{Total release (lysed with detergent)}} \times 100\%$$

As IgE-mediated degranulation (*Total IgE release*) for serum pools were 50–60% of total release for all serum pools and no statistically significant difference was found between groups, results are expressed as percent of maximum biological release:

$$\beta-\textit{hexosamindase release}\ (\%) = \frac{\%\ \text{Specific release}}{\%\ \text{Total IgE release}} \times 100\%$$

### Statistical analysis

Statistical analysis of data was carried out using GraphPad Prism version 4.00 for Windows (GraphPad Software, San Diego, CA, USA). ELISA results expressed as antibody titers or $IC_{50}$ values were examined using non-parametric statistical analysis when distributions were not normal (Kruskal-Wallis test followed by Dunn's multiple comparison test). One-way ANOVA followed by Tukey's multiple comparison test was used for comparison between groups with normal distributions. Differences between experimental groups were regarded as significant when $p \leq 0.05$.

## Results

### Acid hydrolyzed gluten induces the highest level of specific IgE by the i.p. route

Although unmodified gluten induced a statistically significant higher IgG1 response compared to the acid hydrolyzed gluten all three products induced a high level of specific IgG1 in all rats when immunized i.p. (Figure 1*A*). In contrast, the highest level of specific IgE was obtained by immunization with acid hydrolyzed gluten (Figure 1*B*). ELISAs for measurement of specific IgE against the different gluten products are not necessarily comparable as it is uncertain whether biotin has been equally coupled to the mixture of proteins (and hydrolysis products) present in the gluten products. However, acid hydrolyzed gluten also induced the highest level of anti-gliadin IgE (Figure 1*C*).

### Acid hydrolysis of gluten discloses or produces new epitopes

Examination of IgG1-binding capacity showed that sera from rats sensitized to unmodified or enzymatic hydrolyzed gluten had

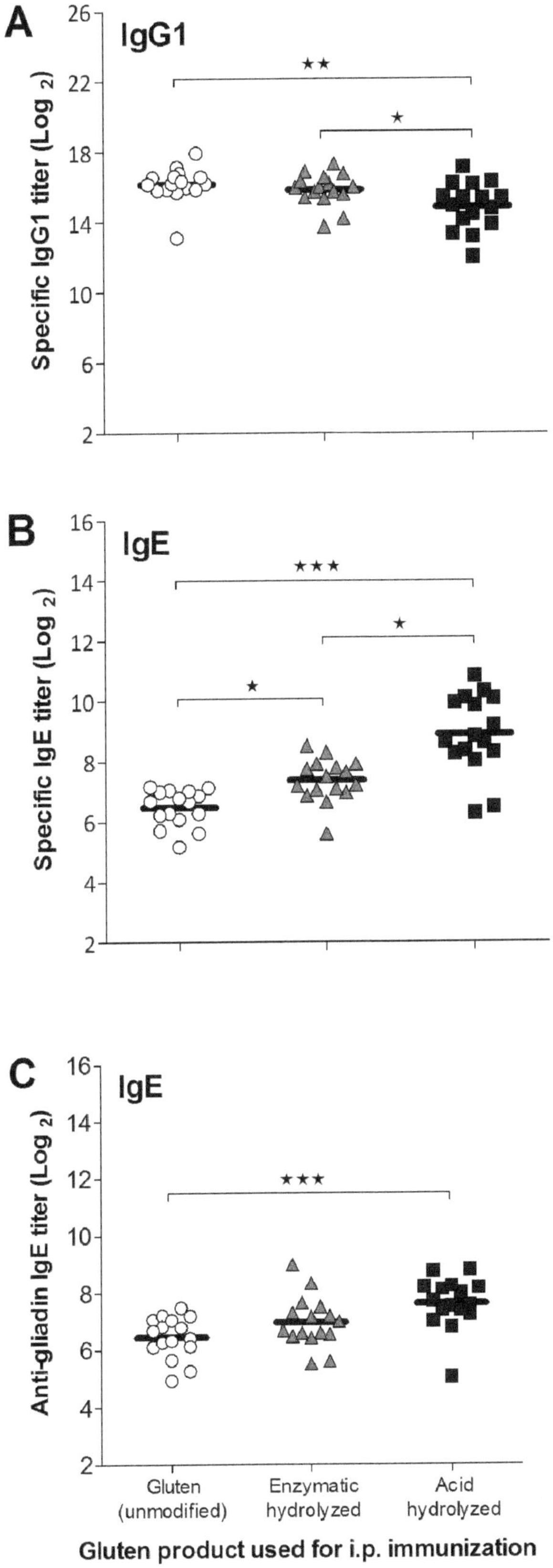


**Figure 1. Specific IgG1 and IgE response in sera from BN rats immunized i.p. with unmodified gluten (open circles), enzymatic hydrolyzed gluten (grey triangles) or acid hydrolyzed gluten (black squares).** Groups of rats were immunized i.p. on day 0, 14 and 28 with 200 µg gluten protein per rat without adjuvant. Serum samples were obtained at sacrifice (day 35) and analyzed by ELISA for specific IgG1 (*A*) and IgE (*B*) against the gluten product used for immunization and for anti-gliadin IgE (*C*). Each symbol represents an animal and horizontal bars indicate mean values. Data were analyzed by one-way ANOVA (IgG1) and non-parametrical test (IgE). Asterisks indicate statistically significant difference between groups; *: $p \leq 0.05$, **: $p \leq 0.01$, ***: $p \leq 0.001$.

equivalent binding capacity with high affinity for unmodified and enzymatic hydrolyzed gluten and significant lower affinity for acid hydrolyzed gluten (Figure 2*D, E*). The opposite was demonstrated for sera from rats sensitized to acid hydrolyzed gluten, which bound remarkably stronger to acid hydrolyzed gluten than to the other gluten products (Figure 2*F*). As shown in Figure 2, inhibition curves were identical when rats were sensitized to unmodified or enzymatic hydrolyzed gluten (2*A, B*). In contrast, for most rats sensitized to acid hydrolyzed gluten, the inhibition curve for acid hydrolyzed gluten was not parallel to the corresponding inhibition curves for unmodified and enzymatic hydrolyzed gluten (2*C*). Sensitization to acid hydrolyzed gluten induced IgG1 with higher avidity (mean IC50: 0.3 µg/mL) than sensitization to unmodified (mean IC50: 2.4 µg/mL) and enzymatic hydrolyzed gluten (mean IC50: 1.2 µg/mL). Together these results demonstrate that acid hydrolysis in contrast to enzymatic hydrolysis alters gluten proteins resulting in formation or disclosure of 'new' IgG-binding epitopes.

## The level of specific IgE does not reflect biological functionality

Although i.p. sensitization to acid hydrolyzed gluten seemed to induce the highest level of specific IgE (Figure 1), a lower IgE functionality was found for sera from rats sensitized to acid hydrolyzed gluten compared to sera from rats sensitized to unmodified or enzymatic hydrolyzed gluten in terms of a lower allergen-specific degranulation of RBL cells (Figure 3). In accordance with IgG1-binding results, IgE-mediated degranulation of cells sensitized with anti-gluten or anti-enzymatic hydrolyzed gluten sera was slightly decreased when stimulated with acid hydrolyzed gluten compared to the two other products. Likewise, the highest allergen-specific degranulation of cells sensitized with anti-acid hydrolyzed gluten sera was found when stimulated with acid hydrolyzed gluten (Figure 3).

## Gluten and hydrolysis products thereof can sensitize via the oral route

Sensitization capacity of unmodified gluten and hydrolysis products by the oral route was examined by dosing BN rats by gavage for 35 days with 'whole' gluten products suspended in PBS. A dose-response study was performed for each of the three gluten products by dosing rats with 0.2, 2 or 20 mg of gluten per rat per day for 35 days. The highest dose corresponds to 0.2% of the daily rat diet (10 gram feed/rat/day). In man eating 1.5 kg food/day, 0.2% corresponds to 3 gram of gluten (30 gram of wheat flour) or gluten product corresponding to 60 gram or 1–2 slices of bread. As shown in Figure 4, a significant IgG1 response were induced for all gluten products in the high dose groups (20 mg/rat/day) whereas at lower doses unmodified and enzymatic hydrolyzed gluten induced higher levels of specific IgG1 compared to acid hydrolyzed gluten. Levels of specific IgG1 and number of responders were clearly dose-related for enzymatic hydrolyzed gluten while unmodified gluten induced comparable IgG1 levels at all tested doses. Acid hydrolyzed gluten only induced a notable IgG1 at the highest dose. Analysis of sera from day 0, 14, 28 and

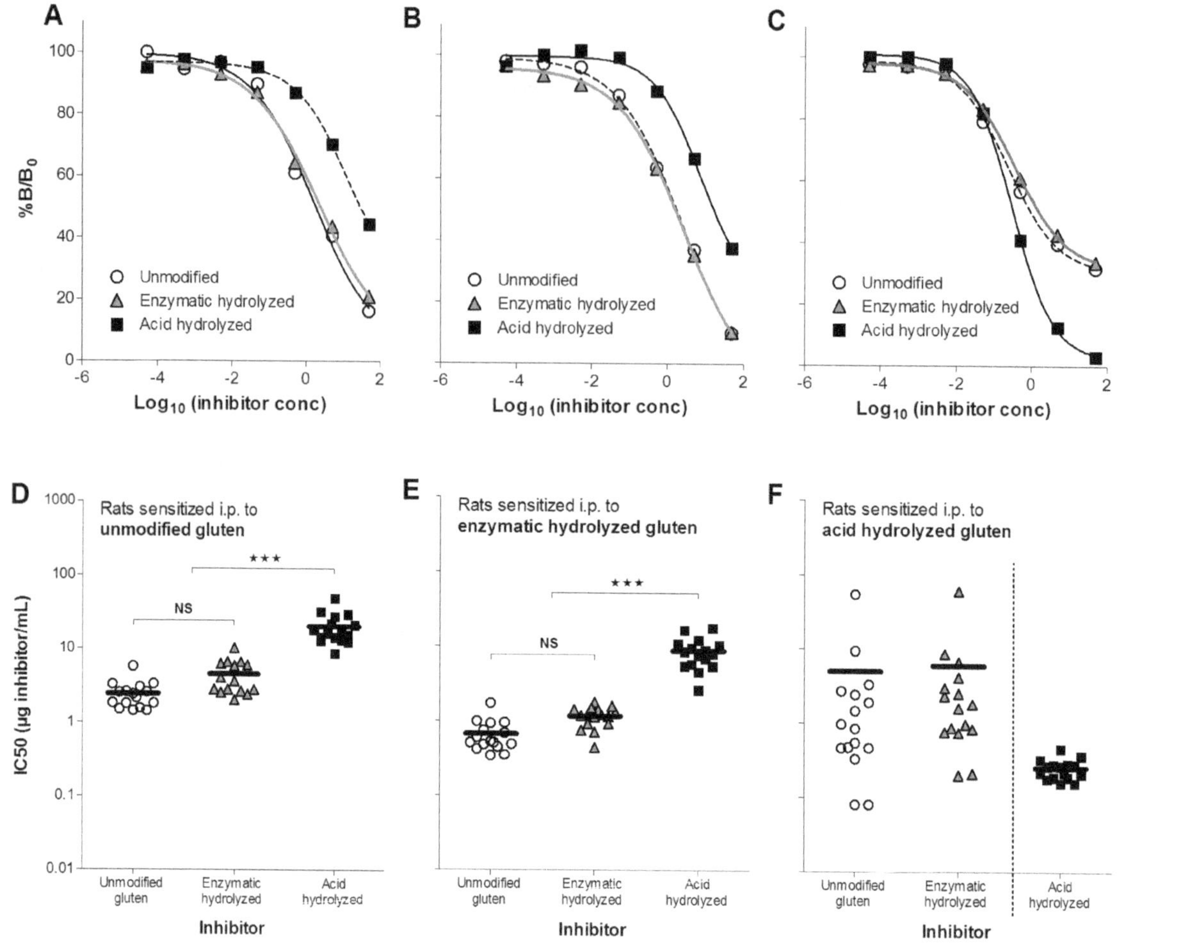


**Figure 2. Comparison of inhibition curves and IC50 values for IgG1-binding capacity.** Rats were immunized i.p. on day 0, 14 and 28 with 200 μg of unmodified gluten (*A, D*), enzymatic hydrolyzed gluten (*B, E*) or acid hydrolyzed gluten (*C, F*). Sera from individual rats obtained at sacrifice were preincubated with tenfold dilutions (50 pg/mL–50 μg/mL) of gluten products (unmodified gluten [open circles], enzymatic hydrolyzed gluten [grey triangles] or acid hydrolyzed gluten [black squares]) before determination of IgG1-binding capacity by addition to ELISA plates coated with the gluten product used for sensitization. Graphs *2A–C* show examples of inhibition curves for individual rats sensitized to unmodified (*2A*, rat no. 12), enzymatic hydrolyzed (*2B*, rat no. 31) or acid hydrolyzed (*2C*, rat no. 35) gluten. Symbols represent triplicates of the same serum/inhibitor mix and bars represent IC50 mean values for each group. Data were analyzed by one-way ANOVA. Asterisks indicate statistically significant difference between groups; ***: $p \leq 0.001$, NS: not significant.

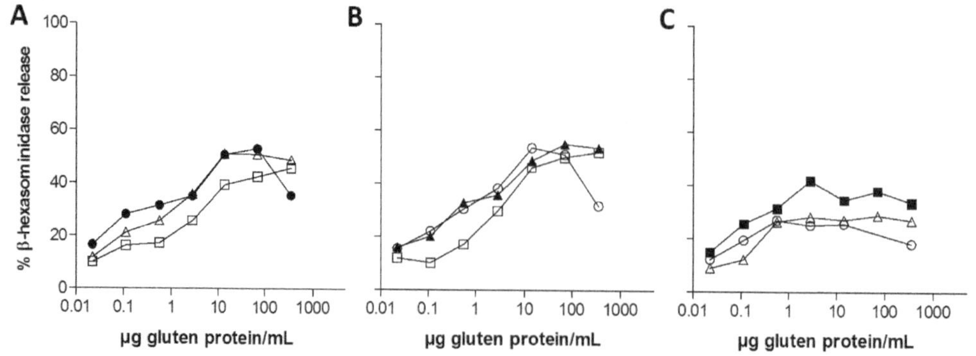


**Figure 3. Allergen-specific degranulation of RBL cells.** RBL cells were passively sensitized with undiluted serum pools of groups sensitized i.p. to unmodified gluten (*A*), enzymatic hydrolyzed gluten (*B*) or acid hydrolyzed gluten (*C*). For degranulation, cells were stimulated with five-fold dilutions of gluten products (unmodified [open circles], enzymatic hydrolyzed [grey triangles] and acid hydrolyzed [black squares] gluten, closed symbols represent the gluten product used for sensitization of rats). Data are presented as percentage allergen-specific *β*-hexosaminidase release of total release. IgE-mediated degranulation for serum pools were 50–60% for all serum pools (data not shown). Symbols represent mean values of duplicates for each serum pool.

42 showed that the magnitude of specific IgG1 and number of responders increased over time for all of the tested gluten products (data not shown). Like the IgG1 response, a dose-related IgE response was only found for enzymatic hydrolyzed gluten. Only enzymatic hydrolyzed gluten induced a significant IgE response. This was at the high dose. A few rats sensitized with low dose unmodified or acid hydrolyzed gluten had remarkably high IgE titers (Figure 4). Direct IgG1 ELISAs for detection of specific IgG1 against the gluten products were based on coating with proteins, which were soluble in PBS (Table 1). To measure specific IgG1 against 'all' gluten proteins, the gliadin and glutenin fractions obtained from unmodified gluten were used for coating in IgG1 ELISAs. The results showed that although only a minor fraction of unmodified gluten is salt soluble the anti-gliadin IgG1 response is comparable to the IgG1 response to unmodified gluten in PBS whereas the response to glutenin is slightly lower. Identical results were found for enzymatic and acid hydrolyzed gluten (Figure 5).

### IgG1-binding after oral sensitization to acid hydrolyzed gluten differs from sensitization to unmodified or enzymatic hydrolyzed gluten

Analysis of IgG1-binding capacity by inhibition ELISAs using sera from orally dosed rats (Figure 6) demonstrated the same pattern as found for sera from the i.p. sensitized rats (Figure 2) namely that acid hydrolysis but not enzymatic hydrolysis of gluten pro-teins generates 'new' epitopes. In addition, unmodified and enzymatic hydrolyzed gluten showed a tendency to produce antibodies with a stronger binding (higher avidity) after oral sensitization than after i.p. sensitization. For acid hydrolyzed gluten IgG1-binding for the two sensitization routes was identical when acid hydrolyzed gluten was used as inhibitor. With unmodified or enzymatic hydrolyzed gluten as inhibitor i.p. immunization induced antibodies with stronger binding (Figure 7).

## Discussion

Using Brown Norway rats kept on a gluten free diet for many generations and therefore naïve to gluten, we have shown that gluten and hydrolyzed gluten products can sensitize i.e. induce specific IgE using either the intraperitoneal or the oral route for dosing without the use of adjuvant. As expected i.p. immunization resulted in more responders and a higher antibody level than dosing by gavage. The i.p. route bypasses the digestive system as well as the gut-associated lymphoid tissue designed to induce tolerance to food antigens.

Using the i.p. route, immunization with the acid hydrolyzed gluten resulted in a significantly higher IgE response than both the unmodified and the enzymatic hydrolyzed gluten. When studying IgE functionality in RBL assay, sera from animals sensitized to acid hydrolyzed gluten had a lower biological activity with all three gluten products compared to sera from animals sensitized to unmodified or enzymatic hydrolyzed gluten. This result is in accordance with previous human and animal studies showing that IgE titer and biological activity may not necessarily correlate

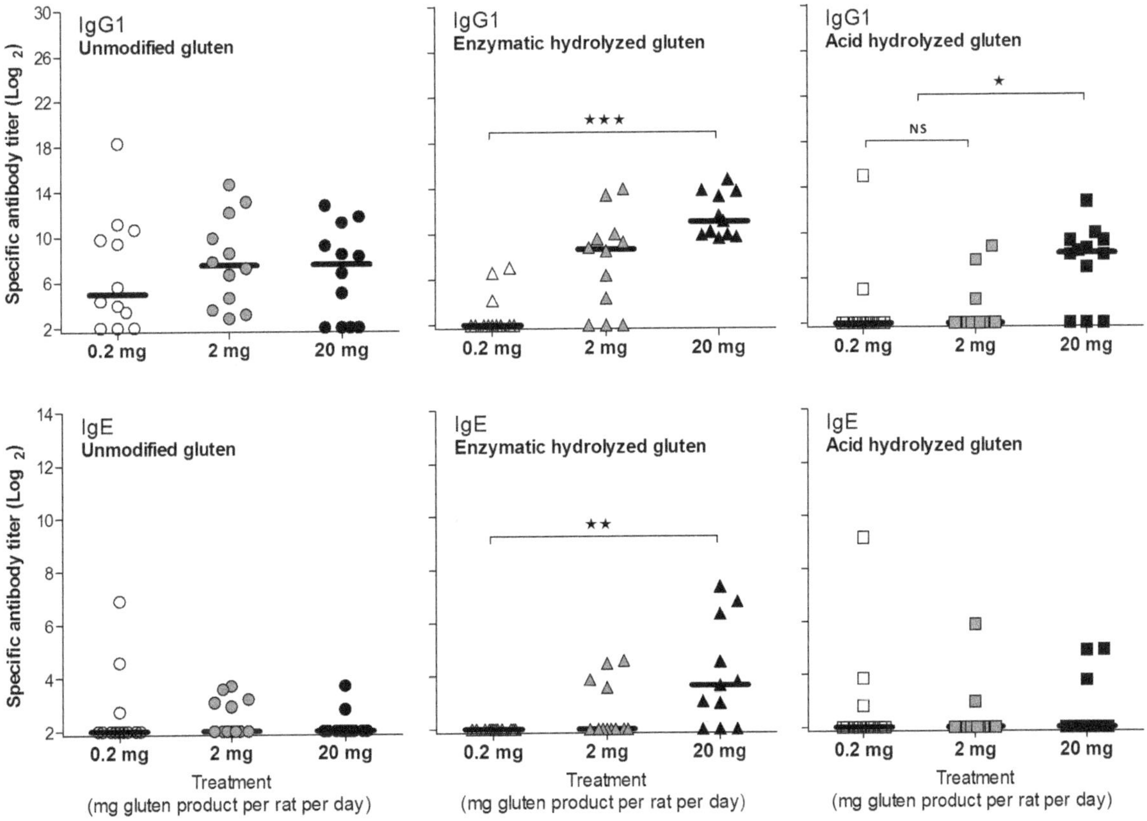


**Figure 4. Specific antibody response in sera from BN rats dosed orally with unmodified or hydrolysis products thereof.** Groups of female rats were dosed by gavage at day 1–35 with 0.2, 2 or 20 mg/rat of unmodified, enzymatic hydrolyzed or acid hydrolyzed gluten. Serum samples were obtained at sacrifice (day 42) and analyzed by ELISA for specific IgG1 and IgE. Each symbol represents an animal and horizontal bars indicate median values. Data were analyzed by non-parametrical test. Asterisks indicate statistically significant difference between groups; *: $p \leq 0.05$, **: $p \leq 0.01$, ***: $p \leq 0.001$, NS: not significant.

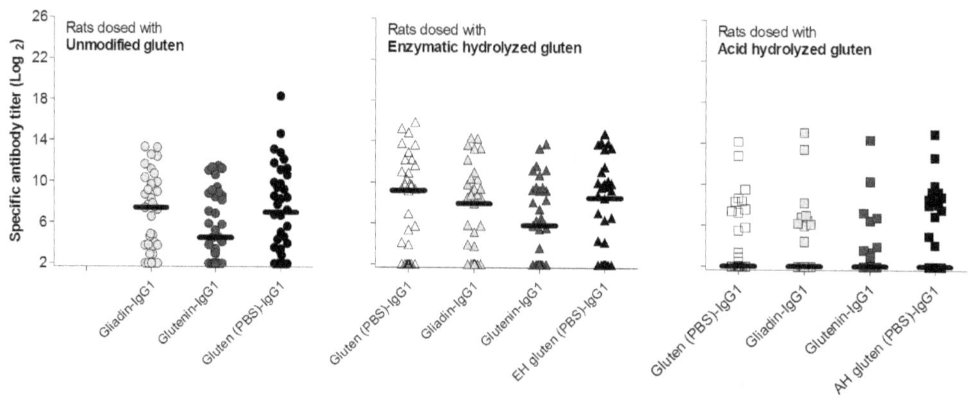


**Figure 5. Cross-reactivity of specific IgG1 in BN rats sensitized orally to gluten products.** Groups of female rats were dosed by gavage at day 1–35 with 0.2, 2 or 20 mg/rat of unmodified gluten or hydrolysis products thereof. Serum samples were obtained at sacrifice (day 42) and analyzed by direct ELISAs for specific IgG1 against unmodified gluten extracted in PBS (white symbols), gliadin fraction (light grey symbols), glutenin fraction (dark grey symbols) and the PBS extracted gluten product rats were sensitized to (black symbols). Each symbol represents an animal and horizontal bars indicate median values for groups (rats dosed with different doses of the same gluten product are shown as one group). Gluten (PBS): unmodified gluten proteins extracted by PBS, EH gluten (PBS): enzymatic hydrolyzed gluten proteins extracted by PBS, AH gluten (PBS): acid hydrolyzed gluten proteins extracted by PBS.

[29,32]. In contrast, the acid hydrolyzed gluten induced an IgG1 response with a stronger binding affinity to the antigen compared to the response induced by the two other antigens. Based on the results we cannot explain this difference, but only speculate that IgE-mediated degranulation is dependent on binding of IgE to two epitopes for cross-linking with the related structural limitations. Binding measured by inhibition ELISA is possible with binding between one antibody per epitope. The results of IgG inhibition ELISAs showed that acid hydrolyzed gluten has epitopes that are not present on either unmodified or enzymatic hydrolyzed gluten. This is in line with results presented by Denery-Papini *et al.* [33] who found that IgE from patients allergic to gluten deamidated by heating and acid treatment reacted strongest with an epitope where two or three glutamines were deamidated to glutamic acid. These data supports our finding, that acid hydrolysis of gluten induces formation of new epitopes.

Gourbeyre *et al.* [6] have studied the sensitizing capacity of acid hydrolyzed gluten proteins. In this study, mice were dosed four times i.p. with 10 μg of native or deamidated gliadin together with adjuvant ($Al(OH)_3$) on day 0, 10, 20 and 30. Results showed that deamidated gliadin induced a higher IgE response and higher histamine release than native gliadin. It was also shown that the native gliadin induced a more Th1 type (not allergic) response compared to deamidated gliadin. The mice used in the Gourbeyre experiments were most likely tolerant to gliadin because they were bred on a wheat-containing diet and only kept on a gluten-free diet from three weeks before experiments were initiated. Generally, rodents should be bred on an 'allergen-free' diet for at least three generations to obtain naïve animals with no immunological memory of the examined allergen [34–36]. Tolerance can be broken when immunizing i.p., but the functionality of the immune response will be influenced by the tolerance [29]. Because of the

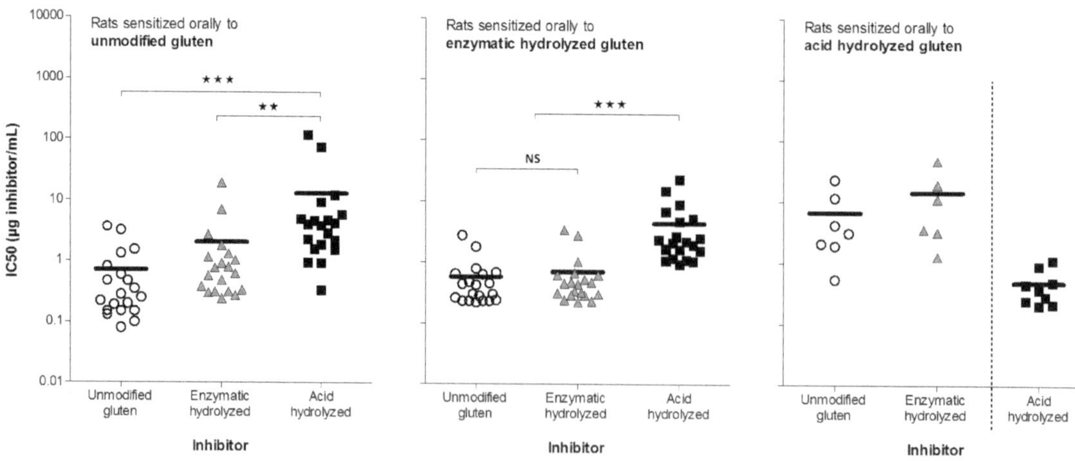


**Figure 6. Comparison of IgG1-binding capacity of sera from oral sensitization studies with gluten products.** Groups of rats were dosed by gavage at day 1–35 with 0.2, 2 and 20 mg/rat of unmodified gluten or hydrolysis products thereof. Sera from individual rats obtained at sacrifice were preincubated with tenfold dilutions of (50 pg/mL–50 μg/mL) of unmodified gluten (open circles), enzymatic hydrolyzed gluten (grey triangles) or acid hydrolyzed gluten (black squares) before measurement of IgG1-binding capacity by addition to ELISA plates coated with the gluten product used for sensitization. Only sera with an IgG1 titer >7 were analyzed by inhibition ELISA. Symbols represent triplicates of the same serum/inhibitor mix and bars represent IC50 median values for each group. Data were analyzed by non-parametrical analysis. Asterisks indicate statistically significant difference between groups; **: $p \leq 0.01$, ***: $p \leq 0.001$, NS: not significant.

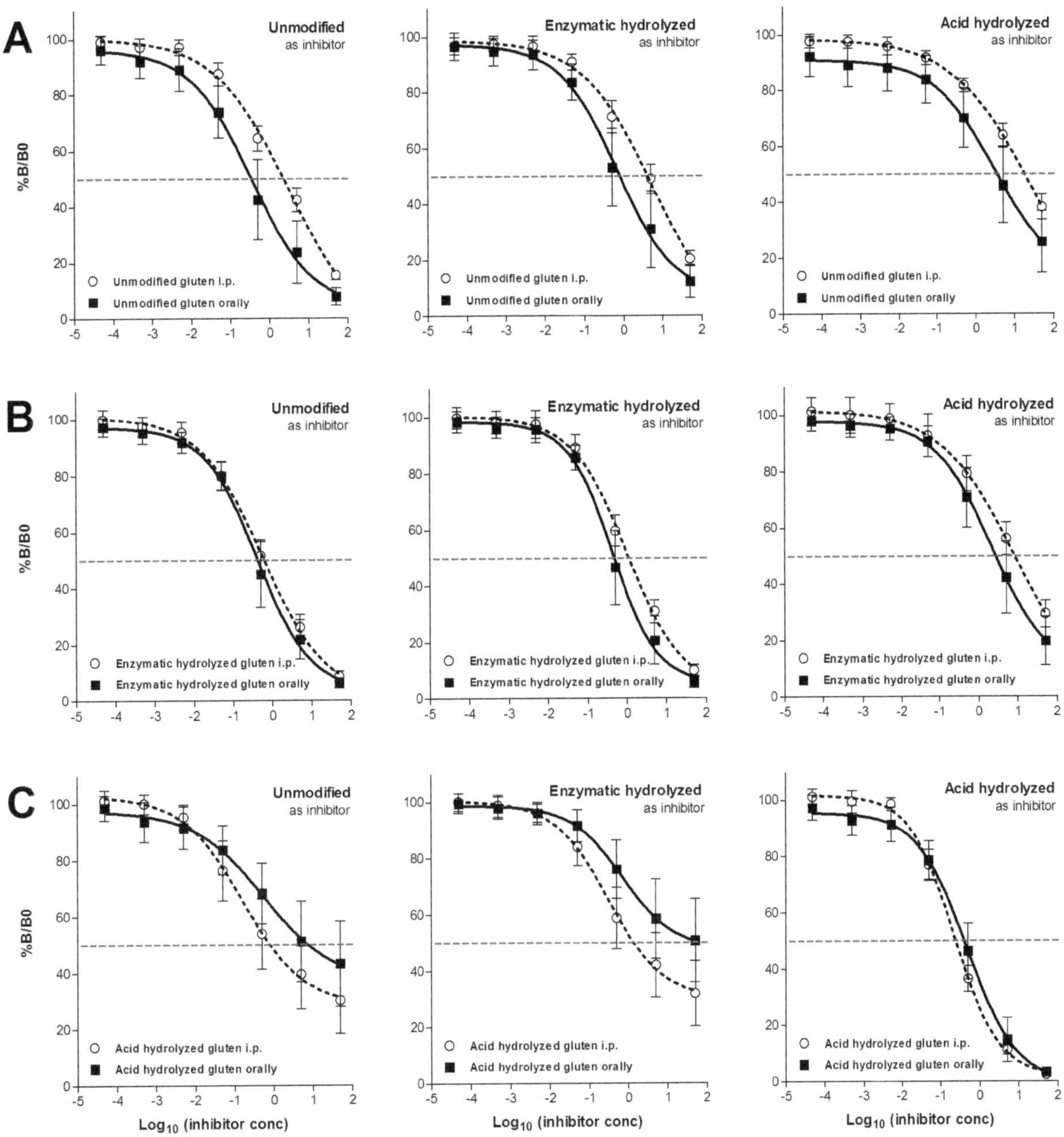


**Figure 7. Comparison of IgG1-binding capacity in rats immunized i.p. or dosed orally with unmodified (*A*), enzymatic hydrolyzed (*B*) or acid hydrolyzed (*C*) gluten.** Rats were immunized i.p. at day 0, 14 and 28 with 200 µg of gluten product per rat for i.p. studies or dosed by gavage at day 1–35 with different concentrations of gluten products for oral sensitization studies. Serum samples obtained at sacrifice were preincubated with tenfold dilutions (50 pg/mL–50 µg/mL) of unmodified, enzymatic hydrolyzed or acid hydrolyzed gluten before measurement of IgG1-binding capacity by addition to ELISA plates coated with the gluten product used for sensitization. Each graph represents mean IgG1 inhibition curves for groups of rats sensitized to the same gluten product by the i.p. (open symbols) or oral (closed symbols) route. Error bars represent ± SD.

likely tolerance and in light of our finding, that acid hydrolysis of gluten proteins creates new epitopes, comparing the results between sensitization to native and deamidated gliadin based on the Gourbeyre results becomes questionable. The underlying tolerance to the native gliadin epitopes will affect the response to gliadin epitopes but not to the deamidated gliadin epitopes. Thus, the results showing that native gliadin seems to induce a Th1 type response may well be explained by the underlying tolerance and not by differences in immunogenicity *per se*. This demonstrates that it is very important to know if the animals are tolerant or not to the protein under investigation or cross-reacting proteins and results must be interpreted carefully in the light of this.

Using the more physiologically relevant oral route we showed that in contrast to the i.p. results, enzymatic hydrolyzed gluten is a better sensitizer in the high dose group than both unmodified and acid hydrolyzed gluten whereas there is no difference in sensitizing capacity between the three proteins in the low and medium group. The IgE response was not high enough to allow testing for functionality in RBL assay.

Recently, Adachi *et al.* [37] showed that mice bred and kept on a standard rodent diet were sensitized to acid hydrolyzed gluten but not to unmodified gluten after transdermal exposure. Administration of gluten together with SDS increased sensitization capacity of gluten thus indicating that an increased solubility or transdermal permeability of gluten may be important for sensitization. In Japan, the use of facial soap containing acid hydrolyzed wheat has resulted in many cases of sensitization pointing to the skin or mucosal surfaces as the likely route of sensitization [20,21]. The most important risk factor for developing wheat allergy in persons using facial soap with acid hydrolyzed wheat was the number of soap bars used [38]. In contrast to the European experience, Japanese patients also developed allergy to wheat as WDEIA [20,21]. In an experiment, Strid *et al.* [39] were able to break oral tolerance in mice when the allergen (peanut) was dosed on tape stripped skin. It seems that in the Japanese patients, allergic skin reactions caused by the acid hydrolyzed wheat protein have contributed to break the oral tolerance to epitopes on native wheat.

We have used commercial enzyme and commercial acid hydrolyzed gluten. Although our results on acid hydrolyzed gluten are supported by others [6,21,24], generalization of results between different enzyme hydrolyzed products or different acid hydrolyzed products may be done with caution. The results by Denery-Papini *et al.* [24] show the degree of deamidation to be crucial for the changed allergenic properties of (acid) hydrolyzed gluten. Our results support these findings.

In conclusion, we have shown that in rats not tolerant to gluten i.p. immunization results in statistically significant difference in the specific IgE response with acid hydrolyzed > enzymatic hydrolyzed > unmodified gluten. This result is not reflected in the biological reactivity where unmodified = nzymatic hydrolyzed > acid hydrolyzed gluten. In the more physiological relevant oral route enzymatic hydrolyzed gluten gives a higher IgE response in the high dose group. There is no difference between the proteins in the low and medium dose groups. As we do not know the dose-response relationship in sensitization it is difficult to interpret the significance of the different dose-response relations in IgE response between unmodified and acid hydrolyzed gluten (no dose response) and enzymatic hydrolyzed gluten (clear dose response).

The results also support the existence of 'new' epitopes formed by deamidation on acid hydrolyzed gluten compared to unmodified and enzymatic hydrolyzed gluten. This makes it possible to be tolerant to gluten (be able to eat wheat products) and develop an allergic reaction to acid hydrolyzed gluten. There are several reports describing sensitization in wheat tolerant humans to hydrolyzed gluten via the skin [7,14,15,18–21]. It is not always very clear whether sensitization in wheat tolerant subjects was caused by acid hydrolyzed or enzyme hydrolyzed gluten because the type of hydrolysis is not always clearly specified. Our results indicate that sensitization to acid hydrolyzed gluten is possible in wheat tolerant subjects because of new epitopes. Likewise our results indicate that sensitization to enzyme hydrolyzed gluten is unlikely in wheat tolerant subjects because of the identical epitopes. As with other proteins, our results show that a sensitization route bypassing the gut is more efficient for all three gluten products tested. This difference is most striking for acid hydrolyzed gluten.

## Acknowledgments

The authors thank Anne Ørngren, Eva Ferdinansen, Elise Navntoft, Maja Danielsen, Eigil Frank and Kenneth Worm (National Food Institute, DTU, Denmark) for excellent technical assistance and Anne Blicher (Enzyme and Protein Chemistry, Department of Systems Biology, DTU, Denmark) for performing amino acid analysis.

## Author Contributions

Conceived and designed the experiments: SK CBM. Performed the experiments: SK NBA TFR. Analyzed the data: SK NBA TFR SJ CBM. Contributed reagents/materials/analysis tools: SJ. Contributed to the writing of the manuscript: SK NBA TFR SJ CBM.

## References

1. Belitz H-D, Grosch W, Schieberle P (2004) Food Chemistry, 3rd revised Edn, Berlin: Springer.
2. Shils ME, Shike M, Ross AC, Caballero B, Cousins RJ (2006) Modern nutrition in health and disease, 10th Edition, 50th anniversary Edition. Philadelphia: Lippincott Williams and Wilkins, Wolters Kluwer.
3. Wieser H (2007) Chemistry of gluten proteins. Food Microbiol 24: 115–119.
4. Tatham AS, Shewry PR (2008) Allergens in wheat and related cereals. Clin Exp Allergy 38: 1712–1726.
5. Mills ENC, Sancho AI, Rigby NM, Jenkins JA, Mackie AR (2009) Impact of food processing on the structural and allergenic properties of food allergens. Mol Nutr Food Res 53: 963–969.
6. Gourbeyre P, Denery-Papini S, Larré C, Gaudin JC, Brossard C, et al. (2012) Wheat gliadins modified by deamidation are more efficient than native gliadins in inducing a Th2 response in Balb/c mice experimentally sensitized to wheat allergens. Mol Nutr Food Res 56: 336–344.
7. Varjonen E, Petman L, Mäkinen-Kiljunen S (2000) Immediate contact allergy from hydrolyzed wheat in a cosmetic cream. Allergy 55: 294–296.
8. Finley JW, Hopkins DT (1985) Digestibility and amino acid availability in cereals and oilseeds. Minnesota, St. Paul: American Association of Cereal Chemists.
9. Mittag D, Niggemann B, Sander I, Reese I, Fiedler E-M, et al. (2004) Immunoglobulin E-reactivity of wheat-allergic subjects (baker's asthma, food allergy, wheat-dependent, exercise-induced anaphylaxis) to wheat protein fractions with different solubility and digestibility. Mol Nutr Food Res 48: 380–389.
10. Kumagai H, Suda A, Sakurai H, Kumagai H, Arai S, et al. (2007) Improvement of digestibility, reduction in allergenicity, and induction of oral tolerance of wheat gliadin by deamidation. Biosci Biotechnol Biochem 71: 977–985.
11. Lauriére M, Pecquet C, Boulenc E, Bouchez-Mahiout I, SnégaroffJ, et al. (2007) Genetic differences in omega-gliadins involved in two different immediate food hypersensitivities to wheat. Allergy 62: 890–896.
12. Palosuo K (2003) Update on wheat hypersensitivity. Curr Opin Allergy Clin Immunol 3: 205–209.
13. Leduc V, Moneret-Vautrin D-A, Guerin L, Morisset M, Kanny G (2003) Anaphylaxis to wheat isolates: immunochemical study of a case proved by means of double-blind, placebo-controlled food challenge. J Allergy Clin Immunol 111: 897–899.
14. Lauriére M, Pecquet C, Bouchez-Mahiout I, SnégaroffJ, Bayrou O, et al. (2006) Hydrolysed wheat proteins present in cosmetics can induce immediate hypersensitivities. Contact Dermatitis 54: 283–289.
15. Bouchez-Mahiout I, Pecquet C, Kerre S, SnégaroffJ, Raison-Peyron N, et al. (2010) High molecular weight entities in industrial wheat protein hydrolysates are immunoreactive with IgE from allergic patients. J Agric Food Chem 58: 4207–4215.
16. Pelkonen AS, Mäkinen-Kiljunen S, Hilvo S, Siltanen M, Mäkelä MJ (2011) Severe allergic reaction to gluten hydrolysate without reaction to wheat. Ann Allergy Asthma Immunol 106: 343–344.
17. Shinoda J, Inomata N, Chinuki Y, Morita E, Ikezawa Z (2012) Case of allergy due to hydrolyzed wheat proteins in commercial boiled pork. J Dermatol 39: 724–726.
18. Pecquet C, Bayrou O, Vigan M, Raison N, Lauriére M (2004) Hydrolysed wheat protein: a new allergen in cosmetics and food. Contact Dermatitis 50: 182–183.
19. Chinuki Y, Murata S, Morita E (2011) A case of wheat-dependent exercise-induced anaphylaxis sensitized with hydrolysed wheat protein in a soap. Contact Dermatitis 65: 55–57.
20. Fukutomi Y, Itagaki Y, Taniguchi M, Saito A, Yasueda H, et al. (2011) Rhinoconjunctival sensitization to hydrolysed wheat protein in facial soap can induce wheat-dependent excersise-induced anaphylaxis. J Allergy Clin Immunol 127: 531–533.
21. Nakamura R, Nakamura R, Sakai S, Adachi R, Hachisuka A, et al. (2013) Tissue transglutaminase generates deamidated epitopes on gluten, increasing reactivity with hydrolysed wheat protein-sensitized IgE. Allergy Clin Immunol 132: 1436–1438.
22. Battais F, Mothes T, Moneret-Vautrin DA, Pineau F, Kanny G, et al. (2005) Identification of IgE-binding epitopes on gliadins for patients with food allergy to wheat. Allergy 60: 815–821.
23. Pastorello EA, Farioli L, Conti A, Pravettoni V, Bonomi S, et al. (2007) Wheat IgE-mediated food allergy in European patients: α-amylase inhibitors, lipid

transfer proteins and low-molecular-weight glutenins. Int Arch Allergy Immunol 144: 10–22.
24. Denery-Papini S, Bodinier M, Pineau F, Triballeau S, Tranquet O, et al. (2011) Immunoglobulin-E-binding epitopes of wheat allergens in patients with food allergy to wheat and in mice experimentally sensitized to wheat proteins. Clin Exp Allergy 41: 1478–1492.
25. Bohle B (2004) T lymphocytes and food allergy. Mol Nutr Food Res 48: 424–433.
26. Berin MC, Sicherer S (2011) Food allergy: mechanisms and therapeutics. Curr Opin Immunol 23: 794–800.
27. Cianferoni A, Spergel JM (2009) Food allergy: review, classification and diagnosis. Allergol Int 58: 457–66.
28. Barkholt V, Jensen AL (1989) Amino acid analysis: determination of cysteine plus half-cysteine in proteins after hydrochloric acid hydrolysis with a disulfide compound as additive. Anal Biochem 177: 318–322.
29. Kroghsbo S, Bøgh KL, Rigby NM, Mills EN, Rogers A, et al. (2011) Sensitization with 7S globulins from peanut, hazelnut, soy or pea induces IgE with different biological activities which are modified by soy tolerance. Int Arch Allergy Immunol 155: 212–224.
30. Pilegaard K, Madsen C (2004) An oral Brown Norway rat model for food allergy: comparison of age, sex, dosing volume, and allergen preparation. Toxicology 196: 247–257.
31. Kroghsbo S, Madsen C, Poulsen M, Schrøder M, Kvist PH, et al. (2008) Immunotoxicological studies of genetically modified rice expressing PHA-E lectin or Bt toxin in Wistar rats. Toxicology 245: 24–34.
32. Shreffler WG, Beyer K, Chu TH, Burks AW, Sampson HA (2004) Microarray immunoassay: association of clinical history, in vitro IgE function, and heterogeneity of allergenic peanut epitopes. J Allergy Clin Immunol 13: 776–782.
33. Denery-Papini S, Bodinier M, Larré C, Brossard C, Pineau F, et al. (2012) Allergy to deamidated gluten in patients tolerant to wheat: specific epitopes linked to deamidation. Allergy 67: 1023–32.
34. Christensen HR, Brix S, Frøkiaer H (2004) Immune response in mice to ingested soya protein: antibody production, oral tolerance and maternal transfer. Br J Nutr 91: 725–732.
35. Brix S, Christensen HR, Barkholt V, Frøkiaer H (2005) Effect of maternal dietary cow's milk on the immune response to beta-lactoglobulin in the offspring: a four-generation study in mice. Int Arch Allergy Immunol 136: 250–257.
36. De Jonge JD, Knippels LM, Ezendam J, Odink J, Penninks AH, et al. (2007) The importance of dietary control in the development of a peanut allergy model in Brown Norway rats. Methods 41: 99–111.
37. Adachi R, Nakamura R, Sakai S, Fukutomi Y, Teshima R (2012) Sensitization to acid-hydrolyzed wheat protein by transdermal administration to BALB/c mice, and comparison with gluten. Allergy 67: 1392–1399.
38. Fukutomi Y, Kishikawa R, Sugiyama A, Minami T, Taniguchi M, et al. (2014) Akiyama K. Risk factors for the development of wheat allergy among individuals who have used a facial soap containing hydrolysed wheat protein: case-control study. EAACI Copenhagen Abstract 1617.
39. Strid J, Hourihane J, Kimber I, Callard R, Strobel S (2005) Epicutaneous exposure to peanut protein prevents oral tolerance and enhances allergic sensitization. Clin Exp Allergy 35: 757–766.

6

# IgE Reactivity of Blue Swimmer Crab (*Portunus pelagicus*) Tropomyosin, Por p 1, and Other Allergens; Cross-Reactivity with Black Tiger Prawn and Effects of Heating

**Jodie B. Abramovitch[1,2]ⓢ, Sandip Kamath[3]ⓢ, Nirupama Varese[1,2], Celia Zubrinich[3], Andreas L. Lopata[3], Robyn E. O'Hehir[1,2], Jennifer M. Rolland[1,2]***

**1** Department of Immunology, Monash University, Melbourne, Victoria, Australia, **2** Department of Allergy, Immunology and Respiratory Medicine, The Alfred Hospital and Monash University, Melbourne, Victoria, Australia, **3** School of Pharmacy and Molecular Science, James Cook University, Townsville, Queensland, Australia

## Abstract

Shellfish allergy is a major cause of food-induced anaphylaxis, but the allergens are not well characterized. This study examined the effects of heating on blue swimmer crab (*Portunus pelagicus*) allergens in comparison with those of black tiger prawn (*Penaeus monodon*) by testing reactivity with shellfish-allergic subjects' serum IgE. Cooked extracts of both species showed markedly increased IgE reactivity by ELISA and immunoblotting, and clinical relevance of IgE reactivity was confirmed by basophil activation tests. Inhibition IgE ELISA and immunoblotting demonstrated cross-reactivity between the crab and prawn extracts, predominantly due to tropomyosin, but crab-specific IgE-reactivity was also observed. The major blue swimmer crab allergen tropomyosin, Por p 1, was cloned and sequenced, showing strong homology with tropomyosin of other crustacean species but also sequence variation within known and predicted linear IgE epitopes. These findings will advance more reliable diagnosis and management of potentially severe food allergy due to crustaceans.

**Editor:** Srinivas Kaveri, Cordelier Research Center, INSERMU872-Team16, France

**Funding:** The Alfred Research Trusts. The funders had no role in study design, data collection and analysis, decision to publish, or preparation of the manuscript.

**Competing Interests:** The authors have declared that no competing interests exist.

* E-mail: jennifer.rolland@monash.edu

ⓢ These authors contributed equally to this work.

## Introduction

Shellfish play an important role in human nutrition and health, but can provoke serious IgE-mediated adverse reactions in susceptible individuals. Shellfish are a major cause of food-induced anaphylaxis [1–3]. Currently, there is no specific therapy for shellfish allergy, with only emergency treatment following accidental exposure [4]. Unlike most food allergies, allergy to shellfish is typically life-long and predominantly affects the adult population [5–6]. A major difficulty in managing shellfish allergy is the lack of reliable diagnostic assays due to limited knowledge of clinically relevant shellfish allergens.

The shellfish group includes crustaceans (phylum arthropoda including prawns, lobsters and crabs) and molluscs (phylum mollusca including oysters, mussels and squid). In the few studies characterizing shellfish allergens to date, including our own, one of the most frequently recognized (major) allergens of species in both shellfish phyla is the abundant muscle protein tropomyosin (TM) [7–11]. Other identified allergens are also derived from muscle tissue: myosin light-chain, arginine kinase, sarcoplasmic Ca-binding protein and troponin C [9,11–14]. However, only a few species have been studied to date, mostly shrimp and prawn, with few reports on crab allergens [11,15]. Prior to our current report, only one crab allergen, TM from the crucifix crab (*Charybdis feriatus*), was published in the International Union of Immunological Societies (IUIS) allergen database (http://www.allergen.org/index.php). Furthermore, there is little information on shellfish from the southern hemisphere or Asia-Pacific region. Patients frequently report clinical reactions to more than one shellfish species, but whether this is a result of multiple sensitivities or from IgE cross-reactivity between allergens of different shellfish species is unknown [5,16]. This information is vital for optimal management of shellfish allergy.

Adding complexity, there are reports of altered stability and allergenicity of food proteins after processing [17–19]. Most members of the TM allergen family are highly heat-stable [20–21]. However, there is a paucity of information on the effects of heating on allergens within whole shellfish extracts [22], with most studies testing heated purified allergens. Heating can enhance allergenicity through several mechanisms including protein denaturation and exposure of new epitopes, aggregation and chemical modification such as the Maillard reaction [23].

We report here the characterization of allergenicity of a commonly eaten crustacean species, the blue swimmer crab (*Portunus pelagicus*), and in particular the identification of the major allergen Por p 1. Evidence of cross-species IgE reactivity with another commonly consumed species, the black tiger prawn (*Penaeus monodon*), was sought and the effect of heating on allergens of both species and their cross-reactivity was assessed. Clinically relevant IgE reactivity to the shellfish extracts was assessed by a whole blood basophil activation assay.

## Materials and Methods

### Ethics Statement

Informed written consent was obtained from all subjects, with ethics approvals from the Alfred Hospital Research Ethics Committee (Project number 192/07) and the Monash University Human Ethics Committee (MUHREC CF08/0225).

### Study Population and Sera

Serum samples were obtained from twenty-four shellfish-allergic subjects (mean age 32±10.5 years; 13/24 female), seven non-atopic controls (mean age 40.3±12.3 years; 4/7 female) and one atopic non-shellfish-allergic subject (age 28 years, female). Allergic subjects were identified from the Alfred Hospital Allergy clinic seafood allergy database on the basis of clinical history of allergy to shellfish and positive shrimp-specific IgE (ImmunoCAP [Phadia Pty Ltd, Uppsala, Sweden] >0.35 $kU_A/L$) (Table 1). Of these subjects, 18/24 (75%) were also positive for crab-specific IgE. Eight control subjects were selected on the basis of no clinical history of shellfish allergy; seven were non-atopic, i.e. had a negative skin prick test response to a panel of common aeroallergens and one was atopic (Bahia grass pollen-sensitized).

### Preparation of Shellfish Extracts

Fresh blue swimmer crab (*Portunus pelagicus*) and black tiger prawn (*Penaeus monodon*) were purchased at Prahran market (Melbourne, Australia). For raw crab (RC) and raw prawn (RP) extracts, the outer shell was removed and muscle collected. Finely cut muscle was blended with PBS pH 7.2 and left overnight at 4°C with constant mixing. The crude extract was centrifuged at 13,000 rpm at 4°C for 20 minutes. Supernatant was collected and filter sterilized before storage at −80°C in aliquots. For cooked crab (CC) and cooked prawn (CP) extracts, the outer shell was kept during the heating process (20 minutes immersed in boiling PBS) before removal and extract preparation as above. The protein concentration of each extract was determined using the Bradford assay kit (Bio-Rad Laboratories, Hercules, CA) using bovine gamma globulin as a standard.

### Sodium Dodecyl Sulfate-Polyacrylamide Gel Electrophoresis (SDS-PAGE)

Proteins of shellfish extracts, 15 μg/lane, were separated by electrophoresis under reducing conditions using 4–12% Bis-Tris gels (NuPage, Carlsbad, CA). Pre-stained standards (1× See Blue

**Table 1.** Clinical features of subjects with allergy to shellfish.

| Subject | Age (yrs) | Sex | Total IgE (IU/mL) | Crab specific IgE ($kU_A/L$) | Shrimp specific IgE ($kU_A/L$) | Clinical presentation to shellfish | |
|---|---|---|---|---|---|---|---|
| | | | | | | Symptoms | Known shellfish species |
| 1 | 19 | F | 242 | 1.17 | 1.32 | As, R, U | Prawn |
| 2 | 45 | M | 136 | 2.77 | 4.54 | O | Prawn |
| 3 | 25 | M | 158 | 0.57 | 0.85 | R, U, An | Prawn |
| 4 | 28 | F | 238 | 6.05 | 5.93 | A, An | Prawn |
| 5 | 23 | M | 283 | 18.1 | 19.7 | As, R, O, U | Prawn |
| 6 | 22 | F | 3401 | 3.36 | 6.65 | As, R, U, An | Prawn |
| 7 | 47 | M | 822 | 2.72 | 5.37 | A, U | Prawn and all crustaceans |
| 8 | 24 | F | 1946 | 9.5 | 2.42 | R, A, O | Prawn, crab |
| 9 | 35 | F | 3887 | 2.94 | 3.33 | O, U | Shrimp |
| 10 | 39 | M | 192 | 0.06 | 1.22 | R, O | Raw prawn |
| 11 | 44 | M | 976 | 8.21 | 9.03 | R, O | Squid |
| 12 | 23 | M | 658 | 4.56 | 5.14 | R, U, An | Prawn |
| 13 | 26 | M | 127 | 0.15 | 1.65 | O | Prawn |
| 14 | 55 | F | 566 | 0.13 | 1.36 | As, R, O | Raw prawn, crab |
| 15 | 37 | M | 194 | 0.2 | 1.41 | R, O | Prawn, lobster, crayfish |
| 16 | 47 | F | 92 | 0.01 | 1.41 | R, O | Prawn, lobster |
| 17 | 32 | F | 28 | 8.42 | 9.82 | O, U | Shellfish |
| 18 | 30 | F | 748 | 0.63 | 2.84 | R, U | Crustaceans |
| 19 | 32 | M | 183 | 3.09 | 6.84 | An, O | Crustaceans |
| 20 | 22 | F | 164 | 0.01 | 1.43 | As, R | Prawn |
| 21 | 17 | F | 1550 | 58.3 | 60.8 | U, An | Prawn |
| 22 | 22 | M | 81 | 2.37 | 2.57 | As, R, U, An, A | Crustaceans |
| 23 | 44 | F | 167 | 22.9 | 32.4 | As, R, U | Prawn |
| 24 | 31 | F | 130 | 6.97 | 8.98 | O | Crab |

F: female, M: male. As: asthma, R: rhinitis, A: anaphylaxis, U: urticaria, An: angioedema, O: oral/facial symptoms.

Plus2, Invitrogen, Carlsbad, CA) were used as molecular weight (MW) markers. Proteins were resolved at 200 V for 35 minutes using an Xcell II mini-cell apparatus (Invitrogen) and the gel was stained with Coomassie brilliant blue.

## IgE ELISA and Inhibition IgE ELISA

Wells of a 96-well EIA/RIA plate (Costar, St. Louis, MO) were coated with 100 μL extract (RC, CC, RP or CP; 1 μg/mL in PBS, or PBS alone for 'no-antigen' control wells), and incubated overnight at 4°C. All of the following incubations were performed for 1 hour unless otherwise stated and the plate was washed 4 times in 0.05% Tween 20/PBS (PBS-T) between steps. Blocking was performed using 5% skim milk powder diluted in PBS-T. Serum, 100 μL diluted 1:10 in 1% skim milk powder/PBS-T, was added to wells and then incubated for 3 hours at room temperature with shaking (45 rpm). Rabbit anti-human IgE antibody (1:4000; Dako, Glostrup, Denmark) and goat anti-rabbit IgG-HRP (1:1000; Promega, Madison, WI) were added sequentially to wells and plates incubated at room temperature for 1 hour with gentle shaking. Plates were then washed 5 times in PBS-T, followed by 3 washes in PBS. IgE binding was detected using TMB (3,3′,5,5′-Tetramethylbenzidine) substrate (Invitrogen). After 5 minutes, the reaction was terminated using 1 M HCl and the absorbance (O.D.) at 450 nm measured by spectrophotometry (Thermo Fisher Scientific, Melbourne, Australia). Sera from seven non-atopic subjects were screened to determine the extent of non-specific binding. 'No-antigen', background values were subtracted from test sera data. Two standard deviations above the mean $O.D._{450\ nm}$ value for the non-atopic subject sera were used to determine the cut-off for positive IgE binding in shellfish-allergic subjects.

For inhibition ELISA experiments, individual subject sera were first titrated (1:10–1:1280) for IgE reactivity with CC or CP to determine the concentration at which the $O.D._{450\ nm}$ was ~1 and within the linear phase of the titration curve. Using this dilution, serum samples were incubated with an equal volume of shellfish extract (RC, CC, RP or CP at 0.16, 0.8, 4, 20 and 100 μg/mL), purified recombinant TM from black tiger prawn (rPen m 1.0101; Kamath et al., unpublished) or purified recombinant TM from blue swimmer crab (rPor p 1) (at 0.048, 0.24, 1.2, 6, and 30 μg/mL) for 1 hour at room temperature and then tested for reactivity with either CC or CP extracts. Percent inhibition was calculated using the following equation: percent inhibition = 100−[($O.D._{450\ nm}$ of serum with inhibitor/$O.D._{450\ nm}$ of serum without inhibitor) X100]. For comparison of inhibition by different extracts, the extract (inhibitor) concentration that caused 50% inhibition was calculated from dose-response curves. To assess non-specific inhibition by extracts, serum from a non-shellfish-allergic, atopic (Bahia grass pollen-sensitized) subject was incubated with the above inhibitors, and then tested for IgE reactivity with Bahia grass pollen extract in comparison with untreated serum.

## IgE Immunoblot and Inhibition IgE Immunoblot

Proteins of each of the four extracts (RC, CC, RP, CP) were separated by SDS-PAGE as above with 3 μg/well loaded into a 10 or 15-well 4–12% Bis-Tris gel (NuPage), or 60 μg protein loaded into a 6 cm 2D well 4–12% Bis-Tris gel (NuPage). Proteins were transferred to a nitrocellulose membrane (0.45 μm; Thermo Scientific, Rockford IL) using an Xcell II blotting apparatus (Invitrogen) at a constant voltage of 30 V for 1 hour. Successful transfer of protein was evaluated by Coomassie brilliant blue staining of the gel as above. The membrane was blocked using 5% skim milk powder/PBS-T for 1 hour at room temperature with gentle rocking. Subject serum (1:40 in 5% SMP/PBS-T) was then applied to the membrane using a Miniblotter apparatus (Immunetics, Boston, MA). To detect IgE binding, the immunoblot was incubated sequentially with rabbit anti-human IgE antibody (Dako; 1:15000) and goat anti-rabbit IgG-HRP conjugated antibody (Promega; 1:15000) each for 1 hour at room temperature with gentle horizontal shaking. Following incubation with chemiluminescent peroxidase substrate (Sigma-Aldrich, St. Louis, MO), proteins were visualized using enhanced chemiluminescence technique [24]. TM bands were identified in parallel immunoblots using a rat anti-TM monoclonal antibody (mAb; 1:6000; Abcam, Cambridge, UK) followed by rabbit anti-mouse IgG-peroxidase antibody (1:80000; Sigma-Aldrich) and development as above.

For inhibition IgE immunoblot experiments, serum samples (final concentration 1:40) were first incubated with whole crude extracts (RC, CC, RP or CP at 4, 20 and 100 μg/mL) or rPen m 1 (1.2 μg/mL) for 1 hour at room temperature and then tested for reactivity with the CC or CP extracts by immunoblotting as described above. In a separate experiment to directly compare rPor p 1 with rPen m 1, serum samples were incubated with rPor p 1 or rPen m 1 at 0.048, 0.24 and 1.2 μg/mL. A 'no inhibitor' control was also included. Complete protease inhibitor (Roche, Basel, Switzerland) was added to the diluent (one tablet in 50 mL of diluent) to prevent non-specific proteolytic degradation of IgE antibodies. Non-specific inhibition was assessed as described for the inhibition IgE ELISA above.

## Sequence Analysis of Blue Swimmer Crab Tropomyosin

A band corresponding to the predominant IgE-reactive 39 kDa protein was excised from the SDS gel for mass spectrometric analysis. The band was de-stained, reduced, alkylated and digested with trypsin as reported previously [9]. Digested protein was injected into a DIONEX Ultimate 3000 liquid chromatography system (Germering, Germany) coupled with a QSTAR XL hybrid quadrupole-quadrupole/time-of-flight tandem mass spectrometer (QqToF-MS/MS; Applied Biosystems/MDS Sciex, Foster City, USA). The resultant tandem spectra were searched using the Matrix Science (Mascot) search engine (precursor and product ion mass tolerance set at 0.1 Da). For cloning and full sequencing of the crab TM, total RNA was extracted from crab pincer muscles using Trizol reagent (Invitrogen) following the manufacturer's instructions. Single stranded cDNA was reverse transcribed from the RNA using RT-PCR with a cDNA synthesis kit (Bioline, Sydney, Australia). Oligo(dT) primers were used for the reverse transcription. Due to the high amino acid sequence identity of the N- and C-terminal regions of TM among crustacean species, the primers were designed based on the amino acid sequence of Rock lobster TM, previously determined by our group (Rock lobster, *Jasus lalandii*, Genbank accession number JX860677.1). The primer pair used was BSC-TM (F) 5′-GCCGGATCC-ATG-GACGCAATCAAGAAGAAGATGCAG-3′ and BSC-TM (R) 5′-GCGGAATTC-TTAGTAGCCAGACAGTTCG-3′. The PCR included one cycle of denaturation at 94°C for 2 minutes, 35 cycles at 94°C for 30 seconds, annealing at 55°C for 45 seconds and elongation at 72°C for 1 minute, and a final elongation step at 72°C for 7 minutes. The amplified full length open reading frame was cloned into the sequencing vector, pCR 2.1 (Invitrogen) using the BamH1 and EcoR1 restriction sites for cloning, and the open reading frame for TM sequenced (Macrogen Inc, Seoul, South Korea) to obtain the construct pCR2.1_TM.

## Expression and Purification of Recombinant Blue Swimmer Crab Tropomyosin

The open reading frame of TM was cross-cloned from the construct, pCR2.1_TM to the expression vector, pProEXHT-B using restriction sites for BamH1 and EcoR1 and ligation was performed using T4 DNA Ligase (Invitrogen, CA, USA). This expression plasmid construct was transformed into chemical-competent NM522 *E.coli* cells using heat-shock for 30 seconds, incubation in SOC medium at 37°C for 1 hour and grown overnight on Luria Bertani (LB) agar plates with 100 µg/mL ampicillin (Amresco, USA) at 37°C. Positive colonies were tested using PCR as described above and selected for protein expression.

For recombinant protein expression, 5 mL of fresh overnight culture from a single colony was used to initiate growth in 1 L LB broth containing 100 µg/mL ampicillin. Recombinant protein expression was induced using 0.6 mM isopropylthio-β-galactoside (Amresco, USA). After expression, the culture was centrifuged at 3500 g for 10 minutes to obtain the bacterial pellet and subsequently resuspended in extraction buffer (25 mM Tris-HCl, 300 mM NaCl, 1 mM imidazole, pH 8). Recombinant blue swimmer crab TM containing the 6xHis tag was extracted from the *E.coli* cells using a French-Pressure Cell, purified using nickel charged metal-chelate affinity chromatography (GE Healthcare, USA) following the manufacturer's instructions and stored at −80°C until further use. The protein concentration of the purified protein was determined by absorbance at 280 nm using a nanodrop spectrophotometer (ND-1000, NanoDrop Technologies Inc., Wilmington, Delaware, USA).

## Whole Blood Basophil Activation Test

Shellfish extracts were tested for basophil activation using our established methodology [25]. Briefly, heparinised peripheral blood samples (100 µL) from five shellfish-allergic subjects, a non-shellfish allergic atopic control and one non-atopic control were incubated with shellfish extracts (0.01–10 µg/ml) or rPen m 1 (0.001–1 µg/mL) for 20 minutes at 37°C and then basophil activation was assessed by flow cytometry by determining the percentage of viable (7-AAD negative), high IgE-positive cells expressing surface CD63. Anti-IgE antibody (cross-linking) and the bacterial peptide f-Met-Leu-Phe (fMLP) were used as positive controls (for IgE-dependent and -independent activation respectively), and stimulation buffer alone was used as a negative control.

## Statistical Analysis

The Wilcoxon matched-pairs signed rank test was used to compare overall serum IgE reactivity between shellfish extracts, and Spearman's correlation test was used to assess correlation between individual specific IgE levels against different extracts or using different assays. Analyses were performed using GraphPad Prism version 5.04 for Windows (GraphPad, San Diego, CA).

# Results

## SDS-PAGE Analysis of Shellfish Extracts

Analysis of raw and cooked shellfish extracts by SDS-PAGE and Coomassie brilliant blue staining (Figure 1) revealed an array of proteins ranging from ≈6 to 188 kDa. A prominent protein band at 37–39 kDa was seen in all extracts, consistent with TM (34–39 kDa). Other bands were observed at positions consistent with the known shellfish allergens arginine kinase (≈42 kDa), myosin light chain, sarcoplasmic calcium binding protein and troponin C (≈21 kDa), but several other bands were also apparent at positions that do not correspond to known shellfish allergens. Some differences could be seen between the RC and RP extracts, most notably the band at 69 kDa seen strongly in the RC but only weakly in the RP. In addition, there was only one major protein band in the TM region in RC, whilst there were two bands in RP. More pronounced differences were seen when raw and cooked extracts of both species were compared. For both CC and CP extracts, the higher MW proteins seen in the raw extracts were not present, most likely due to protein degradation during the cooking process. This is supported by the appearance of lower (<35 kDa) MW proteins only present in the cooked extracts. The actual sizes of these lower proteins differed between the crab and prawn extracts. The MW of the prominent TM region band for the prawn extract decreased from 39 kDa to 37 kDa on cooking, but did not change for the CC extract, remaining at 39 kDa.

## ELISA for Serum IgE Reactivity to Shellfish Extracts

Quantitation of serum IgE binding to the shellfish extracts by ELISA (Figure 2) showed that the cooked extracts have markedly higher IgE reactivity than the corresponding raw extracts. Median O.D. values for CC and RC were 0.86 and 0.41 respectively (CC vs RC $p<0.001$) and for CP and RP were 0.51 and 0.08 respectively (CP vs RP $p<0.001$). The RC extract was significantly more IgE reactive than RP ($p<0.001$), but there was no overall difference between the two cooked extracts. Of the 24 shellfish-allergic subjects, 5 (21%) had positive IgE reactivity to RC, 15 (63%) to CC (including 4 of the 5 RC positives), none to RP, and 11 (46%) to CP. A similar pattern of reactivity was observed between the CC and CP extracts. All subjects who were positive to CP were also positive to CC, and of those positive to CC but not to CP, reactivity was only weak (10, 14, 15 and 16). These same four subjects had a negative crab ImmunoCAP. Overall there was a significant correlation between IgE levels by ELISA for the CC and CP and the relevant ImmunoCAP values ($p<0.01$), but not for the raw extracts. However, several subjects showed a lack of concordance of positive or negative result for ELISA with cooked extracts and ImmunoCAP.

## IgE Immunoblotting of Shellfish Extracts

Sera from 12 subjects with IgE positivity to RC and/or CC by ELISA, and where sufficient serum was available, were used for immunoblotting to visualize IgE-reactive proteins in the shellfish extracts (Figure 3). Immunoblotting showed markedly increased IgE binding to cooked compared with raw extracts, in terms of number of proteins recognized and intensity of binding. In

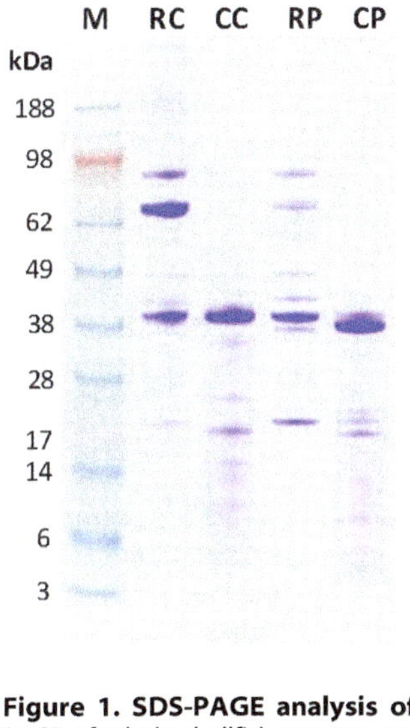


**Figure 1. SDS-PAGE analysis of shellfish extracts.** 4–12% SDS-PAGE of whole shellfish extracts stained with Coomassie brilliant blue. M, MW markers; RC, raw blue swimmer crab; CC, cooked blue swimmer crab; RP, raw black tiger prawn; CP, cooked black tiger prawn.

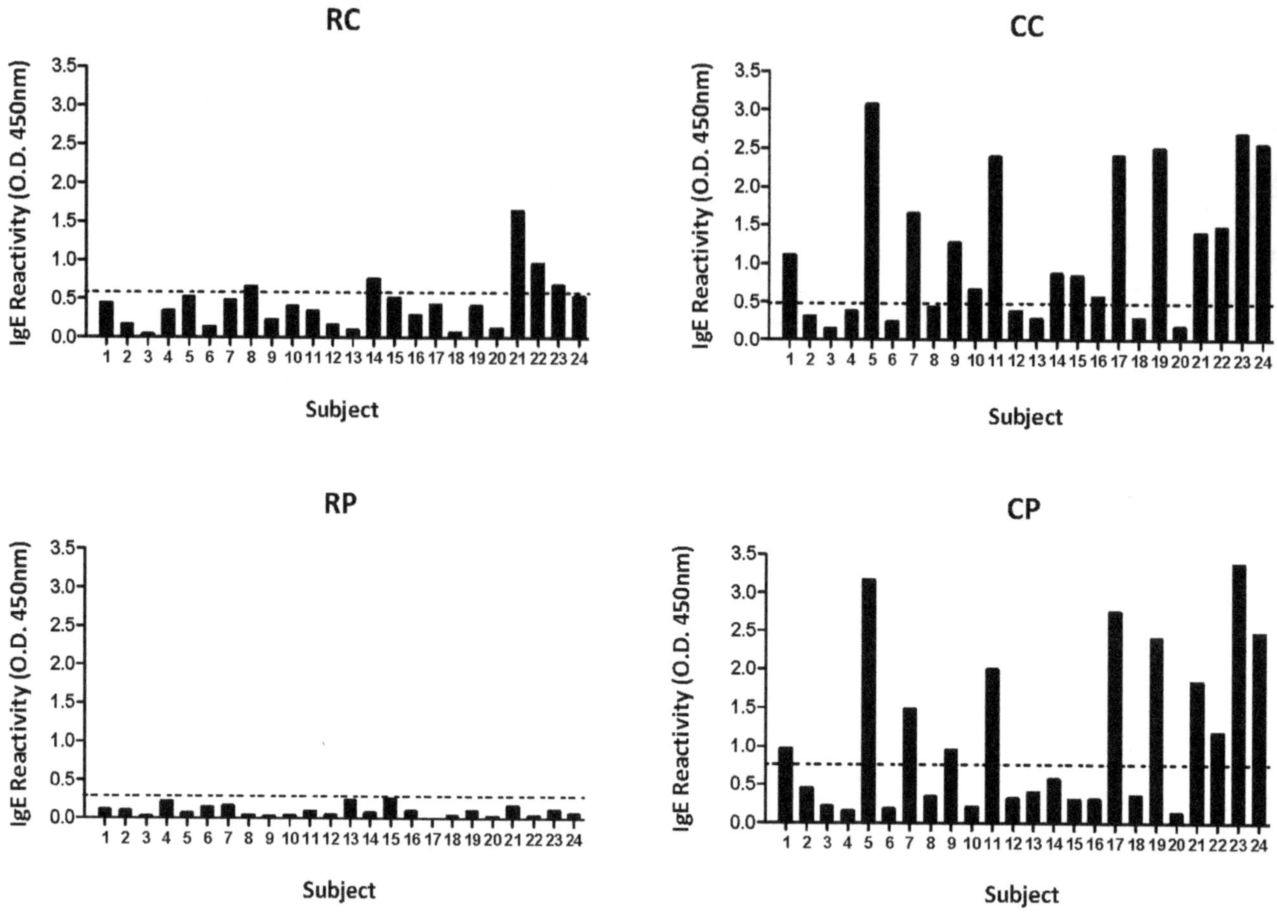


**Figure 2. ELISA for serum IgE reactivity to shellfish extracts.** ELISA for serum IgE reactivity to raw blue swimmer crab (RC), cooked blue swimmer crab (CC), raw black tiger prawn (RP) and cooked black tiger prawn (CP) for 24 shellfish-allergic subjects. The cut-off of two standard deviations above mean reactivity of 7 non-atopic subjects to each of the extracts is indicated by the dotted line (0.56 for RC, 0.49 for CC, 0.29 for RP and 0.75 for CP).

particular there was increased IgE binding to proteins within the TM region (37–39 kDa); 9 (75%) subjects showed IgE binding within this region for CC (7 in RC) and 7 (58%) subjects for CP (3 in RP). The identity of the protein(s) within this region was confirmed as TM using an anti-TM mAb (data not shown). An increase in IgE-reactive lower MW proteins (<39 kDa) was observed in the CC extract and to a lesser extent in the CP extract. A protein of ≈62 kDa was recognized by 5/12 (42%) subjects in the RP extract but showed little or no reactivity in the RC or cooked extracts. For both the raw and cooked extracts, IgE-reactive proteins were observed at 40 kDa and 20–28 kDa that could correspond to other documented allergens i.e. arginine kinase, and sarcoplasmic calcium binding protein, myosin light chain and troponin C, respectively.

## Sequence Analysis of Blue Swimmer Crab Tropomyosin

Following analysis of allergenic proteins using IgE immunoblot, the highly IgE-reactive 39 kDa protein of the blue swimmer crab was identified as TM by peptide mass fingerprinting analysis (Table 2). The blue swimmer crab TM was subsequently cloned and the complete sequence derived from cDNA and published in Genbank under accession number JX874982.1 (Figure 4). Based on the allergen sequence and patient serum IgE reactivity (see below), this allergen has been designated Por p 1.0101 by the IUIS allergen nomenclature subcommittee (http://www.allergen.org/index.php). The most similar TMs were from the American lobster (*Homarus americanus*) and the black tiger prawn (*Penaeus monodon*) which both showed 98% sequence identity. Sequence identity with other *Portunus* species TM, and the only crab TM, Cha f 1, listed within the IUIS allergen database was 92%. There were no amino acid differences between relevant regions in the blue swimmer crab TM and published linear IgE epitopes described for *Penaeus aztecus* (Pen a 1) [26–27] and *Penaeus monodon* (Pen m 1) [28] TMs, except for the last epitope (amino acid 266 to 280) where two amino acid substitutions were identified. Another region (amino acid 43 to 56) of known and predicted IgE epitope specificity for other crustacean species showed several amino acid differences for the blue swimmer crab (Figure 4).

## IgE Reactivity of Recombinant Blue Swimmer Crab Tropomyosin, rPor p 1

Recombinant blue swimmer crab TM, rPor p 1, was successfully expressed and purified with approximately 95% purity. Coomassie brilliant blue staining of SDS-PAGE of rPor p 1 under denaturing conditions showed a single band with a MW of approximately 41 kDa (Figure 5A). The higher MW of the rPor p 1 band compared to that for the natural blue swimmer crab TM in whole extract is due to the attached linker chain and 6-histidine

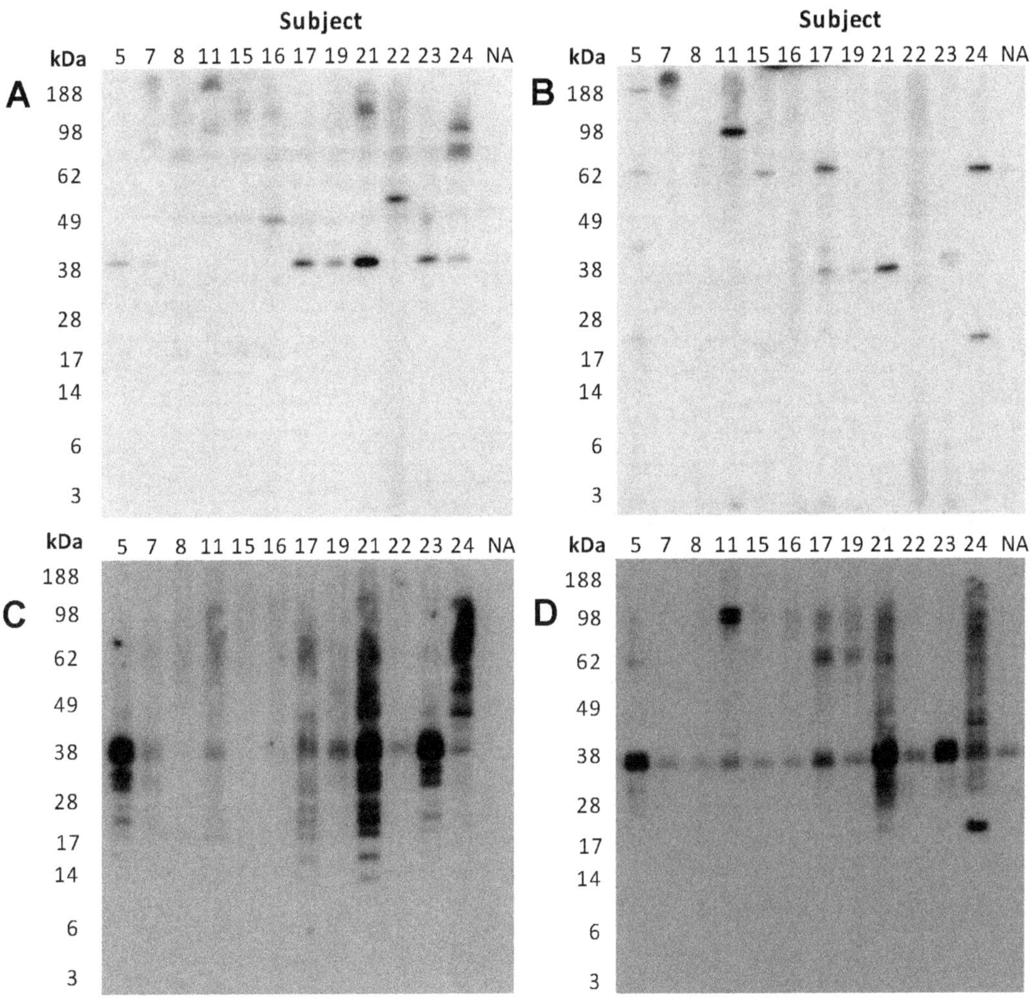


**Figure 3. Immunoblotting for serum IgE reactivity against shellfish extracts.** Sera from 12 shellfish-allergic subjects (5–24) and one non-atopic (NA) subject were tested for IgE reactivity to shellfish extract proteins separated by 4–12% SDS-PAGE. **A.** RC, **B.** RP, **C.** CC, **D.** CP.

tag. When an immunoblot was probed with sera from shellfish-allergic patients, rPor p 1 was shown to be highly IgE reactive (Figure 5B). There was strong IgE binding to the 41 kDa band for 75% of the patient sera tested, but no reactivity by a control non-atopic donor serum. Sera that showed IgE reactivity with rPor p 1 were those that reacted with the prominent TM band in the IgE immunoblots of the whole blue swimmer crab extract (Figure 3). Additional IgE-reactive higher MW bands observed in the rPor p 1 preparation are most likely multimers of rPor p 1 since their reactivity paralleled that for the major 41 kDa band.

## Basophil Activation Test

To assess biologically relevant shellfish allergen-specific IgE antibody reactivity, the ability of the different extracts to activate basophils from five shellfish-allergic subjects (7, 8, 19, 22, 24) was analyzed by flow cytometry. Activated basophils were identified by high IgE expression and up-regulation of surface CD63 (Figure 6A, B). No non-allergen specific activation of basophils or toxicity was caused by the different shellfish extracts, as determined by incubating extracts with the basophils from a non-shellfish allergic, atopic subject and a non-atopic subject (data not shown).

Dose-dependent basophil activation to the crab and prawn extracts was observed, with a range of sensitivities for the subjects, consistent with their different crab- and prawn-specific IgE reactivities by ImmunoCAP and our ELISA and immunoblotting assays (Figure 6C). When subject basophil sensitivities were compared by examining the extract concentration required for 50% maximal stimulation, three subjects (19, 22, 24) showed markedly higher basophil activation by the cooked extracts than the raw extracts, with little difference between the two crustacean species. Subjects 7 and 8 showed lower basophil activation with similar sensitivity to the four extracts. rPen m 1 was shown to induce strong basophil activation in those subjects with high reactivity to the whole extracts (Figure 6D).

## Inhibition IgE ELISA

Inhibition ELISA was used to quantitate the degree of IgE cross-reactivity between the two shellfish species and the effects of cooking. No non-specific inhibition of IgE reactivity by the shellfish extracts, rPen m 1 or rPor p 1 was evident using serum IgE from a Bahia grass pollen-sensitized control subject and Bahia grass pollen extract (data not shown). Using shellfish-allergic subjects, both cooked extracts showed greater inhibition of IgE binding than the corresponding raw extracts (Table 3). For most subjects, the lowest concentration of cooked extract (0.16 μg/mL) resulted in >50% inhibition of IgE binding to both CC and CP.

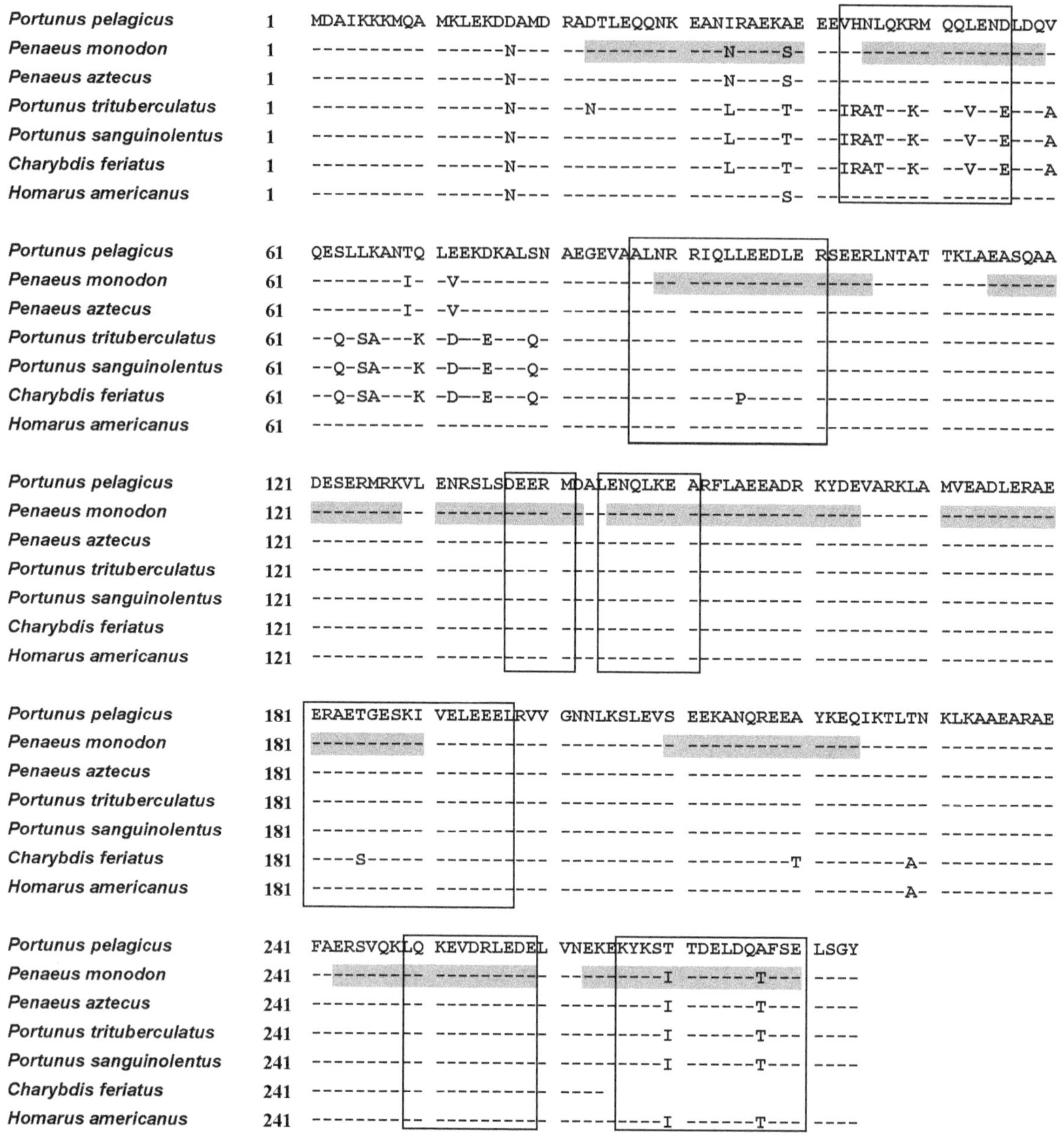


**Figure 4. Tropomyosin sequence alignment.** Alignment of TM sequences with *Portunus pelagicus* (blue swimmer crab) TM, Por p 1 (Genbank accession number JX874982.1), as reference using NCBI Protein BLAST. Species include *Penaeus monodon* (NCBI protein database accession number: A1KYZ2.1), *Portunus trituberculatus* (ABL89183.1), *Portunus sanguinolentus* (ABS12234.1), *Charybdis feriatus* (Q9N2R3.1) and *Homarus americanus* (AAC48288.1). Sequences that correlate with known linear epitopes of *Penaeus aztecus* TM (Pen a 1) [26–27] are boxed. Predicted linear IgE epitopes based on studies with *Penaeus monodon* TM (Pen m 1) [28] are shaded grey.

RC was a more efficient inhibitor of IgE binding to the cooked extracts than RP. Both rPen m 1 and rPor p 1 inhibited >50% serum IgE reactivity to CC and CP at the lowest concentration (0.048 µg/mL) for all except three subjects (11, 19, 24). In these cases, higher concentrations were required, but these were still well below the maximum tested except for serum 11. It was noted that this serum showed marked IgE reactivity to allergens other than TM by immunoblotting.

## Inhibition IgE Immunoblotting

Inhibition immunoblotting was used to examine the proteins responsible for cross-reactivity of IgE antibodies between the different extracts, and in particular whether there were potentially unique allergens within the blue swimmer crab. Again, non-specific inhibition by the extracts was excluded by testing for inhibition of the binding of serum IgE from a Bahia grass pollen-allergic control subject to Bahia grass pollen extract (data not shown). Four shellfish-allergic subjects (5, 19, 21 and 24) with IgE reactivity to TM (39 kDa) were selected for this assay. For all subjects, rPen m 1 markedly inhibited IgE binding to the TM band, further confirming the identity of this protein as TM (Figure 7). The CC and CP extracts also strongly inhibited IgE binding to TM in both species. However, the raw extracts inhibited IgE binding to TM only at higher concentrations, with

**Table 2.** List of generated peptides of blue swimmer crab tropomyosin using trypsin and mass spectroscopy analysis.

| Residue numbers * | Peptide sequence |
|---|---|
| 77–90 | ALQNAEGEVAALNR |
| 92–101 | IQLLEEDLER |
| 141–149 | MDALENQLK |
| 168–178 | KLAMVEADLER |
| 190–198 | IVELEEELR |
| 252–264 | EVDRLEDELVNEK |

*Residue numbers corresponding to the full sequence of blue swimmer crab tropomyosin, Por p 1 (Genbank accession number JX874982).

RC showing greater inhibition than RP. Similarly, reactivity with the low MW proteins in both CC and CP was inhibited by the cooked extracts and RC, but poorly with RP. rPen m 1 could also inhibit the reactivity to the low MW bands, suggesting that they were predominantly breakdown products of TM.

When the IgE inhibitory reactivity of rPor p 1 and rPen m 1 were compared over a concentration range using two shellfish-allergic patient sera, rPor p 1 showed slightly greater inhibition of IgE reactivity with the TM band in CC than rPen m 1, and rPen m 1 inhibited reactivity with CP TM slightly better than rPor p 1(Figure 8). Neither recombinant TM preparation inhibited IgE reactivity with the higher MW bands.

## Discussion

Shellfish allergy is a serious and increasing health issue, with current limitations in accurate diagnosis and management due to lack of information regarding clinically relevant allergens and IgE cross-reactivity between shellfish species. Crustaceans, especially crabs and prawns, are a common cause of shellfish allergy worldwide. This study examined the IgE-reactive components of a commonly eaten crustacean species, the blue swimmer crab, compared with those of a well characterized species, the black tiger prawn. In particular, the effects of heating on IgE reactivity and cross-reactivity of the crab allergens were investigated. In addition, the major TM allergen of the blue swimmer crab was cloned and sequenced and its IgE reactivity characterized.

When shellfish-allergic subject serum IgE reactivity with whole extracts was compared, the raw crab extract showed greater IgE reactivity compared with the raw prawn extract by both ELISA and immunoblotting. Whether this was due to inherent differences between the proteins of the blue swimmer crab and black tiger prawn, or to differences in sensitizing species or route of sensitization is not clear. We and others have shown previously that inhalation during commercial processing can result in sensitization to seafood [29–32]. In the present study, although some subjects identified food handling as a cause of adverse reaction, this route could not be distinguished in all subjects and the majority reported ingestion-related allergic episodes. More strikingly, we found that cooked extracts were more IgE reactive than raw for both species. This may be due to the more common ingestion of cooked crab and prawn or to chemical modification of the crustacean proteins on heating as discussed below. That the IgE reactivity of the crustacean extracts observed in our study was clinically relevant was demonstrated by the functional, basophil activation test, again confirming higher allergenicity of the cooked extracts.

IgE immunoblotting studies were performed to examine individual IgE-reactive proteins. As for other crustacean species, TM is a major allergen of the blue swimmer crab. Over 50% of shellfish-allergic subjects showed IgE-reactivity to proteins corre-

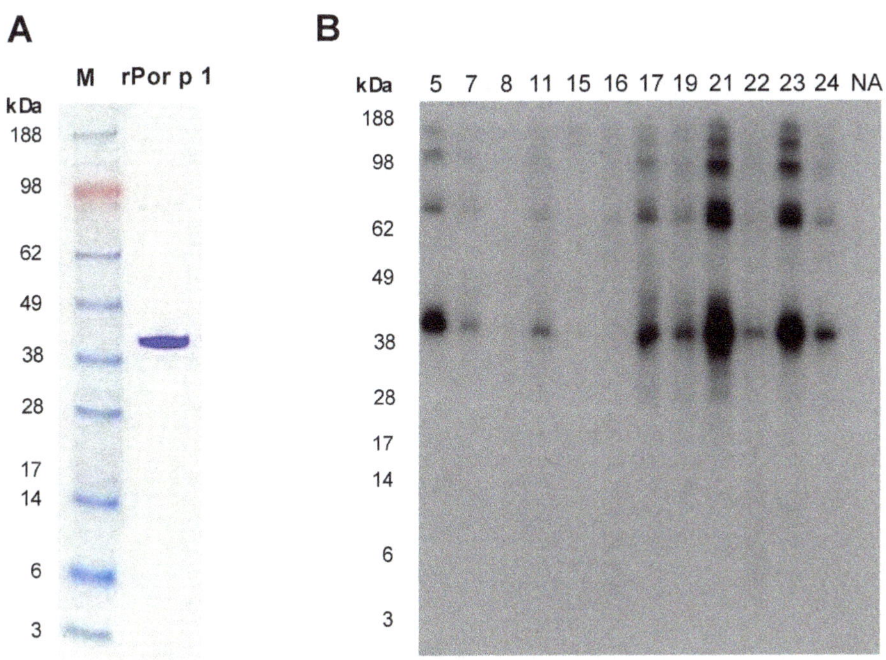


**Figure 5. Characterization of recombinant blue swimmer crab tropomyosin, rPor p 1. A.** 4–12% SDS-PAGE of recombinant blue swimmer crab TM, rPor p 1 stained with Coomassie brilliant blue. M, MW markers. **B.** Sera from 12 shellfish-allergic subjects (5–24) and one non-atopic (NA) subject were tested for IgE reactivity to rPor p 1 using direct IgE immunoblotting.

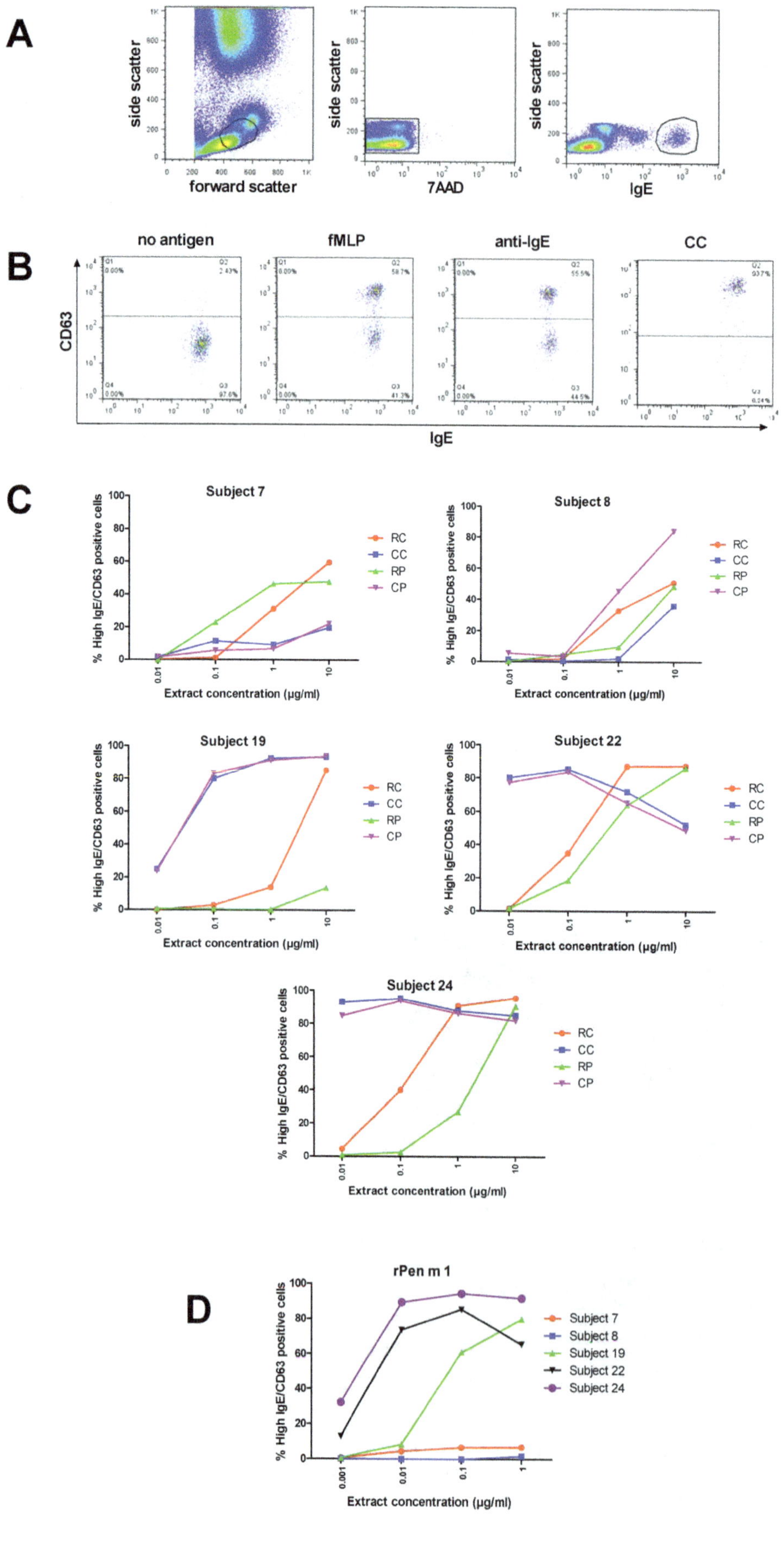
A
side scatter
forward scatter
side scatter
7AAD
side scatter
IgE
B
no antigen
fMLP
anti-IgE
CC
CD63
IgE
C
Subject 7
Subject 8
Subject 19
Subject 22
Subject 24
% High IgE/CD63 positive cells
Extract concentration (μg/ml)
RC
CC
RP
CP
D
rPen m 1
% High IgE/CD63 positive cells
Extract concentration (μg/ml)
Subject 7
Subject 8
Subject 19
Subject 22
Subject 24

**Figure 6. *In vitro* basophil activation by shellfish extracts and rPen m 1. A.** Representative dot plots showing gating of viable basophils (7AAD$^{-}$, high IgE positive). **B.** Representative dot plots (subject 19) showing analysis of activated basophils (up-regulation of cell surface CD63) for negative and positive controls, and CC (10 μg/mL). **C.** Dose-dependent activation of basophils from shellfish-allergic subjects (7, 8, 19, 22, 24) by shellfish extracts. **D.** Dose-dependent activation of basophils from shellfish-allergic subjects (7, 8, 19, 22, 24) by rPen m 1.

sponding to TM in both raw and cooked crab extracts and TM identity was confirmed by TM-specific mAb reactivity and peptide mass fingerprinting of the highly IgE-reactive 39 kDa protein. We report here for the first time the cloning and full sequence analysis of the *Portunus pelagicus* TM, Por p 1. This revealed strong homology of the blue swimmer crab TM with other crustacean TMs, but regions of amino acid sequence difference at sites of known and predicted linear IgE epitopes support the need for crustacean species-specific diagnostic reagents. The purified rPor p 1 showed high IgE reactivity by direct immunoblotting, but in agreement with sequence differences, IgE inhibition immunoblotting showed differential reactivity of rPor p 1 and rPen m 1. When compared for inhibition of IgE reactivity with TM in shellfish extracts, rPor p 1 could better inhibit reactivity with the cooked blue swimmer crab TM and rPen m 1 was the better inhibitor of reactivity with black tiger prawn TM. Several other allergenic proteins of the blue swimmer crab were recognized at lower frequency. For some subjects, these proteins were recognized in the absence of TM reactivity. Testing of a larger subject cohort is required to assess the clinical importance and cross-reactivity of these proteins and hence define an appropriate panel of defined allergens for refined diagnostic assays.

In view of potential food matrix-associated effects on the outcome of heating of allergens [33], we chose to examine heating of whole extracts rather than purified allergens. For both the crab and prawn species studied, ELISA and immunoblotting showed markedly increased IgE reactivity of cooked extracts compared with raw. In particular, IgE immunoblotting demonstrated increased IgE-reactivity of TM within the cooked extracts. Although all sera including the non-atopic serum bound weakly to the TM band in the CP extract suggesting non-specific binding due to glycosylation for example, if this reactivity was used as a background reference, stronger binding of some shellfish-allergic sera was observed. The higher non-specific reactivity of the CP extract in this assay is consistent with the higher cut-off value for the IgE ELISA for this extract. Several higher MW bands with smearing, also typically a feature of glycosylated proteins, were observed in the cooked extracts. Some of these may represent heat-modified TM multimers. In addition, a range of highly IgE-reactive lower MW proteins was observed following heating, presumably largely TM fragments since this was especially notable for sera that reacted with the single TM band in the raw extracts. Investigation of the mechanisms responsible for the increase in allergenicity of TM and other allergens within the whole shellfish extracts following cooking is warranted as most shellfish is heat processed before consumption. Potential mechanisms include denaturation of protein with exposure of neo-epitopes and the Maillard reaction. In this heat-dependent reaction, sugars, both endogenous and exogenous, are non-enzymatically attached at different locations on the protein molecule generating advanced glycation end products [23,34]. The Maillard reaction has not been well explored in the context of shellfish allergy, although found to play a role in the IgE reactivity of other allergens, particularly peanut allergens [35–36]. Our findings support the inclusion of thermally-processed whole extract as well as defined allergen preparations in commercial diagnostic tests for shellfish allergy.

Cross-reactivity between crustacean species is essential to understand in order for shellfish-allergic subjects to receive the best clinical advice on food avoidance. There are limited studies of crustacean cross-reactivity to date, often with small subject cohorts [15,37–39]. Our study showed that IgE cross-reactivity between the blue swimmer crab and black tiger prawn was high, especially between the cooked extracts. Cross-reactivity between the cooked extracts was symmetric as both were able to effectively inhibit IgE binding to each other to a similar extent [40]. This means that the sensitizing species is unable to be determined in most cases without accurate clinical history. As shown by inhibition ELISA, except for serum 11, the capacity of cooked whole extracts to inhibit IgE binding to the cooked crab extract was similar to that for rPor p 1, consistent with allergenicity in the cooked blue swimmer crab being largely due to cross-reactive TM. TM has previously been documented as the major allergen of the black tiger prawn [9]. Our sequence analysis of the blue swimmer crab TM, Por p 1, and alignment with black tiger prawn TM, Pen m 1, provides a molecular basis for the high IgE cross-reactivity observed between these species in our study. The different reactivity seen with serum

**Table 3.** Inhibitor concentration (μg/mL) required for 50% inhibition of IgE binding to cooked blue swimmer crab (CC) extract or cooked black tiger prawn (CP) extract.

| | Coating antigen: CC | | | | | | Coating antigen: CP | | | | | |
|---|---|---|---|---|---|---|---|---|---|---|---|---|
| | Inhibitor | | | | | | Inhibitor | | | | | |
| Subject | RC | CC | RP | CP | rPen m 1 | rPor p 1 | RC | CC | RP | CP | rPen m 1 | rPor p 1 |
| 5 | 12 | <0.16 | >100 | <0.16 | <0.05 | <0.05 | 60 | 0.64 | >100 | <0.16 | <0.05 | <0.05 |
| 11 | 2.4 | <0.16 | 16 | <0.16 | 1.2 | >30 | 18 | <0.16 | 20 | <0.16 | 1.2 | 0.3 |
| 17 | 1.3 | <0.16 | 36 | <0.16 | <0.05 | <0.05 | 1.6 | <0.16 | 47 | <0.16 | <0.05 | <0.05 |
| 19 | 0.8 | <0.16 | 60 | <0.16 | <0.05 | <0.05 | 2.4 | <0.16 | 47 | <0.16 | <0.05 | 0.12 |
| 21 | 1.3 | <0.16 | 47 | <0.16 | <0.05 | <0.05 | 2.9 | <0.16 | 47 | <0.16 | <0.05 | <0.05 |
| 23 | 4 | <0.16 | 87 | <0.16 | <0.05 | <0.05 | 20 | <0.16 | 90 | <0.16 | <0.05 | <0.05 |
| 24 | >100 | 14 | 84 | 20 | 0.14 | <0.05 | 2.1 | <0.16 | 20 | <0.16 | <0.05 | <0.05 |

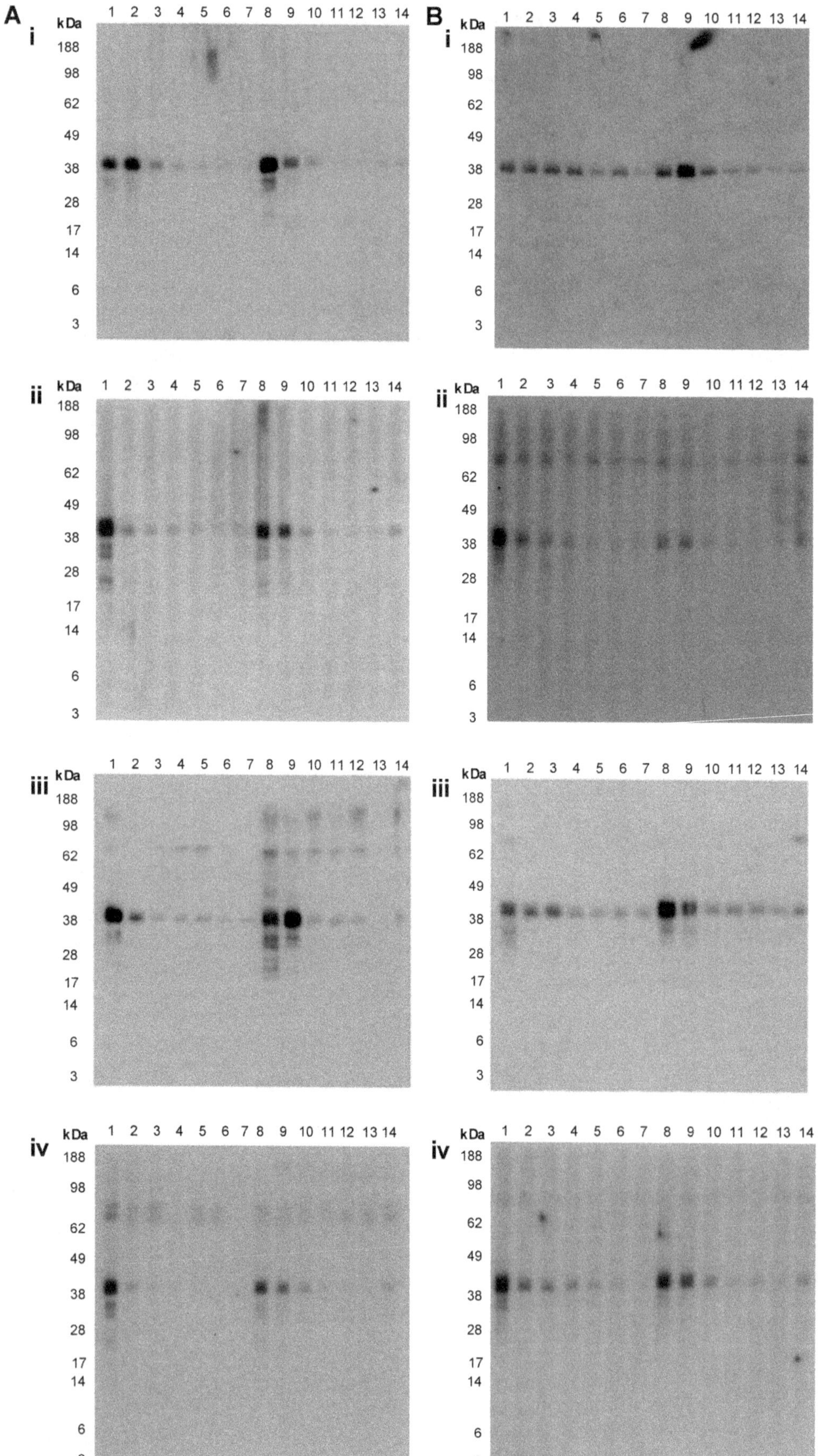
A
B
i
ii
iii
iv
kDa
1 2 3 4 5 6 7 8 9 10 11 12 13 14
188
98
62
49
38
28
17
14
6
3

**Figure 7. Inhibition IgE immunoblotting with shellfish extracts.** Inhibition of serum IgE reactivity to CC (A) and CP (B) by shellfish extracts for subjects 5 (i), 19 (ii), 21 (iii) and 24 (iv). Lanes 1: No inhibitor, 2: 4 μg/ml RC, 3: 20 μg/ml RC, 4: 100 μg/ml RC, 5: 4 μg/ml CC, 6: 20 μg/ml CC, 7: 100 μg/ml CC, 8: 4 μg/ml RP, 9: 20 μg/ml RP, 10: 100 μg/ml RP, 11: 4 μg/ml CP, 12: 20 μg/ml CP, 13: 100 μg/ml CP, 14: 1.2 μg/ml rPen m 1.

11 is consistent with its stronger reactivity with a higher MW band than with TM by IgE immunoblotting.

Screening of shellfish-allergic subjects by IgE ELISA against raw and cooked extracts gave insight into whether the current diagnostic ImmunoCAP for crab is relevant in a southern hemisphere clinical setting. Although a double-blind placebo-controlled food challenge can confirm diagnosis of food allergy, this procedure has a high risk of anaphylaxis for adults with shellfish allergy who may have other comorbidities, and is not routinely performed in our hospital [41]. Similarly, skin prick testing of these patients is also not routine practice. For these reasons, in this study only ImmunoCAP data together with a careful clinical history were collected. In most cases, subjects were unable to identify clearly which individual crustacean species had provoked their clinical reaction. However, for the three subjects who did identify crab as an offending species (Table 1), only two of these had positive ImmunoCAP scores for crab-specific IgE. The third subject (14) had a negative crab ImmunoCAP but tested positive for both raw and cooked blue swimmer crab in our IgE ELISA. We found a significant correlation between the cooked, but not raw, crustacean extract ELISA results and ImmunoCAP scores, but in addition to the subject mentioned above, a small number of subjects with a negative crab ImmunoCAP result showed IgE reactivity to the crab extracts in both the IgE ELISA and immunoblot. This finding suggests either greater sensitivity of our assays, and/or lack of appropriate crab species or preparation method in the ImmunoCAP allergen preparation (*Cancer pagurus* or brown crab, a northern hemisphere species). All subjects with IgE-reactivity to crab or prawn TM by immunoblot had moderate to high levels of allergen-specific IgE (≥2.37 $kU_A/L$) as determined by ImmunoCAP to shrimp and/or crab. These subjects were also more likely to have had severe allergic symptoms, such as angioedema and anaphylaxis, upon contact with shellfish. However, there were some subjects who had a strong ImmunoCAP result to shrimp and/or crab and clinical history of severe reactions but showed low or no IgE reactivity by ELISA or immunoblot. These subjects may have species-specific IgE with limited or no cross-reactivity with the crustacean species in our study [42–43], likely due to ingestion of different species.

Previous studies have concluded that specific-IgE to TM is an accurate predictor of shrimp allergy [44–45]. Our study supports the importance of TM as a major allergen of the blue swimmer crab, but several other crab proteins were shown to be allergenic and subjects exhibited different allergen reactivity profiles, several with no TM IgE reactivity. Component-resolved allergen-microarray technology would allow the simultaneous screening of serum IgE reactivity to a full panel of shellfish allergens, including whole allergen extracts, purified native and recombinant allergens, allergen fragments, and cooked and raw preparations. This would be of great advantage for the sensitive and specific diagnosis of shellfish allergy, and more information regarding the correlation between allergen-sensitization and severity of clinical symptoms could be gathered.

In conclusion, heating causes a marked increase in clinically relevant IgE reactivity of blue swimmer crab extract. In particular, we identified and characterized the blue swimmer crab TM, Por p 1, as a heat-stable major cross-reactive allergen. Other IgE-reactive blue swimmer crab proteins were observed, some corresponding to molecular weights of documented shellfish allergens, but others currently unidentified, some potentially unique to the blue swimmer crab. Our findings will advance reliable diagnosis and management of shellfish allergy.

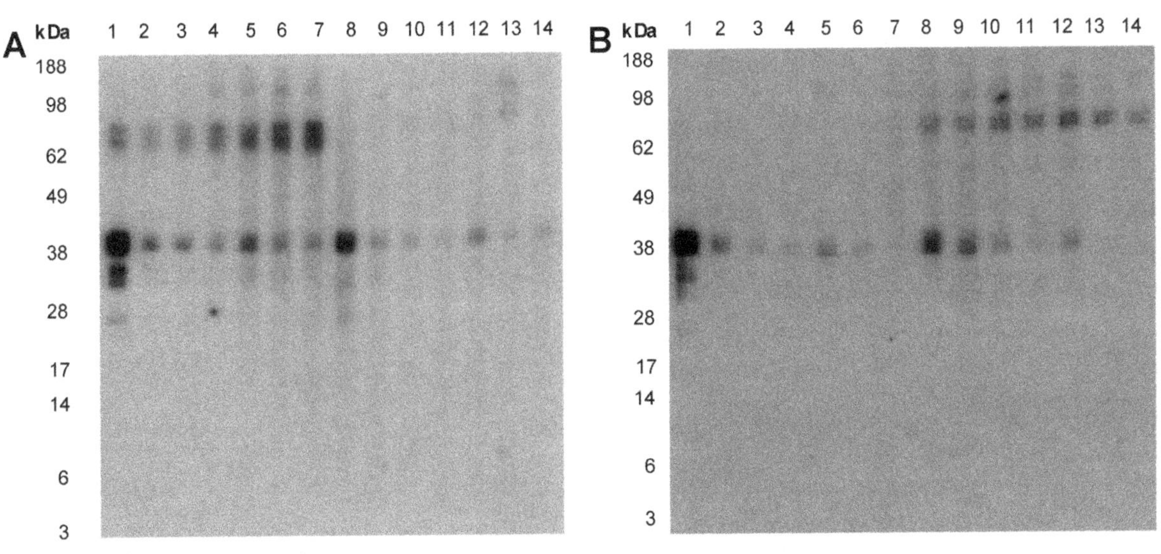


**Figure 8. Inhibition IgE immunoblotting with recombinant tropomyosin preparations.** Inhibition of serum IgE reactivity to CC (A) and CP (B) by rPor p 1 and rPen m 1 using subjects 24 (lanes 1–7) and 19 (lanes 8–14). Lanes 1: No inhibitor, subject 24, 2: 0.048 μg/ml rPor p 1, 3: 0.24 μg/ml rPor p 1, 4: 1.2 μg/ml rPor p 1, 5: 0.048 μg/ml rPen m 1, 6: 0.24 μg/ml rPen m 1, 7: 1.2 μg/ml rPen m 1, 8: No inhibitor, subject 19, 9: 0.048 μg/ml rPor p 1, 10: 0.24 μg/ml rPor p 1, 11: 1.2 μg/ml rPor p 1, 12: 0.048 μg/ml rPen m 1, 13: 0.24 μg/ml rPen m 1, 14: 1.2 μg/ml rPen m 1.

## Acknowledgments

We thank Karen Symons and Kirsten Deckert for subject recruitment and collection of blood samples, and Astrid Voskamp for technical advice regarding the basophil activation test.

## Author Contributions

Conceived and designed the experiments: JA SK RO JR CZ AL. Performed the experiments: JA SK NV. Analyzed the data: JA SK JR NV AL. Contributed reagents/materials/analysis tools: SK AL. Wrote the paper: JA JR SK RO. Critically revised the paper for important intellectual content: JA SK NV CZ AL RO JR. Provided clinical assessment of subjects: RO CZ.

## References

1. Ross MP, Ferguson M, Street D, Klontz K, Schroeder T, et al. (2008) Analysis of food-allergic and anaphylactic events in the National Electronic Injury Surveillance System. J Allergy Clin Immunol 121:166–171.
2. Boyce JA, Assa'ad A, Burks AW, Jones SM, Sampson HA, et al. (2010) Guidelines for the diagnosis and management of food allergy in the United States: Summary of the NIAID-sponsored expert panel report. J Allergy Clin Immunol 126:1105–1118.
3. Lopata AL, O'Hehir RE, Lehrer SB (2010) Shellfish allergy. Clin Exp Allergy 40:850–858.
4. Lieberman P, Nicklas RA, Oppenheimer J, Kemp SF, Lang DM, et al. (2010) The diagnosis and management of anaphylaxis practice parameter: 2010 Update. J Allergy Clin Immunol 126:477–480+e471–e442.
5. Skypala I (2011) Adverse Food Reactions-An Emerging Issue for Adults. J Am Diet Assoc 111:1877–1891.
6. Crespo JF, Rodriguez J (2003) Food allergy in adulthood. Allergy 58:98–113.
7. Lopata AL, Lehrer S (2009) Seafood Allergen Overview: Focus on Crustacean. In: LJaHJ W, Chemical and Biological Properties of Food Allergens: CRC Press. 233–257.
8. Emoto A, Ishizaki S, Shiomi K (2009) Tropomyosins in gastropods and bivalves: Identification as major allergens and amino acid sequence features. Food Chem 114:634–641.
9. Abdel Rahman AM, Kamath S, Lopata AL, Helleur RJ (2010) Analysis of the allergenic proteins in black tiger prawn (Penaeus monodon) and characterization of the major allergen tropomyosin using mass spectrometry. Rapid Commun Mass Spectrom 24:2462–2470.
10. Lopata AL, Lehrer SB (2009) New insights into seafood allergy. Curr Opin Allergy Clin Immunol 9:270–277.
11. Rosmilah M, Shahnaz M, Zailatul HM, Noormalin A, Normilah I (2012) Identification of tropomyosin and arginine kinase as major allergens of Portunus pelagicus (blue swimming crab). Trop Biomed 29:467–478.
12. Ayuso R, Grishina G, Bardina L, Carrillo T, Blanco C, et al. (2008) Myosin light chain is a novel shrimp allergen, Lit v 3. J Allergy Clin Immunol 122:795–802.
13. Garcia-Orozco KD, Aispuro-Hernandez E, Yepiz-Plascencia G, Calderon-de-la-Barca AM, Sotelo-Mundo RR (2007) Molecular characterization of arginine kinase, an allergen from the shrimp Litopenaeus vannamei. Int Arch Allergy Immunol 144:23–28.
14. Shiomi K, Sato Y, Hamamoto S, Mita H, Shimakura K (2008) Sarcoplasmic calcium-binding protein: Identification as a new allergen of the black tiger shrimp Penaeus monodon. Int Arch Allergy Immunol 146:91–98.
15. Motoyama K, Suma Y, Ishizaki S, Nagashima Y, Shiomi K (2007) Molecular cloning of tropomyosins identified as allergens in six species of crustaceans. J Agric Food Chem 55:985–991.
16. Sicherer SH (2001) Clinical implications of cross-reactive food allergens. J Allergy Clin Immunol 108:881–890.
17. Wickham M, Faulks R, Mills C (2009) In vitro digestion methods for assessing the effect of food structure on allergen breakdown. Mol Nutr Food Res 53:952–958.
18. Mandalari G, Adel-Patient K, Barkholt V, Baro C, Bennett L, et al. (2009) In vitro digestibility of beta-casein and beta-lactoglobulin under simulated human gastric and duodenal conditions: a multi-laboratory evaluation. Regul Toxicol Pharmacol 55:372–381.
19. Bublin M, Radauer C, Knulst A, Wagner S, Scheiner O, et al. (2008) Effects of gastrointestinal digestion and heating on the allergenicity of the kiwi allergens Act d 1, actinidin, and Act d 2, a thaumatin-like protein. Mol Nutr Food Res 52:1130–1139.
20. Shanti KN, Martin BM, Nagpal S, Metcalfe DD, Rao PVS (1993) Identification of tropomyosin as the major shrimp allergen and characterization of its IgE-binding epitopes. J Immunol 151:5354–5363.
21. Leung PSC, Chu KH, Chow WK, Ansari A, Bandea CI, et al. (1994) Cloning, expression, and primary structure of Metapenaeus ensis tropomyosin, the major heat-stable shrimp allergen. J Allergy Clin Immunol 94:882–890.
22. Samson KTR, Chen FH, Miura K, Odajima Y, Iikura Y, et al. (2004) IgE binding to raw and boiled shrimp proteins in atopic and nonatopic patients with adverse reactions to shrimp. Int Arch Allergy Immunol 133:225–232.
23. Clare Mills EN, Sancho AI, Rigby NM, Jenkins JA, Mackie AR (2009) Impact of food processing on the structural and allergenic properties of food allergens. Mol Nutr Food Res 53:963–969.
24. Lopata AL, Jeebhay MF, Reese G, Fernandes J, Swoboda I, et al. (2005) Detection of fish antigens aerosolized during fish processing using newly developed immunoassays. Int Arch Allergy Immunol 138:21–28.
25. Drew AC, Eusebius NP, Kenins L, De Silva HB, Suphioglu C, et al. (2004) Hypoallergenic variants of the major latex allergen Hev b 6.01 retaining human T lymphocyte reactivity. J Immunol 173:5872–5879.
26. Ayuso R, Lehrer SB, Reese G (2002) Identification of continuous, allergenic regions of the major shrimp allergen pen a 1 (Tropomyosin). Int Arch Allergy Immunol 127:27–37.
27. Reese G, Viebranz J, Leong-Kee SM, Plante M, Lauer I, et al. (2005) Reduced allergenic potency of VR9-1, a mutant of the major shrimp allergen Pen a 1 (tropomyosin). J Immunol 175:8354–8364.
28. Zheng LN, Lin H, Pawar R, Li ZX, Li MH (2011) Mapping IgE binding epitopes of major shrimp (Penaeus monodon) allergen with immunoinformatics tools. Food Chem Toxicol 49:2954–2960.
29. Kalogeromitros D, Makris M, Gregoriou S, Chliva C, Katoulis A, et al. (2006) IgE-mediated sensitization in seafood processing workers. Allergy Asthma Proc 27:399–403.
30. Gautrin D, Cartier A, Howse D, Horth-Susin L, Jong M, et al. (2010) Occupational asthma and allergy in snow crab processing in Newfoundland and Labrador. Occup Environ Med 67:17–23.
31. Jeebhay MF, Robins TG, Miller ME, Bateman E, Smuts M, et al. (2008) Occupational allergy and asthma among salt water fish processing workers. Am J Ind Med 51:899–910.
32. Jeebhay MF, Robins TG, Lehrer SB, Lopata AL (2001) Occupational seafood allergy: A review. Occup Environ Med 58:553–562.
33. Thomas K, Herouet-Guicheney C, Ladics G, Bannon G, Cockburn A, et al. (2007) Evaluating the effect of food processing on the potential human allergenicity of novel proteins: international workshop report. Food Chem Toxicol 45:1116–1122.
34. Davis PJ, Smales CM, James DC (2001) How can thermal processing modify the antigenicity of proteins? Allergy 56:56–60.
35. Vissers YM, Iwan M, Adel-Patient K, Stahl Skov P, Rigby NM, et al. (2011) Effect of roasting on the allergenicity of major peanut allergens Ara h 1 and Ara h 2/6: The necessity of degranulation assays. Clin Exp Allergy 41:1631–1642.
36. Chung SY, Champagne ET (2001) Association of end-product adducts with increased IgE binding of roasted peanuts. J Agric Food Chem 49:3911–3916.
37. DeWitt ÅM, Mattsson L, Lauer I, Reese G, Lidholm J (2004) Recombinant tropomyosin from Penaeus aztecus (rPen a 1) for measurement of specific immunoglobulin E antibodies relevant in food allergy to crustaceans and other invertebrates. Mol Nutr Food Res 48:370–379.
38. Leung PSC, Wing Kuen C, Duffey S, Hoi Shan K, Gershwin ME, et al. (1996) IgE reactivity against a cross-reactivity allergen in crustacea and mollusca: Evidence for tropomyosin as the common allergen. J Allergy Clin Immunol 98:954–961.
39. Zhang Y, Matsuo H, Morita E (2006) Cross-reactivity among shrimp, crab and scallops in a patient with a seafood allergy. Journal of Dermatology 33:174–177.
40. Aalberse RC, Akkerdaas J, Van Ree R (2001) Cross-reactivity of IgE antibodies to allergens. Allergy 56:478–490.
41. Asero R, Ballmer-Weber BK, Beyer K, Conti A, Dubakiene R, et al. (2007) IgE-mediated food allergy diagnosis: Current status and new perspectives. Mol Nutr Food Res 51:135–147.
42. Jirapongsananuruk O, Sripramong C, Pacharn P, Udompunturak S, Chinratanapisit S, et al. (2008) Specific allergy to Penaeus monodon (seawater shrimp) or Macrobrachium rosenbergii (freshwater shrimp) in shrimp-allergic children. Clin Exp Allergy 38:1038–1047.
43. Morgan JE, O'Neil CE, Daul CB, Lehrer SB (1989) Species-specific shrimp allergens: RAST and RAST-inhibition studies. J Allergy Clin Immunol 83:1112–1117.
44. Gámez C, Sánchez-García S, Ibáñez MD, López R, Aguado E, et al. (2011) Tropomyosin IgE-positive results are a good predictor of shrimp allergy. Allergy 66:1375–1383.
45. Yang AC, Arruda LK, Santos ABR, Barbosa MCR, Chapman MD, et al. (2010) Measurement of IgE antibodies to shrimp tropomyosin is superior to skin prick testing with commercial extract and measurement of IgE to shrimp for predicting clinically relevant allergic reactions after shrimp ingestion. J Allergy Clin Immunol 125:872–878.

7

# Variable Food-Specific IgG Antibody Levels in Healthy and Symptomatic Chinese Adults

**Qiang Zeng[1*], Sheng-Yong Dong[1], Liu-Xin Wu[2], Hong Li[3], Zhi-Jian Sun[4], Jing-Bo Li[5], Hong-Xia Jiang[6], Zhi-Heng Chen[7], Qi-Bin Wang[8], Wei-Wei Chen[9*]**

**1** International Medical Center, Chinese PLA General Hospital, Beijing, China, **2** The Second Laboratory, PLA Air Force Institute of Aviation Medicine, Beijing, China, **3** Health Management Center, Fujian Provincial Hospital, Fuzhou, Fujian, China, **4** Health Management Center, Shandong Provincial Hospital, Jinan, Shandong, China, **5** Health Management Center, Southwest Hospital, The Third Military Medical University, Chongqing, China, **6** Health Management Center, Xiangya Hospital, Central South University, Changsha, Hunan, China, **7** Health Management Center, The Third Xiangya Hospital of Central South University, Changsha, Hunan, China, **8** Health Management Center, Shandong Electric Power Center Hospital, Jinan, Shandong, China, **9** Treatment and Research Center for Infectious Diseases, 302 Hospital of PLA, Beijing, China

## Abstract

***Background:*** The presence of food-specific IgG antibodies in human serum may be useful for diagnosis of adverse food reactions. However, the clinical utility of tesing for such antibodies remains very controversial. The aim of this study was to evaluate the serum levels and population distribution of food-specific IgGs and their association with chronic symptoms in a large-scale Chinese population.

***Methodology/Principal Findings:*** A total of 21305 adult participants from different regions of China had 14 type of food-specific serum IgG antibodies that were measured by enzyme-linked immunosorbent assay. Amongthese, 5,394 participants were randomly chosen to complete follow-up questionnaire surveys on their dietary characteristics and chronic symptoms. The concentrations of food-specific IgGs against 14 foods ranged from a median (interquartile range) of 7.3 (3.8, 12.6) U/mL of pork-specfic IgG to 42.3 (28.8, 60.2) U/mL of crab-specific IgG. The concentration of food-specific IgGs was closely related to gender; after adjustment for region and age, women had higher concentrations of food-specific IgGs against all of the 14 foods except chicken (regression coefficient (95% CI): 0.01 (−0.003, 0.023); $P = 0.129$) and corn (0.002 (−0.013, 0.016); $P = 0.825$). Similar results were also found in the relationship of geographic region to the food-specific IgG concentrations for the 14 foods. Chronic symptoms were negatively associated with the concentrations of a few food-specific IgGs, and were positively associated with the concentrations of other food-specific IgGs.

***Conclusions:*** The levels of food-specific IgGs were variable both in healthy and in symptomatic Chinese adults. These findings raise awareness that demographic factors, the type of food and specific chronic symptoms should be considered before food elimination treatment based on IgG testing in patients with chronic symptoms is used in clinical practice.

**Editor:** Susanne Krauss-Etschmann, Ludwig-Maximilians-University Munich, Germany

**Funding:** This study was supported by the State Science and Technology Support Program (No. 2012BAI37B04). The funders had no role in study design, data collection and analysis, decision to publish, or preparation of the manuscript.

**Competing Interests:** The authors have declared that no competing interests exist.

* E-mail: zq301@hotmail.com (QZ); cww302@126.com (WC)

These authors contributed equally to this work.

## Introduction

The prevalence of migraine, asthma, allergic dermatitis and irritable bowel syndrome has been continuously increasing. Etiological studies suggest that these diseases may be related to adverse food reactions (food hypersensitivity) [1,2,3,4,5]. According to a recent report of an expert panel sponsored by the U.S. National Institute of Allergy and Infectious Diseases [6], adverse food reactions include food allergies and food intolerances, and the gold standard for the diagnosis of adverse food reactions remains the double-blind, placebo-controlled food challenge (DBPCFC). However, DBPCFC is difficult to use in large population studies due to the tedious, inconvenient, and costly procedures involved [7]. Other diagnostic tests such as skin prick tests, serum food-specific IgE tests, and atopy patch tests lack specificity and may lead to the unnecessary exclusion of foods from the patient's diet [6].

Previous studies have found that the levels of food-specific IgGs and IgG subclasses in blood serum were significantly higher in individuals with food hypersensitivity [8,9,10], and that IgG-mediated immunologic responses may play an important role in the pathogenesis of adverse food reactions [11,12,13]. However, other studies indicate that the serum level of food-specific IgGs may also be elevated in healthy individuals, suggesting that the elevation of food-specific IgGs and IgG subclasses may merely reflect the presence of immunological tolerance to food-specific antigens, i.e., that it may only reflect a history of exposure to a certain food [14,15]. Therefore, it was determined that food-specific IgGs and IgG subclasses lack diagnostic value for food allergy/intolerance [15,16,17].

Although the diagnostic utility of the presence of food-specific IgGs in patients with adverse food reactions remain controversial, serum food-specific IgG tests have been used in patients with chronic symptoms because of their convenience [18,19]. In addition, selective food elimination based on the results of food-specific IgG testing has been suggested to be effective in the treatment of irritable bowel syndrome and migraine [4,5]. However, the distribution of food-specific IgG concentrations, and the relationship of food-specific IgGs to chronic symptoms has not been reported in any large-scale population studies [18]. The aim of this study was to investigate the factors related to the presence of food-specific IgGs and their association with diet characteristics and chronic symptoms in a large adult population from various regions of China.

## Materials and Methods

### Study Population

The study population was recruited as patients presented to the clinic and underwent routine physical examination in general hospitals in 23 provinces in China (Figure S1), beginning in August 2008. Participation in the study was voluntary. Individuals aged 18–75 years were randomly selected using a single-blind method;, patients who were pregnancy or had a history of anaphylactic shock, secondary chronic symptoms caused by other known cardiovascular diseases, chronic kidney diseases or organic intestinal diseases were excluded. The concentrations of serum IgGs that reacted with 14 foods that are commonly consumed in China were measured in these individuals. By October 2010, a total of 21305 participants were included after excluding those with incomplete data. From this population, 6000 subjects were randomly selected and contacted for a questionnaire survey. Informed written consent was obtained from all participants, and the study protocol was approved by the Institution Review Board of the Chinese PLA General Hospital, Beijing, China.

### Questionnaire Design

A questionnaire was designed with questions adapted to Chinese adults. The questions included consumption frequencies of 14 common foods: beef, chicken, codfish, corn, crab, eggs, mushrooms, cow's milk, pork, rice, shrimp, soybeans, tomatoes and wheat. Regular consumption referred to a consumption frequency of ≥3 times/week, and rare consumption referred to a consumption frequency ≤ one time/3 months; moderate consumption was defined as a consumption frequency that fell between these two extremes. The questionnaire also included information about perceived connections between ingestion of specific foods and chronic symptoms, such as gastrointestinal symptoms (abdominal pain, diarrhea or nausea), eczema, urticaria, rhinitis, asthma, arthritis, migraine headaches or other chronic symptoms (chest pain, or heart discomfort).

### Food-specific Serum IgG Assays

Participants' sera were collected and sent, with only numerical identifiers, to authorized hospital laboratories, where enzyme-linked immunosorbent assays (ELISA) were performed to measure the concentrations of 14 different food-specific IgGs using a commercially available kit (Biomerica, Inc. USA). This assay has been described in a previous study [20]. Briefly, the serum samples were diluted 100-fold, and added to reaction wells coated with one of 14 food-specific allergens. After the plate was sealed, incubated at room temperature for 1 hour, washed and patted dry, anti-human IgG antibody conjugated to horseradish peroxidase was added to the wells. After another incubation at room temperature for 30 minutes, washing and patting dry, 100 µl of a substrate mixture consisting of equal proportions of 3,3′,5,5′-tetramethylbenzidine and hydrogenperoxide was added. The reaction was stopped after 10 minutes, and absorbance was measured at 450 nm. The concentrations of food-specific IgGs (U/mL; 1 U = 1.47 ng) were calculated using the standard curves of 14 types of food-specific IgGs provided by the manufacture. The detection limit was 0.01 U/mL. All authorized laboratories were asked to satisfy several standards of quality assurance for the determinations of these 14 types of food-specific IgGs. The quality assurance standards were as follows: the optical density of the negative controls should be <0.2, the concentrations of IgG in the positive quality controls should be >100 U/mL and the optical density in 50 U/mL, 100 U/mL, 200 U/mL and 400 U/mL standard wells should be 1.2 times more than in negative 50 U/mL, 100 U/mL and 200 U/mL standard wells, respectively. For the great majority of clinically relevant allergens, no standardized reference allergens are available for comparisons between methods. To ensure the reproducibility and accuracy of the ELISA kit assays, each serum sample was tested in duplicate parallel tests, all ELISA kits were required to be used within 10 days of their delivery from the factory, and all testing was performed using an automated spotting system that was supervised by well-trained medical laboratory technologists who were blinded to the clinical data. On average, the intra- and inter-assay coefficients of variant were 2.7% and 5.3%, respectively, in the Chinese PLA General Hospital laboratory, and 8.5% and 12.1% in other authorized laboratories. Before the study, all participating laboratories calibrated food-specific IgG measurements according to the quality control results distributed from the Chinese PLA General Hospital laboratory.

### Statistical Analysis

All data were entered into an Epidata 3.0 database through double-blinded entry, followed by automatic check and verification. Continuous variables are reported as median values with the corresponding 25th and 75th percentiles. Discrete variables are summarized in terms of frequencies and percentages. Because the data demonstrated a skewed distribution, serum concentrations of food-specific IgGs were logarithmically transformed; undetectable specific IgG concentrations (<0.01 U/mL) were considered 0.005 U/mL. Maximum likelihood estimation was performed to evaluate the means and standard deviations of food-specific IgG concentrations using R 2.15.2. To visualize the distribution of food-specific IgG concentrations in all subjects and demographic subgroups (sex, geographic region and age group), histograms or line graphs were generated, and one-way analysis of variance (ANOVA) and post-hoc Tukey tests were used for comparison of the resultings curves. *P*-values for trends were calculated when age group-related differences in food-specific IgG concentrations were examined. Pearson correlation was performed to analyze the relationship of food-specific IgG concentrations among the 14 foods. Differences in food consumption frequencies in demographic subgroups were tested using the Pearson chi-square test and *P* values for trends were calculated when differences in the food consumption frequencies of different age group were examined. Differences in food-specific IgG concentrations between subjects with chronic symptoms and subjects without chronic symptoms were also examined with ANOVA. Multivariate linear regression models were applied to evaluate the association of food-specific IgG concentrations of each of the 14 foods with demographic factors and food consumption frequencies. Logistic regression models were performed to analyze the association of chronic symptoms with food-specific IgG concentrations of the 14 foods, and odd ratios (OR) and 95% CI were calculated. All statistical analyses were performed with SPSS 10.0 (SPSS Inc., Chicago, IL, USA). Two-tailed P values <0.05 were considered significant.

## Results

### Study Population Characteristics

Of the 21305 subjects (mean age: 46.63±10.52 years; 13,426 men and 7,879 women), most (74.0%) were northern Chinese. Questionnaire replies were received from 5394 individuals (89.9% of the randomly selected subjects); of the 5394 individuals who responded to the questionnaire, 32.2% were women and 77.2% were northern Chinese. In the 2353 subjects who reported having chronic symptoms, the most common chronic symptoms were gastrointestinal symptoms (23.6%), rhinitis (11.8%) and migraine (9.5%) (Table 1).

### Distribution of Food-specific IgG Concentrations

The distributions of the serum concentrations of food-specific IgG against the 14 foods tested varied significantly (Figure 1). The log-distributed curves for food-specific IgG concentrations of crab, codfish, egg and shrimp are shifed slightly to the right; the medians (interquartile range) of the IgG concentrations against these foods were 42.3 (28.8, 60.2) U/mL, 27.5 (16.9, 44.2) U/mL, 26.6 (11.4, 72.5) U/mL and 22.8 (14.9, 35.2) U/mL, respectively. For pork-specific IgG, the log-distributed curve is shifted slightly to the left; the median and interquartile range of the concentration of pork-specific IgG is 7.3 and 3.8 to 12.6 U/mL. The means and standard deviations of log-transformed food-specific IgG concentrations that were calculated using maximum likelihood estimation are shown in Table S1.

The distribution of food-specific IgG concentration against egg varied more than for other foods. For example, a total of 61 subjects had levels of egg-specific IgG above 1000 U/mL, and the proportion of subjects who had egg-specific IgG levels above 200 U/mL was 8.4%, the highest od the 14 foods. The proportion of subjects who had the egg-specific IgG levels less than 10 U/mL was 21.7%; this level was higher than for other foods against which subjects had similar IgG levels, such as codfish (only 8.8% of the subjects had codfish-specific IgG levels that were less than 10 U/mL). Interestingly, the food-specific IgG levels against the 14 foods tested were all correlated with each other. The strongest relationship between food-specific IgG levels were found for beef and chicken (correlation coefficient, 0.691; $P<0.01$); the next strongest was for codfish and crab (correlation coefficient, 0.561; $P<0.01$) (Table S2).

### Relationship of Demographic Factors and Food-specific IgG Concentrations

Compared to the log-distributed curves of the frequencies of food-specific IgG concentrations in men, the log-distributed curves of the frequencies of food-specific IgG concentrations in women were shifted to the right for 10 of the 14 foods; the exceptions were chicken (median (interquartile) men vs. women: 11.5 (7.1, 17.3) U/mL vs. 11.8 (7.4, 17.9) U/mL; $P=0.052$), corn (men vs. women: 11.3 (6.5, 18.5) U/mL vs. 12.0 (6.9, 19.0) U/mL; $P=0.378$), mushrooms (men vs. women: 14.5 (8.1, 22.4) U/mL vs. 14.9 (8.1, 23.9) U/mL; $P=0.065$) and pork (men vs. women: 7.3 (3.8, 12.4) U/mL vs. 7.4 (3.8, 12.8) U/mL; $P=0.432$). When the subjects were grouped according to sex, the greatest difference in food-specific IgG concentrations between men and women was found for egg (men vs. women: 22.4 (10.3, 61.2) U/mL vs. 36.8 (14.2, 93.6) U/mL; $P<0.001$); the next greatest differences were for cow's milk (men vs. women: 14.9 (8.5, 26.2) U/mL vs. 18.2 (10.1,

**Table 1.** Baseline characteristics of the study population.

| | Overall subjects, n = 21305 Number (%) | Subjects with questionnaire survey, n = 5394 Number (%) |
|---|---|---|
| Women | 7879 (37.0) | 1735 (32.2) |
| Age (year) | | |
| 18–34 | 1585 (7.4) | 462 (8.6) |
| 35–44 | 7526 (35.3) | 1751 (32.5) |
| 45–54 | 8268 (38.8) | 2025 (37.5) |
| 55–64 | 2849 (13.4) | 733 (13.6) |
| ≥65 | 1077 (5.1) | 423 (7.8) |
| Region | | |
| South China | 5547 (26.0) | 1231 (22.8) |
| North China | 15758 (74.0) | 4163 (77.2) |
| Chronic symptoms | | |
| Gastrointestinal | -- | 1274 (23.6) |
| Rhinitis | -- | 636 (11.8) |
| Migraine | -- | 511 (9.5) |
| Arthritis | -- | 392 (7.3) |
| Eczema | -- | 310 (5.7) |
| Urticaria | -- | 259 (4.8) |
| Asthma | -- | 153 (2.8) |
| Other | -- | 721 (13.4) |

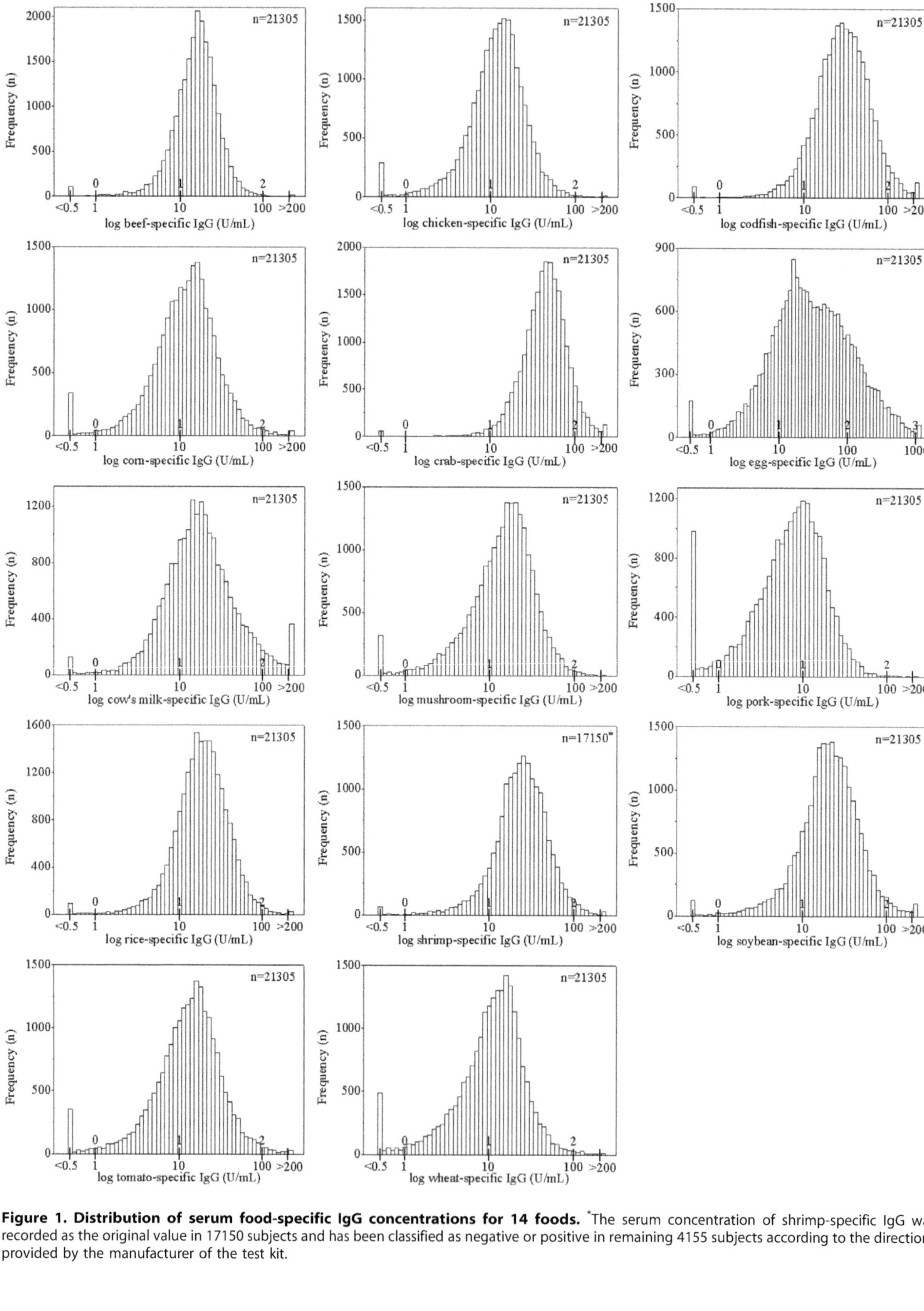


**Figure 1. Distribution of serum food-specific IgG concentrations for 14 foods.** *The serum concentration of shrimp-specific IgG was recorded as the original value in 17150 subjects and has been classified as negative or positive in remaining 4155 subjects according to the directions provided by the manufacturer of the test kit.

34.3) U/mL; $P<0.001$) and soybean (men vs. women: 18.7 (11.7, 30.1) U/mL vs. 22.4 (13.9, 36.8) U/mL; $P<0.001$) (Figure S2).

Region subgroup histograms also showed that the log-distributed curves for almost all of the 14 foods shifted slightly for South Chinese compared to North Chinese subjects; the exceptions were chicken (south vs. north: 10.7 (7.1, 16.4) U/mL vs. 11.9 (7.3, 17.9) U/mL; $P=0.333$) and soybean (south vs. north: 18.7 (11.5, 30.8) U/mL vs. 20.5 (12.8, 33.0) U/mL; $P=0.062$) (Figure S3). Compared to subjects in North China, subjects in South China had higher mean concentrations of beef-specific IgG (south vs. north: 16.3 (11.6, 22.8) U/mL vs. 14.6 (9.9, 20.1) U/mL; $P<0.001$), corn-specific IgG (south vs. north: 11.7 (6.9, 19.7) U/mL vs. 11.5 (6.5, 18.3) U/mL; $P<0.001$) and shrimp-specific IgG (south vs. north: 24.9 (16.5, 37.6) U/mL vs. 22.6 (14.8, 35.0) U/mL; $P<0.001$). The mean concentrations of food-specific IgG against the other 9 foods were higher in North China than in South China, especially mushroom (south vs. north: 9.9 (5.1, 18.5) U/mL vs. 15.9 (9.6, 24.1) U/mL; $P<0.001$), pork (south vs. north: 4.8 (2.4, 9.1) U/mL vs. 8.3 (4.5, 13.6) U/mL; $P<0.001$) and wheat (south vs. north: 7.8 (4.1, 13.9) U/mL vs. 12.3 (7.3, 18.3) U/mL; $P<0.001$).

With increasing age of the subjects, the mean concentrations of food-specific IgG for almost all of the 14 foods increased. The exceptions were corn (11.9 (6.6, 19.4) U/mL, 11.4 (6.5, 18.7) U/mL, 11.3 (6.6, 18.3) U/mL, 11.8 (6.7, 18.5) U/mL and 13.2 (7.9, 21.7) U/mL for 20–34, 35–44, 45–54, 55–64 and ≥65 years age group, respectively; $P$ for trend = 0.092) and wheat (12.1 (6.5, 20.0) U/mL, 10.5 (5.6, 17.2) U/mL, 10.9 (6.2, 17.3) U/mL, 11.6 (6.8, 17.5) U/mL and 13.4 (8.0, 18.8) U/mL for 20–34, 35–44, 45–54, 55–64 and ≥65 years age groups, respectively; $P$ for trend = 0.115). Although food-specific IgG concentrations for the other 12 foods showed an increasing trend with age, the concentrations of egg-specific IgG and cow's milk-specific IgG were significantly higher in the 18–34 years age group than in the 35–44, 45–54 and 55–64 years age groups (Figure S4).

Multivariate analysis showed that women had higher food-specific IgG concentrations than men against all of the 14 foods except chicken (regression coefficient (95% CI): 0.01 (−0.003, 0.023); $P=0.129$) and corn (0.002 (−0.013, 0.016); $P=0.825$) after adjustment for region and age. Of the other 12 foods, egg-specific IgG concentration showed the strongest relationship to sex (0.184 (0.166, 0.202); $P<0.001$). After adjustment for sex and age, subjects in South China had higher concentrations of beef-specific IgG (−0.079 (−0.089, −0.068); $P<0.001$), corn-specific IgG (−0.047 (−0.063, −0.031); $P<0.001$) and shrimp-specific IgG (−0.052 (−0.071, −0.033); $P<0.001$) than subjects in North China, whereas they had similar chicken-specific IgG concentration (−0.009 (−0.023, 0.005); $P=0.210$) as subjects in North China; food-specific IgG concentrations against the other 11 foods were higher in subjects in North China. After adjustment for sex and region, age also showed strong relationship with to the food-specific IgG concentrations against all foods except corn (0.001 (0, 0.001); $P=0.083$), cow's milk (0.001 (0, 0.001); $P=0.065$) and wheat (0 (−0.001, 0.001); $P=0.910$). Age was inversely associated with egg-specific IgG concentration (−0.002 (−0.003, −0.001); $P<0.001$) and positively associated with food-specific IgG concentrations for the other 10 foods (Figure 2).

## Relationship between Consumption Frequency and Food-specific IgG

Of the 5394 subjects who responded to the questionnaire, the majority regularly consumed (≥3 times/week) rice and pork (83.8% and 70.1%, respectively); a minority of subjects regularly consumed shrimp and crab (15.4% and 6.9%, respectively). Men showed higher diet frequencies of codfish and meat, while more women regularly consumed cow's milk and non-meat foods. The proportions of subjects who regularly consumed rice, crab, shrimp and codfish were higher in South than in North China, while the proportion of subjects who regularly consumed wheat was higher in North China population (69.7% vs. 35.4%, respectively; $P<0.001$).Shrimp, chicken, beef and pork were consumed most frequently by the 18–34 yearold age group, and the consumption of egg, cow's milk, soybeans, corn, tomatoes and wheat increased with age ($P$ for trend $<0.001$) (Table S3).

After adjustment for sex, region and age, the diet frequencies of 9 of the tested foods were not significantly associated with the corresponding food-specific serum IgG concentrations. Dietary consumption frequencies of egg, cow's milk and rice were inversely associated with egg-specific IgG (regression coefficient (95%CI): −0.052 (−0.088, −0.016); $P=0.005$), cow's milk-specific IgG (−0.039 (−0.062, −0.015); $P=0.001$) and rice-specific IgG concentrations (−0.03 (−0.059, −0.002); $P=0.038$), respectively; whereas, the dietary consumption frequencies of chicken and tomato were positively associated with chicken-specific IgG (0.028 (0.001, 0.054); $P=0.042$) and tomato-specific IgG concentrations (0.034 (0.004, 0.064); $P=0.028$), respectively (Figure 3).

## Relationship between Food-specific IgGs and Chronic Symptoms

Compared to subjects who reported having no gastrointestinal symptoms, subjects who reported having chronic symptoms had higher concentrations of codfish-specific IgG (median (interquartile) gastrointestinal symptom, yes vs. no: 23.8 (14.3, 45.1) U/mL vs. 20.9 (14.4, 37.9) U/mL; $P=0.013$) and rice-specific IgG (16.7 (9.4, 28.0) U/mL vs. 15.4 (10.9, 22.0) U/mL; $P=0.032$); and lower concentrations of mushroom-specific IgG (8.9 (4.3, 16.0) U/mL vs. 12.0 (6.5, 16.9) U/mL; $P=0.026$), tomato-specific IgG (10.1(5.1, 17.7) U/mL vs. 13.1 (7.2, 18.4) U/mL; $P=0.018$) and wheat-specific IgG (6.8 (3.0, 13.3) U/mL vs. 9.9 (4.6, 15.7) U/mL; $P=0.010$). Subjects who reported having migraine also had lower concentrations of mushroom-specific IgG (8.4 (4.1, 15.7) U/mL vs. 11.8 (6.2, 16.9) U/mL; $P=0.007$) and tomato-specific IgG (9.8 (4.6, 16.2) U/mL vs. 13.0 (7.0, 18.5) U/mL; $P=0.003$) than subjects who reported having no migraine. Subjects who reported having eczema had higher concentrations of crab-specific IgG (44.8 (24.8, 66.5) U/mL vs. 37.3 (21.4, 58.5) U/mL; $P=0.038$) and rice-specific IgG (17.0 (11.7, 27.2) U/mL vs. 15.5 (10.5, 22.9) U/mL; $P=0.009$) than subjects who reported having no eczema. Rice-specific IgG concentration was higher in subjects who reported having urticaria than in subjects who reported having no urticaria (20.9 (13.0, 31.2) U/mL vs. 15.4 (10.5, 22.7) U/mL; $P=0.006$); whereas, cow's milk-specific IgG concentration was lower in subjects who reported having asthma than in subjects who reported having no asthma (14.2 (6.6, 23.7) U/mL vs. 15.3 (9.0, 27.7) U/mL; $P=0.042$). The concentrations of food-specific IgG for cow's milk, pork and wheat were also lower in subjects who reported having other symptoms than in those who reported having no other symptoms (Figure S5).

The association of chronic symptoms with serum levels of specific IgGs against the 14 foods tested is shown in Figure 4. After adjustment for sex, region and age, gastrointestinal symptom were inversely associated with mushroom-specifi (OR (95% CI): 0.85 (0.72, 0.99); $P=0.048$), tomato-specific (0.82 (0.70, 0.97); $P=0.020$) and wheat-specific (0.84 (0.73, 0.95); $P=0.007$) IgG levels; and positively associated with codfish-specific (1.47 (1.11, 1.94); $P=0.007$), rice-specific (1.45 (1.08, 1.95); $P=0.015$) and shrimp-specific (1.40 (1.06, 1.85); $P=0.017$) IgG levels. Rhinitis was inversely associated with the serum concentration of tomato-

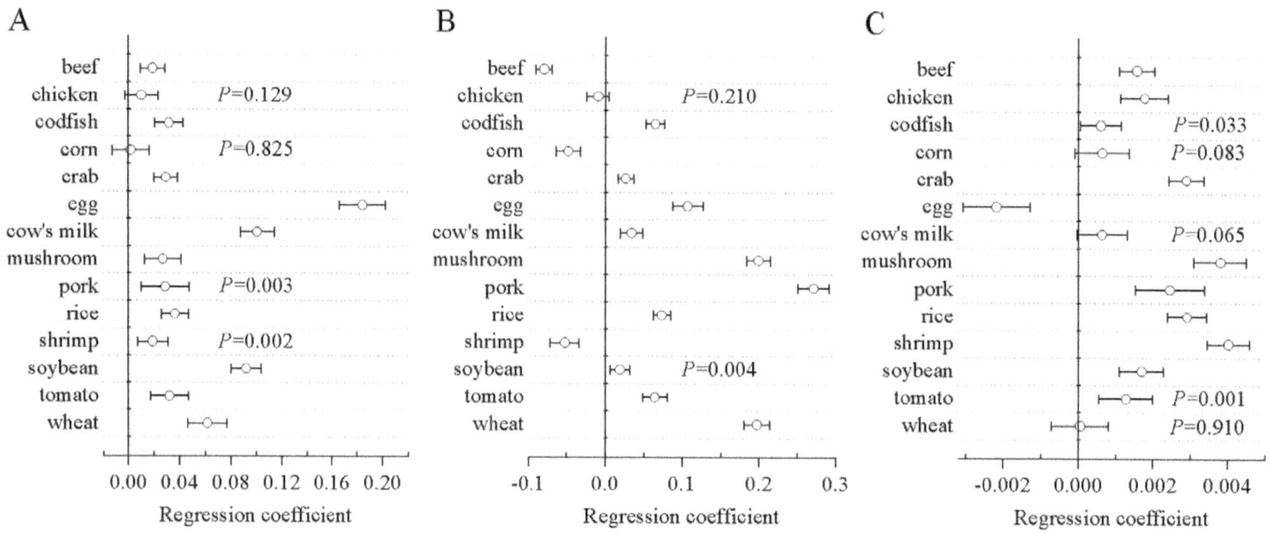


**Figure 2. Association of demographic subgroups with serum food-specific IgG concentrations for 14 foods.** (A) sex, (B) geographic region, (C) age. Regression coefficients and *P* values were derived from multivariate linear regression models that set sex (men, 0; women, 1), geographic region (South China, 0; North China, 1) and age as independent variables and the logarithmically transformed serum food-specific IgG concentrations for 14 foods as dependent variables. The food items for which *P* values are not shown yielded mean *P* values less than 0.001.

specific IgG (0.82 (0.66, 0.99); $P=0.049$) and positively associated with the concentration of rice-specific IgG (1.49 (1.01, 2.19); $P=0.044$). Migraine was inversely associated with mushroom-specific (0.78 (0.64, 0.95); $P=0.016$) and tomato-specific IgG levels (0.74 (0.61, 0.91); $P=0.004$) and positively associated with rice-

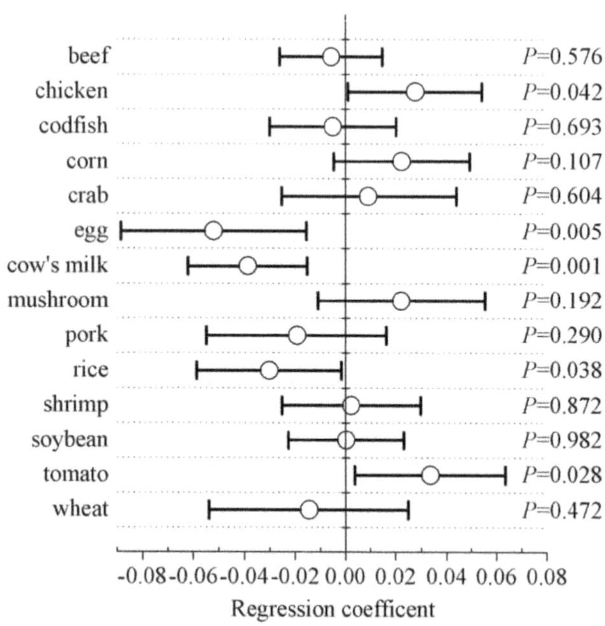


**Figure 3. Association of various dietary frequencies of 14 foods with corresponding serum food-specific IgG concentrations.** Regression coefficients and *P* values were derived from multivariate linear regression models in which the dietary frequencies of 14 foods (rare, 0; moderate, 1; regular, 2) were used as independent variables and the corresponding and logarithmically transformed serum food-specific IgG concentrations for 14 foods were the dependent variables. Demographic factorsincluding sex, region and age were adjusted for in these models.

specific IgG levels (1.57 (1.01, 2.43); $P=0.043$). Arthritis was inversely associated with wheat-specific IgG levels (079 (0.63, 0.98); $P=0.035$). Eczema was positively associated with food-specific concentrations of beef-specific (2.01 (1.07, 3.75); $P=0.030$), crab-specific (1.90 (1.12, 3.20); $P=0.017$) and rice-specific (2.23 (1.27, 3.93); $P=0.005$) IgG levels. Urticaria was positively associated with rice-specific (3.71 (1.76, 7.86); $P=0.001$) and shrimp-specific (2.15 (1.11, 4.18); $P=0.024$) IgG levels. Asthma was inversely associated with milk-specific IgG levels (0.63 (0.41, 0.98); $P=0.042$). Other symptoms were inversely associated with pork-specific (075 (0.64, 0.89); $P=0.001$) and wheat-specific (0.80 (0.69, 0.93); $P=0.004$) IgG levels and positively associated with crab-specific IgG levels (1.53 (1.07, 2.17); $P=0.019$).

## Discussion

Although commercial laboratories worldwide are currently offering broad-scale = testings for serum levels of food-specific IgGs to the public, to our knowledge, the study described here is the first representative cross-sectional study to address the distribution of food-specific IgGs and its relationship to chronic symptoms in a large population. Previous studies have either involved \ research on the potential involvement of various IgG subclasses in food allergy/intolerance [9,21] or have addressed food elimination based on IgG testing [4,5].

Although testing for the presence of food-specific IgGs has been regarded as a potential tool for the diagnosis of food allergy/intolerance, it's the accuracy and clinical utility of such testing remain unclear. In our study, serum concentrations of food-specific IgGs against the 14 foods tested varied widely. Different foods have different proteins and components, and this may induce different immune reactions and lead to the presence of variable amounts of food-specific IgG. The completeness of extraction of different food proteins and other components of the 14 foods tested and the relative coupling efficiency of different extracted food components/antigens to the ELISA plate would also be expected to influence the accuracy of measurement of serum concentrations of food-specific IgGs. Although the levels of

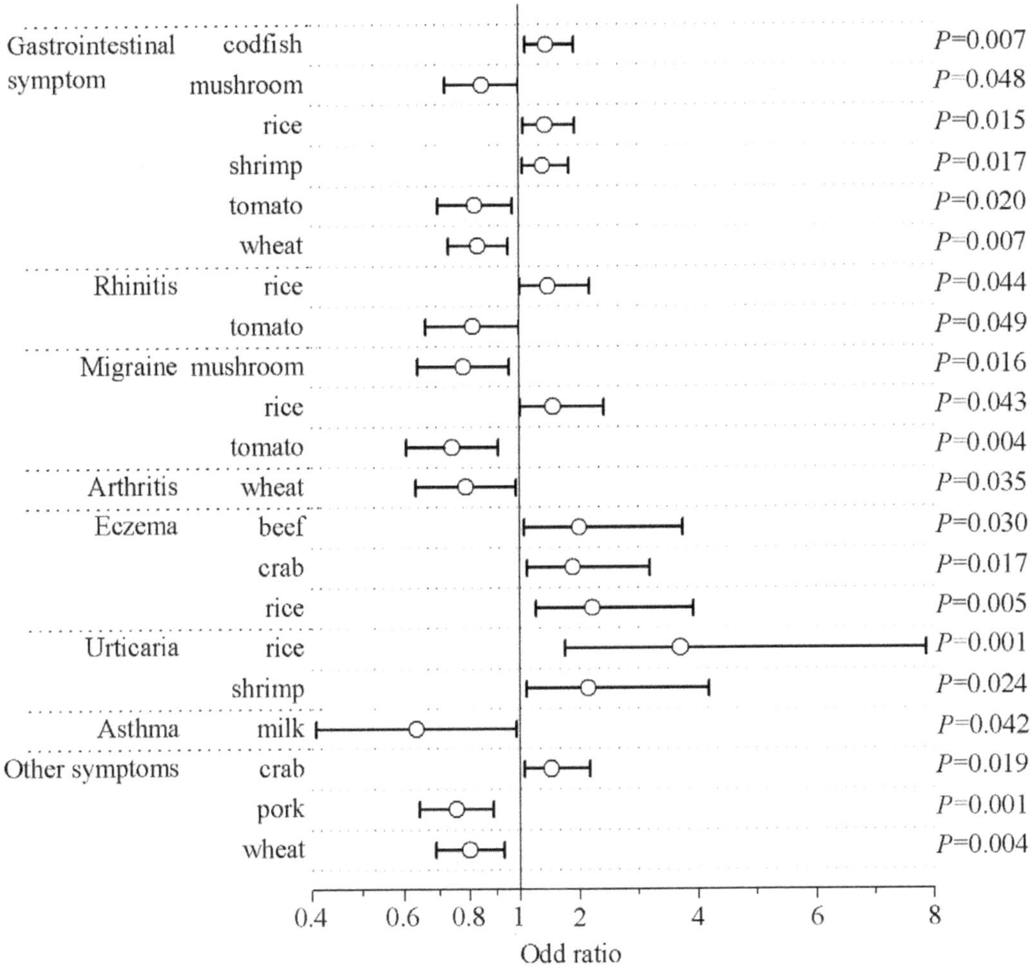


**Figure 4. Association of chronic symptoms with food-specific IgG concentrations for 14 foods.** Only the foods for which food-specific IgG levels were significantly associated with certain chronic symptoms ($P<0.05$) are listed. Odds ratios and *P* values were derived from logistic regression models that set logarithmically transformed serum food-specific IgG concentrations for the 14 foods as the independent variables and the presence of various chronic symptoms (No, 0; Yes, 1) as the dependent variables. Demographic factors including sex, region and age were adjusted for in these models.

food-specific IgG against the 14 tested foods were significantly different, the concentrations of all 14 food-specific IgGs, especially IgGs directed against beef and chicken, were correlated with one another. Similar results were reported by Kanagawa et al [22] in an analysis of food antigens in 6549 subjects; the results of that study suggested that the appearance of food antigens clusters may be a result of immune cross-reaction between similar food antigens [6].

In our study, the distribution of food-specific IgG levels varied as a function of demographic subgroups (sex, region and age). Women had higher concentrations offood-specific IgGs against almost all of the tested foods than men. It has been consistently reported that the prevalence of food allergy/intolerance is significantly higher in women than in men [23,24,25]. In childhood, boys suffer from asthma, urticaria, anaphylaxis and food allergies to eggplant and peanuts more frequently than girls, while the sex difference is reversed after puberty [26,27,28,29]. Studies suggest that some female sex steroids are pro-inflammatory and increase the susceptibility of atopy, while testosterone is a powerful inhibitor of histamine and known to inhibit mast cell degranulation [26,30]. Moreover, for the first time, our study demonstrated that the distribution of food-specific IgGs against almost all of the 14 foods tested were significantly different between Southern and Northern Chinese. In the present study, this difference is not related to the subject's gender, age or dietary habits; however, it may be due to the different genetic backgrounds of subjects of different ethnicities [31,32]. Our study also showed that the serum concentrations of all food-specific IgGs except egg-specific IgG were positively associated with age. Previous studies have suggested that older people may be more likely than younger people to experience allergic reactions to foods [33]. It is not clear whether the higher levels of foods-specific IgGs in older persons indicates a higher probability of food allergies with increasing age. It is also unclear why egg-specific IgG concentrations were highest in the 20–34-year-old subjects and lowest in the 35–44-yearold subjects.

Previous studies have shown that abdominal discomforts self-attributed to food hypersensitivity is not related to eating habits or meal patterns [34]. Our study also showed that although the dietary frequencies of the 14 foods differed significantly in the demographic subgroups, only the dietary frequencies of chicken, egg, cow's milk, rice and tomato were associated with the corresponding food-specific IgG serum levels after adjustment for demographic factors. The immunological mechanism responsible for the association of chicken, egg, cow's milk, rice and tomato eating patterns with food-specific serum IgG concentrations is unclear, and further studies of this phenomenon are needed.

Previous studies have shown that chronic symptoms are closely related to food hypersensitivity [2,6]. In our study, we found the food-specific concentrations of a few IgGs to be associated with a variety of chronic symptoms; the levels of some food-specific IgG were inversely associated with chronic symptoms, while the levels of other food-specific IgG were positively associated with chronic symptoms. Chronic symptoms were positively related to the serum levels of certain food-specific IgG. This may be a result of chronic inflammatory responses induced by elevated IgG or IgG subclasses in highly sensitive individuals [5]. For instance, gliadins and glutenins in wheat may increase specific IgG levels and may lead to chronic symptoms [35]. Our study also revealed negative associations between the level of rice-specific IgG and gastrointestinal symptoms, rhinitis, migraine, urticaria and eczema; such associations may result from different (protective or negative) roles of different IgG antibodies. Similarly, Tay et al [36] found that strong IgG responses to ovalbumin may be a normal physiological response to protein ingestion frequently shown in infancy, whereas up-regulated IgG responses that occur in peanut allergy may be indicative of a dysregulated immune response to peanut allergens. The normal physiological response reflected by the presence of food-specific IgG subclasses may be immunological tolerance due to the secretion of IL-10 by the activation of regulatory T cells upon prolonged exposure to food antigen [37].

The present study has several limitations. First, because food-specific IgG antibody testing is popular in China, we only tested for the presence of IgGs against commonly consumed foods, and did not measure levels of specific IgGs against pollen, fruits, nuts or food additives [1,24,25]. However, it should be kept in mind that self-reported chronic symptoms may result from the presence of IgGs specific for the latter foods and substances rather than from the presence of IgGs against the 14 tested food allergens. Second, in our study, the prevalence of chronic symptoms was determined by self-reporting of such symptoms on a questionnaire. The chronic symptoms reported by the patients in this study have not been confirmed by the adjudication of professional doctors. Thus, misclassification of chronic symptoms is possible, and the conclusions of the study regarding the associations of specific chronic symptoms with certain food-specific IgG levels should be regarded cautiously. Third, children and adolescents 0–17 years of age were not included in our study. It has been reported that the presence of food-specific IgGs in serum is more common in children and adolescents than in adults [15]. In children and adolescents, high levels of specific IgG are not significantly associated with clinical symptoms, and are likely to represent a protective mechanism that can result in immune tolerance to the corresponding foods later in life [38]. However, a similar protective role of food-specific IgG and IgG subclasses in adults has not been confirmed [15,21]. Finally, the study does not provide an answer to the question of whether food-specific IgGs play a protective role or an allergic role in adults. The immunological mechanisms by which food-specific IgGs are induced are also unclear. A complete understanding of the importance of the presence of food-specific IgGs requires further accumulation of epidemiologic and experimental data.

In summary, the present study demonstrates for the first time that food-specific IgG serum concentrations are variable in both healthy and symptomatic Chinese adults. These findings raise awareness that demographic factors, types of food and the presence or absence of specific chronic symptoms should be considered before food elimination treatment based on IgG testing in patients with chronic symptoms is used in clinical practice. Further elucidation of the role played by food-specific IgGs in food allergies and tolerance should be an objective of future studies.

## Supporting Information

**Figure S1 Map of China with participating sites and numbers of subjects.** The middle line represents the boundary between southern China and northern China. The dots and triangles represent the participating sites in northern China and southern China, respectively.
(TIF)

**Figure S2 Distribution of serum food-specific IgG concentrations for 14 foods in subgroups according to sex.** The white and gray columns represent men and women, respectively. * See Figure 1.
(TIF)

**Figure S3 Distribution of serum food-specific IgG concentrations for 14 foods in subgroups according to geographic region.** The white and gray columns represent participants in South China and North China, respectively. * See Figure 1.
(TIF)

**Figure S4 Distribution of serum food-specific IgG concentrations for 14 foods according to age group.** CI, confidence interval.
(TIF)

**Figure S5 Differences in serum food-specific IgG concentrations in subjects with and without chronic symptoms.** * *P* value <0.05. CI, confidence interval.
(TIF)

**Table S1 Means and standard deviations of log-transformed food-specific IgG concentrations.** *The means and standard deviations of log-transformed food-specific IgG concentrations were calculated after the undetectable food-specific IgG concentrations were set as the half-value of the limit of detection. †The means and standard deviations of log-transformed food-specific IgG concentrations were calculated using maximum likelihood estimation.
(DOC)

**Table S2 Correlation of food-specific IgG concentrations among 14 foods*.** *The Pearson correlation was used to analyze possible correlations among the food-specific IgG concentrations for 14 foods. **Indicates that the correlation is significant at the 0.01 level (2-tailed).
(DOC)

**Table S3 Regular intake (≥3 times/week) of 14 foods in 5394 subjects (number (%)).**
(DOC)

## Acknowledgments

We thank the staffs of China Health Management Association, Medical Center of the First Affiliated Hospital of China Medical University, Medical Center of Sichuan Provincial People's Hospital, Medical Center of the Health Ministry Beijing Hospital, Beijing Xiaotangshan Hospital, The First Affiliated Hospital of Chongqing Medical University, Bethune International Peace Hospital, Xinjiang Uygur Autonomous Region People's Hospital, Zhongshan Hospital Xiamen University, General Hospital of Guangzhou Military Command of PLA, and Shuguang

Hospital Affiliated to Shanghai University of Traditional Chinese Medicine for their commitment, and all subjects who participated in the study.

## Author Contributions

Conceived and designed the experiments: QZ WC. Performed the experiments: LW HL ZS JL HJ. Analyzed the data: SD WC. Contributed reagents/materials/analysis tools: QZ LW ZC QW. Wrote the paper: QZ SD.

## References


1. Sicherer SH (2011) Epidemiology of food allergy. J Allergy Clin Immunol 127: 594–602.
2. Sampson HA (2004) Update on food allergy. J Allergy Clin Immunol 113: 805–819; quiz 820.
3. Penard-Morand C, Raherison C, Kopferschmitt C, Caillaud D, Lavaud F, et al. (2005) Prevalence of food allergy and its relationship to asthma and allergic rhinitis in schoolchildren. Allergy 60: 1165–1171.
4. Atkinson W, Sheldon TA, Shaath N, Whorwell PJ (2004) Food elimination based on IgG antibodies in irritable bowel syndrome: a randomised controlled trial. Gut 53: 1459–1464.
5. Alpay K, Ertas M, Orhan EK, Ustay DK, Lieners C, et al. (2010) Diet restriction in migraine, based on IgG against foods: a clinical double-blind, randomised, cross-over trial. Cephalalgia 30: 829–837.
6. Boyce JA, Assa'ad A, Burks AW, Jones SM, Sampson HA, et al. (2010) Guidelines for the diagnosis and management of food allergy in the United States: report of the NIAID-sponsored expert panel. J Allergy Clin Immunol 126: S1–58.
7. Chafen JJ, Newberry SJ, Riedl MA, Bravata DM, Maglione M, et al. (2010) Diagnosing and managing common food allergies: a systematic review. JAMA 303: 1848–1856.
8. Host A, Husby S, Gjesing B, Larsen JN, Lowenstein H (1992) Prospective estimation of IgG, IgG subclass and IgE antibodies to dietary proteins in infants with cow milk allergy. Levels of antibodies to whole milk protein, BLG and ovalbumin in relation to repeated milk challenge and clinical course of cow milk allergy. Allergy 47: 218–229.
9. Zar S, Benson MJ, Kumar D (2005) Food-specific serum IgG4 and IgE titers to common food antigens in irritable bowel syndrome. Am J Gastroenterol 100: 1550–1557.
10. Dreskin SC, Tripputi MT, Aubrey MT, Mustafa SS, Atkins D, et al. (2010) Peanut-allergic subjects and their peanut-tolerant siblings have large differences in peanut-specific IgG that are independent of HLA class II. Clin Immunol 137: 366–373.
11. Crowe SE, Perdue MH (1992) Gastrointestinal food hypersensitivity: basic mechanisms of pathophysiology. Gastroenterology 103: 1075–1095.
12. Shreffler WG, Lencer DA, Bardina L, Sampson HA (2005) IgE and IgG4 epitope mapping by microarray immunoassay reveals the diversity of immune response to the peanut allergen, Ara h 2. J Allergy Clin Immunol 116: 893–899.
13. Scott-Taylor TH, J OBH, Strobel S (2010) Correlation of allergen-specific IgG subclass antibodies and T lymphocyte cytokine responses in children with multiple food allergies. Pediatr Allergy Immunol 21: 935–944.
14. Johansson SG, Bieber T, Dahl R, Friedmann PS, Lanier BQ, et al. (2004) Revised nomenclature for allergy for global use: report of the Nomenclature Review Committee of the World Allergy Organization, October 2003. J Allergy Clin Immunol 113: 832–836.
15. Stapel SO, Asero R, Ballmer-Weber BK, Knol EF, Strobel S, et al. (2008) Testing for IgG4 against foods is not recommended as a diagnostic tool: EAACI Task Force Report. Allergy 63: 793–796.
16. Ahrens B, Lopes de Oliveira LC, Schulz G, Borres MP, Niggemann B, et al. (2010) The role of hen's egg-specific IgE, IgG and IgG4 in the diagnostic procedure of hen's egg allergy. Allergy 65: 1554–1557.
17. Hochwallner H, Schulmeister U, Swoboda I, Twaroch TE, Vogelsang H, et al. (2011) Patients suffering from non-IgE-mediated cow's milk protein intolerance cannot be diagnosed based on IgG subclass or IgA responses to milk allergens. Allergy 66: 1201–1207.
18. Hunter JO (2005) Food elimination in IBS: the case for IgG testing remains doubtful. Gut 54: 1203; author reply 1203.
19. Pelsser LM, Frankena K, Toorman J, Savelkoul HF, Dubois AE, et al. (2011) Effects of a restricted elimination diet on the behaviour of children with attention-deficit hyperactivity disorder (INCA study): a randomised controlled trial. Lancet 377: 494–503.
20. Zuo XL, Li YQ, Li WJ, Guo YT, Lu XF, et al. (2007) Alterations of food antigen-specific serum immunoglobulins G and E antibodies in patients with irritable bowel syndrome and functional dyspepsia. Clinical and experimental allergy : journal of the British Society for Allergy and Clinical Immunology 37: 823–830.
21. Antico A, Pagani M, Vescovi PP, Bonadonna P, Senna G (2011) Food-Specific IgG4 Lack Diagnostic Value in Adult Patients with Chronic Urticaria and Other Suspected Allergy Skin Symptoms. Int Arch Allergy Immunol 155: 52–56.
22. Kanagawa Y, Matsumoto S, Koike S, Imamura T (2009) Association analysis of food allergens. Pediatr Allergy Immunol 20: 347–352.
23. Young E, Stoneham MD, Petruckevitch A, Barton J, Rona R (1994) A population study of food intolerance. Lancet 343: 1127–1130.
24. Schafer T, Bohler E, Ruhdorfer S, Weigl L, Wessner D, et al. (2001) Epidemiology of food allergy/food intolerance in adults: associations with other manifestations of atopy. Allergy 56: 1172–1179.
25. Zuberbier T, Edenharter G, Worm M, Ehlers I, Reimann S, et al. (2004) Prevalence of adverse reactions to food in Germany - a population study. Allergy 59: 338–345.
26. Harish Babu BN, Mahesh PA, Venkatesh YP (2008) A cross-sectional study on the prevalence of food allergy to eggplant (Solanum melongena L.) reveals female predominance. Clinical and experimental allergy : journal of the British Society for Allergy and Clinical Immunology 38: 1795–1802.
27. Poulos LM, Waters AM, Correll PK, Loblay RH, Marks GB (2007) Trends in hospitalizations for anaphylaxis, angioedema, and urticaria in Australia, 1993–1994 to 2004–2005. J Allergy Clin Immunol 120: 878–884.
28. Sicherer SH, Munoz-Furlong A, Sampson HA (2003) Prevalence of peanut and tree nut allergy in the United States determined by means of a random digit dial telephone survey: a 5-year follow-up study. J Allergy Clin Immunol 112: 1203–1207.
29. Chen Y, Stewart P, Johansen H, McRae L, Taylor G (2003) Sex difference in hospitalization due to asthma in relation to age. J Clin Epidemiol 56: 180–187.
30. Zaitsu M, Narita S, Lambert KC, Grady JJ, Estes DM, et al. (2007) Estradiol activates mast cells via a non-genomic estrogen receptor-alpha and calcium influx. Molecular immunology 44: 1977–1985.
31. Hong X, Wang G, Liu X, Kumar R, Tsai HJ, et al. (2011) Gene polymorphisms, breast-feeding, and development of food sensitization in early childhood. J Allergy Clin Immunol 128: 374–381 e372.
32. Campos Alberto EJ, Shimojo N, Suzuki Y, Mashimo Y, Arima T, et al. (2008) IL-10 gene polymorphism, but not TGF-beta1 gene polymorphisms, is associated with food allergy in a Japanese population. Pediatr Allergy Immunol 19: 716–721.
33. Harduar-Morano L, Simon MR, Watkins S, Blackmore C (2011) A population-based epidemiologic study of emergency department visits for anaphylaxis in Florida. The Journal of allergy and clinical immunology 128: 594–600 e591.
34. Carvalho RV, Lorena SL, Almeida JR, Mesquita MA (2010) Food intolerance, diet composition, and eating patterns in functional dyspepsia patients. Dig Dis Sci 55: 60–65.
35. Battais F, Pineau F, Popineau Y, Aparicio C, Kanny G, et al. (2003) Food allergy to wheat: identification of immunogloglin E and immunoglobulin G-binding proteins with sequential extracts and purified proteins from wheat flour. Clin Exp Allergy 33: 962–970.
36. Tay SS, Clark AT, Deighton J, King Y, Ewan PW (2007) Patterns of immunoglobulin G responses to egg and peanut allergens are distinct: ovalbumin-specific immunoglobulin responses are ubiquitous, but peanut-specific immunoglobulin responses are up-regulated in peanut allergy. Clin Exp Allergy 37: 1512–1518.
37. Satoguina JS, Weyand E, Larbi J, Hoerauf A (2005) T regulatory-1 cells induce IgG4 production by B cells: role of IL-10. J Immunol 174: 4718–4726.
38. Skripak JM, Nash SD, Rowley H, Brereton NH, Oh S, et al. (2008) A randomized, double-blind, placebo-controlled study of milk oral immunotherapy for cow's milk allergy. J Allergy Clin Immunol 122: 1154–1160.

8

# Induction of Allergic Responses to Peanut Allergen in Sheep

**Jenna L. Van Gramberg[1], Michael J. de Veer[1], Robyn E. O'Hehir[2], Els N. T. Meeusen[1], Robert J. Bischof[1]***

**1** Biotechnology Research Laboratories, Department of Physiology, Monash University, Clayton, Australia, **2** Department of Allergy, Immunology and Respiratory Medicine, Alfred Hospital and Monash University, Melbourne, Australia

## Abstract

Peanut allergy is the leading cause of deaths due to food-induced anaphylaxis but despite continued research, there are currently no specific treatments available. Challenge testing is limited in patients due to the high risk of adverse reactions, emphasising the need for an appropriate animal model. In the present study we examine the induction of allergic responses in a sheep model for peanut allergy. Sheep were sensitised with peanut (PN) extract and in separate injections with ovalbumin (OVA) or house dust mite (HDM) extract. Serum PN-specific IgE responses were detected in 40–50% of immunised sheep, while only 10% (1 of 10 sheep) showed detectable OVA-specific IgE. All PN-allergic sheep tested showed an Ara h 1-specific IgE response, while four out of five allergic sheep showed an Ara h 2-specific IgE response. Animals with high serum IgE levels to HDM were also PN IgE-positive. Of the PN-sensitised animals with high PN-specific IgE, 80% also showed an immediate hypersensitivity reaction following an intradermal PN injection. This new large animal model of peanut allergy may provide a useful tool for future investigations of allergen-associated immune mechanisms and specific immunotherapy.

**Editor:** Marco Idzko, University Hospital Freiburg, Germany

**Funding:** This work was supported by a grant from the Australian Research Council (ARC). The funders had no role in study design, data collection and analysis, decision to publish, or preparation of the manuscript.

**Competing Interests:** The authors have declared that no competing interests exist.

* E-mail: rob.bischof@monash.edu

## Introduction

'Food allergy' can be described as an exaggerated immune response to certain ingredients present in food and chiefly characterised by the production of immunoglobulin E (IgE) antibodies [1,2]. These IgE antibodies have been shown to have high affinity to receptors on immune cells such as mast cells and basophils [3] and interactions with these cells can lead to the release of potent mediators and the development of allergy symptoms [4,5]. The symptoms of allergy can range from mild reactions (e.g. swelling, wheezing, vomiting/diarrhoea) to life threatening systemic anaphylaxis [6]. Adverse reactions to food account for 30–50% of emergency anaphylactic cases in North America, Europe, Asia and Australia, however, these rates are said to be even higher in paediatric patients [7].

The establishment of food allergies has been found to be more prevalent in the first two years of life. A 2011 study by Osborne *et al* [8], found that 10% of a sample of Australian infants had IgE-mediated food allergy, a rate they consider as being "higher than expected". Food allergy sufferers also frequently experience other atopic conditions such as asthma, dermatitis (eczema) and rhinitis [9,10]. This trend is consistent in peanut (*Arachis hypogaea*) allergy, with approximately 1% of children affected. However, unlike hypersensitivities to milk and egg, peanut allergies typically persist with age, becoming a lifelong burden on health and management [11].

Since peanut allergy is so prevalent and peanuts are the leading cause of deaths due to food-induced anaphylaxis globally [12,13], considerable effort has been made to identify the major peanut allergens. As many as eleven peanut proteins have been categorised (Ara h 1–Ara h 11) [2] and, of these, Ara h 1 [14] and Ara h 2 [15] have been classified as major allergens, as they are recognised by serum IgE from more than 90% of peanut allergic subjects [16]. Further studies have reported that Ara h 2 is functionally more potent than Ara h 1 [17,18] when comparing specific IgE and the ability of the protein to induce histamine release from basophils in sensitised subjects [19].

The use of animal models for the study of food allergens has continued to gain interest, since many key mechanisms and the observed responses mimic processes commonly seen in human allergic disease states [20–23]. Peanut allergy has been investigated in mice [21,23,24] as well as larger animals including dogs [22,25] and pigs [20]. While animal models have furthered our understanding of the phenomenon that is allergy, larger animals are thought to reflect the human allergic state more closely due to their large size and outbred nature.

We have previously established a sheep model of allergic asthma based on house dust mite (HDM), that represents many features of the human disease including allergen-specific IgE responses, local and systemic inflammation and remodelling of the airways [26,27]. The aim of the present study was to examine the induction of allergic responses to crude peanut allergens in sheep and establish the potential for this model in future studies of peanut allergy predisposition.

## Materials and Methods

### Experimental sheep and allergen sensitisations

All experimental animal procedures and the collection of tissues and cells were approved by the Animal Experimental Ethics Committee of Monash University, following guidelines set by the National Health and Medical Research Council (NH&MRC) of Australia. Merino cross ewes were treated with anthelminthic to eliminate any parasites prior, then housed in indoor pens and fed lucerne chaff for the duration of the experiment.

### Allergens

Crude peanut (PN) extract was prepared from commercial unsalted, dry-roasted peanuts as described [28], dialysed against phosphate-buffered saline (PBS) and filter-sterilised. Ara h 1 and Ara h 2 were each separated from crude peanut extract based on published methodology [29,30] and kindly provided by Dr. Sara Prickett (Department of Immunology, Monash University). Ovalbumin (OVA) was purchased from Sigma. House dust mite extract (HDM; *Dermatophagoides pteronyssinus*; CSL Limited, Parkville, Australia) was prepared as previously described [26].

### Experimental Protocol

In Study 1 (n = 10) sheep were sensitised separately with a crude PN extract and OVA. The immunisation protocol involved 3 subcutaneous (s.c.) injections at 2-week intervals and a 4$^{th}$ 'boost' injection after a rest period of 4 weeks. Each injection comprised either 100 μg of solubilised crude PN extract or 100 μg of OVA prepared in a total of 1 ml sterile saline with 50 μl of a commercial aluminium adjuvant (alum); Rehydragel ® LV- Aluminium hydroxide (Reheis Inc/NJ, USA). This protocol was derived from previous studies involving animal models that were immunised s.c. with allergen in alum [22,26]. The PN injection was administered s.c. in the foreleg, whilst OVA was injected s.c. into the hindleg.

In Study 2 (n = 10), sheep were simultaneously immunised with PN allergen (as for Study 1) and HDM (50 μg/injection) allergen [26], prepared in 1 ml sterile saline with aluminium hydroxide as adjuvant. The immunisation protocol was similar to Study 1, with the PN and HDM injections administered s.c. at two different sites.

### Measuring antibody responses

Blood samples were collected from the jugular vein prior to the first immunisation (this served as a control for each individual sheep), as well as 4, 7, 14 and 21 days following the last injection. Serum samples were stored at −20°C prior to being assayed.

For the detection of PN-, HDM- or OVA-specfic total Ig by enzyme-linked immunosorbent assay (ELISA), ELISA plates were coated with 2.5 μg of the selected antigen in PBS, then washed, blocked and incubated with serum (1/200) for 1 hr at 37°C. After washing, plates were incubated with polyclonal rabbit anti-sheep horse-radish peroxidase (HRP; Dako, CA, USA) for 1 hr at 37°C, then washed and developed with 3′, 3′, 5′, 5′- tetramethylbenzidine dihydrochloride hydrate (TMB; Invitrogen, VIC, Australia). Plates were read at 450 nm on a Molecular Devices SPECTRAmax PLUS spectrophotometer. All samples were tested in duplicate.

PN-, HDM- or OVA-specific IgE was determined by ELISA of $NH_4SO_4$-treated serum samples as described previously [26]. Briefly, equal volumes of serum and 60% $NH_4SO_4$ solution were mixed and the sample centrifuged after 30 min in a microcentrifuge (13000 rpm for 10 min). The supernatants (diluted 1:1 with 0.1% Tween 20/$dH_20$) were added to 2.5 μg (PN/HDM/OVA) or 1 μg (Ara h 1/h 2) antigen-coated plates and incubated overnight at 4°C, followed by washing and incubation with anti-IgE mAb (clone XB6-YD3) [31]. Plates were then washed and incubated with HRP-conjugated (γ-chain specific) goat anti-mouse IgG (Sigma, NSW, Australia), then washed and developed with TMB-substrate. Plates were read at 450 nm on a Molecular Devices SPECTRAmax PLUS spectrophotometer. All samples were tested in duplicate.

### Skin testing

Immediate hypersensitivity responses were assessed following intra-dermal injections of 100 μl (1 μg/ml in saline) of PN, HDM and OVA; saline alone served as a negative control and histamine (1 μg/ml in saline) as a positive control. Injections were administered on the inner thigh of the animal. Thirty minutes after injection, wheal size was calculated as a mean of two measurements recorded using digital callipers [32].

## Results

### Serum Ig responses to PN extract and ovalbumin immunisations

In Study 1, sheep were sensitised s.c. with crude PN extract and at a separate site with OVA, a commonly used model antigen. ELISAs were performed to determine PN/OVA-specific total and IgE levels in serum samples collected before (pre) and 7 days after the final injection. Sera collected prior to sensitisation served as a control for each animal. Sheep were classified as sensitised (allergic) on the basis of a 50% increase in PN-specific serum IgE levels. From the 10 sheep immunised, 5 animals developed a high PN-specific IgE response and were referred to as allergic sheep (Figure 1A, solid bars). Only 1 of the 10 immunised sheep developed a specific-IgE response to OVA (Figure 1A, sheep 6); this sheep was also allergic to PN. OVA, however, showed a greater percentage change for total specific-Ig levels in post-sensitisation sera, with 8 out of the 10 animals displaying an OVA-specific total Ig percentage change greater than 50% (Figure 1B). No change greater than 50% was seen in PN-specific total Ig responses (Figure 1B).

In order to track the specific IgE antibody response in the PN responders more closely, blood serum was also collected at days 4, 7, 14 and 21 after the final (boost) injection of PN extract. PN-specific IgE levels began to increase by the earliest time-point examined (day 4), with levels peaking at day 7 post boost and declining thereafter; these levels, however, remained higher than baseline levels as shown in Figure 2. A significant difference was seen in IgE levels between pre and day 7 sera levels ($p<0.01$).

In order to test reproducibility, an additional 10 sheep were immunised for Study 2. Sheep in study 2 were simultaneously sensitised with crude PN extract and HDM (s.c. injections in a separate site) to compare antibody responses to different allergens. A similar trend to Study 1 was seen with 40% of the sensitised sheep developing a PN-specific IgE response (Figure 1A), with no significant difference in the level of sensitisation to PN allergen comparing animals in Study 1 vs 2. Interestingly, while PN-specific IgE levels were similar to Study 1, the relative change in PN-specific total Ig levels appeared greater in Study 2 (Figure 1B). Sheep in Study 2 were also immunised with HDM allergen; 9 of 10 sheep became sensitised to HDM, and two sheep that showed the highest HDM-specific IgE levels were also positive for PN-specific IgE (data not shown).

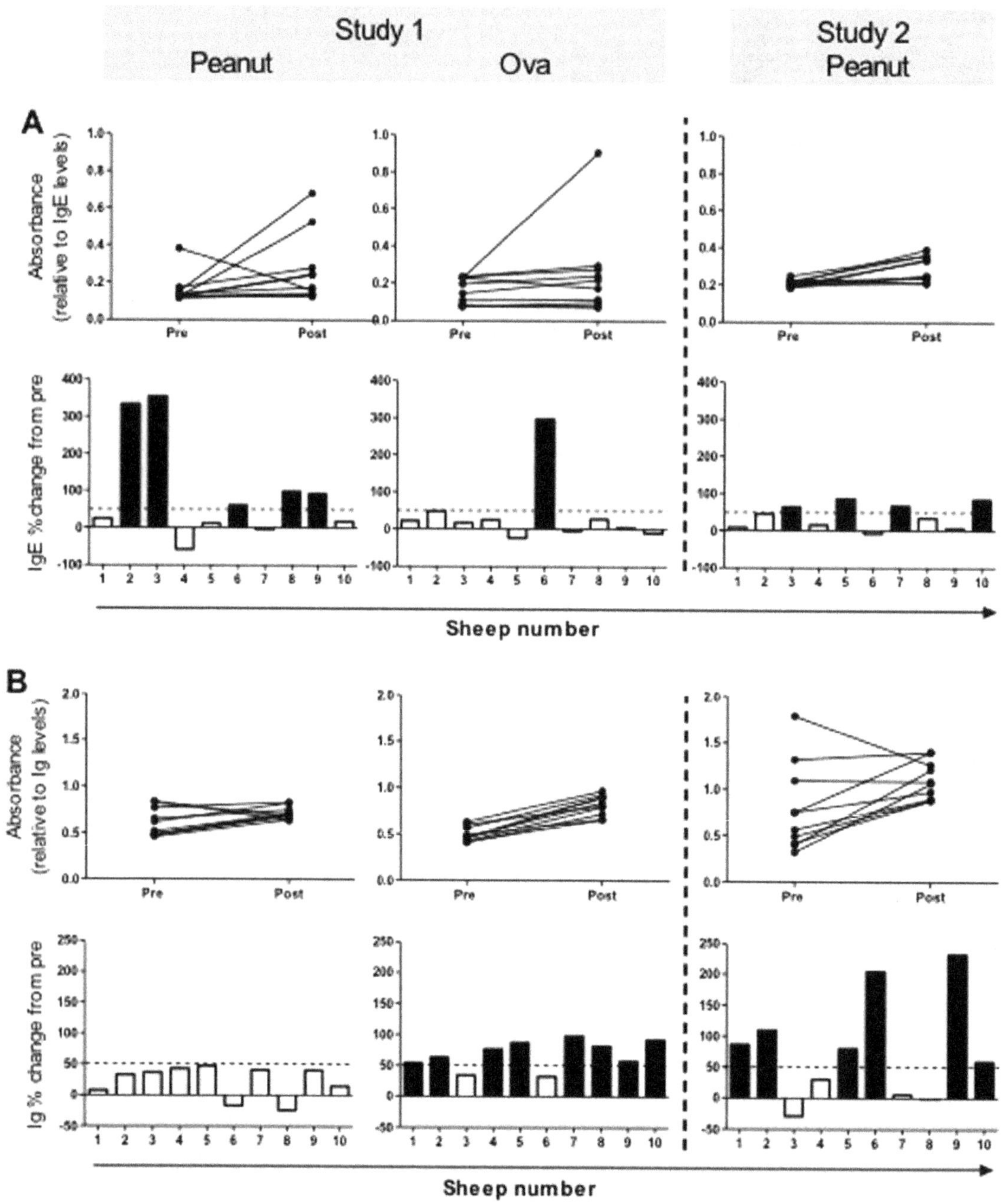


**Figure 1. Serum Ig responses to peanut (PN) and ovalbumin (OVA) immunisations.** Peripheral blood serum samples were collected at baseline (pre) and 7 days after the final PN/OVA immunisation (post). Line graphs depict allergen-specific IgE (A) and total Ig (B) levels (absorbance read at 450 nm) for individual sheep. Percentage change from baseline for each animal is presented in the bar graphs for allergen-specific IgE (A) and total Ig (B) levels. Solid bars illustrate a percentage change greater than 50%.

## Serum IgE responses to the major peanut allergens Ara h 1 and Ara h 2

To detect whether the IgE antibodies raised against the PN extract were specific to the major PN allergens Ara h 1 and Ara h 2, further allergen-specific ELISAs were conducted. For PN-allergic sheep (n = 5) and one non-responder sheep (sheep 7), pre and 7 day post serum samples were tested for the presence of Ara h 1- and Ara h 2-specific IgE. All 5 PN-allergic sheep showed an Ara h 1-specific IgE response, while 4 out of 5 allergic sheep showed an Ara h 2-specific IgE response. The non-responder control (sheep 7) did not show an increased percentage change for either Ara h 1 or Ara h 2 (Figure 3).

## Skin wheal responses to crude PN and ovalbumin

Skin reactions following intradermal injections of PN extract and OVA were assessed in sheep of study 1 before (pre) and after (post) sensitisation. Saline served as a negative and histamine as a positive control. Immediate skin wheal reactions were observed and recorded at 30 minutes post injection in all sheep (Figure 4). Several sheep showed an unexpected wheal response to each of the

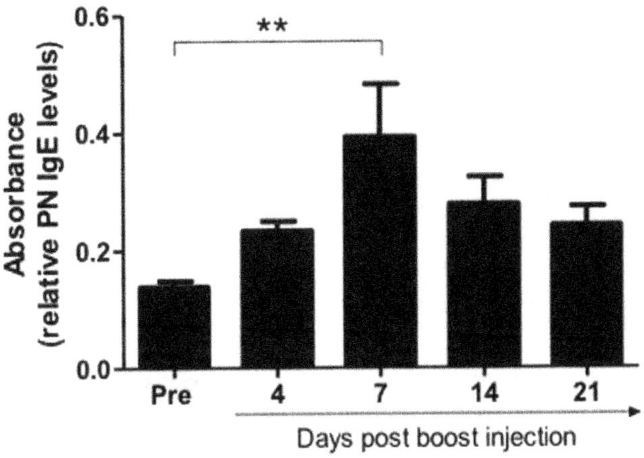


**Figure 2. PN-specific IgE responses overtime in allergic sheep.** Blood serum samples were collected before sensitisation (pre) and on days 4, 7, 14 and 21 after the final (boost) injection of PN extract, in order to track the peanut specific IgE antibody response overtime. Values are shown as the mean +/− SEM, n = 5 (data was analysed using a one-way ANOVA on repeated measures, Gaussian approximation); ** indicates a significant difference ($p<0.01$) comparing samples collected before and after PN exposure.

injections at the pre-sensitisation stage. Three out of four sheep that showed a wheal response to OVA post sensitisation were also strong PN IgE responders. Four out of five animals that showed a strong IgE response to PN allergen (see Figure 1A) also gave a positive wheal response to PN post sensitisation.

## Discussion

In the present study we report the induction of allergic responses to peanut (PN) allergen in sheep, whereby sensitisation with a crude extract of PN induced high levels of PN-specific IgE in 40–50% of animals. Significantly, PN-allergic sheep showed strong IgE reactivity to two of the major peanut allergens, Ara h 1 and Ara h 2, which feature prominently in PN allergy in humans [14–16]. In addition to the systemic induction of PN-specific IgE, 80% of PN-allergic animals (4 of 5 sheep in Study 1) also displayed post-sensitisation wheal responses to PN allergen.

In a second study conducted here (Study 2), sheep were simultaneously sensitised with crude PN extract and a non-food allergen, house dust mite (HDM). The number of animals that displayed an elevated PN-specific IgE response (ie atopic for PN) was similar to that seen in Study 1, however, a more robust total Ig (presumably IgG1) response to PN allergen was observed in sheep in Study 2; most likely this was due to different genetic backgrounds of the sheep in each study and reflective of the outbred nature of this species (similar to humans). Sensitisation to HDM allergen is known to be a major contributing factor towards the development of allergic asthma in humans. In previous studies

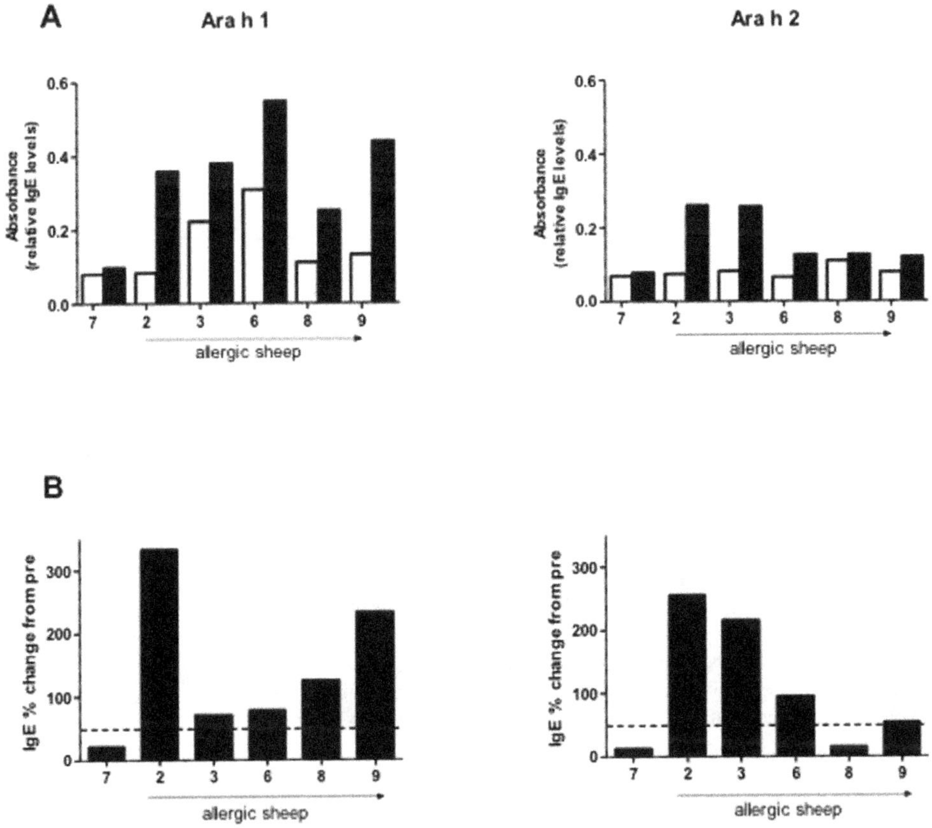


**Figure 3. PN allergic sheep respond to the major peanut allergens Ara h 1 and Ara h 2.** Blood serum collected before sensitisation (pre) and 7 days after the final (boost) injection of PN from allergic sheep (numbers 2, 3, 6, 8 and 9) and one non-responder (number 7) were tested for the presence of Ara h 1- and Ara h 2-specific IgE by ELISA. (A) Illustrates the individual differences between pre IgE (open bars) and day 7 post boost IgE levels (solid bars) whilst (B) shows the IgE percentage change from pre. Dashed line delineates greater than 50% change.

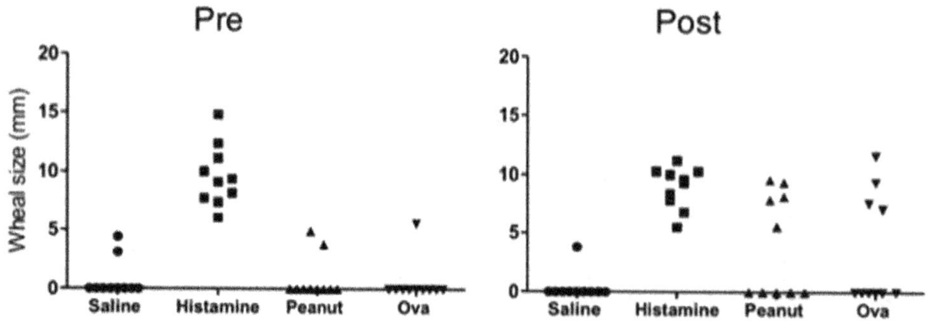


**Figure 4. Skin wheal responses before and after allergen sensitisation.** Mean wheal reaction size measured at 30 minutes post injection in Study 1 (n = 10). Saline alone served as a negative and histamine as a positive control.

we used sheep as a model to characterise humoral and cellular immune responses after sensitisation with HDM extract and reported sensitisation rates of 50–60% [32], a rate similar to that seen in the present study using PN as the allergen. Comparing the sensitisation responses to PN and HDM allergen in the present study, we found that strong HDM-specific IgE responders were also positive for PN-specific IgE. This is in agreement with human studies, where it has been found that patients with asthma show an increased likelihood of sensitivity to other allergens including food allergens [33]. In individuals who experience anaphylaxis, a large proportion also display an asthmatic phenotype [7,12,34,35] indicating a strong association (genetic predisposition) between these conditions.

The effects of sensitisation with PN allergen were also compared to ovalbumin (OVA), a common antigen used in murine allergy studies. In stark contrast to PN allergen, it was shown that OVA had a poor capacity for specific IgE induction (10% of immunised animals); this finding is supported in our own subsequent studies with 7 out of 76 animals showing Ova-specific IgE after sensitisation (Bischof *et al*, unpublished data). The discordance in the allergic response to PN compared with OVA may be due to inherent structural/protein differences between PN and OVA since it is well documented that peanuts have strong allergenic properties compared to other proteins. PN-induced allergic reactions are more severe compared to other food allergies [36] and are also a principal cause of IgE-mediated food allergy in humans, resolving infrequently and remaining a major source of morbidity in approximately 80% of allergic patients [2]. Interestingly, the present study showed that OVA immunisations result in elevated total OVA-specific Ig levels (80% of animals), despite the poor induction of OVA-specific IgE. Treatment success in immunotherapy trials is accompanied by increased IgG levels [37], suggesting that allergen-specific IgG may be able to block IgE-mediated reactions. Support for this was found in a murine model that showed antigen-specific IgG can block IgE mediated reactions through direct competition and signalling via the inhibitory IgG receptor FcγRIIb [38]. We showed in the present study that sheep can be sensitised concurrently with several food allergens (PN and OVA) and display differing levels of sensitivity/reactivity to these allergens, similar to previous studies in a dog model of food allergy [22].

In the present study we report that 2 of the 10 sheep tested showed a positive intradermal skin test to PN allergen at baseline (before PN sensitisation). False positive skin allergen tests have also been documented in other animal studies [20], as well as with human patients [4]. The existence of common carbohydrate cross-reactive determinants between PN-specific allergens and natural 'environmental' allergens may provide an explanation for the occurrence of false positive allergen sensitivity tests [39,40]. Similarly, this may account for the revelation that 2 animals showed basal IgE reactivity to the peanut allergen Ara h1. In the clinical setting, intradermal skin tests for food allergy at times display poor specificity; positive skin reactions routinely require confirmation using other methods including blood testing or, where appropriate, food challenge [4].

A distinct advantage of large animals is their outbred status, which translates into a similar diversity of responses as seen in humans. The sheep model of PN allergy outlined here relies on sensitisation through subcutaneous injections of allergen in adjuvant (aluminium hydroxide), a protocol used widely in a range of animal models of allergy to induce significant levels of sensitisation and allow relevant studies on disease progression and responses to allergen provocation. While sensitisation to food allergens such as peanut is thought to principally occur via the oral route, other modes of sensitisation are likely, including respiratory and dermal routes [41].

Animal models have served to increase our understanding of the mechanisms responsible for allergy and have the potential to facilitate the development of safer therapeutic approaches. This study describes a new large animal model of peanut allergy that shows systemic IgE-responsiveness to peanut allergen and provides a robust system for investigative studies on allergen-associated immune mechanisms.

## Author Contributions

Conceived and designed the experiments: JVG MDV RO EM RB. Performed the experiments: JVG RB. Analyzed the data: JVG MDV EM RB. Contributed reagents/materials/analysis tools: RO EM RB. Wrote the paper: JVG MDV RO EM RB.

## References

1. Boyce JA, Assa'ad A, Burks AW, Jones SM, Sampson HA, et al. (2010) Guidelines for the diagnosis and management of food allergy in the United States: report of the NIAID-sponsored expert panel. Journal of Allergy & Clinical Immunology 126: S1–58.
2. Otsu K, Dreskin SC (2011) Peanut Allergy: An Evolving Clinical Challenge. Discovery Medicine 12: 319–328.
3. Kawakami T, Galli SJ (2002) Regulation of mast-cell and basophil function and survival by IgE. Nature Reviews Immunology 2: 773–786.

4. Loza C, Brostoff J (1995) Peanut Allergy. Clinical & Experimental Allergy 25: 493–502.
5. Comeau MR, Ziegler SF (2010) The influence of TSLP on the allergic response. Mucosal Immunology 3: 138–147.
6. Valenta R, Ball T, Focke M, Linhart B, Mothes N, et al. (2004) Immunotherapy of Allergic Disease. Advances in Immunology 82: 105–153.
7. Wang J, Sampson HA (2007) Food anaphylaxis. Clinical & Experimental Allergy 37: 651–660.
8. Osborne NJ, Koplin JJ, Martin PE, Gurrin LC, Lowe AJ, et al. (2011) Prevalance of challenge-proven IgE-mediated food allergy using population-based sampling and predetermined challenge criteria in infants. Journal of Allergy & Clinical Immunology 127: 668–676.
9. Prioult G, Nagler-Anderson C (2005) Mucosal immunity and allergic responses: lack of regulation and/or lack of microbial stimulation? Immunological Reviews 206: 204–218.
10. Morar N, Willis-Owen SAG, Moffatt MF, Cookson WOCM (2006) The genetics of atopic dermatitis. Journal of Allergy & Clinical Immunology 118: 24–34.
11. de Leon MP, Rolland JM, O'Hehir RE (2007) The peanut allergy epidemic: allergen molecular characterisation and prospects for specific therapy. Expert Reviews in Molecular Medicine 9: 1–18.
12. Pumphrey RSH (2000) Lessons for management of anaphylaxis from a study of fatal reactions. Clinical & Experimental Allergy 30: 1144–1150.
13. Sicherer SH, Sampson HA (2010) Food Allergy. Journal of Allergy & Clinical Immunology 125: S116–S125.
14. Burks AW, Williams LW, Helm RM, Connaughton C, Cockrell G, et al. (1991) Identification of a major peanut allergen, Ara h I, in patients with atopic dermatitis and positive peanut challenges. Journal of Allergy & Clinical Immunology 88: 172–179.
15. Burks AW, Williams LW, Connaughton C, Cockrell G, O'Brien TJ, et al. (1992) Identification and characterization of a second major peanut allergen, Ara h II, with use of sera of patients with atopic dermatitis and positive peanut challenge. Journal of Allergy & Clinical Immunology 90: 962–969.
16. Burks AW, Cockrell G, Stanley JS, Helm RM, Bannon GA (1995) Recombinant peanut allergen Ara h I expression and IgE binding in patients with peanut hypersensitivity. The Journal of Clinical Investigation 96: 1715–1721.
17. Palmer GW, Dibbern Jr DA, Burks AW, Bannon GA, Bock SA, et al. (2005) Comparative potency of Ara h 1 and Ara h 2 in immunochemical and functional assays of allergenicity. Clinical Immunology 115: 302–312.
18. de Leon MP, Drew AC, Glaspole IN, Suphioglu C, O'Hehir RE, et al. (2007) IgE cross-reactivity between the major peanut allergen Ara h 2 and tree nut allergens. Molecular Immunology 44: 463–471.
19. Koppelman SJ, Wensing M, Ertmann M, Knulst AC, Knol EF (2004) Relevance of Ara h1, Ara h2 and Ara h3 in peanut-allergic patients, as determined by immunoglobulin E Western blotting, basophil-histamine release and intracutaneous testing: Ara h2 is the most important peanut allergen. Clinical & Experimental Allergy 34: 583–590.
20. Helm RM, Furuta GT, Stanley JS, Ye J, Cockrell G, et al. (2002) A neonatal swine model for peanut allergy. Journal of Allergy & Clinical Immunology 109: 136–142.
21. Li X-M, Serebrisky D, Lee S-Y, Huang C-K, Bardina L, et al. (2000) A murine model of peanut anaphylaxis: T- and B-cell responses to a major peanut allergen mimic human responses. Journal of Allergy & Clinical Immunology 106: 150–158.
22. Teuber SS, del Val G, Morigasaki S, Jung HR, Eisele PH, et al. (2002) The atopic dog as a model of peanut and tree nut food allergy. Journal of Allergy & Clinical Immunology 110: 921–927.
23. Morafo V, Srivastava K, Huang C-K, Kleiner G, Lee S-Y, et al. (2003) Genetic susceptibility to food allergy is linked to differential $T_H2$-$T_H1$ responses in C3H/HeJ and BALB/c mice. Journal of Allergy & Clinical Immunology 111: 1122–1128.
24. Fischer R, McGhee JR, Vu HL, Atkinson TP, Jackson RJ, et al. (2005) Oral and nasal sensitization promote distinct immune responses and lung reactivity in a mouse model of peanut allergy. American Journal of Pathology 167: 1621–1630.
25. Ermel RW, Kock M, Griffey SM, Reinhart GA, Frick OL (1997) The atopic dog: a model for food allergy. Laboratory Animal Science 47: 40–49.
26. Bischof RJ, Snibson K, Shaw R, Meeusen ENT (2003) Induction of allergic inflammation in the lungs of sensitized sheep after local challenge with house dust mite. Clinical & Experimental Allergy 33: 367–375.
27. Meeusen EN, Snibson KJ, Hirst SJ, Bischof RJ (2009) Sheep as a model species for the study and treatment of human asthma and other respiratory diseases. Drug Discovery Today: Disease Models 6: 101–106.
28. de Leon MP, Glaspole IN, Drew AC, Rolland JM, O'Hehir RE, et al. (2003) Immunological analysis of allergenic cross-reactivity between peanut and tree nuts. Clinical & Experimental Allergy 33: 1273–1280.
29. De Jong EC, Van Zijverden M, Spanhaak S, Koppelman SJ, Pellegrom H, et al. (1998) Identification and partial characterization of multiple major allergens in peanut proteins. Clinical & Experimental Allergy 28: 743–751.
30. Prickett SR, Voskamp AL, Dacumos-Hill A, Symons K, Rolland JM, et al. (2011) Ara h 2 peptides containing dominant CD4+ T-cell epitopes: Candidates for a peanut allergy therapeutic. Journal of Allergy & Clinical Immunology 127: 608–615.
31. Shaw RJ, McNeill MM, Gatehouse TK, Douch PGC (1997) Quantification of total sheep IgE concentration using anti-ovine IgE monoclonal antibodies in an enzyme immunoassay. Veterinary Immunology and Immunopathology 57: 253–265.
32. Bischof RJ, Snibson KJ, Van Der Velden J, Meeusen ENT (2008) Immune response to allergens in sheep sensitized to house dust mite. Journal of Inflammation 5: 16.
33. Gillman A, Douglass JA (2010) What do asthmatics have to fear from food and additive allergy? Clinical & Experimental Allergy 40:1295–1302.
34. Sampson HA, Mendelson L, Rosen JP (1992) Fatal and near-fatal anaphylactic reactions to food in children and adolescents. The New England Journal of Medicine 327: 380–384.
35. Bock S, Munoz-Furlong A, Sampson HA (2001) Fatalities due to anaphylactic reactions to foods. Journal of Allergy & Clinical Immunology 107: 191–193.
36. Breiteneder H, Clare Mills EN (2005) Plant food allergens - structural and functional aspects of allergenicity. Biotechnology Advances 23: 395–399.
37. Lack G, Nelson HS, Amran D, Oshiba A, Jung T, et al. (1997) Rush Immunotherapy results in allergen-specific alterations in lymphocyte function and interferon-$\gamma$ production in $CD4^+$ T cells. Journal of Allergy & Clinical Immunology 99: 530–538.
38. Strait RT, Morris SC, Finkelman FD (2006) IgG-blocking antibodies inhibit IgE-mediated anaphylaxis in vivo through both antigen interception and Fc$\gamma$RIIb cross-linking. The Journal of Clinical Investigation 116: 833–841.
39. Aalberse RC, Koshte V, Clemens JG (1981) Immunoglobulin E antibodies that crossreact with vegetable foods, pollen, and *Hymenoptera* venom. Journal of Allergy & Clinical Immunology 68: 356–364.
40. Sicherer SH (2001) Clinical implications of cross-reactive food allergens. Journal of Allergy & Clinical Immunology 108: 881–890.
41. Lack G, Fox D, Northstone K, Golding J (2003) Factors associated with the development of peanut allergy in childhood. The New England Journal of Medicine 348: 977–985.

9

# High Prevalence of Lipid Transfer Protein Sensitization in Apple Allergic Patients with Systemic Symptoms

**Francisca Gomez[1☯], Ana Aranda[2☯], Paloma Campo[1], Araceli Diaz-Perales[3], Natalia Blanca-Lopez[4], James Perkins[2], Maria Garrido[3], Miguel Blanca[1], Cristobalina Mayorga[1,2¶], Maria José Torres[1*¶]**

**1** Allergy Service, IBIMA, Regional University Hospital of Malaga, UMA, Malaga, Spain, **2** Research Laboratory, IBIMA, Regional University Hospital of Malaga, UMA, Malaga, Spain, **3** Biotechnology Department, Center for Plant Biotechnology and Genomics, Pozuelo de Alarcon, Madrid, Spain, **4** Allergy Service, Infanta Leonor Hospital, Madrid, Spain

## Abstract

***Background:*** Apple allergy manifests as two main groups of clinical entities reflecting different patterns of allergen sensitization: oral allergy syndrome (OAS) and generalized symptoms (GS).

***Objective:*** We analysed the sensitization profile to a wide panel of different components of food allergens (rMal d 1, Mal d 2, rMal d 3, rMal d 4, rPru p 3, rBet v 1 and Pho d 2) for a population of Mediterranean patients with OAS and GS to apple.

***Methods:*** Patients (N = 81) with a history of apple allergy that could be confirmed by positive prick-prick test and/or double-blind-placebo-controlled food challenge (DBPCFC), were included. Skin prick test (SPT) and ELISA were performed using a panel of inhalant, fruit and nut allergens. ELISA and ELISA inhibition studies were performed in order to analyse the sensitization patterns.

***Results:*** Thirty-five cases (43.2%) had OAS and 46 (56.8%) GS. SPT showed a significantly higher number of positive results with peach, cherry and hazelnut in those with GS. ELISA showed a significantly high percentage of positive cases to rMal d 3, rMal d 4, rPru p 3 and Pho d 2 in patients with OAS and GS compared to controls, and to rBet v 1 in patients with OAS vs controls and between OAS and GS patients. Three different patterns of recognition were detected: positive to LTP (rMal d 3 or rPru p 3), positive to profilin (rMal d 4 and Pho d 2), or positive to both. There were also patients with rMal d 1 recognition who showed cross-reactivity to rBet v 1.

***Conclusion:*** In an apple allergy population with a high incidence of pollinosis different patterns of sensitization may occur. LTP is most often involved in those with GS. Profilin, though more prevalent in patients with OAS, has been shown to sensitise patients with both types of symptoms.

**Editor:** Simon Patrick Hogan, Cincinnati Children's Hospital Medical Center, University of Cincinnati College of Medicine, United States of America

**Funding:** The study was funded by the FIS-Thematic Networks and Co-operative Research Centres: RIRAAF (RD07/0064) and ISCIII PI12/02481. The funders had no role in study design, data collection and analysis, decision to publish, or preparation of the manuscript.

**Competing Interests:** The authors have declared that no competing interests exist.

* Email: mjtorresj@gmail.com

☯ These authors contributed equally to this work.

¶ These authors also contributed equally to this work.

## Introduction

In adults and older children Rosacea fruits are the plant foods most often responsible for allergic reactions [1–3]. Of these, apple allergy is a prevalent entity in Central and Northern Europe and the sensitization pattern has been studied in detail [4,5]. Although also important in Southern Europe, it is less frequent and has thus received less attention [1,6,7]. Four apple allergens have been identified so far: Mal d 1, a pathogenesis-related protein (PR-10) [8]; Mal d 2, a thaumatin-like protein (TLP) [9]; Mal d 3, a lipid transfer protein (LTP) [10]; and Mal d 4, a profilin [11].

Two major groups of entities have been described according to the patterns of allergen sensitization [1,4–7]: oral allergy syndrome (OAS) and generalized symptoms (GS) that include urticaria and anaphylaxis. In Central and Northern Europe, apple sensitization has been associated with initial sensitization to an aeroallergen, with Betula pollen allergen the most often involved [4,5,7]. Patients sensitized to Bet v 1 also respond to Mal d 1 because of the structural homology [4,5,7]. In fact, over 60% of Betula sensitized patients have mild symptoms after apple ingestion, usually OAS [4,5,7]. By contrast, in Southern European countries, apple allergic patients more frequently have GS, no association with Betula sensitization and cross-reactions to other fruits, especially peach [1,6,7,12]. In this situation peach LTP, Pru p 3, is the strongest candidate for these sensitizations [1,6,7,12]. Moreover, atopic patients allergic to peach and apple may have OAS in an environment where the prevalence of Betula pollen sensitization is low. In this situation, profilin is an important sensitizer [13–15].

As mentioned earlier, in the Mediterranean area, the origin of apple allergy is generally attributed to LTP sensitization [1,6,7,12], although the relevance of sensitization to other allergens has not yet been fully established, particularly for patients with pollen allergy. Therefore OAS can be caused both by labile (such as PR-10 and profilins), as well as stable allergens (such as LTPs), whereas systemic symptoms are associated with the latter and seldom with labile allergens. The aim of this study was to undertake a detailed analysis of allergen sensitization profiles in an important number of patients diagnosed as allergic to apple from a Mediterranean population. A clinical questionnaire was used to record the allergic response or tolerance to other fruits and vegetables. Inhibition ELISA was performed using the four apple allergens identified, as well as other important related allergens such as rBet v 1, rPru p 3 and Pho d 2 (equivalent to rMal d 1, rMal d 3 and rMal d 4, respectively).

## Materials and Methods

### Patients and controls

Patients referred to the Allergy Unit of Malaga Hospital (south of Spain area) with a history of apple allergy that could be confirmed by positive prick-prick test and/or double-blind-placebo-controlled food challenge (DBPCFC), were included. Patients were classified according to symptoms: OAS when they were restricted to the skin or mucosal sites of direct contact with the allergen (itching of the oral mucosa and lips with or without angioedema immediately after eating apple), and GS when reactions involved organs far from the site of initial contact with the food (urticaria, with or without angioedema, and anaphylaxis) accompanied or not to OAS. A control group, from the same geographical area, comprised 25 non-allergic subjects with tolerance to apple. All participants completed a written informed consent and the ethical committee of our institution approved the study (CEI Provincial of Malaga).

### Diagnostic work-up

The allergological evaluation included an examination of the patient's clinical history, a detailed questionnaire, skin test, specific IgE determination and DBPCFC.

The skin test was performed according to European guidelines [16] using Golden Delicious apples for the prick-prick technique with peel and pulp tested separately, and by SPT using commercialized extract from *Phleum*, *Olea*, *Betula*, *Platanus*, *Cupressus*, *Parietaria* and *Artemisia* pollen and apple, peach, cherry and hazelnut from ALK-Abelló (Madrid, Spain). The SPT response was considered positive if the diameter of the wheal area was 3 mm greater than that induced by the negative control.

Specific IgE antibodies to apple were measured by Immuno-CAP following the manufacturers recommendations (Phadia, Uppsala, Sweden). A positive result was defined as a value > 0.35 kUA/l.

DBPCFC was performed as described [17], except in cases with a recent history (<1 year) of anaphylaxis after apple ingestion and SPT positive to apple. Briefly, meals containing 5, 40, and 120 g of fresh ground apple with a mixture of yogurt, orange juice, coffee dried, and oatmeal flakes were freshly prepared 5 minutes before administration to prevent the loss of allergenicity. Placebo meals consisted of the same ingredients, without fresh apple. If cutaneous and/or respiratory symptoms or alterations in vital signs appeared, the procedure was stopped and the symptoms were evaluated and treated.

### Purification and quality controls

The LTPs was purified following the method previous published by Diaz-Perales [18]. Briefly, LTP was purified from defatted peel peach or apple fruit by RP-HPLC on a Vydac-C4 column (22×250 mm; particle size 10 mm; The Separations Group, Hesperia, CA, USA), followed by RP-HPLC Nucleosil 300-C4 column (8×250 mm; particle size 5 mm; Sugelabor, Madrid, Spain). Finally, proteins were analyzed by mass spectrometry, SDS-PAGE and immunoblotting.

Mal d 2 was purified from apple fruit by cation-exchange chromatography on a Bio-ScaleTM Mini Macro-Preps High S

**Table 1.** Comparison of demographic and clinical characteristics of the patients evaluated with OAS and GS. Statistical significance is indicated (P).

| CHARACTERISTICS | OAS N = 35 | GS N = 46 | P |
|---|---|---|---|
| **Age in years (median, IR)** | 30 (24–38) | 32 (25–39) | 0.583 |
| **Sex (N, % female)** | 25 (71.42) | 37 (80.43) | 0.430 |
| **Apple prick by prick positive (N, %)** | 27 (77.14) | 41 (89.13) | 0.145 |
| **Apple commercial skin test positive (N, %)** | 20 (57.14) | 35 (76.08) | 0.094 |
| **Specific IgE to apple (N,%)** | 27 (77.14) | 38 (82.60) | 0.072 |
| **Pollen sensitization (N, %)** | 31 (88.57) | 40 (86.95) | 0.553 |
| **Pollen allergy (N, %)** | 26 (74.28) | 28 (60.86) | 0.151 |
| **Foods involved (N, %)** | | | 0.399 |
| Peach | 32 (91.42) | 45 (97.82) | |
| Hazelnut | 13 (37.14) | 17 (36.95) | |
| **Age at symptom onset in years (median, IR)** | | | |
| Pollen | 18 (5.75–32.25) | 15 (8.25–24.25 | 0.690 |
| Apple | 19 (12.75–29.52) | 15 (11–26) | 0.252 |
| Peach | 15 (11–26) | 14 (9.25–24.52) | 0.383 |
| Hazelnut | 23 (16–31) | 15 (12.25–24.75) | 0.151 |

**Table 2.** Skin test results to inhalant and food allergens in patients with OAS and GS. Statistical significance is indicated (P).

| ALLERGEN SOURCE | OAS N (%) | GS N (%) | P |
|---|---|---|---|
| *Phleum* pollen | 24 (68.57) | 25 (54.34) | 0.340 |
| *Olea* pollen | 27 (77.14) | 27 (58.69) | 0.204 |
| *Betula* pollen | 16 (45.71) | 14 (30.43) | 0.220 |
| *Platanus* pollen | 17 (48.57) | 27 (58.69) | 0.476 |
| *Cupressus* pollen | 20 (57.14) | 21 (45.62) | 0.474 |
| *Parietaria* pollen | 15 (42.85) | 23 (50) | 0.636 |
| *Artemisia* pollen | 14 (40) | 21 (45.62) | 0.811 |
| Peach | 13 (37.14) | 33 (71.73) | **0.004** |
| Cherry | 10 (28.57) | 24 (52.17) | **0.05** |
| Hazelnut | 8 (22.85) | 24 (52.17) | **0.016** |

column (BioRad, Hercules,CA, USA). Following this, its purity and reactivity was analyzed by mass spectrometry, SDS-PAGE and immunoblotting.

rMal d 1 and Pho d 2 was obtained from Biomay (Vienna, Austria) and ALK-Abello (Madrid, Spain), respectively.

rMal d 4 was prepared using the protocol described by Scheurer S [19]. Briefly, the protein was cloned by polymerase chain reaction and produced in *Escherichia coli* BL21. The profilin was purified as non-fusion proteins by affinity chromatography on poly-(L-proline)-Sepharose and its purity and IgE reactivity was analyzed by SDS-PAGE and immunoblotting.

rBet v 1 was produced in *Escherichia coli* BL21 (DE3). This protein was purified under denaturing conditions from inclusion bodies and subsequently subjected to Immobilized Metal Affinity Chromatography (IMAC) followed by ion-exchange chromatography (IEC). Finally, His-Tagged rBet v 1 was analyzed by SDS PAGE and Immunoblotting using an anti-His-Tag antibody, anti-Bet v 1 monoclonal antibody and sera from patients with IgE-reactivity to Bet v 1.

## Specific IgE and inhibition studies by ELISA

ELISA assays were performed as described [18]. Costar plates (Corning, NY, USA) were coated with 5 μg/mL of rMal d 1 (Biomay, Vienna, Austria), Mal d 2, rMal d 3 and rPru p 3 (Dra Díaz-Perales, Polytechnical University of Madrid), rMal d 4 and rBet v 1 (Dr Vieths, Paul-Ehrlich Institut) and Pho d 2 (ALK-Abelló). After, the plates were blocked with blocking solution (Sigma, St. Louis,USA) for 1 h. Individual serum from patients and controls at 1:5 dilution was added to each well. We used two negative controls, a pool of sera from non-allergic subjects and blocking buffer, and as positive controls we used patients sera with known specific IgE to proteins. The assay was completed with rabbit anti-human IgE antibody (1:3000, DAKO, Denmark) conjugated to horseradish peroxidase (HRP). IgE binding was detected using o-phenylenediamine (OPD, DAKO). Results are expressed as absorbance units, measured at 490 nm. They were considered positive when >0.18 (mean OD + 3xSD to blocking).

For ELISA inhibition, sera were pre-incubated with different inhibitors (rMal d 3, rMal d 4, rPru p 3, Pho d 2) at final concentrations of 20, 2, and 0.2 μg/mL or with phosphate buffer for the non-inhibited serum for 3 h at room temperature. Subsequently, the inhibitor mixtures were added to plates coated

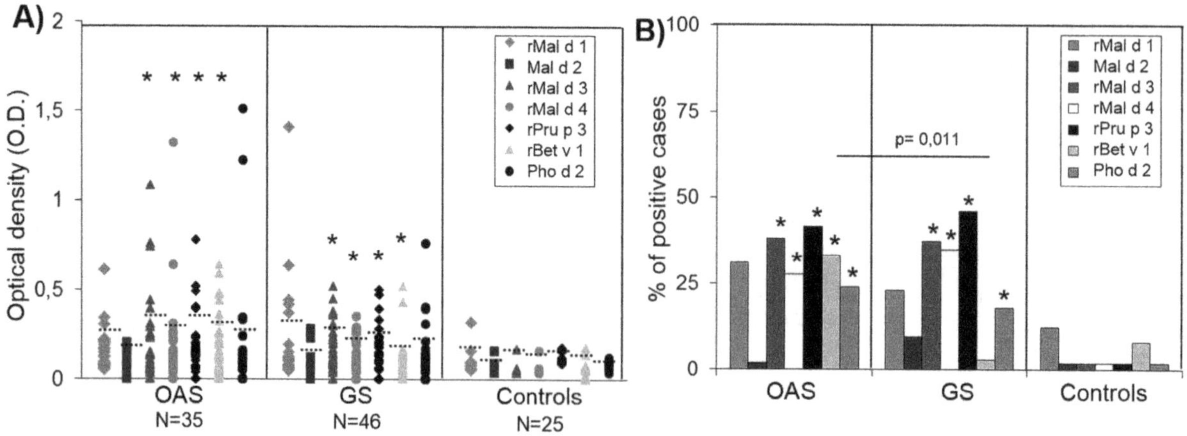


**Figure 1. ELISA results to allergens (Mal d 1, Mal d 2, rMal d 3, rMal d 4, rPru p 3, rBet v 1 and Pho d 2) in sera from patients with OAS (N = 35) and GS (N = 46) and a control group with tolerance to apple (N = 25).** (**A**) Results are expressed as individual O.D. values and median represented as a dotted line. (**B**) Results are expressed as the percentage of positive cases. (*p<0.05) represents a significant difference compared to healthy controls.

**Table 3.** Percentages of ELISA positive cases combining allergens from LTP and profilin family in patients allergic to apple with OAS or GS.

| GROUPS | PATTERN SENSITIZATION | OAS | GENERALIZED | P |
|---|---|---|---|---|
| 1 | LTP | 10 (28.57%) | 16 (34.78%) | 0.635 |
| 2 | PROFILIN | 8 (22.85%) | 7 (15.21%) | 0.402 |
| 3 | LTP-PROFILIN | 1 (2.85%) | 11 (23.91%) | **0.010** |
| 4 | Negative | 16 (45.71%) | 12 (26.08%) | 0.098 |

with rMal d 3, rMal d 4, rPru p 3 or Pho d 2, followed by the ELISA protocol described above.

To analyse the sensitization of patients positive to rMal d 1 and rBet v 1, sera from specific IgE positive patients were pre-incubated with rMal d 1, Mal d 2, rMal d 3, rMal d 4 and rBet v 1 and added in solid phases with rMal d 1 and rBet v 1.

Percentage inhibition of IgE binding was calculated as follows: % Inhibition = (serum not inhibited-serum inhibited/serum not inhibited) x100.

### Statistical studies

Quantitative variables are shown as medians and interquartile ranges (IR), while qualitative variables are shown as frequencies. Medians between groups were compared using Mann-Whitney or Kruskal-Wallis tests, while $\chi^2$ was used to compare proportions. Differences with a $p<0.05$ were considered significant.

## Results

### Patient characteristics

The study included 81 patients with a diagnosis of hypersensitivity to apple. Their median age was 31 (IR:25–38) years and 62 (76.44%) were female. Thirty-five patients (43.20%) had OAS and 46 (56.79%) had GS (22 anaphylaxis (47.82%) and 24 (52.12%) urticaria). Sixty-eight cases (83.95%) showed positive prick by prick skin tests with apple peel and pulp and 55 (67.90%) positive skin test with the commercial extract for 77.14% of cases tested using prick by prick and for 57.14% with skin test. In GS patients we found that 76.08% showed skin test positivity with commercial extract and 89.13% with prick by prick. Moreover, we did not find any patient who was positive with commercial extracts and negative with prick by prick. In addition, 65 (80.24%) had serum specific IgE to apple and 62 a positive DBPCFC to apple. DBPCFC was not performed in 19 cases who had recent apple-related anaphylaxis (<1 year) and a positive skin test to apple.

Seventy-one (87.65%) were sensitized to pollen and from these 54 (76.05%) had clinical symptoms consisting of rhinitis and/or asthma; 77 (95.06%) presented symptoms with peach and 31 (38.27%) with hazelnut. The median age at symptom onset was 15 (IR:10–25) years to peach, 17 (IR:11–27) to apple, 17.5 (IR:7.75–25) to pollen and 18 (IR:13–25) to hazelnut.

Comparisons between patients with OAS and GS (Table 1) showed that although the percentage of cases with a positive SPT and specific IgE to apple was higher in those with GS, there were no significant differences between the groups in any of the variables evaluated.

Comparisons of clinical symptoms between patients with (N = 54, 66.66%) and without pollen allergy (N = 27, 33.33%) showed that in those with pollen allergy 24 (44.44%) developed GS and 30 (55.55%) OAS, whereas in those without pollen allergy, 18 (66.66%) developed GS and 9 (33.33%) OAS (Data not shown).

### Skin prick test results

Analysis of the SPT showed that 49 (60.49%) cases were positive to *Phleum*, 54 (66.67%) to *Olea*, 30 (65.22%) to *Betula*, 44 (54.32%) to *Platanus*, 41 (50.62%) to *Cupressus*, 38 (46.91%) to *Parietaria*, 35 (43.21%) to *Artemisa*, 46 (56.79%) to peach, 34 (41.97%) to cherry and 32 (39.51%) to hazelnut. Comparison between patients with OAS and those with GS showed a significantly higher percentage of positive results only with peach, cherry and hazelnut in those with GS (Table 2).

### Specific IgE results by ELISA

Comparisons of specific IgE determinations (Figure 1A) in OAS, GS, and controls showed significant differences between the three groups for rMal d 3 ($p<0.001$), rMal d 4 ($p<0.001$), rPru p 3 ($p = 0.015$) and rBet v 1 ($p = 0.02$). In more detail, there was an increase in levels of IgE to four allergens in OAS when compared to controls (rMal d 3: $p<0.001$, rMal d 4: $p<0.001$, rPru p 3: $p = 0.007$, and rBet v 1: 0.010) and in GS compared to controls (rMal d 3: $p<0.001$, rMal d 4: $p = 0.001$, rPru p 3: $p = 0.013$, and rBet v 1: $p = 0.041$), with no differences between OAS and GS. Comparisons in terms of positive percentage (Figure 1B) showed significant differences between OAS and controls for rMal d 3 ($p = 0.036$), rMal d 4 ($p = 0.042$), rPru p 3 ($p = 0.009$), rBet v 1 ($p = 0.038$) and Pho d 2 ($p = 0.021$) and between GS and controls for rMal d 3 ($p = 0.005$), rMal d 4 ($p = 0.009$), rPru p 3 ($p = 0.007$) and Pho d 2 ($p = 0.045$). Moreover, rBet v 1 was higher in OAS compared to GS ($p = 0.011$).

### Sensitization frequencies to apple allergens

We detected that 27% of the patients recognized Mal d 1, 5% to Mal d 2, 37% to Mal d 3 and 30% to Mal d 4. When we analyzed the sensitization percentages taking into account symptoms we observed no significant differences between OAS and GS. In patients with OAS, 31% of them had specific IgE to Mal d 1, 2% to Mal d 2, 38% to Mal d 3 and 28% to Mal d 4. In patients with GS, 23% had specific IgE to Mal d 1, 9% to Mal d 2, 37.50% to Mal d 3 and 35% to Mal d 4.

Based on the IgE response to allergens from LTP and profillin families, the patients were classified in three groups (Table 3): Group 1 (LTP pattern), positive to rMal d 3 and/or rPru p 3; Group 2 (Profilin pattern), positive to rMal d 4 and/or Pho d 2; and Group 3 (LTP-Profilin pattern), positive to both. We found a significant increase in the percentage of patients positive to LTP-profilin in the group with GS. Moreover, if we consider all those with an LTP response, regardless of the profilin results, there were 11 (31.42%) positive cases in the OAS group and 27 (58.69%) in the GS ($p = 0.024$). On the other hand, considering all those who were positive to profilin, regardless of the LTP results, 9 (25.71%) were positive in the OAS group and 18 (39.13%) in the GS group ($p = 0.240$).

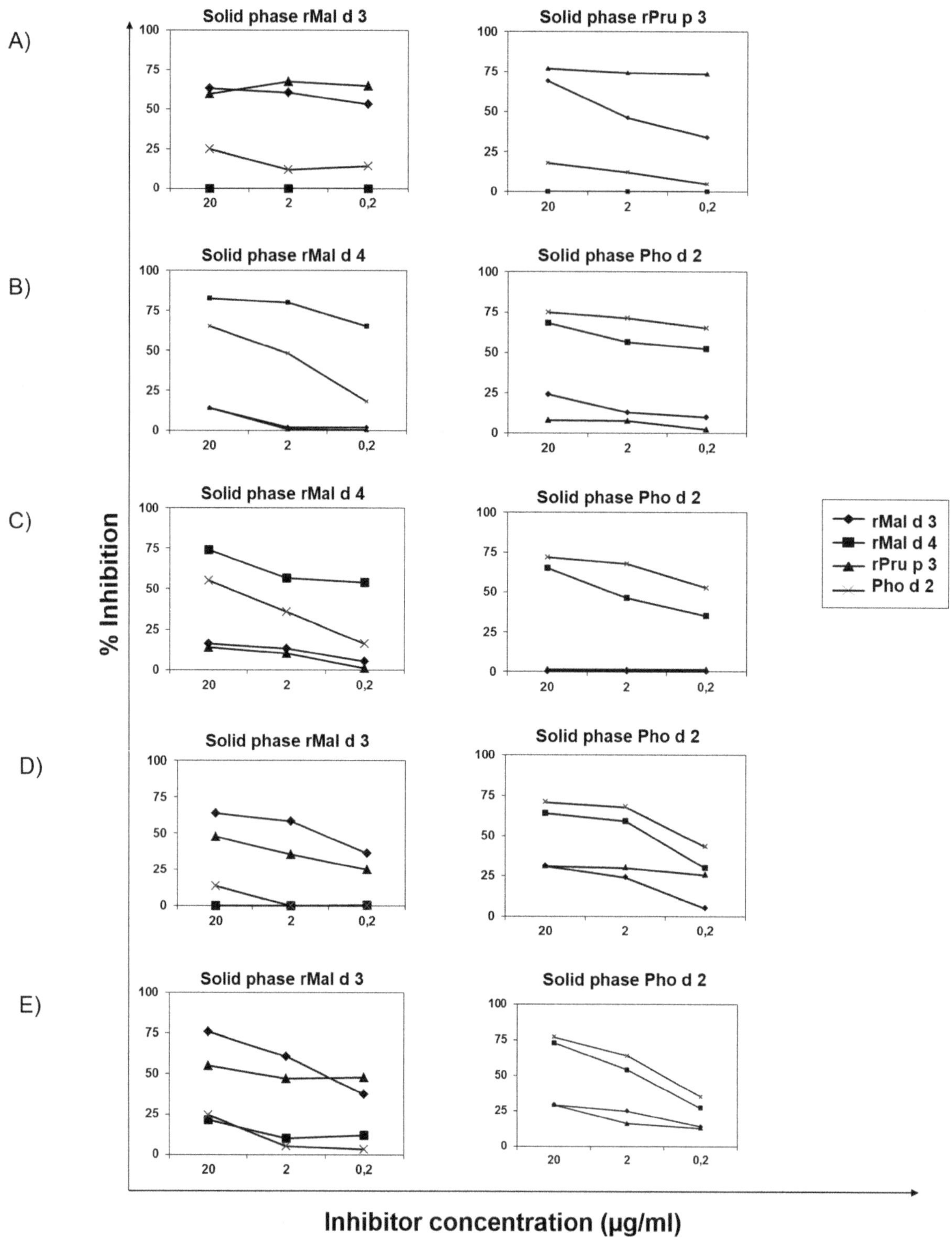


**Figure 2. ELISA Inhibition results using rMal d 3 and rPru p 3 in the solid phase for a representative case from Group 1 with GS (A); Mal d 4 and Pho d 2 in a representative case from Group 2 with OAS (B) and a case with GS (C); and Mal d 3 and Pho d 2 in a representative case from Group 3 with OAS (D) and a case with GS (E).** Sera were preincubated with decreasing concentrations (20–0.2 µg/ml) of rMal d 3, rMal d 4, rPru p 3, and Pho d 2, before they were added to the solid phase. Results are expressed as percentage inhibition.

## IgE recognition pattern to different allergens

ELISA inhibition was performed for all cases showing a sIgE level greater than 0.5 of O.D. Figure 2 shows the ELISA inhibition pattern for representative cases from each group of patients. Results from the Group 1, patients with GS, showed that using either rMal d 3 or rPru p 3 in the solid phase the strongest

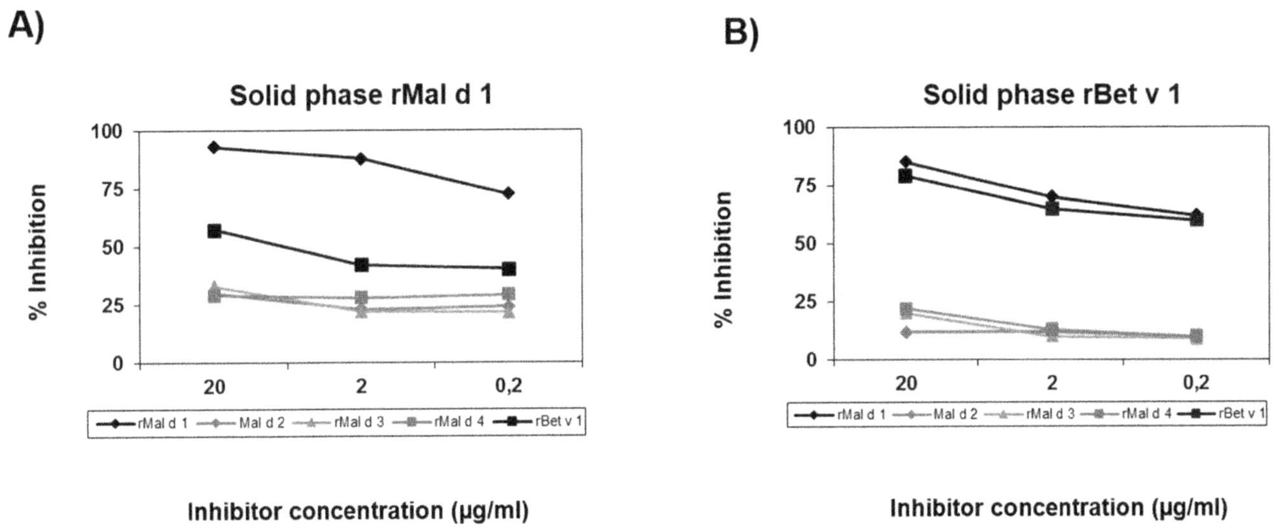


**Figure 3. ELISA Inhibition results using in the solid phase rMal d 1 (A) and rBet v 1 (B) with different concentrations (20–0.2 μg/ml) of rMal d 1, Mal d 2, rMal d 3, rMal d 4 and rBet v 1 in a representative OAS patient with high recognition of Betv1.**

inhibitor was rPru p 3, followed by rMal d 3, with no inhibition by the other allergens (Figure 2A).

In Group 2, patients with either OAS or GS, using rMal d 4 in the solid phase, the highest inhibition was found with itself followed by Pho d 2; similar results were seen using Pho d 2 in the solid phase (Figure 2B and C).

Figures 2D and 2E show sera from Group 3 for patients with OAS or GS, respectively. In both cases, when using rMal d 3 in the solid phase the highest inhibition was found with rMal d 3 followed by rPru p 3. Using Pho d 2 in the solid phase we detected the highest inhibition with itself and rMal d 4.

In order to further analyse sensitization to Bet v 1 observed in the patients allergic to apple, ELISA inhibition studies were performed by analyzing the IgE recognition to the PR-10 proteins, rMal d 1 and rBet v 1 (Figure 3). Data showed that rMal d 1 was the most potent inhibitor regardless of the solid phase used (rMal d 1 or rBet v 1). However, rBet v 1 only showed high inhibition when the same allergen was used in the solid phase. Moreover, no inhibition was detected with Mal d 2, rMal d 3 or rMal d 4.

## Discussion

In this study we compared the sensitization pattern and IgE recognition for a wide panel of relevant purified proteins from inhalant and fruit allergens in a population of Mediterranean patients allergic to apple. Patients were selected based on a consistent clinical history, skin test, specific IgE and/or DBPCFC. Considering the clinical symptoms, in our population over 50% of patients developed GS, with almost half developing anaphylaxis. This is contrary to what occurs in Central and Northern European countries, where OAS is the most frequent clinical entity [2,3,5,7]. This case series differs from a previously published study of a Spanish population, which reported a lower percentage of patients with GS (35%) [7].

For patients with GS we found that 58.69% of cases had IgE antibodies to LTP (rMal d 3 or rPru p 3), independently of profilin sensitization; thus confirming previous data showing that proteins from the LTP family are the most relevant sensitizers in apple allergy in southern Europe [6,7,15,10,20,21]. Moreover, these patients had higher sensitization to peach, cherry and hazelnut, where LTPs are also relevant allergens [18,22], therefore confirming that in apple allergic patients, LTP sensitization is related with more severe symptoms [7].

Considering profilin sensitization (rMal d 4 and Pho d 2), we found that 38.06% of cases were positive to these allergens only, with no differences between patients with OAS and GS (22.85% and 15.21% of cases respectively). These results indicate that when all patients with apple allergy are analysed together the picture is more complex than previously thought [6,7], and that in some cases profilin may be the sole agent responsible for the symptoms. Nevertheless, our results are in agreement with some studies detecting a high association between profilin sensitization and OAS in peach and/or apple allergic patients [13,14,23].

Importantly, this study confirmed different patterns of IgE recognition through the use of detailed inhibition studies. Our data indicate the recognition of Mal d 3 with high cross-reactivity with Pru p 3 in those with LTP sensitization and of Mal d 4 with high cross-reactivity with Pho d 2 in those sensitized to profilin.

Another important point is that in our population 87.65% of all cases were sensitized to pollen with 76.05% of all cases having clinical symptoms of asthma or rhinitis. When we consider apple allergy in the context of pollen sensitization we found that those positive to these inhalant allergens had less severe symptoms as have been described by Pastorello in peach allergy where patients positive to Pru p 3 were significantly less likely to develop severe symptoms when also sensitised to Pru p 1 and Pru p 4 [23]. More specifically, among those with GS, 66.7% did not have pollen allergy compared to 44.6% who did have pollen allergy.

Although *Betula* is not normally encountered in our area we detected positive SPT to *Betula* pollen and specific IgE antibodies to Bet v 1 in 43.41% and 20.29% of cases, respectively, with no differences between patients with OAS and with GS. Differences were also observed between the *Betula* major allergen Bet v 1 and the homologous Mal d 1, with higher percentages of specific IgE antibodies in patients with OAS (33.32% and 31%, respectively) compared with GS (3% and 23.14%, respectively). These figures, although lower than those detected in central and northern Europe [7,24], are nevertheless higher than those previously detected in a Spanish population allergic to apple [7]. In our geographical area, people are not exposed to *Betula* and the clinical expression of this sensitization is not relevant. Other, *Betula* related species, such as such as hazel and oak from the Fagales order, have been shown to cause cross-reactivity in *Betula*-free areas [25,26]. However, in our study the inhibition results indicate that *Betula* recognition in our population could be due to cross-reactivity with Mal d 1, the latter being the primary sensitizer.

Finally, we detected a low frequency of Mal d 2 sensitization, 2% in those with OAS and 9% in those with GS. These results are similar to those detected throughout Europe [7,27,28].

Summarizing, we have analysed a population of patients with apple allergy and a high percentage of pollinosis. Within this population we have seen various patterns of sensitization, with LTP being the most prevalent sensitizer for patients with GS while profilin, though more prevalent for those with OAS, is an important sensitizer for patients with both type of symptoms. Moreover, Mal d 1 was also detected and associated with mild symptoms. All these results indicate that, given the different recognition patterns, it would be desirable to include profillin, LTP and also PR-10 allergens in routine diagnosis of apple allergic patients.

## Acknowledgments

We thank to Stefan Vieths (Paul-Ehrlich-Institut, Federal Institute for Vaccines and Biomedicines, Division of Allergology, Langen, Germany) for the provision of different allergens necessary for the study. We also thank Ian Johnstone for help with the English language version of the manuscript and Luisa Galindo for the technical assistance in the diagnostic studies.

## Author Contributions

Conceived and designed the experiments: MJT CM MB. Performed the experiments: AA CM ADP MG. Analyzed the data: AA CM. Contributed reagents/materials/analysis tools: MJT CM MB. Wrote the paper: MJT FG AA CM. Collected patients' sera: MJT FG NBL PC MB. Corrected the manuscript and suggested important contributions to define the final version: MJT CM JP MB.

## References

1. Cuesta Herranz J, Lazaro M, Figueredo E, Igea JM, Umpierrez A, et al. (2000). Allergy to plant derived fresh foods in a birch and ragweed free area. Clin Exp Allergy; 30: 1411–1416.
2. Kanny G, Moneret-Vautrin DA, Flabee J, Beaudouin E, Morisset M, et al. (2001). Population study of food allergy in France. J Allergy Clin Immunol; 108: 133–140.
3. Kivity S, Dunner K, Marian Y (1994). The pattern of food hypersensitivity in patients with onset after 10 years of age. Clin Exp Allergy; 24: 19–22.
4. Eriksson NE, Formgren H, Svenonius E (1982). Food hypersensitivity in patients with pollen allergy. Allergy; 37: 437–443.
5. Ortolani C, Ispano M, Pastorello EA, Bigi A, Ansaloni R (1988). The oral allergy syndrome. Ann Allergy; 61: 47–52.
6. Fernandez Rivas M, van Ree R, Cuevas M (1997). Allergy to Rosaceae fruits without related pollinosis. J Allergy Clin Immunol; 100: 728–733.
7. Fernandez Rivas M, Bolhaar S, Gonzalez-Mancebo E, Asero R, van Leeuwen A, et al. (2006). Apple allergy across Europe: How allergen sensitization profiles determine the clinical expression of allergies to plant foods. J Allergy Clin Immunol; 118: 481–488.
8. Vanek-Krebitz M, Hoffmann-Sommergruber K, Laimer da Camara Machado M, Susani M, Ebner C, et al. (1995). Cloning and sequencing of Mal d 1, the major allergen from apple (Malus domestica), and its immunological relationship to Bet v 1, the major birch pollen allergen. Biochem Biophys Res Commun; 214: 538–551.
9. Krebitz M, Wagner B, Ferreira F, Peterbauer C, Campillo N, et al. (2003). Plant-based heterologous expression of Mal d 2, a thaumatin-like protein and allergen of apple (*Malus domestica*), and its characterization as an antifungal protein. J Mol Biol; 329: 721–730.
10. Garcia-Selles FJ, Diaz-Perales A, Sanchez-Monge R, Alcántara M, Lombardero M, et al. (2002). Patterns of reactivity to lipid transfer proteins of plant foods and Artemisia pollen: an in vivo study. Int Arch Allergy Immunol; 128: 115–122.
11. Ma Y, Zuidmeerw L, Bohle B, Bolhaar ST, Gadermaier G, et al. (2006). Characterization of recombinant Mal d 4 and its application for component resolved diagnosis of apple allergy. Clin Exp Allergy; 36: 1087–1096.
12. González-Mancebo E, Fernández-Rivas M (2008). Outcome and safety of double-blind, placebo-controlled food challenges in 111 patients sensitized to lipid transfer proteins. J Allergy Clin Immunol; 121: 1507–1508.
13. Cuesta-Herranz J, Barber D, Blanco C, Cistero-Bahíma A, Crespo JF, et al. (2010). Differences among pollen-allergic patients with and without plant food allergy. Int Arch Allergy Immunol; 153: 182–192.
14. Asero R, Monsalve R, Barber D (2008). Profilin sensitization detected in the office by skin prick test: a study of prevalence and clinical relevance of profilin as a plant food allergen. Clin Exp Allergy; 38: 1033–1037.
15. Andersen MB, Hall S, Dragsted LO (2011). Identification of european allergy patterns to the allergen families PR-10, LTP, and profilin from Rosaceae fruits. Clin Rev Allergy Immunol; 41: 4–19.
16. Dreborg S, Frew A (1993). Allergen Standardization and skin tests. Allergy; 48: 49–54.
17. Bolhaar STHP, van de Weg WE, van Ree R, Gonzalez-Mancebo E, Zuidmeer L, et al. (2005). In vivo assessment with prick-to-prick testing and double-blind, placebo-controlled food challenge of allergenicity of apple cultivars. J Allergy Clin Immunol; 116: 1080–1086.
18. Diaz Perales, Lombardero M, Sánchez-Monge R, García-Selles FJ, Pernas M, et al. (2000). Lipid-transfer proteins as potential plant panallergens: cross-reactivity among proteins of Artemisia pollen, Castanea nut and Rosaceae fruits, with different IgE-binding capacities. Clin Exp Allergy; 30: 1403–1410.
19. Scheurer S, Wangorsch A, Nerkamp J, Skov PS, Ballmer-Weber B, et al. (2001).Cross-reactivity within the profilin panallergen family investigated by comparison of recombinant profilins from pear (Pyr c 4), cherry (Pru av 4) and celery (Api g 4) with birch pollen profilin Bet v 2. J Chromatogr B Biomed Sci Appl.; 756(1–2): 315–25.
20. Pastorello EA, Pravettoni V, Farioli L, Gonzalez-Mancebo E, Zuidmeer L, et al. (1999). Clinical role of a lipid transfer protein that acts as a new apple-specific allergen. J Allergy Clin Immunol; 104: 1099–1106.
21. Barber D, de la Torre F, Feo F, Florido F, Guardia P, et al. (2008). Understanding patient sensitization profiles in complex pollen areas: a molecular epidemiological study. Allergy; 63: 1550–1558.
22. Asero R, Mistrello G, Roncarolo D, de Vries SC, Gautier MF, et al. (2000). Lipid transfer protein: a pan-allergen in plant-derived foods that is highly resistant to pepsin digestion. Int Arch Allergy Immunol; 122: 20–32.
23. Pastorello EA, Farioli L, Pravettoni V, Scibilia J, Mascheri A, et al. (2011). Pru p 3-sensitised Italian peach-allergic patients are less likely to develop severe symptoms when also presenting IgE antibodies to Pru p 1 and Pru p 4. Int Arch Allergy Immunol; 156: 362–372.
24. Ebner C, Hirschwehr R, Bauer L, Breiteneder H, Valenta R, et al. (1995). Identification of allergens in fruits and vegetables: IgE cross-reactivities with the important birch pollen allergens Bet v 1 and Bet v 2 (birch profilin). J Allergy Clin Immunol; 95: 962–969.
25. Mari A, Wallner M, Ferreira F (2003). Fagales pollen sensitization in a birch-free area: a respiratory cohort survey using Fagales pollen extracts and birch recombinant allergens (rBet v 1, rBet v 2, rBet v 4). Clin Exp Allergy; 33: 1419–28.
26. Mari A (2001). Multiple pollen sensitization: a molecular approach to the diagnosis. Int Arch Allergy Immunol; 125: 57–65.
27. Palacin A, Tordesillas L, Gamboa P, Sanchez-Monge R, Cuesta-Herranz J, et al. (2010). Characterization of peach thaumatin-like proteins. Clin Exp Allergy; 40: 1422–1430.
28. Palacín A, Rivas LA, Gómez-Casado C, Aguirre J, Tordesillas L, et al. (2012). The involvement of thaumatin-like proteins in plant food cross-reactivity: a multicenter study using a specific protein microarray. PLoS One; (9): e44088.

# The Major Cow Milk Allergen Bos d 5 Manipulates T-Helper Cells Depending on Its Load with Siderophore-Bound Iron

**Franziska Roth-Walter[1], Luis F. Pacios[2], Cristina Gomez-Casado[2], Gerlinde Hofstetter[1], Georg A. Roth[3], Josef Singer[4], Araceli Diaz-Perales[2], Erika Jensen-Jarolim[1,4]***

**1** Comparative Medicine, Messerli Research Institute of the University of Veterinary Medicine Vienna, Medical University Vienna and University Vienna, Vienna, Austria, **2** Biotechnology Department, Center for Plant Biotechnology and Genomics, Technical University of Madrid, Madrid, Spain, **3** Department of Anesthesiology, General Intensive Care and Pain Medicine, Medical University of Vienna, Austria, **4** Comparative Immunology and Oncology, Department of Pathophysiology and Allergy Research, Center of Pathophysiology, Infectiology and Immunology, Medical University of Vienna, Vienna, Austria

## Abstract

The mechanisms of allergic sensitization to milk are still elusive. The major allergen Bos d 5 belongs to the lipocalin-family and thus is able to transport numerous ligands. In this study we investigated its ability to bind to iron-siderophore complexes and tested the immune-modulatory properties of Bos d 5 in either forms. Structural and *in silico* docking analysis of Bos d 5 revealed that Bos d 5 is able to bind to iron via catechol-based flavonoids (quercetin, myricetin, luteolin) that act as siderophores as confirmed by spectral-analysis and iron staining. Calculated dissociation constants of docking analyses were below 1 μM by virtual addition of iron. When incubated with human peripheral blood mononuclear cells (PBMCs), only the *apo*-form of Bos d 5 led to an increase of CD4+positive cells and significantly elevated IL13 and IFNγ-levels. In contrast, *holo*-Bos d 5 decreased numbers of CD4 expressing cells and induced apoptosis. Taken together, our data give evidence that Bos d 5 is capable of binding iron via siderophores. Moreover, our data support for the first time the notion that the form of application (*apo*- or *holo*-form) is decisive for the subsequent immune response. The *apo*-form promotes Th2 cells and inflammation, whereas the *holo*-form appears to be immunosuppressive.

**Editor:** Lax Devireddy, Case Western Reserve University, United States of America

**Funding:** This work was supported by the F4606-B19 of the Austrian Science Fund FWF. CGC was financially supported with the grant BES-2010-034628of the FPI Programme from the Spanish Government (MICINN/MINECO). JS was financially supported by FWF grants W1205-B09 (PhD program CCHD) and P23398-B11. The funders had no role in study design, data collection and analysis, decision to publish, or preparation of the manuscript.

**Competing Interests:** The authors provide an amended statement of Competing Interests to declare that a patent was filed based on part of the data provided (Method and means for diagnosing and treating allergy, Patent #14150965.3-1408). There exist no other relevant declarations relating to employment, consultancy, patents, products in development or modified products etc.

* Email: Erika.jensen-jarolim@meduniwien.ac.at

## Introduction

Cow milk allergy represents one of the most common food allergies affecting between 1.8 to 7.5% of infants during the first year of life [1]. In the majority of cases (85-90%) milk allergy resolve, however, children, who have outgrown milk allergy, still have a higher risk in developing atopic eczema, egg allergy or allergic asthma [2] Almost all known symptoms of food allergy (skin, gastrointestinal, respiratory) [3] including anaphylaxis have been reported after consumption of cow milk. Cow milk contains approximately 35 grams proteins per liter. About 80% of these proteins are caseins (80%) comprising αS1-, αS2-, β-, and κ-casein and the remaining 20% is present in the whey fractions consisting mainly of β-lactoglobulin (Bos d 5), α-lactalbumin and serum albumin. Caseins and β-lactoglobulin are regarded as the major allergens in milk. Because a Bos d 5 homologue is lacking in human milk, it has long been considered the most important cow's milk allergen.[4]

Bos d 5 belongs to the lipocalins, which are a functionally diverse family of proteins that in generally bind small, hydrophobic ligands. Despite their low sequence homology the core structure is highly conserved with an antiparallel-β barrel that defines the calyx [5]. Bos d 5, like most lipocalins, is thought to modulate cellular processes by binding to ligands. Numerous ligands have been reported to bind to Bos d 5 including fatty acids like palmitic acid with a dissociation constant, $K_d$ of 0.6 μM or retinol having different affinities ranging from 0.6 μM [6] to 10 μM [7,8]. Interestingly, Bos d 5 binds with similar or higher affinity to flavonols ($K_d$ 0.3–1.5 μM) [9] with many possessing a catechol-core structure [6].

In this study, we aimed to investigate the immune-modulatory properties of Bos d 5. The fact that Bos d 5 is a major allergen implicates that at some point it is in contact with our immune system. Interestingly, also our human body harbors a great number of lipocalin proteins, some of which do have immune-regulatory function. In particular, the immune-modulatory protein human lipocalin-2, LCN2, draw our attention, by the facts that 1) it is highly expressed in sites exposed to the environment like the lung and the gut [10] and 2) that its immune-regulatory properties depend whether it carries iron via siderophores or not [11-13].

Siderophores are small, high-affinity iron chelating compounds and are amongst the strongest soluble iron(III) binding agents known, which usually are secreted by bacteria, fungi and grasses. The major groups of siderophores include the catecholates (phenolates), hydroxamates and carboxylates (e.g. derivates of citric acid) [14].

In this respect, we investigated the potential functions of the major allergen Bos d 5 to likewise bind to iron via siderophores and to act on primary human immune cells.

## Materials and Methods

### Materials

Bovine beta-lactoglobulin, deferoxamine mesylate, ammonium iron (III) citrate, potassium ferrocyanide, dihidroxybenzene (catechol), dihydroxybenzoic acid (DHBA) were all purchased from Sigma (Sigma Aldrich, Steinheim, Germany). Ficoll-Paque PLUS was obtained from GE Healthcare (Uppsala, Sweden). IFNγ and IL13 ELISA kits were from ebiosciences (Santa Clara, CA). Antibodies were either purchased by ebioscience (CD3-APC clone SK7; 7AAD) or BD Bioscience (CD4-PE-Cy7, clone SK3; CD8-PE, clone SK1; Annexin V FITC).

### Structural and Docking Analysis

Bos d 5 structure was taken from the complex with retinoic acid, PDB entry 1GX9 [15]. The geometries of ligand molecules were obtained upon energy minimization with the MM2 force field of structures drawn using the ChemBioDraw/ChemBio3D Ultra 12.0 package. Docking input files for protein and ligands were prepared with AutoDockTools [16]. A grid box of 22 Å x 22 Å x 22 Å with origin at a point corresponding to the C6 atom in the retinoic acid molecule in the 1GX9 structure was used for docking calculations which were performed with AutoDock Vina [17]. In all cases, the docking geometry with the lowest affinity energy $E_{af}$ was selected. Estimates of dissociation equilibrium constants $K_d$ were then calculated for the protein-ligand complexes by assuming Eaf ~ ΔG with Kd = exp(-ΔG/RT) at $T$ = 298.15 K. Structural comparison of Bos d 5 with human NGAL (PDB entry 1L6M) was performed using FATCATflex (Flexible structure AlignmenT by Chaining Aligned Fragment Pairs) [18],

### Generation of *apo*-Bos d 5

Commercially available bovine beta-lactoglobulin was prior use three-times dialyzed against 10 μM deferoxamine mesylate solution. Subsequently, another dialyzation against deionized water was performed.

### Generation of *holo*-Bos d 5

*Apo*-Bos d 5 was incubated with an equimolar concentration of ammonium iron (III) citrate and a three-fold molar concentration of catechol.

### Binding assays

Optical spectra of siderophore-iron complex containing 375 μM iron and 1.125 mM were monitored in the presence or absence of 362 μM Bos d 5 in Tris-buffer at pH 7. Control spectra only contained Bos d 5. Absorbance was measured between 280 and 950 nm in 5 nm increments in quarz cuvettes using the spectrophotometer (TECAN infinite200Pro, Tecan, Crailsheim, Germany).

For iron staining 5 μl of the above-mentioned solutions (*apo*- and *holo*-Bos d 5, Fe-DHBA-complex as well as buffer control) were dotted on a nitrocellulose membrane. After rigorous washing in 20 mM Tris-buffer containing 0.5% Tween-20, membrane was stained with 5% potassium ferrocyanide in 1 M HCl for 20 minutes. Membrane was washed with water and iron-staining (Prussian blue) on dry membrane was visualized using incident light with a FluorChem FC3 apparatus (proteinsimple, Santa Clara, California).

### Isolation of PBMCs

The study was approved by the institutional ethics committee of the Medical University of Vienna and conducted in accordance with the Helsinki Declaration of 1975. Twenty-five volunteers donated 15 ml blood. All subjects gave their full written informed consent.

Blood was mixed with equal volumes of PBS containing 2% fetal calf serum (FCS) before applying onto 10 ml Ficoll-Paque PLUS, centrifugation at 400 g for 30 min without brake and washing the cells twice with 0,89% sodium chloride solution. Cells were then diluted to a concentration of 1 Mio cells/ml in RPMI medium containing 10% FCS. Throughout the study FCS of the same lot was used.

### Stimulation of PBMCs

Isolated PBMCs (0.5 Mio/test) were incubated with a final concentration of 0.75 ng/ml PMA, 100 μg/ml *apo*-Bos d 5 in the presence or absence of 30 μM catechol and 10 μM iron. Controls included PMA alone or in the presence of 30 μM catechol and 10 μM iron. PMA concentration was determined in pre-experiments and considered optimal when cells were slightly downregulating surface CD4+ expression [19]. After 18 h supernatants were collected and stored at -80°C until further analysis.

Cells were stained for 30 min at 4°C with CD3-APC, CD4-PE-Cy7, CD8-PE in PBS containing 2% FCS, followed by 10 min incubation of Annexin V FITC and 7AAD in Binding buffer (10 mM Hepes, 140 mM NaCl, 2.5 mM $CaCl_2$) at room temperature. Acquisition and analysis was performed on a FACS Canto II machine (BD Bioscience, San Jose, CA, USA) using the FACSDiva Software 6.0. Living Cells were gated by forward and sideward scatter. Further gating was performed on CD3 cells, before plotting towards CD4 and CD8 were performed. For Annexin V staining, living cells were plotted for CD4 and Annexin V without further gating to CD3.

### Determination of Cytokines

IL13 and IFNγ were detected with commercially available kits according to the manufacturers' protocol using undiluted supernatants. ELISAs for human IL13 and IFNγ have a reported sensitivity of 4 pg/ml.

### Statistical Analysis

Statistical analyses were conducted with repeated measures ANOVA following Newman-Keuls Multiple Comparison test was calculated using GraphPad Prism 5 software (GraphPad, San Diego, CA, USA). $P<0.05$ was considered statistically significant.

## Results

### Bos d 5 is able to bind to iron-siderophore complexes

Structural alignment using the FATCATflex approach revealed a high structural homology of Bos d 5 (PDB entry 1GX9) with human LCN2 (PDB entry 1L6M) as demonstrated by FATCAT-

**Table 1.** Calculated affinities energies and dissociation constants of ligands to Bos d 5.

| Ligand | Affinity energy (kcal/mol) | Dissociation constant $K_d$ (μM) |
|---|---|---|
| Quercetin | −7.9 | 1.4 |
| Fe-(Quercetin) | −8.5 | 0.51 |
| Fe-(Quercetin)$_2$ | −9.4 | 0.11 |
| Luteolin | −8.1 | 1.0 |
| Fe-(Luteolin) | −8.4 | 0.61 |
| Fe-(Luteolin)$_2$ | −9.6 | 0.078 |
| Myricetin | −8.1 | 1.0 |
| Fe-(Myricetin) | −8.3 | 0.72 |
| Fe-(Myricetin)$_2$ | −9.0 | 0.22 |
| DHBA | −5.9 | 43 |
| Fe-(DHBA) | −6.1 | 31 |
| Fe-(DHBA)$_2$ | −8.2 | 0.85 |
| Fe-(DHBA)$_3$ | −7.0 | 6.6 |
| retinol | −8.5 | 0.51 |
| retinoic acid | −7.8 | 1.7 |

flex superposition parameters ($p = 7.64 \times 10^{-12}$, Score 310.66. RMSD: 3.14, data not shown).

For docking experiments same crystal structure of Bos d 5 was taken for protein while the following compounds were selected for the ligands: DHBA chosen as a simple model of catechol-based siderophores and flavonoids quercetin, luteolin and myricetin known to be present in fruits, vegetables, leaves and grains [20,21]. Retinol and retinoic acid were also taken as control ligands (Table 1). Docking analyses were also performed with virtual addition of Fe to DHBA and flavonoids [22]. Indeed, we were able

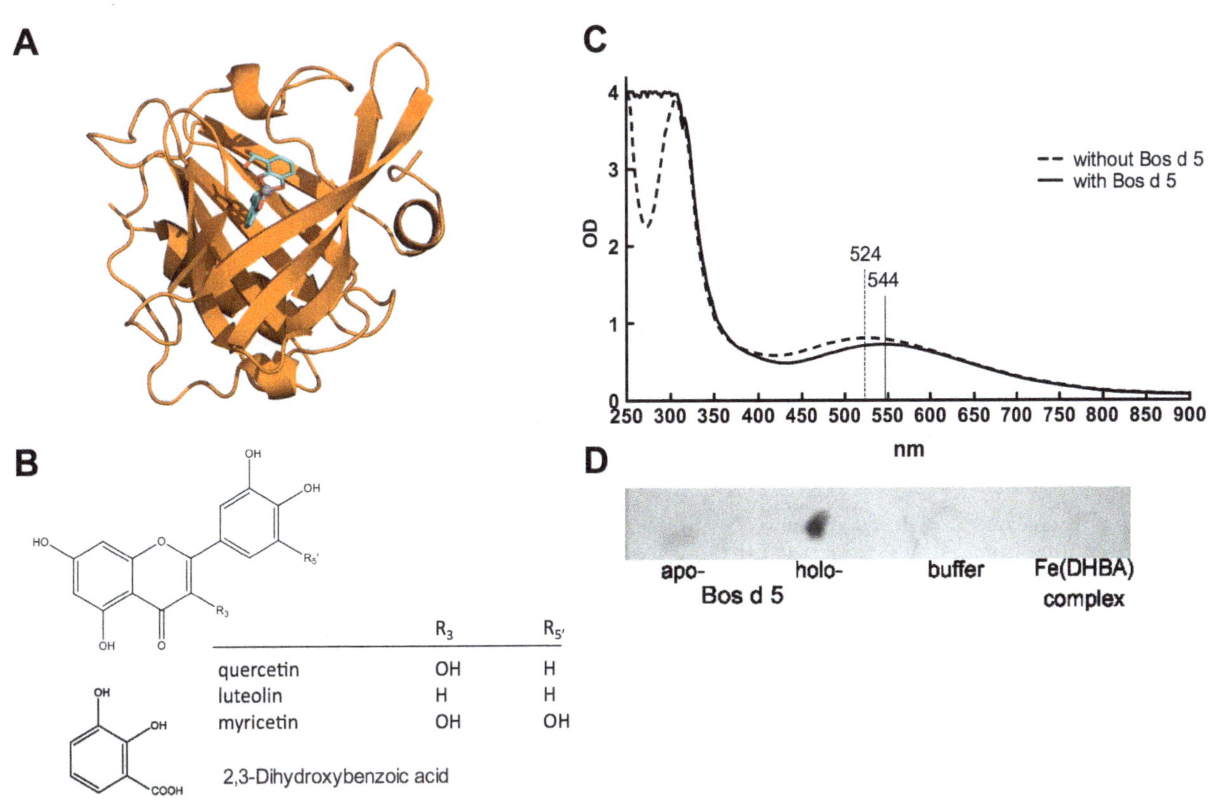


**Figure 1. Bos d 5 is able to bind iron via siderophores.** (A) Bos d 5 (1GX9) with Fe(DHBA)$_2$ (B) chemical structure of siderophores (C) UV-VIS spectra of Fe(DHBA) complex in the presence or absence of Bos d 5 or with Bos d 5 alone. (D) Iron-staining of *apo-* or *holo-*Bos d 5 as well as controls (buffer and iron-siderophore-complex) dotted on nitrocellulose-membrane.

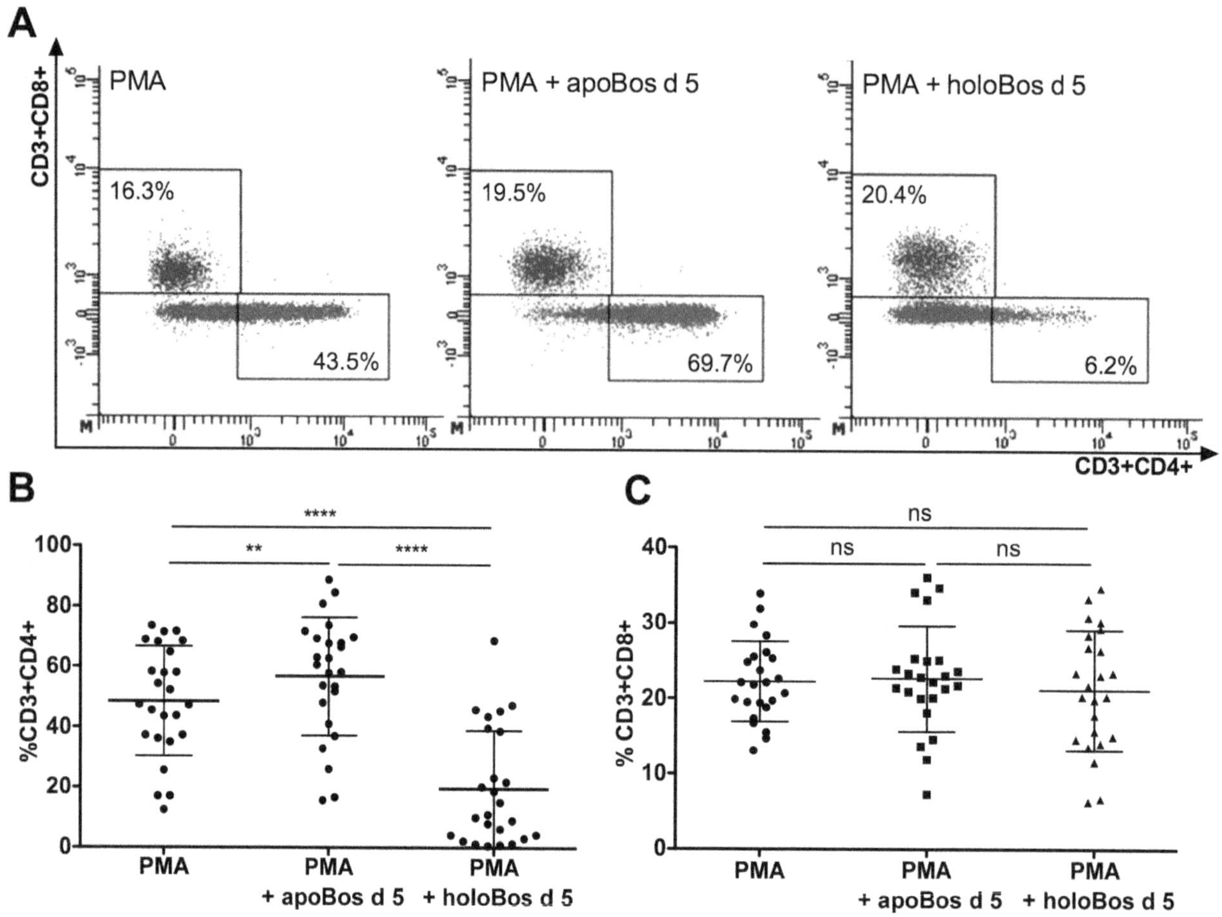


**Figure 2.** ***Apo-*, but not *holo*-Bos d 5 promotes CD4 cells.** PBMCs were treated with PMA alone or in the presence of *apo*- or *holo*-Bos d 5. (A) Living cells were gated on forward and side scatter, before gating on CD3 positive cells were performed. CD3 gated cells were then analyzed for their CD4 and CD8 expression.Representative pictograms of CD3 gated PBMCs plotted for CD4 and CD8 (B) Percentage of CD3+CD4+ cells. (C) Percentage of CD3+CD8+ cells. Statistical analyses were conducted with repeated measures ANOVA following Newman-Keuls Multiple Comparison test. $^{**}P<0.01$, $^{****}P<0.0001$, ns not significant.

to support the notion that flavonoids are siderophores and that affinities of Bos d 5 actually improved by virtual addition of Fe. Dissociation constants estimated for quercetin from docking results changed from 1.4 μM in the absence of Fe to 0.51 and 0.11 μM for one and two quercetin molecules ligating iron, respectively. For luteolin these variations were 1.0 to 0.61 to 0.078 μM, myricetin 1.0 to 0.72 to 0.22 μM. DHBA affinities also improved from 43 μM for isolated DHBA to 31 for Fe(DHBA) to 0.85 μM for $Fe(DHBA)_2$. In comparison the known ligands of Bos d 5 retinol and retinoic acid displayed dissociation constants of 0.51 and 1.7 μM, respectively. Hence, our results suggest that Bos d 5 is able to transport iron via flavonoids with affinities exceeding the binding of retinol and retinoic acid (Table 1).

Iron-binding capacity of Bos d 5 was also monitored by acquisition of UV-visible spectra of the siderophore-iron complex alone or in the presence of Bos d 5. Binding of the siderophore-iron-complex to Bos d 5 resulted in a shift in the visible spectra from 524 to 544 nm (Fig. 1C). Moreover, iron staining with Prussian blue revealed that indeed iron was found bound to Bos d 5 (Fig. 1D). For excluding unspecific binding of the siderophore-iron complex alone to the membrane, complex and buffer controls were included. Hence, our *in vitro* and *in silico* data suggest that Bos d 5 has the potential to bind iron via catechol-based siderophores.

## *Apo-* but not *holo-* Bos d 5 promote Th2 cells

LCN2 is able to drive immune responses dependent on its iron-loading state [11]. Consequently, in our next approach we investigated whether primary human immune cells discerned between the *apo-* (without iron-siderophore) and the *holo*-state (with iron-siderophore) of Bos d 5. Indeed, activation of peripheral blood mononuclear cells, PBMCs, from healthy individuals with low concentration of phorbol12-myristate13-acetate, PMA, and *apo-* or *holo*-Bos d 5 for 18 h *in vitro* resulted in a completely different CD4 expression pattern of CD3+ cells as well as cytokine profiles. Stimulation of immune cells with *apo*-Bos d 5 promoted expression of CD3+CD4+ lymphocytes, whereas introduction of the *holo*-form further decreased CD4+ expression in lymphocytes (Fig. 2A,B). Interestingly, Bos d 5 only had an impact on CD4, but not on the CD8 expression (Fig. 2C). To further determine which type of Thelper cells were promoted by stimulation of human immune cells with the *apo*-form of Bos d 5, cytokine contents in supernatants were analyzed for typical Th1 (IFNγ) and Th2 (IL13) cytokines. Indeed, we were able to detect IL13 already after 18 h stimulation with *apo*-Bos d 5 in PMA-activated PBMCs suggesting that Th2-cells were generated (Fig.3), which was not seen when cells were incubated with the *holo*-form. However, also IFNγ were generated upon addition of *apo*-Bos d 5, but not upon addition of

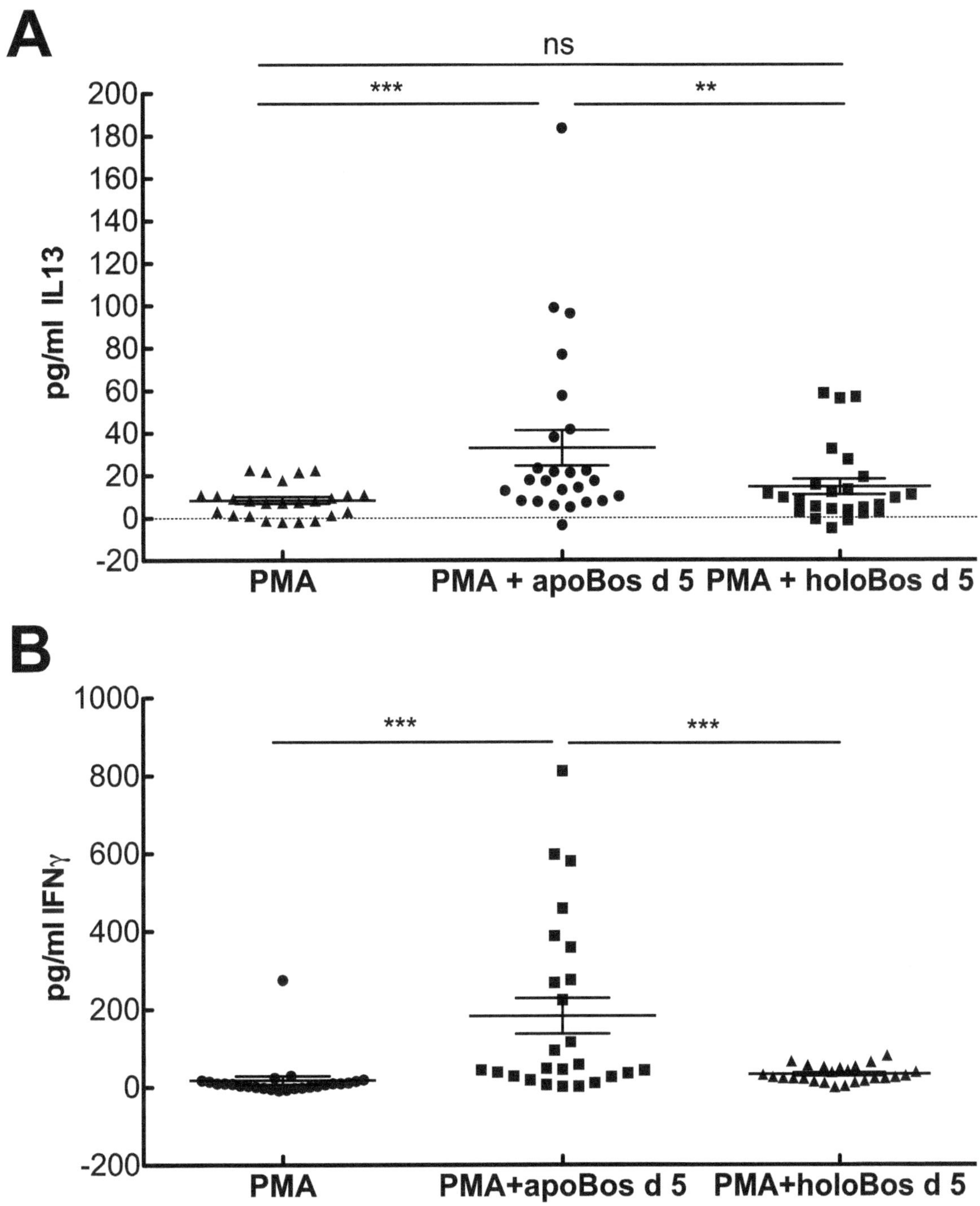


**Figure 3. Bos d 5 devoid of iron promotes IL13 and IFNγ secretion.** (A) IL13 levels and (B) IFNγ levels of stimulated PBMCs. Statistical analyses were conducted with repeated measures ANOVA following Newman-Keuls Multiple Comparison test. **$P<0.01$, *** $P<0.001$, ns not significant.

the *holo*-form, suggesting that Th1-cells were the source of IFNγ (Fig. 3).

Cells were also stained for Annexin V. Careful analysis revealed that no significant changes in Annexin V staining could be observed in untreated (media) or with iron-catechol incubated controls. In contrast significant more CD4+, but not CD4-negative cells could be stained for Annexin V upon incubation with PMA (Fig. 4). Further addition of *apo*-Bos d 5 did not alter Annexin V-staining of PMA-stimulated cells. In contrast addition of *holo*-Bos d 5 to PMA-stimulated PBMCs rendered significantly less Annexin V+ and CD4+ positive cells than Annexin V+ CD4-negative cells (Fig. 4). Hence, cells appeared to downregulate CD4-expression before undergoing apoptosis upon incubation with the *holo*-version of Bos d 5 (Fig.4). Thus, Bos d 5 was able to mount a Th2-response in its *apo*-form, but it abrogated an immune response partly by induction of apoptosis when introduced to immune cells in its *holo*-form.

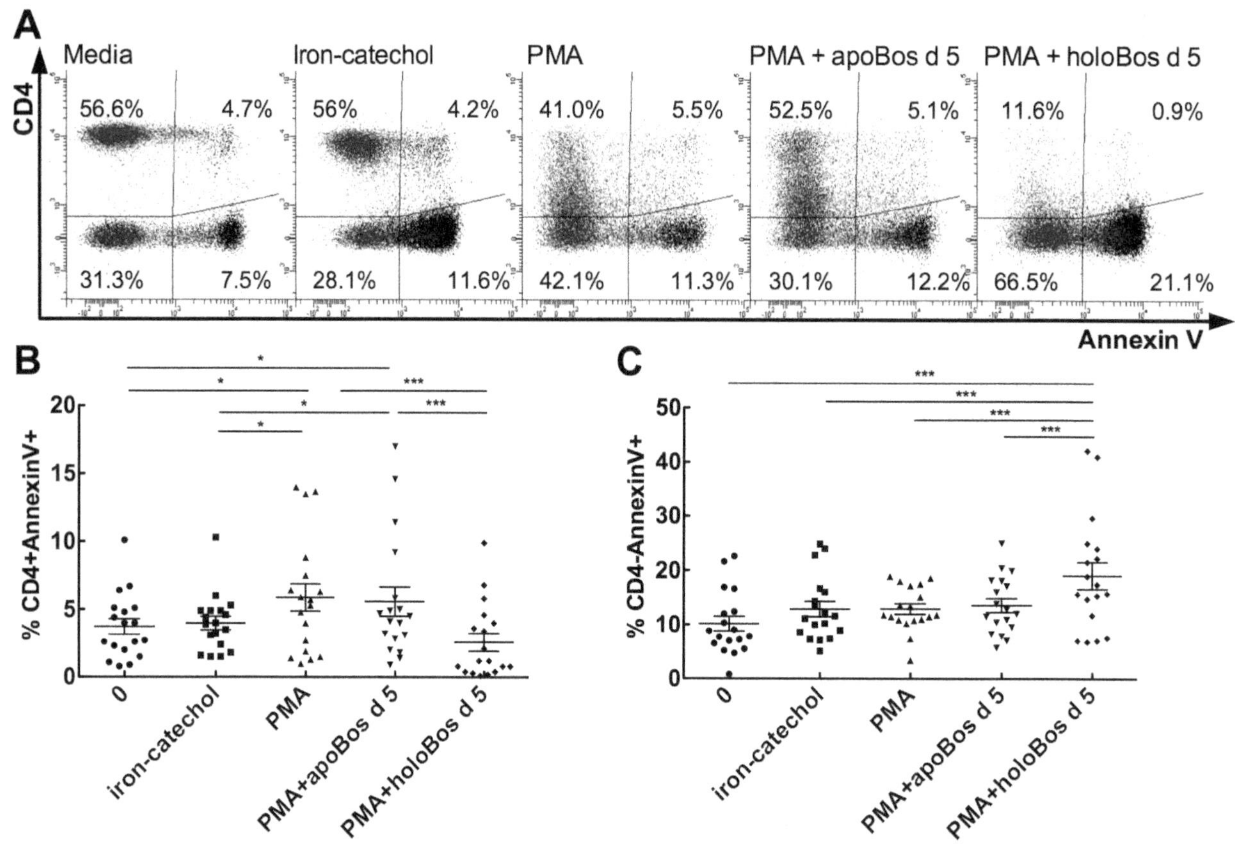


**Figure 4. Annexin V staining of PBMCs.** PBMCs were left unstimulated or treated with iron-catechol alone or with PMA alone or in the presence of *apo*- or *holo*-Bos d 5. Living cells were gated on forward and side scatter and then plotted for CD4 and Annexin V. (A) Representative pictograms of PBMCs plotted for CD4 and Annexin V. (B) Summary of percentage of CD4+Annexin V+ cells. (C) Summary of percentage of CD4-Annexin V+ cells. Statistical analyses were conducted with repeated measures ANOVA following Newman-Keuls Multiple Comparison test. ***$P<0.001$, *$P<0.05$.

## Discussion

Milk allergy is one of the most common food allergies. Most children will outgrow their allergy within the first years, however they pertain a greater risk to develop respiratory allergies like hay fever or asthma. Indeed, between 50-80% of milk allergic infants will develop respiratory allergies before puberty [23].

This is interesting, because most respiratory allergens deriving from mammalians, and recently also the major birch pollen allergen Bet v 1 [24], were identified to belong to the same protein family as the major milk allergen Bos d 5, namely the lipocalins. Lipocalins share a common tertiary structure consisting of a β-barrel enclosing an internal ligand binding sites, but have very low sequence homology [25]. They are extracellular proteins whose expression is confirmed in bacteria, protoctists, plants, arthropods and chordates [26]. The humans homologue is termed LCN2. In respect to xenogenous lipocalins in general, one striking feature that they do seem to have in common is their very low immunogenicity, despite their high allergenic potential [27].

Thus, we hypothesized that normally Bos d 5 harbors immune-suppressive qualities, but under certain conditions could be able to interfere with immune-regulatory proteins like human LCN2, thereby skewing the system towards Th2.

The biological function of Bos d 5 in milk is still not clear. It is known to bind to retinol and retinoic acid in the μM range, but interestingly docking analysis revealed similar or even stronger binding to flavonols from plants ($K_d = 0.2–0.6$ μM) with many possessing a catechol-core structure. The possible transfer of flavonols to milk was confirmed in a recent study showing that phenolic compounds from plants were found in the milk of grazing cows [28]. An important aspect hereby is that flavonoids are known metal-chelators and thus have stronger free radical scavenging properties than free flavonoids [29]. Support of Bos d 5 carrying iron also comes from research using β-lactoglobulin hydrolysate-iron complexes as a vehicle for iron supplementation [30] and showing that iron-binding properties of Bos d 5 *per se* exceeded that of α-lactalbumin [31].

Thus, binding of Bos d 5 to plant-derived flavonoids and polyphenols complexed with iron is a possible scenario happening under steady-state situations in the milk.

Our *in silico* as well as *in vitro* data moreover support the notion that Bos d 5 is able to bind to siderophores in conjunction with iron in affinities similarly seen with retinol. It is unlikely that retinol itself is able to bind iron due to the lack of neighboring hydroxyl-groups or of a hydroxyl-group adjacent to a carbonyl-group, even though a thorough search in the literature revealed that retinol, which itself is important during immune-homeostasis and inflammation, is linked with iron-metabolisms [32–34]. Moreover, it is striking to note that many lipocalin-proteins bind to retinol [35] and only in recent years their ability to bind siderophores has been discovered. We were however methodologically unable to address whether a direct connection between retinol and ferric ions exists.

Analogously, there are multiple studies showing that the human counterpart LCN2 binds to catechol-based structures, when they are complexed with iron [22,36]. Moreover, for LCN2 the biological function clearly is dictated whether it binds iron or not [11,12,37,38].

In this respect, we deprived commercially available Bos d 5 of iron (*apo*-form) and on purpose loaded part of it with iron, before adding it in their *apo*- or *holo*-form to activated isolated immune cells of human subjects.

Indeed, we show here for the first time that Bos d 5 acts distinctly on immune cells dependent whether it is introduced in its *apo*- or *holo*-form. *Apo*-Bos d 5 per se was able to mount a Th2 response leading to increased numbers of CD4+ cells and the secretion of IL13 as well as IFNγ. Since we analyzed serum of a mixed immune cells population, we cannot exclude that the cytokines derived from other immune cell population, e.g. IFNγ from NK cells, Th1 and cytotoxic T cells and IL13 from Th2 cells, but also group 2 innate lymphoid cells including natural helper cells and nuocytes [39]. The parallel induction of a Th1 as well as a Th2 response is a common phenomenon [27,40,41]. Moreover, in allergics the ratio between Th1/Th2 cells seems rather to reflect the allergic status than the presence of Th1 cells alone [41]. Importantly, in our study the *holo*-version of Bos d 5 had an antagonistic effect to the *apo*-form and resulted in a reduction of CD4+ cell numbers and their increased cell death, without any significant cytokine secretion.

The obtained results have significant implications in understanding the pathophysiological mechanisms leading to allergic sensitization. These results suggest that Bos d 5 - under natural conditions - is found in its *holo*-form and as such generally suppresses an immune response. We speculate that in situations in which the local mucosal environment has an increased need for iron, e.g. during bacterial infections by bacterial siderophores or during inflammation, Bos d 5 can display all its allergenic properties in turning into its *apo*-form.

Indirect evidence is given in a study linking maternal illnesses during pregnancy with an increased risk of asthma at 5 years [42]. Further, cow feed, organic farming, or milk processing and formula production may have significant impact on the allergenicity of Bos d 5 by influencing its iron load. For instance, milk from cows fed fresh green forage will have a higher proportion of unsaturated fatty acids [43] as well increased phenolic compounds [28] compared to cows on silage diet. Moreover, homogenization not only reduces the milk fat globules size to less than 1.0 μm, but has been shown to lead to denaturation of whey proteins in particular in pasteurized and in a lesser extend also in raw milk [44]. Similary, pasteurization has been shown to cause aggregtion of whey proteins [27], as well as to decrease copper and iron content [45] in milk.

In this respect, it is also noteworthy to mention that farm milk consumption is inversely associated with asthma and allergy and was independent of farm-related co-exposures in a cross sectional multi-center study including 14893 children aged 5–13 years [46]. Hence, the overall composition as well as food processing procedure will influence the allergenic potential of milk allergens.

In conclusion, we provide evidence that Bos d 5 is capable of binding iron via siderophores with similar or higher affinities as retinol. Moreover, our data attest that the iron load of Bos d 5 is decisive for the subsequent immune response with the *apo*-form skewing the system towards Th2, whereas the *holo*-form being immunosuppressive.

## Acknowledgments

We thank Anna Willensdorfer, Anna Moskovskich and Lukas Einhorn for help in the experimental set-up and technical assistance.

## Author Contributions

Conceived and designed the experiments: FRW. Performed the experiments: FRW CGC LFP GH JS. Analyzed the data: LFP FRW EJJ. Contributed reagents/materials/analysis tools: CGC ADP JS GAR EJJ LFP. Contributed to the writing of the manuscript: FRW EJJ ADP.

## References


1. Luyt D, Ball H, Makwana N, Green MR, Bravin K, et al. (2014) BSACI Guideline for the Diagnosis and Management of Cow's Milk Allergy. Clinical and experimental allergy: journal of the British Society for Allergy and Clinical Immunology.
2. Jarvinen KM, Beyer K, Vila L, Chatchatee P, Busse PJ, et al. (2002) B-cell epitopes as a screening instrument for persistent cow's milk allergy. The Journal of allergy and clinical immunology 110: 293–297.
3. Host A (1994) Cow's milk protein allergy and intolerance in infancy. Some clinical, epidemiological and immunological aspects. Pediatric allergy and immunology: official publication of the European Society of Pediatric Allergy and Immunology 5: 1–36.
4. Fiocchi A, Brozek J, Schunemann H, Bahna SL, von Berg A, et al. (2010) World Allergy Organization (WAO) Diagnosis and Rationale for Action against Cow's Milk Allergy (DRACMA) Guidelines. The World Allergy Organization journal 3: 57–161.
5. Goetz DH, Holmes MA, Borregaard N, Bluhm ME, Raymond KN, et al. (2002) The neutrophil lipocalin NGAL is a bacteriostatic agent that interferes with siderophore-mediated iron acquisition. Molecular cell 10: 1033–1043.
6. Keppler JK, Sonnichsen FD, Lorenzen PC, Schwarz K (2014) Differences in heat stability and ligand binding among beta-lactoglobulin genetic variants A, B and C using H NMR and fluorescence quenching. Biochimica et biophysica acta.
7. Belatik A, Kanakis CD, Hotchandani S, Tarantilis PA, Polissiou MG, et al. (2012) Locating the binding sites of retinol and retinoic acid with milk beta-lactoglobulin. Journal of biomolecular structure & dynamics 30: 437–447.
8. Muresan S, van der Bent A, de Wolf FA (2001) Interaction of beta-lactoglobulin with small hydrophobic ligands as monitored by fluorometry and equilibrium dialysis: nonlinear quenching effects related to protein—protein association. Journal of agricultural and food chemistry 49: 2609–2618.
9. Riihimaki LH, Vainio MJ, Heikura JM, Valkonen KH, Virtanen VT, et al. (2008) Binding of phenolic compounds and their derivatives to bovine and reindeer beta-lactoglobulin. Journal of agricultural and food chemistry 56: 7721–7729.
10. Cowland JB, Borregaard N (1997) Molecular characterization and pattern of tissue expression of the gene for neutrophil gelatinase-associated lipocalin from humans. Genomics 45: 17–23.
11. Devireddy LR, Gazin C, Zhu X, Green MR (2005) A cell-surface receptor for lipocalin 24p3 selectively mediates apoptosis and iron uptake. Cell 123: 1293–1305.
12. Devireddy LR, Teodoro JG, Richard FA, Green MR (2001) Induction of apoptosis by a secreted lipocalin that is transcriptionally regulated by IL-3 deprivation. Science 293: 829–834.
13. Kehrer JP (2010) Lipocalin-2: pro- or anti-apoptotic? Cell biology and toxicology 26: 83–89.
14. Hider RC, Kong X (2010) Chemistry and biology of siderophores. Natural product reports 27: 637-657.
15. Kontopidis G, Holt C, Sawyer L (2002) The ligand-binding site of bovine beta-lactoglobulin: evidence for a function? Journal of molecular biology 318: 1043–1055.
16. Morris GM, Huey R, Lindstrom W, Sanner MF, Belew RK, et al. (2009) AutoDock4 and AutoDockTools4: Automated docking with selective receptor flexibility. Journal of computational chemistry 30: 2785–2791.
17. Trott O, Olson AJ (2010) AutoDock Vina: improving the speed and accuracy of docking with a new scoring function, efficient optimization, and multithreading. Journal of computational chemistry 31: 455–461.
18. Ye Y, Godzik A (2003) Flexible structure alignment by chaining aligned fragment pairs allowing twists. Bioinformatics 19 Suppl 2: ii246–255.
19. Kaldjian E, McCarthy SA, Sharrow SO, Littman DR, Klausner RD, et al. (1988) Nonequivalent effects of PKC activation by PMA on murine CD4 and CD8 cell-surface expression. FASEB journal: official publication of the Federation of American Societies for Experimental Biology 2: 2801–2806.

20. Miean KH, Mohamed S (2001) Flavonoid (myricetin, quercetin, kaempferol, luteolin, and apigenin) content of edible tropical plants. Journal of agricultural and food chemistry 49: 3106–3112.
21. Shimoi K, Okada H, Furugori M, Goda T, Takase S, et al. (1998) Intestinal absorption of luteolin and luteolin 7-O-beta-glucoside in rats and humans. FEBS letters 438: 220–224.
22. Gomez-Casado C, Roth-Walter F, Jensen-Jarolim E, Diaz-Perales A, Pacios LF (2013) Modeling iron-catecholates binding to NGAL protein. Journal of molecular graphics & modelling 45: 111–121.
23. Saarinen KM, Pelkonen AS, Makela MJ, Savilahti E (2005) Clinical course and prognosis of cow's milk allergy are dependent on milk-specific IgE status. The Journal of allergy and clinical immunology 116: 869–875.
24. Roth-Walter F, Gomez-Casado C, Pacios LF, Mothes-Luksch N, Roth GA, et al. (2014) Bet v 1 from Birch Pollen is a Lipocalin-like Protein acting as Allergen only when devoid of Iron by promoting Th2 lymphocytes. The Journal of biological chemistry.
25. Parviainen S, Kinnunen T, Rytkonen-Nissinen M, Nieminen A, Liukko A, et al. (2013) Mammal-derived respiratory lipocalin allergens do not exhibit dendritic cell-activating capacity. Scandinavian journal of immunology 77: 171–176.
26. Sanchez D, Ganfornina MD, Gutierrez G, Marin A (2003) Exon-intron structure and evolution of the Lipocalin gene family. Molecular biology and evolution 20: 775–783.
27. Roth-Walter F, Berin MC, Arnaboldi P, Escalante CR, Dahan S, et al. (2008) Pasteurization of milk proteins promotes allergic sensitization by enhancing uptake through Peyer's patches. Allergy 63: 882–890.
28. Kuhnen S, Moacyr JR, Mayer JK, Navarro BB, Trevisan R, et al. (2014) Phenolic content and ferric reducing-antioxidant power of cow's milk produced in different pasture-based production systems in southern Brazil. Journal of the science of food and agriculture.
29. Symonowicz M, Sykula-Zajac A, Lodyga-Chruscinska E, Rumora I, Straukas M (2012) Evaluation of polyphenols and anthocyanins contents in black chockeberry—Photinia melanocarpa (Michx.) fruits extract. Acta poloniae pharmaceutica 69: 381–387.
30. Zhou J, Wang X, Ai T, Cheng X, Guo HY, et al. (2012) Preparation and characterization of beta-lactoglobulin hydrolysate-iron complexes. Journal of dairy science 95: 4230–4236.
31. Wang X, Ai T, Meng XL, Zhou J, Mao XY (2014) In vitro iron absorption of alpha-lactalbumin hydrolysate-iron and beta-lactoglobulin hydrolysate-iron complexes. Journal of dairy science.
32. Jang JT, Green JB, Beard JL, Green MH (2000) Kinetic analysis shows that iron deficiency decreases liver vitamin A mobilization in rats. The Journal of nutrition 130: 1291-1296.
33. Suharno D, West CE, Muhilal, Karyadi D, Hautvast JG (1993) Supplementation with vitamin A and iron for nutritional anaemia in pregnant women in West Java, Indonesia. Lancet 342: 1325–1328.
34. Rosales FJ, Jang JT, Pinero DJ, Erikson KM, Beard JL, et al. (1999) Iron deficiency in young rats alters the distribution of vitamin A between plasma and liver and between hepatic retinol and retinyl esters. The Journal of nutrition 129: 1223–1228.
35. Akerstrom B, Flower DR, Salier JP (2000) Lipocalins: unity in diversity. Biochimica et biophysica acta 1482: 1–8.
36. Bao G, Clifton M, Hoette TM, Mori K, Deng SX, et al. (2010) Iron traffics in circulation bound to a siderocalin (Ngal)-catechol complex. Nature chemical biology 6: 602–609.
37. Srinivasan G, Aitken JD, Zhang B, Carvalho FA, Chassaing B, et al. (2012) Lipocalin 2 deficiency dysregulates iron homeostasis and exacerbates endotoxin-induced sepsis. Journal of immunology 189: 1911–1919.
38. Xu G, Ahn J, Chang S, Eguchi M, Ogier A, et al. (2012) Lipocalin-2 induces cardiomyocyte apoptosis by increasing intracellular iron accumulation. The Journal of biological chemistry 287: 4808–4817.
39. Neill DR, Wong SH, Bellosi A, Flynn RJ, Daly M, et al. (2010) Nuocytes represent a new innate effector leukocyte that mediates type-2 immunity. Nature 464: 1367–1370.
40. Van Hemelen D, Oude Elberink JN, Bohle B, Heimweg J, Nawijn MC, et al. (2011) Flow cytometric analysis of cytokine expression in short-term allergen-stimulated T cells mirrors the phenotype of proliferating T cells in long-term cultures. Journal of immunological methods 371: 114–121.
41. Tordesillas L, Cuesta-Herranz J, Gonzalez-Munoz M, Pacios LF, Compes E, et al. (2009) T-cell epitopes of the major peach allergen, Pru p 3: Identification and differential T-cell response of peach-allergic and non-allergic subjects. Molecular immunology 46: 722–728.
42. Illi S, Weber J, Zutavern A, Genuneit J, Schierl R, et al. (2014) Perinatal influences on the development of asthma and atopy in childhood. Annals of allergy, asthma & immunology: official publication of the American College of Allergy, Asthma, & Immunology 112: 132–139 e131.
43. Elgersma A, Tamminga S, Ellen G (2006) Modifying milk composition through forage. Animal Feed Science and Technology 131: 207–225.
44. Escobar D, Clark S, Ganesan V, Repiso L, Waller J, et al. (2011) High-pressure homogenization of raw and pasteurized milk modifies the yield, composition, and texture of queso fresco cheese. Journal of dairy science 94: 1201–1210.
45. Zurera-Cosano G, Moreno-Rojas R, Amaro-Lopez MA (1994) Effect of processing on contents and relationships of mineral elements of milk. Food Chemistry 51: 75–78.
46. Waser M, Michels KB, Bieli C, Floistrup H, Pershagen G, et al. (2007) Inverse association of farm milk consumption with asthma and allergy in rural and suburban populations across Europe. Clinical and experimental allergy: journal of the British Society for Allergy and Clinical Immunology 37: 661–670.

11

# Elevated Antigen-Driven IL-9 Responses Are Prominent in Peanut Allergic Humans

**Jungang Xie[1¤], Larisa C. Lotoski[1], Rishma Chooniedass[2], Ruey-Chyi Su[1], F. Estelle R. Simons[1,2], Joel Liem[3], Allan B. Becker[1,2], Jude Uzonna[1], Kent T. HayGlass[1,2*]**

1 Department of Immunology, University of Manitoba, Winnipeg, Canada, 2 Department of Pediatrics and Child Health, University of Manitoba, Winnipeg, Canada, 3 Windsor Allergy Asthma Education Centre, Ontario, Canada

## Abstract

Food allergies, and peanut allergy in particular, are leading causes of anaphylactic fatalities worldwide. The immune mechanisms that underlie food allergy remain ill-defined and controversial, in part because studies in humans typically focus on analysis of a limited number of prototypical Th1/Th2 cytokines. Here we determine the kinetics and prevalence of a broad panel of peanut-driven cytokine and chemokine responses in humans with current peanut allergy vs those with stable, naturally occurring clinical tolerance to peanut. Our primary focus is identification of novel indicators of immune dysregulation. Antigen-specific cytokine mRNA and protein responses were elicited in primary culture via peanut or irrelevant antigen (*Leishmania* extract, milk antigens) mediated stimulation of fresh peripheral blood cells from 40 individuals. Peanut extract exposure in vitro induced a broad panel of responses associated with Th2/Th9-like, Th1-like and Th17-like immunity. Peanut-dependent Type 2 cytokine responses were frequently found in both peanut allergic individuals and those who exhibit clinical tolerance to peanut ingestion. Among Th2/Th9-associated cytokines, IL-9 responses discriminated between allergic and clinically tolerant populations better than did commonly used IL-4, IL-5 or IL-13 responses. Comparison with responses evoked by unrelated control antigen-mediated stimulation showed that these differences are antigen-dependent and allergen-specific. Conversely, the intensity of IL-12, IL-17, IL-23 and IFN-γ production was indistinguishable in peanut allergic and peanut tolerant populations. In summary, the ability to generate and maintain cytokine responses to peanut is not inherently distinct between allergic and peanut tolerant humans. Quantitative differences in the intensity of cytokine production better reflects clinical phenotype, with optimally useful indicators being IL-9, IL-5, IL-13 and IL-4. Equivalent, and minimal, Ag-dependent pro-inflammatory cytokine levels in both healthy and peanut allergic volunteers argues against a key role for such cytokines in maintenance of clinical tolerance to food antigens in humans.

**Editor:** Jörg Hermann Fritz, McGill University, Canada

**Funding:** Supported by Canadian Institutes of Health Research (CIHR), AllerGen NCE, the Manitoba Institute of Child Health (MICH), and the Canada Research Chairs program. JX held a MICH postdoctoral fellowship and LL a joint AllerGen/CIHR studentship. KH holds the Canada Research Chair in Immune Regulation. The funders had no role in study design, data collection and analysis, decision to publish, or preparation of the manuscript.

**Competing Interests:** Operating support for this study was obtained from the Canadian Institutes of Health Research (CIHR), the Canada Reserch Chairs (CRC) Program and AllerGen NCE.

* E-mail: hayglass@cc.umanitoba.ca

¤ Current address: Department of Respiratory Disease, Tongji Medical College, Huangzhong University of Science and Technology, Wuhan, PR China

## Introduction

Food allergies, and peanut allergy in particular, are leading causes of anaphylaxis. While their natural history, epidemiology and social consequences are increasingly well defined [1–4], validated gains in diagnosis, prevention or management are generally viewed as modest [5–7]. One key roadblock hindering development of improved prophylactic and therapeutic interventions is our limited understanding of which immune responses are differentially expressed in humans with food allergy vs those exhibited by individuals who maintain clinical tolerance to common foods.

Several factors contribute to this challenge. Logistical difficulties associated with eliciting, detecting and quantifying food antigen-driven cytokine responses in humans using primary culture often leads investigators to make use of polyclonal activators as surrogates for biologically relevant ligands, notwithstanding the fact that such approaches lead to activation of a much larger proportion of the immune repertoire than does antigen-dependent activation. Secondly, despite recognition of the large number of cytokines involved in immune regulation, the research focus in human food allergy research to date has primarily been on a rather restricted panel of cytokines. IFNγ plus IL-5 and/or IL-13 as indicators of Th1-like and Th2-like responses are frequently the main or only readouts examined. While Th2-skewed Ag-specific responses are obviously common to many allergic disorders, identification of or comparison between other Th1 or Th2-immunity cytokines, or those linked to Th9 or Th17-like phenotypes remains speculative in humans. With a broad variety of innovative therapeutic approaches under consideration to modulate hypersensitivity [8–12], better understanding of characteristic human cytokine responses to common foods is key to progress. Murine models provide excellent tools, but with few exceptions [13,14], most require adjuvant and have other characteristics that may limit their ability to directly extrapolate their findings.

Here, we utilized short term antigen-stimulated primary culture of peripheral blood mononuclear cells (PBMC) directly ex vivo to assess peanut dependent cytokine and chemokine production in humans of distinct clinical phenotypes. Experimental conditions were identified to allow examination of a broad panel of cytokine mRNA targets that we hypothesized are differentially expressed in peanut allergic humans versus in those humans who exhibit sustained naturally occurring clinical tolerance to peanut. We map the kinetics of mRNA expression for this panel of established and novel Th2-associated (IL-4, IL-5, IL-9, IL-13), proinflammatory/Th17 related (IL-17, IL-23) and Th1-immunity associated cytokine (IFNγ, IL-12, IL-23) responses in humans following acute in vitro re-stimulation with peanut, then apply this strategy to 40 clinically well characterized individuals. The data reveal that differences in food-Ag driven IL-9 mRNA and protein responses are superior to most extensively used, "classical" Th2 markers. Peanut dependent IL-17 mRNA responses are frequent and intense but do not differ between clinical phenotypes. Indeed, none of the Th1 or Th17-associated indicators examined revealed differential expression of pro-inflammatory cytokine gene expression between the two populations. Collectively, the data reveal ubiquitous CD4 T cell dependent responses to peanut allergen in the population as a whole, identify novel cytokine responses and reveal quantitatively distinct patterns of peanut Ag-driven responses between peanut allergic individuals and those who maintain clinical tolerance to this common food antigen. The findings argue for their utilization in future investigations of the complex mechanisms that underlie food allergy vs clinically apparent, functional tolerance.

## Materials and Methods

### Subjects

Following University of Manitoba Research Ethics Board approval, written informed consent was obtained before enrollment. Twenty peanut allergic and 20 individuals exhibiting clinical tolerance to peanut were recruited. Peanut allergic individuals had (i) convincing histories of anaphylaxis (defined [6] as a serious allergic reaction that may cause death taking place within the previous five years despite stringent efforts to avoid dietary peanut, (ii) clearly positive epicutaneous tests via the prick-through drop technique using 1:20 w/v peanut/glycerin extract, (Omega Laboratories, Montreal Canada) and (iii) elevated peanut specific IgE ImmunoCAP results. Several of these peanut allergic individuals exhibited positive skin tests, clinical symptoms to additional allergens, allergic rhinitis and/or asthma. Peanut non-allergic individuals were recruited on the basis of (i) a detailed allergy history consistent with a lack of clinical reactivity to peanut, ever, (ii) negative epicutaneous tests (<3 mm wheals) and (iii) peanut specific IgE ImmunoCAP results <0.35 kU/L. These participants took no precautions to avoid peanut, and ingested it without developing any symptoms or signs. Table 1 provides more detailed information on these populations. Due to local research ethics board constraints, screening for individuals exhibiting peanut sensitization alone was not possible.

### Peripheral blood mononuclear cell isolation and culture

All studies were carried out with fresh samples directly ex vivo. 20–50 ml whole blood was collected into 2 ml 2.7% EDTA. Whole peanut antigen extract was prepared from roasted peanut extracted for 72 h in aqueous buffer (borate pH 8.4) with the protein concentration determined by BCA Protein Assay (Pierce,

**Table 1.** Demographic and Clinical Characteristics of Participants.*

| | Peanut allergic | Peanut tolerant |
|---|---|---|
| No. of individuals | 20 | 20 |
| Males | 14/20 | 11/20 |
| Age (y) | 18.6 (2–54) | 21.1 (12–33) |
| Wheal diameter (mm) | 9.2 (4–20) | 0 (0) |
| Peanut specific IgE ($kU_A/L$) | 17.3 ( 0.5–63) | <0.35 (<0.35) |
| Other food allergy | 11/20 | 1/20 |
| Asthma | 12/20 | 1/20 |
| Allergic rhinitis | 15/20 | 4/20 |

*Values are expressed as median (range) or absolute numbers within the population.

Rockford, IL). Endotoxin levels of complete medium and peanut antigen were assessed by LAL assay (Associates of Cape Cod, East Falmouth MA). All reagents and antigens used exhibited levels <0.01 EU/ml in culture.

Culture systems were established and optimized using peanut extract titrated in culture from 10–200 μg/ml. Briefly, fresh PBMC were cultured in 10% pre-selected FBS-RPMI containing L-glutamine and antibiotic/antimycotic at $5\times10^5$/well in 96 well round bottom plates with 6 replicate wells for each time point harvested. In independent experiments, Ag-specificity requirements for cytokine production were assessed using SLA (soluble *Leishmania* antigen, 10 μg/ml) or semi-purified milk antigens. SLA was prepared as described [15] with minor modifications. Briefly, 7-day stationary phase promastigotes were washed in cold PBS, sonicated and viewed microscopically to ensure that all parasites were disrupted. The parasite lysate was then centrifuged, dialyzed against PBS, sterilized by passage through a 0.22 um filter and stored at −80 C. Whole bovine casein ( a mixture of alpha-S1-casein, alpha-S2-casein, beta-casein, k-casein) and whey ( a source of α-lactalbumin and β-lactoglobulin) were isolated from fresh milk as described [16] and used for stimulation at final protein concentrations of 100 to 900 ug/ml. Anti-CD80 and anti-CD86 Abs (BDBiosciences) were added to some cultures at a final concentration of 5 ug/ml each to assess costimulatory requirements for IL-9 production.

Culture supernatants were collected and stored at −20 C until analyzed by ELISA while cell pellets were stored at −80 C in RNAlater (Qiagen) until analysis. Unstimulated time 0 samples were also prepared from $3–5\times10^6$ PBMC directly ex vivo.

### RNA isolation, Reverse Transcription and Quantitative PCR

Total RNA was isolated from PBMC. cDNA was prepared with first strand synthesis using random hexamers and SuperScript III reverse transcriptase (Invitrogen, Carlsbad, CA). The reaction mix was incubated at 25°C for 5 minutes, 42°C for 1.5 hours for reverse transcription, and finally at 85°C for 5 minutes for reverse transcriptase inactivation. mRNA levels of the cytokines examined were determined by Q-PCR (Applied Biosystems, USA) using primers we designed and validated (Table S1). PCR products were detected in 96-well plates in duplicate using SYBR Green Master Mix (Stratagene, CA). For each cytokine, the "fold change" in mRNA expression was calculated using Delta-Delta Ct Analyses (ABI Data Analysis Software) with 18 s rRNA as for input normalization and paired unstimulated cells as comparison point for each stimulated sample.

### Cytokine ELISA

Primary culture supernatant cytokine levels were determined with reagents from BioLegend (San Diego, CA) for IL-5, IL-9, IL-13 and IFNγ as described [17,18]. Sensitivity was 5.86, 9.38, 5.86 pg/ml and 0.625 IU/ml, respectively, with inter-assay variability generally of 5–10%.

### Statistical analysis

Analyses were carried out with Prism 5 software (GraphPad, San Diego, CA). Where data sets exhibited a Gaussian distribution, Student's t tests were used with matched or unmatched pairs as appropriate. Nonparametric analyses were conducted with validated Wilcoxon matched or unmatched pairs, as appropriate. Two-tailed P values are reported, with differences considered significant if $p<0.05$.

## Results

### Optimization of peanut antigen concentration and kinetics of cytokine production by fresh PBMC

The twenty peanut allergic individuals studied exhibited convincing clinical histories of anaphylaxis within the previous 5 years, strong epicutaneous tests to peanut challenge (mean 18.6 mm wheal diameter) and elevated peanut specific IgE levels (9.2 kU/L). The 20 control individuals with clinical tolerance to peanut had a reported lack of clinical reactivity to peanut ever, negative epicutaneous tests, negative peanut specific IgE ImmunoCAP results and regular dietary peanut exposure (Table 1).

To identify optimal experimental conditions to elicit and quantify Ag-stimulated human cytokine mRNA responses for the range of cytokines being examined, freshly isolated PBMC were cultured without stimulation and in the presence of a range of low endotoxin peanut antigen extract concentrations. PBMC were used in preference to highly enriched CD4 T cell populations because multiple cell types, including but not limited to CD4 T cells, contribute to the net cytokine response evoked by allergen exposure. mRNA levels of representative cytokines associated with Th1, Th2 and Th17-like immune responses were quantified after 3 h, and again at days one through six of culture. No statistically significant differences were observed between the three antigen concentrations in their capacity to elicit responses, so the 100 ug/ml peanut concentrations were used for all subsequent experiments. Peanut allergic individuals exhibited indistinguishable kinetics from those with clinical tolerance to peanut. Illustrative data from three representative experiments of 12 performed are shown in Figure S1.

Recognizing that Q-PCR analysis only increases the sensitivity of detection if paired with detailed knowledge of expression for the genes of interest, we individually determined kinetics for each cytokine to be examined. Peak IL-33 mRNA responses to peanut antigen were exhibited at d.1 and IL-4 at d.3 whereas IL5, IL-9 and IL-13 were maximal at d.5 (Figure 1). Among pro-inflammatory Th1 and Th17 associated cytokines, IL-12/23 p40 expression peaked at day 1 whereas IL-23 p19, IL-12 p35 and IFNγ levels did not exhibit increases in response to peanut stimulation at any of the times studied. IL-17A mRNA was strongly stimulated upon peanut antigen exposure, peaking at d.5. These optimum time points were used for all subsequent analyses.

Given the extensive diversity in human versus inbred murine populations, hence the inherent challenges in identifying differences between highly heterogeneous populations, it was important to assess the extent of experimental reproducibility in QPCR within individuals. Inter-assay reproducibility of QPCR data are not frequently reported. To assess variance, mRNA from multiple samples were independently reanalyzed in separate experiments. Values agreed closely, demonstrating the reproducibility of the technique employed and the data obtained (Table S2). Similarly, while inter-individual variation in the intensity of responses was substantial between individuals, characteristic of most immune responses in human populations, differences in the kinetics of production in different individuals for each of the cytokines examined was minimal. Collectively, these data indicate that while it is clearly essential to examine each cytokine at the time of its peak expression (rather than a single arbitrary time point for logistical convenience), optimal Ag-driven production of, for instance, IL-4 and IL-13 was consistently at days 3 and 5 respectively, regardless of the participant examined or their clinical status.

### Differential cytokine mRNA expression in peanut allergic vs clinically tolerant individuals

These conditions for short term Ag-driven stimulation of fresh cells in primary culture were used to seek qualitative or quantitative differences in cytokine responses between groups clinically tolerant to peanut versus those with clear clinical histories of allergic symptoms and signs after peanut ingestion. Fresh PBMC were cultured with peanut then cell pellets and supernatants harvested at the optimal time point for each candidate cytokine. In the absence of peanut stimulation, cytokine mRNA production ex vivo was usually extremely low in culture (Figure 2). As anticipated, upon peanut stimulation IL-5 was produced by virtually all peanut allergic individuals studied. Importantly, a high proportion of clinically tolerant individuals also exhibited significant responses (Figure 3). Median Ag-dependent IL-5 mRNA up-regulation in the clinically tolerant group was 21-fold (range: 0–174×) whereas the peanut allergic group had median 165-fold enhancement (range: 4–600×). This reflects an approximately eight times stronger intensity of IL-5 responses by peanut allergic individuals (ie 21-fold vs 165-fold increased, $p<0.0005$). IL-13 exhibited a similar pattern, with median 7.8 vs 66-fold increases upon Ag re-exposure, an 8.4× more intense response in the peanut allergic group ($p<0.0001$). Peak IL-4 mRNA levels (d.3) differed significantly between groups ($p<0.0001$, $n=40$) but the intensity of that difference was quite limited (median 2.7 vs 4.9 fold increases, a 1.8 times differential). In contrast, IL-9 responses were discovered to be the most robust discriminator between clinical phenotypes with median 2.1 vs 59 fold enhancement in tolerant vs allergic groups, a 28 times more intense response by peanut allergics.

Assessment of IL-33 responses, a potent promoter of type 2 immune responses [19,20], also revealed a strong association with clinical phenotype. Clinically tolerant individuals generated median 3.4 fold increases in IL-33 mRNA following peanut re-stimulation whereas responses in peanut allergic individuals were 8.6 fold enhanced. This 2.5 fold differential between phenotypes ($p<0.0001$) indicates that widespread and differential intensities of not only Th2-associated effector cytokines (IL-4, 5, 9 and 13) but also of cytokines associated with induction (or perpetuation) of allergic disorders is (i) a characteristic of peanut allergic individuals and (ii) occurs in both peanut allergic and peanut tolerant individuals upon exposure to this common food antigen.

Th1 and Th17-immunity associated cytokines (IL-12, IL-23, IFNγ, IL-17), considered by some to be contributors to oral tolerance in food allergy, reveal a markedly different picture from that seen for type 2 immunity responses (Figure 4). Increased IL-

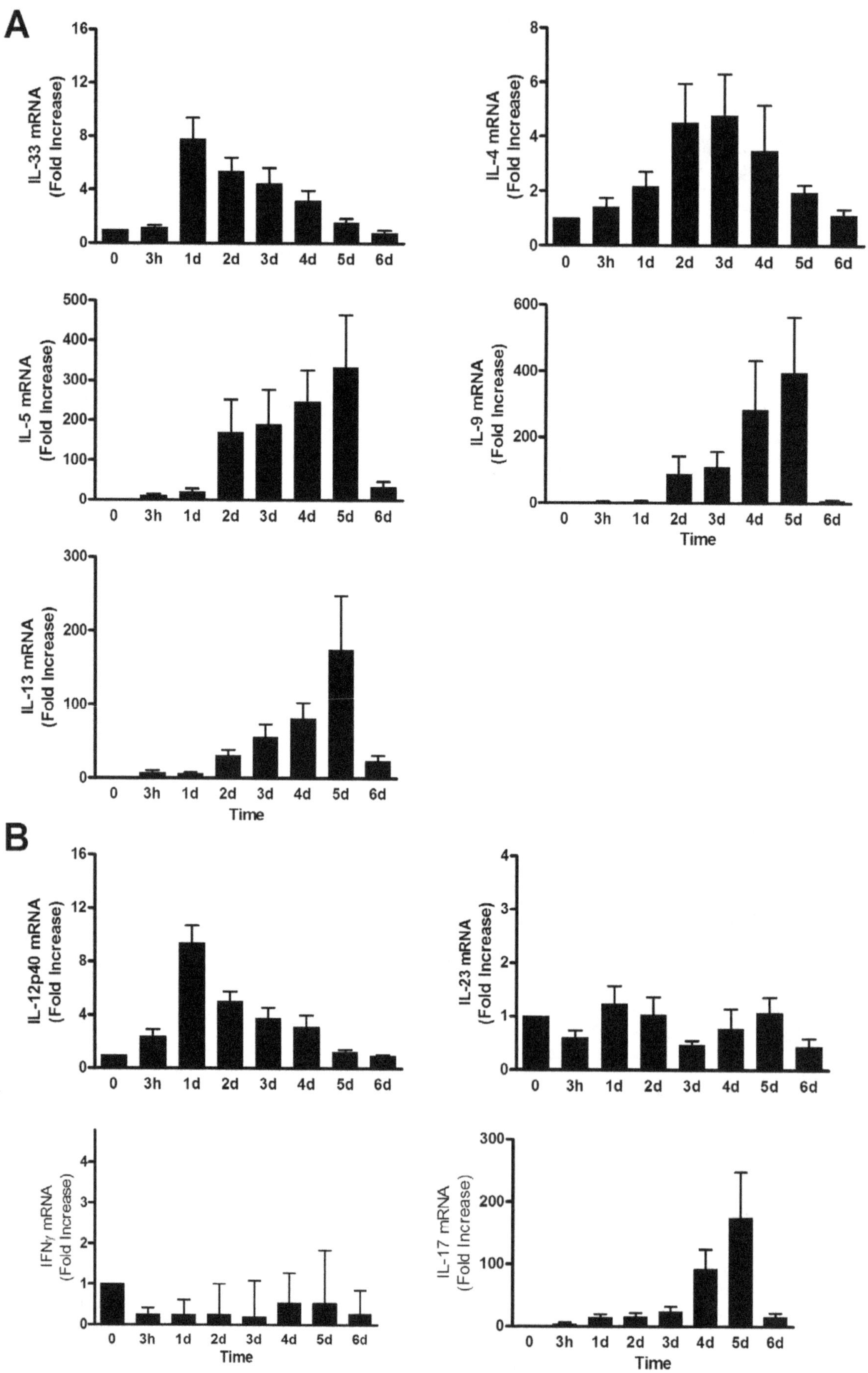
A
IL-33 mRNA (Fold Increase)
IL-4 mRNA (Fold Increase)
IL-5 mRNA (Fold Increase)
IL-9 mRNA (Fold Increase)
IL-13 mRNA (Fold Increase)
0 3h 1d 2d 3d 4d 5d 6d
Time
B
IL-12p40 mRNA (Fold Increase)
IL-23 mRNA (Fold Increase)
IFNγ mRNA (Fold Increase)
IL-17 mRNA (Fold Increase)

**Figure 1. Kinetic characterization of peanut antigen stimulated cytokine mRNA responses.** PBMC from 12 individuals were cultured with 100 µg/ml peanut Ag with cells then harvested at each time point shown. Results are expressed as mean (±SEM) fold changes in mRNA levels normalized against un-stimulated controls. **Panel A:** Th2/Th9 associated cytokines. **Panel B:** Th1/Th17-associated cytokines.

12/23 p40 was detected relative to un-stimulated control cultures but the intensity of these responses did not differ between peanut allergic and tolerant populations. Enhanced IL-23 (p19) mRNA was seen in response to in vitro peanut stimulation in only two of 40 individuals examined. Similarly, median IFNγ mRNA levels were very low and did not differ between groups. Interestingly, while four (of 40) individuals did exceed the threshold of 2-fold enhancement in mRNA levels widely used to define a positive response, both were in the peanut allergic rather the clinically tolerant group. These data argue against a pivotal role for IFNγ in clinical tolerance to peanut.

IL-17 mRNA was strongly induced in both clinically tolerant and peanut allergic populations. As seen in Figure 4, comparable increases of 46 and 85 fold (medians, $p = 0.57$) were elicited following peanut stimulation. Thus, among the panel of cytokines assessed, no qualitative or quantitative differences were evident between clinically tolerant and allergic populations in pro-Th1/pro-inflammatory/Th17-like activation.

## Recall cytokine protein secretion in response to peanut antigen

Because mRNA expression and cytokine protein assessment have different experimental caveats, we quantified levels of representative cytokines in culture supernatants by ELISA. Elevated IL-5, IL-9 (Figure 5) production was readily demonstrable at the protein level, and recapitulated mRNA data. Similarly, as seen for mRNA levels, IFNγ protein levels elicited by peanut Ag were weak and indistinguishable between the two clinical phenotypes.

## Peanut- driven cytokine expression is Ag-specific

To confirm that the mRNA and cytokine protein responses quantified were truly peanut Ag dependent and not due to contaminants, polyclonal activators or spontaneous activation, we utilized three approaches. Endotoxin was ruled out as a contributor to cytokine production because LPS levels in both medium and peanut Ag were <0.01 EU/ml, well below the levels of LPS required to elicit production of these cytokines. Secondly, to assess peanut Ag-independent activation, we incorporated antigens that are highly stimulatory of cytokine production in exposed humans [21] but to which these volunteers had almost certainly not been exposed. Soluble *Leishmania antigen extract* (SLA) was used to stimulate PBMC from both groups, following which cell lysates and supernatants were harvested. IL-5, IL-9, IL-13 and IFN-γ mRNA and protein responses were quantified in eight independent experiments . Figure 6 demonstrates that these individuals respond to peanut but failed to produce any of these cytokines when stimulated with *Leishmania*. As a third approach, we recalled individuals with particularly strong peanut-stimulated IL-9 responses in order to assess the impact of stimulation with unrelated food antigens and, separately, of the capacity of in vitro addition of anti-CD80 and anti-CD86 Ab to block peanut stimulated IL-9 production. As shown in Figure 7, peanut extract stimulated IL-9 production is strictly dependent on costimulation. It was also found that peanut allergic and peanut non-allergic individuals (not allergic to milk) exhibited low level or undetectable IL-9 responses when stimulated with major milk allergens. Collectively these data highlight the antigenic specificity of the peanut-driven cytokine production assessed.

## Relative expression levels of cytokine mRNA

The data presented above assess mRNA responses for each individual cytokine upon stimulation relative to expression of that cytokine in the absence of peanut antigen. To directly compare responses *between* cytokines, we calculated fold changes in mRNA after peanut stimulation, with each expressed relative to 18 s rRNA (Figure 8). As such, the data provide an indication of the relative utility of each cytokine as a potential tool to differentiate between populations with peanut allergy and those exhibiting clinical tolerance upon peanut exposure. . The cytokines exhibiting the most intense differential responses, hence greatest potential utility, when comparing clinical phenotypes were, in order, IL-9, IL-33, IL-5, IL-13 and IL-4.

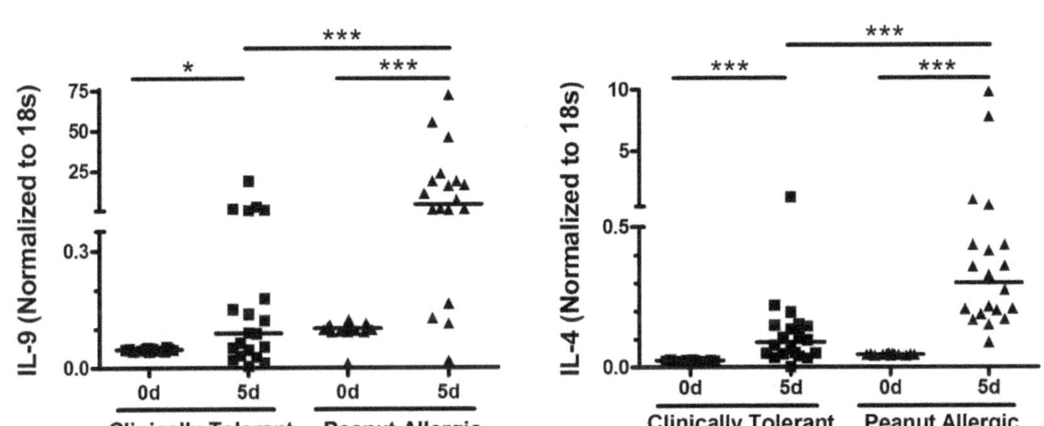


**Figure 2. Antigen-dependent activation of cytokine mRNA expression.** Matched pair analyses of IL-9 and IL-4 expression was assessed relative to 18 s rRNA in the presence and absence of peanut stimulation. Note break in y axis. n = 40. * p<0.05; *** p<0.0001.

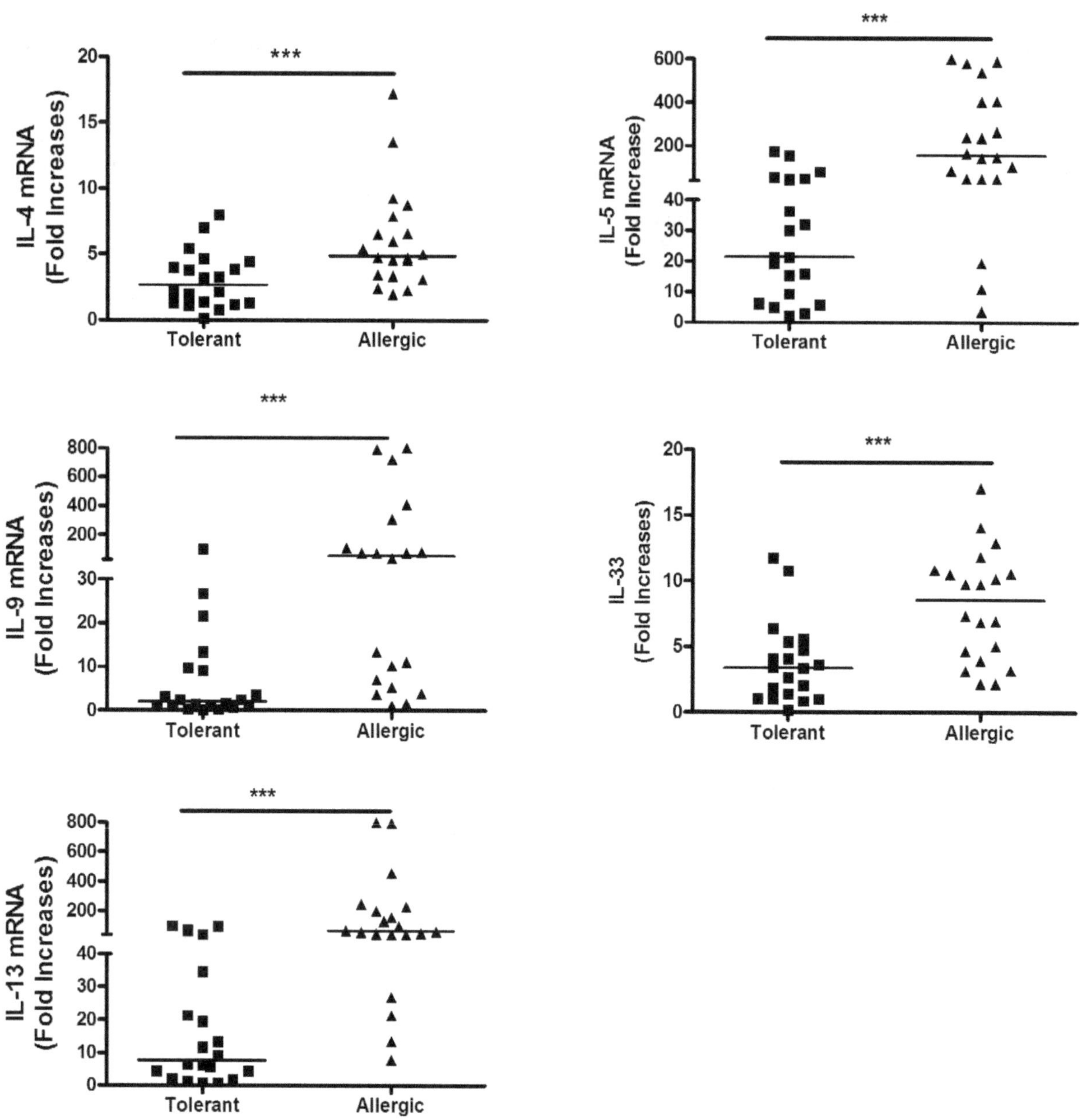


**Figure 3. Comparison of peanut-dependent Type 2 mRNA profiles elicited in peanut allergic and peanut clinically tolerant individuals.** Following in vitro PBMC stimulation (100 ug/ml), RNA was isolated from cells harvested at day 1 (IL-33), day 3 (IL-4), or day 5 (IL-5, IL-9, IL-13), times of optimal Ag-driven cytokine production. Results are expressed as fold-increased levels relative to matched un-stimulated controls. Bars indicate median responses. *** $p<0.0001$.

## Discussion

Two important barriers to increasing understanding of the basic biology of food allergy have been a focus on a small number of prototypic cytokines in humans and the widespread use of antigen non-specific activation protocols to assess food allergen-specific human immune responses. While broadly similar, antigen-driven and polyclonally stimulated responses can yield very different conclusions about immune status [22–24]. To guide future experimental design into mechanisms that underlie food allergy vs clinical tolerance in humans, as well as to further spur development of novel multi-parameter diagnostic and management approaches for food allergy, we assessed a broad panel of cytokines characteristic of human Th1, Th2, Th9 and Th17-like functional phenotypes.

This is the first report of the importance of IL-9 in the human response to food allergens. Importantly, as for the other type 2 immunity cytokines examined here, its production in response to acute food Ag restimulation was not restricted to individuals who exhibit demonstrable clinical sensitivity upon peanut exposure. Indeed, each of the Th2/Th9-like cytokines was frequently stimulated by peanut re-exposure in peanut tolerant as well as in peanut allergic populations. Thus, just as the presence of food-specific serum IgE does not in itself reflect clinical sensitivity [25], expression of peanut-dependent Th2/Th9-like cytokine production in clinically tolerant humans is not indicative of clinical

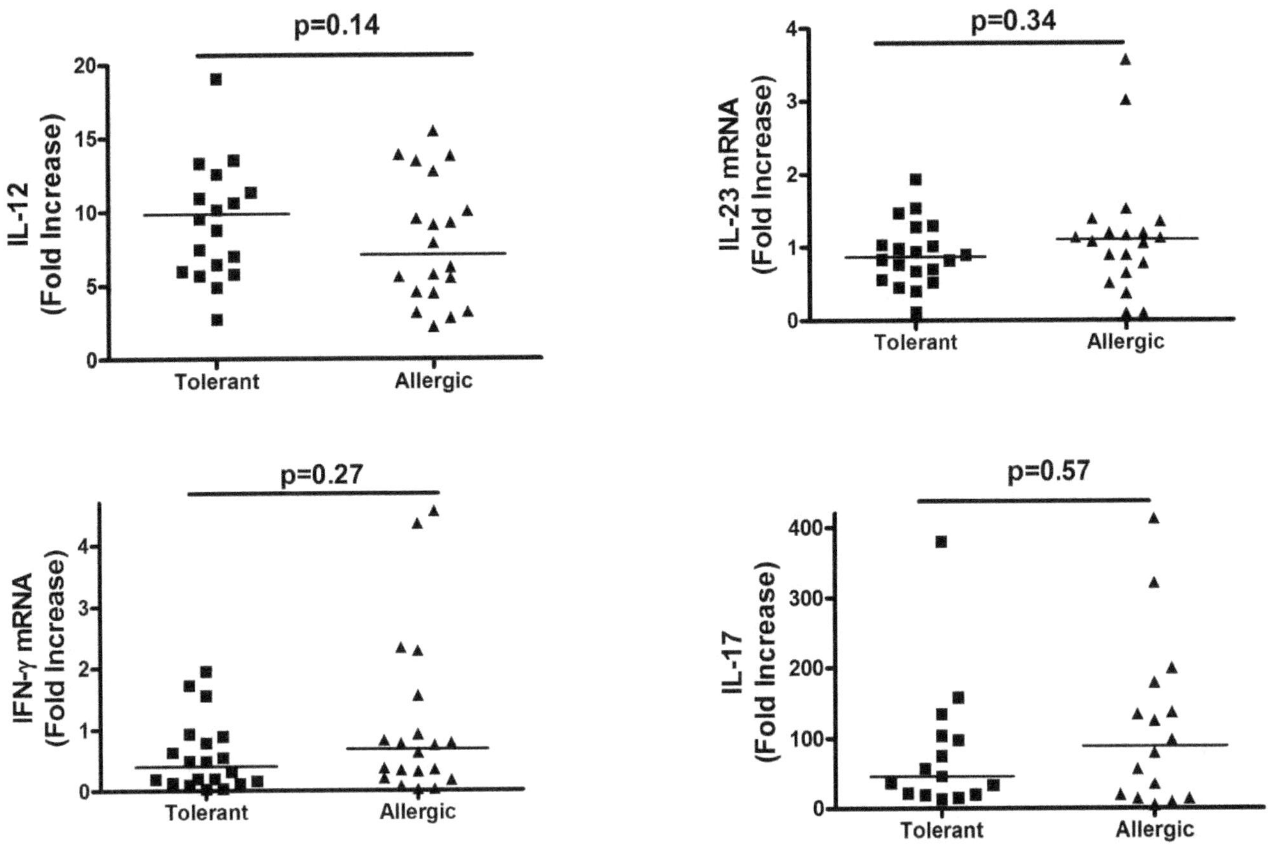


**Figure 4. Peanut-driven stimulation does not elicit differential Th1/Th17-associated cytokine responses in peanut allergic vs. clinically tolerant individuals.** PBMC were cultured as described for Figure 3 and comparisons of the intensity of the Ag-stimulated response (Wilcoxon) were made for each cytokine at the time of its peak antigen-driven response. Results are expressed as fold-increased levels relative to matched antigen un-stimulated controls. Bars indicate median responses. *** $p<0.0001$.

sensitivity. The capacity to generate and maintain cytokine production to this common food allergen is not inherently distinct between allergic and peanut tolerant humans as such responses are clearly ubiquitous in both populations. Rather, quantitative differences in the intensity of several of these responses offer potential for more compelling biomarkers. Given the many economic, logistical, safety and even interpretative concerns associated with food challenges [26], development of improved biomarkers continues to be a major goal [27].

For over two decades, IL-9 has been recognized as a cytokine whose elevated expression is linked to asthma and some related allergic disorders [28–29]. The extensive roles played by IL-9 in immune regulation [30] and effector mechanisms in humans are beyond the scope of this report but we note murine studies indicating that IL-9 can promote systemic anaphylaxis [31,32]. Indeed, among all cytokines examined in the present report, that which exhibits most clear cut differential expression between clinical phenotypes was IL-9. More focus on this understudied cytokine may offer insight into immuno-regulatory events that distinguish food allergic from clinically tolerant humans. While cytokine selective therapeutic strategies have proven to be problematic in most studies [33], ongoing Phase II studies of the impact of blocking IL-9 function are underway in asthma [34].

This is also the first report of Ag-stimulated IL-33 in food allergy. IL-33 mediates its biological effects via ST2, a receptor selectively expressed on Th2 but not Th1 cells [19,20,35]. Here, IL-33 mRNA levels were found to differ quantitatively, with clinically tolerant individuals exhibiting a median 3.4 fold increase and allergic individuals 8.6 fold enhancement upon food Ag stimulation. This 2.5 fold differential in the intensity of responses between clinical phenotypes reveals that elevated production of cytokines associated with induction (or perhaps renewal) of allergic disorders, as well as that of classical Type 2 effector cytokines, occurs in both food allergic and non-allergic individuals, and at quantitatively distinct levels.

The role of pro-inflammatory responses in maintenance of clinical tolerance to food antigens remains controversial. Some groups argue for IFNγ in establishing and maintaining clinical tolerance to food antigens [36–38]. Others, including ourselves, argue that "protective" induction of pro-inflammatory cytokine production by food antigens would be highly hazardous and that alternative mechanisms of oral tolerance are more likely. Evidence exists for both perspectives. Here, upon examination of a panel of cytokines associated with induction (IL-12, IL-23) or expression (IL-17, IFNγ) of pro-inflammatory responses in humans, substantive and equivalent IL-17 mRNA responses were elicited by peanut in both groups, with undetectable levels of IL-17A protein by ELISA (data not shown). No evidence was found for peanut-dependent Th1-associated mRNA or protein production. By comparison, Reovirus, a ubiquitous viral agent that infects cells in respiratory and enteric tracts without causing clinically apparent disease, typically elicits IFNγ recall responses from 10 to >200 IU/ml when PBMC were cultured under virtually identical conditions [39]. Most importantly, none of the pro-inflammatory

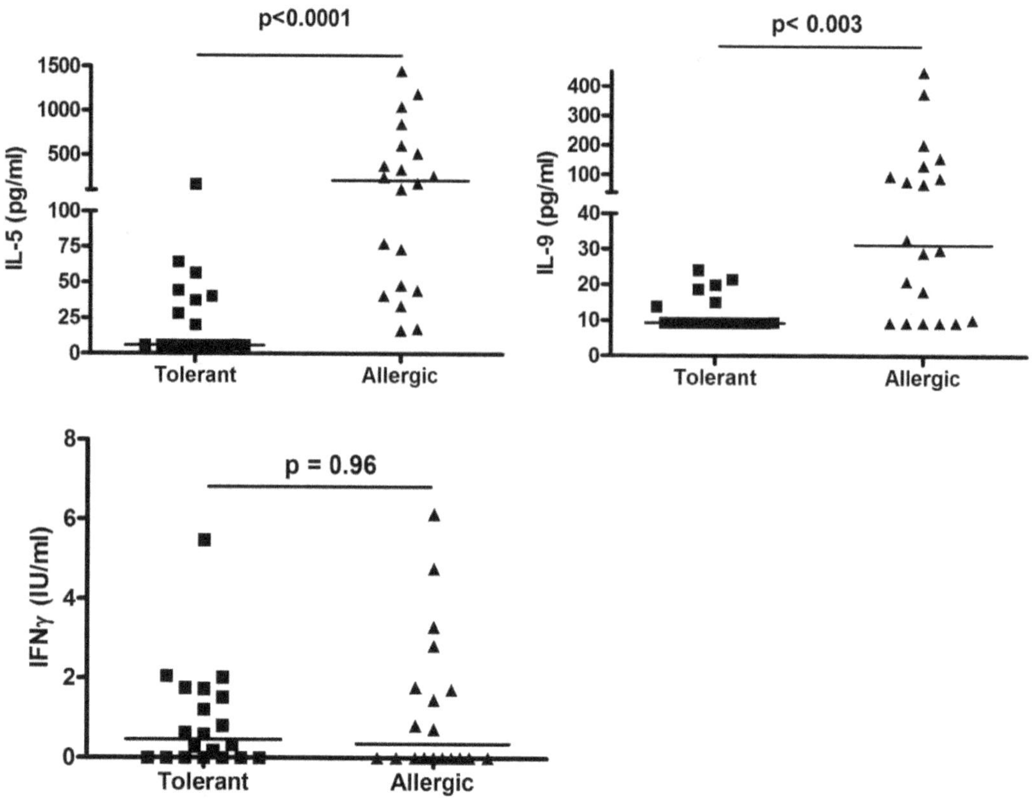


**Figure 5. Cytokine protein profiles in culture supernatants of peanut allergic individuals and those exhibiting clinical tolerance to peanut.** Culture supernatants harvested after five days of peanut Ag (100 ug/ml) stimulation were analyzed by ELISA, with median values shown for each population (Wilcoxon). In most instances, cytokine levels in unstimulated medium controls were at or below the limits of detection detailed at Materials and Methods.

Th1 or Th17 associated cytokines are differentially induced in the groups studied. Thus while pro-inflammatory cytokines clearly play important, usually undesirable, roles in asthma and other allergic disorders [40,41], neither elevated Ag-dependent Th1-associated nor Th17-associated activation appears to be associated with inhibition of food allergy in humans.

Multiple other pathways have been implicated in oral tolerance. Among these, elevated IDO, CTLA4/CD152, IL-10 and/or TGFb activity and enhanced Treg (of which multiple non-overlapping phenotypes and diverse mechanisms have been implicated ) are widely considered as key candidates [42–49]. None are the focus of this report. However, recent evidence

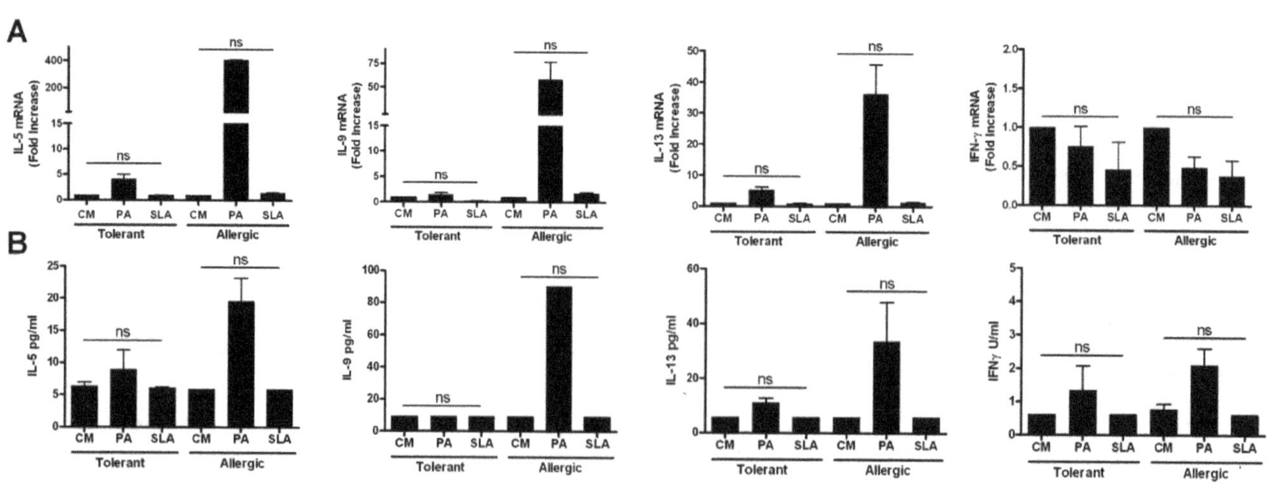


**Figure 6. Antigen-specificity of mRNA expression.** mRNA (panel A) and protein (panel B) responses elicited following culture in the presence of control medium, peanut Ag or soluble *Leishmania* antigen extract (SLA). Values given reflect responses of four individuals examined for each clinical phenotype.

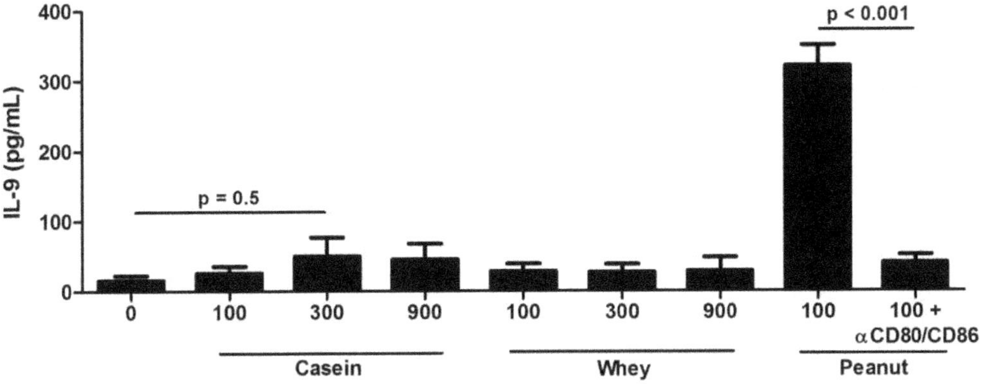


**Figure 7. PBMC from peanut allergic individuals do not exhibit IL-9 responses to unrelated food antigens. Peanut stimulated IL-9 responses require costimulation.** PBMC were stimulated for 5 days with 100 ug/ml peanut extract plus/minus anti-CD80/86 mAbs (each at 5 ug/ml) to assess costimulatory requirements for cytokine production *or* with unrelated the food antigen preparations bovine casein and whey at 100–900 ug/ml. Data reflect responses from triplicate analyses of culture supernatants obtained in nine independent experiments carried out using PBMC from highly peanut allergic (but milk non-allergic) individuals.

(Lotoski et al, manuscript in preparation) indicates that IL-10 plays a key role in limiting the intensity of peanut Ag-driven cytokine responses among individuals with ongoing peanut allergy. Further studies on what mechanisms are responsible for development and maintenance of oral tolerance in humans exposed to ubiquitous food antigens are clearly needed.

An experimental limitation of this study applies to virtually all studies of human immune capacity to foods. Use is made of PBMC rather than gut derived lymphoid tissues. The ethical and logistical concerns that prevent gut biopsies in food allergic and healthy human controls, let alone in sufficient numbers of subjects with sufficient numbers of cells for functional studies in humans, are obvious. Aside from logistical arguments, there is also a good intellectual rationale for use of systemic cells to assess immune responses that are (sometimes) initiated in the gut. Food allergy is a systemic disease. Upon ingestion, food derived peptides have been reported to be systemically available [6]. Here, we find that systemic Ag-dependent responses are evident in a large proportion of healthy and food allergic humans. Clinical reactions by peanut allergic individuals are of course systemic, not restricted to the gut.

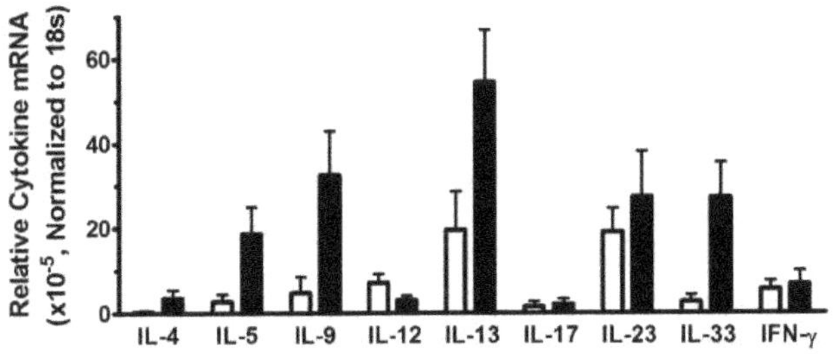


**Figure 8. Relative utility of individual cytokine mRNA responses to differentiate between peanut allergic individuals and those with clinical tolerance to peanut.** Total RNA was isolated from PBMC of peanut tolerant (open bars) and peanut allergic (closed bars) following in vitro stimulation with 100 ug/ml peanut extract for the time period leading to maximal Ag-driven cytokine production. mRNA levels were assessed by Q-PCR and are expressed relative to housekeeping gene 18 s rRNA rather than unstimulated medium controls, to enable comparison across cytokines, thereby identifying which cytokines exhibit the greatest differential response between peanut tolerant and peanut allergic populations.

Analysis of systemic immune responses is the best currently available tool to obtain insight in well powered groups as to how immune systems of food allergic and clinically tolerant individuals differentially respond to food re-exposure.

In summary, we identified optimal conditions for analysis of a broad panel of cytokines of relevance to food allergy in humans, directly ex vivo. While peanut antigen-dependent cytokine responses are common in the general population, clearly differential intensities of response are found for Th2/Th9-associated activation whereas Th1 or Th17-like responses are minimal. Ag-driven IL-9 responses offer a novel, more promising biomarker of dysregulated immunity to differentiate peanut allergic from peanut tolerant individuals. These findings will facilitate a broader approach to investigating immune (in)activation mechanisms linked to food allergy and clinical tolerance in humans.

## Supporting Information

**Figure S1 Determination of optimal peanut antigen concentrations for eliciting cytokine mRNA responses.** Mean mRNA levels in sextuplicate PBMC cultures are shown for three individuals following stimulation with 50 μg/ml (squares) 100 μg/ml (triangles) or 200 μg/ml (circles). Results are expressed as mean (± SEM) fold change in mRNA levels relative to expression at time zero in paired un-stimulated medium controls. (TIF)

**Table S1 Primers validated for assessment of mRNA levels by Q-PCR.**
(DOCX)

**Table S2 Reproducibility of Replicate Q-PCR Analyses.**
(DOCX)

## Acknowledgments

We thank the volunteers who participated in this study and Bill Stefura for excellent technical assistance.

## Author Contributions

Conceived and designed the experiments: KH FERS ABB JU. Performed the experiments: JX LL RC RS. Analyzed the data: JX LL KH. Contributed reagents/materials/analysis tools: RC JL FERS ABB JU. Wrote the paper: JX KH.

## References


1. Berin MC, Sicherer S (2011) Food allergy: mechanisms and therapeutics. Curr Opin Immunol 23:794–800.
2. Vickery BP, Chin S, Burks AW (2011) Pathophysiology of food allergy. Pediatr Clin North Am 58:363–376.
3. Madsen CB, Hattersley S, Allen KJ, Beyer K, Chan CH, et al. (2012) The role of genetics and environment in the rise of childhood food allergy. Clin Exp Allergy 42:30–37.
4. Tan TH, Ellis JA, Saffery R, Allen KJ (2012) Can we define a tolerable level of risk in food allergy? Report from a EuroPrevall/UK Food Standards Agency workshop. Clin Exp Allergy 42:20–29.
5. Diesner SC, Untersmayr E, Pietschmann P, Jensen-Jarolim E (2011) Food Allergy: Only a Pediatric Disease? Gerontology 57:28–32.
6. Sicherer SH, Sampson HA (2009) Food allergy: recent advances in pathophysiology and treatment. Annu Rev Med 60:261–277.
7. Thyagarajan A, Varshney P, Jones SM, Sicherer S, Wood R, et al. (2010) Peanut oral immunotherapy is not ready for clinical use. J Allergy Clin Immunol 126:31–32.
8. Akdis M, Akdis CA (2009) Therapeutic manipulation of immune tolerance in allergic disease. Nat Rev Drug Discov 8:645–660.
9. Scurlock AM, Vickery BP, Hourihane JO, Burks AW (2010) Pediatric food allergy and mucosal tolerance. Mucosal Immunol 3:345–54.
10. Allen KJ, O'Hehir RE (2011) The evolution of oral immunotherapy for the treatment of peanut allergy. Clin Exp Allergy 41:1172–4.
11. Nowak-Węgrzyn A, Sampson HA (2011) Future therapies for food allergies. J Allergy Clin Immunol 127:558–573.
12. Prickett SR, Voskamp AL, Dacumos-Hill A, Symons K, Rolland JM, et al. (2011) Ara h 2 peptides containing dominant CD4+ T-cell epitopes: candidates for a peanut allergy therapeutic. J Allergy Clin mmunol 127:608–615.
13. Swoboda I, Bugajska-Schretter A, Linhart B, Verdino P, Keller W, et al. (2007) A recombinant hypoallergenic parvalbumin mutant for immunotherapy of IgE-mediated fish allergy. J Immunol 178:6290–6296.
14. Gonipeta B, Parvataneni S, Paruchuri P, Gangur V (2010) Long-term characteristics of hazelnut allergy in an adjuvant-free mouse model. Int Arch Allergy Immunol 152:219–225.
15. Muleme HM, Reguera RM, Berard A, Azinwi R, Jia P, et al. (2009) Infection with Arginase-Deficient Leishmania major Reveals a Parasite Number-Dependent and Cytokine-Independent Regulation of Host Cellular Arginase Activity and Disease Pathogenesis. J Immunol 183:8068–8076.
16. Blanc F, Bernard H, Alessandri S, Bublin M, Paty E, et al. (2008) Update on optimized purification and characterization of natural milk allergens. Mol Nutr Food Res 52 Suppl 2: S166–S175.
17. Stinson M, Douville R, Lissitsyn Y, Blanchard M, Stefura W, et al. (2008) Quantification of human chemokine production in TLR-stimulated and antigen-specific recall responses. Methods Mol Med 138:121–131.
18. Stefura WP, Campbell JD, Douville R, Stinson MJ, Simons FE, et al. (2008) Ultrasensitive ELISA for measurement of human cytokine responses in primary culture. Methods Mol Med 138:107–119.
19. Schmitz J, Owyang A, Oldham E, Song Y, Murphy E, et al. (2005) IL-33, an interleukin-1-like cytokine that signals via the IL-1 receptor-related protein ST2 and induces T helper type 2-associated cytokines. Immunity 23:479–490.
20. Liew FY, Pitman NI, McInnes IB (2010) Disease-associated functions of IL-33: the new kid in the IL-1 family. Nat Rev Immunol 10:103–10.
21. Sassi A, Largueche-Darwaz B, Collette A, Six A, Laouini D, et al. (2005) Mechanisms of the natural reactivity of lymphocytes from noninfected individuals to membrane-associated *Leishmania infantum* antigens. J Immunol 174:3598–3607.
22. Imada M, Simons FE, Jay FT, HayGlass KT (1995) Antigen mediated and polyclonal stimulation of human cytokine production elicit qualitatively different patterns of cytokine gene expression. Int Immunol 7:229–237.
23. Sims P, Coffman RL, Hessel EM (2009) Biomarkers measuring the activity of Toll-like receptor ligands in clinical development programs. Methods Mol Biol 517:415–440.
24. Paul WE, Zhu J (2010) How are T(H)2-type immune responses initiated and amplified? Nat Rev Immunol 10:225–35.
25. Sampson HA (2001) Utility of food-specific IgE concentrations in predicting symptomatic food allergy. J Allergy Clin Immunol 107:891–896.
26. Niggemann B (2010) When is an oral food challenge positive? Allergy 65:2–6.
27. HayGlass KT (2011) The quest for predictive immune biomarkers. Clin Exp Allergy 41:1656–9.
28. Noelle RJ, Nowak EC (2010) Cellular sources and immune functions of interleukin-9. Nat Rev Immunol 10:683–687.
29. Goswami R, Kaplan MH (2011) A brief history of IL-9. J Immunol 186:3283–3288.
30. Wilhelm C, Turner JE, Van Snick J, Stockinger B (2012) The many lives of IL-9: a question of survival? Nat Immunol 13:637–641.
31. Forbes EE, Groschwitz K, Abonia JP, Brandt EB, Cohen E, et al. (2008) IL-9 and mast cell-mediated intestinal permeability predisposes to oral antigen hypersensitivity. J Exp Med 205:897–913.
32. Osterfeld H, Ahrens R, Strait R, Finkelman FD, Renauld JC, et al. (2010) Differential roles for the IL-9/IL-9 receptor alpha-chain pathway in systemic and oral antigen-induced anaphylaxis. J Allergy Clin Immunol 125:469–476.
33. Holgate ST (2011) Pathophysiology of asthma: what has our current understanding taught us about new therapeutic approaches? J Allergy Clin Immunol 128:495–505.
34. Oh CK, Raible D, Geba GP, Molfino NA (2011) Biology of the interleukin-9 pathway and its therapeutic potential for the treatment of asthma. Inflamm Allergy Drug Targets 10:180–186.
35. Liew FY (2012) IL-33: a Janus cytokine. Ann Rheum Dis 71: i101–i104.
36. Turcanu V, Maleki SJ, Lack G (2003) Characterization of lymphocyte responses to peanuts in normal children, peanut-allergic children, and allergic children who acquired tolerance to peanuts. J Clin Invest 111:1065–72.
37. Srivastava KD, Qu C, Zhang T, Goldfarb J, Sampson HA, et al. (2009) Food Allergy Herbal Formula-2 silences peanut-induced anaphylaxis for a prolonged posttreatment period via IFN-gamma-producing CD8+ T cells. J Allergy Clin Immunol 123:443–51.
38. Morafo V, Srivastava K, Huang CK, Kleiner G, Lee SY, et al. (2003) Genetic susceptibility to food allergy is linked to differential TH2-TH1 responses in C3H/HeJ and BALB/c mice. J Allergy Clin Immunol 111:1122–8.
39. Douville RN, Su RC, Coombs KM, Simons FE, HayGlass KT (2008) Reovirus serotypes elicit distinctive patterns of recall immunity in humans. J Virol 82:7515–7523.
40. Wang YH, Wills-Karp M (2011) The potential role of interleukin-17 in severe asthma. Curr Allergy Asthma Rep 11:388–394.
41. Besnard AG, Togbe D, Couillin I, Tan Z, Zheng SG, et al. (2012) Inflammasome-IL-1-Th17 response in allergic lung inflammation. J Mol Cell Biol 4:3–10.
42. Zhou Y, Kawasaki H, Hsu SC, Lee RT, Yao X, et al. (2010) Oral tolerance to food-inducedsystemic anaphylaxis mediated by the C-type lectin SIGNR1. Nat Med 16:1128–1133.
43. Marcondes Rezende M, Hassing I, Bol-Schoenmakers M, Bleumink R, Boon L, et al. (2011) CD4(+) CD25(+) T regulatory cells do not transfer oral tolerance to peanut allergens in a mouse model of peanut allergy. Clin Exp Allergy 41:1324–1333.
44. van Wijk F, Nierkens S, de Jong W, Wehrens EJ, Boon L, et al. (2007) The CD28/CTLA-4-B7 signaling pathway is involved in both allergic sensitization and tolerance induction to orally administered peanut proteins. J Immunol 178:6894–6900.
45. Saraiva M, O'Garra A (2010) The regulation of IL-10 production by immune cells. Nat Rev Immunol 10:170–81.
46. Duan W, So T, Mehta AK, Choi H, Croft M (2011) Inducible CD4+LAP+– Foxp3- regulatory T cells suppress allergic inflammation. J Immunol 187:6499–6507.
47. Palomares O, Yaman G, Azkur AK, Akkoc T, Akdis M, et al. (2010) Role of Treg in immune regulation of allergic diseases. Eur J Immunol 40:1232–1240.
48. Rachid R, Umetsu DT (2012) Immunological mechanisms for desensitization and tolerance in food allergy. Semin Immunopathol 34:689–702.
49. Shevach EM (2011) Biological functions of regulatory T cells. Adv Immunol 112:137–176.

12

# Serological Investigation of Food Specific Immunoglobulin G Antibodies in Patients with Inflammatory Bowel Diseases

**Chenwen Cai, Jun Shen, Di Zhao, Yuqi Qiao, Antao Xu, Shuang Jin, Zhihua Ran, Qing Zheng***

Key Laboratory of Gastroenterology & Hepatology, Ministry of Health, Division of Gastroenterology and Hepatology, Ren Ji Hospital, School of Medicine, Shanghai Jiao Tong University, Shanghai Institute of Digestive Diseases, 145 Middle Shandong Road, Shanghai 200001, China

## Abstract

***Objective:*** Dietary factors have been indicated to influence the pathogenesis and nature course of inflammatory bowel diseases (IBD) with their wide variances. The aim of the study was to assess the prevalence and clinical significance of 14 serum food specific immunoglobulin G (sIgG) antibodies in patients with IBD.

***Methods:*** This retrospective study comprised a total of 112 patients with IBD, including 79 with Crohn's disease (CD) and 33 with ulcerative colitis (UC). Medical records, clinical data and laboratory results were collected for analysis. Serum IgG antibodies against 14 unique food allergens were detected by semi-quantitative enzyme linked immunosorbent assay (ELISA).

***Results:*** Food sIgG antibodies were detected in 75.9% (60/79) of CD patients, 63.6% (21/33) of UC patients and 33.1% (88/266) of healthy controls (HC). IBD patients showed the significantly higher antibodies prevalence than healthy controls (CD *vs.* HC, $P=0.000$; UC *vs.* HC, $P=0.001$). However no marked difference was observed between CD and UC groups ($P=0.184$). More subjects were found with sensitivity to multiple antigens (≥3) in IBD than in HC group (33.9% vs.0.8%, $P=0.000$). Egg was the most prevalent food allergen. There was a remarkable difference in the levels of general serum IgM ($P=0.045$) and IgG ($P=0.041$) between patients with positive and negative sIgG antibodies. Patients with multiple positive allergens (≥3) were especially found with significant higher total IgG levels compared with sIgG-negative patients ($P=0.003$). Age was suggested as a protective factor against the occurrence of sIgG antibodies ($P=0.002$).

***Conclusions:*** The study demonstrates a high prevalence of serum IgG antibodies to specific food allergens in patients with IBD. sIgG antibodies may potentially indicate disease status in clinical and be utilized to guide diets for patients.

**Editor:** David L Boone, University of Chicago, United States of America

**Funding:** The work was supported by grants from the National Key Technology R&D Program of China (No. 2012BAI06B03), http://kjzc.jhgl.org/and National Natural Science Foundations of China (No. 81170362, 81200280 and 81370508), http://isisn.nsfc.gov.cn. The funders had no role in study design, data collection and analysis, decision to publish, or preparation of the manuscript.

**Competing Interests:** The authors have declared that no competing interests exist.

* Email: qingzheng101@163.com

## Introduction

Inflammatory bowel diseases (IBD) include two main types, Crohn's disease (CD) and ulcerative colitis (UC), both characterized by mucosal ulceration in gut. Patients with IBD suffer from abdominal pain, diarrhea, weight loss and fatigue. As diseases progress, they can cause perianal lesion, abdominal abscess, intestinal perforation or even canceration as diverse complications. Extraintestinal manifestations including oral ulcer, arthritis, iritis and cholangitis may also occur simultaneously [1]. The tendentiousness of the constant alternation of relapses and remissions seriously affects the quality of life in IBD patients [2]. For the moment the mechanisms involved in the pathogenesis can be summarized that the influence of environmental factors to genetically susceptible individuals triggers abnormal mucosal immune reaction in gut with the involvement of intestinal flora and eventually leads to the bowel inflammation and ulceration [3].

IBD has long been regarded as a problem threatening public health in the Western world. However in recent decades the rising incidence of it in developing nations has made IBD a global issue. In Asia, according to an epidemiological survey, the rapid westernization and modernization may attribute to the condition [4]. Among various environmental factors, diet has been implicated to play a considerable role in the course of IBD [5–8]. A Japanese study suggested the intake of a high fat diet and sweets may associate with CD and UC [9]. Another research also pointed an increased consumption of alcohol and red meat might cause higher incidence of relapse in UC patients [10]. Meanwhile food intolerance, which is defined as a reproducible adverse reaction to specific food or food ingredients, has become more common in recent years [11–12]. Banai J. considered all kinds of

**Table 1.** Demographic data of all subjects.

| Clinicopathological features | CD (N=79) | UC (N=33) | HC (N=266) |
|---|---|---|---|
| Male (*n*, %) | 47(59.5) | 18(54.5) | 146(54.9) |
| Female (*n*, %) | 32(40.5) | 15(45.5) | 120(45.1) |
| Age (yr) (mean, 95% CI) | 36.5(33.6–39.4) | 40.7 (35.9–45.7) | 46.4(45.2–47.6) |
| Age range (yr) | 18–68 | 17–73 | 24–71 |
| Duration of disease (yr) (*n*, %) | | | |
| <1 | 21 (26.6) | 13 (39.4) | / |
| 1–5 | 38 (48.1) | 11 (33.3) | / |
| 5–10 | 16 (20.3) | 7 (21.2) | / |
| >10 | 4 (5.1) | 2 (6.1) | / |
| Disease activity (*n*, %) | | | |
| Remission | 7 (8.9) | 0 (0) | / |
| Mild | 16 (20.3) | 12 (36.4) | / |
| Moderate | 33 (41.8) | 14 (42.4) | / |
| Severe | 23 (29.1) | 7 (21.2) | / |
| Localization of disease (*n*, %) | | | |
| L1 (terminal ileum) | 40 (50.6) | / | / |
| L2 (colon) | 10 (12.7) | / | / |
| L3 (ileocolon) | 29 (36.7) | / | / |
| E1 (rectum) | / | 1 (3.0) | / |
| E2 (left-sided colon) | / | 14 (42.4) | / |
| E3 (entire colon) | / | 18 (54.5) | / |
| Complications of disease (*n*, %) | | | |
| None | 32 (40.5) | 31 (93.9) | / |
| 1 item | 42 (53.2) | 2 (6.1) | / |
| 2 items | 5 (6.3) | / | / |
| Extraintestinal manifestations (*n*, %) | | | |
| None | 60 (75.9) | 26 (78.8) | / |
| 1 item | 18 (22.8) | 7 (21.2)) | / |
| 2 items | 1 (1.3) | / | / |
| Intestinal surgery | 15 (19.0) | 0 (0.0) | / |

CD: Crohn's disease; UC: ulcerative colitis; HC: healthy controls; yr: year; 95% CI: 95% confidence interval; L1,L2,L3: disease localization of Crohn's disease by Montreal Classification; E1,E2,E3: disease localization of ulcerative colitis by Montreal Classification.

food could be antigenic properties to cause chronic mild inflammation in gut and eventually lead to ulcerative colitis [13]. For example, intolerance to milk has long been believed involving in the pathogenesis of IBD [14,15]. Glassman *et al* reported during infancy stage the frequency of symptoms compatible with milk protein sensitivity was greater in UC compared with control population ($P<0.03$) [16]. Furthermore patients who underwent milk intolerance were found to develop UC at an earlier age compared to those without a history of hypersensitivity to milk ($P<0.02$) [16]. The statistics suggested the early antigenic stimuli might play a role in development of IBD at a later age [17]. However the causality of food intolerance and IBD still remains controversial and needs further researches to figure out.

Studies on food adverse reactions mediated by immunoglobulin G (IgG) in certain intestinal diseases, such as irritable bowel syndrome (IBS), have been increasingly reported [18–19]. Researchers used to mainly focus on food intolerance classically by the presence of serous IgE antibodies but it seemed that the characteristically immediate allergic reactions were quite rare in some conditions [20–21]. By contrast, the circulating IgG antibodies provide a more delayed or even asymptomatic response after the exposure to a unique food antigen [22]. Considering that IBD patients mostly suffer a long course of the chronic disease, we hypothesize IgG may have a stronger relevance with IBD than IgE.

Food is a complicated field to study because of its enormous varieties. In another way this feature also makes it a resource palace for us researchers to explore. In this study we aimed to identify the prevalence and significance of 14 food specific IgG antibodies in IBD patients through serological investigation. We expected the results may provide a more clear and detailed connection between food intolerance and IBD in our patient population as well as a supporting evidence for the antibody test to serve the clinical.

## Subjects and Methods

### Ethics Statement

This study was approved by Medical Ethics Committee of Ren Ji Hospital of Shanghai Jiao Tong University School of Medicine.

**Table 2.** Prevalence of food specific IgG antibodies in patients with Crohn's disease (CD), ulcerative colitis (UC) and healthy controls (HC).

| Group | *N* | Seropositive Degree (*n*) | | | | Antibodies (−) | Antibodies (+) |
|---|---|---|---|---|---|---|---|
| | | 0 | +1 | +2 | +3 | (*n*, %) | (*n*, %) |
| CD | 79 | 19 | 10 | 14 | 36 | 19 (24.1) | 60 (75.9) |
| UC | 33 | 12 | 9 | 4 | 8 | 12 (36.4) | 21 (63.6) |
| HC | 266 | 178 | 41 | 24 | 23 | 178 (66.9) | 88 (33.1) |

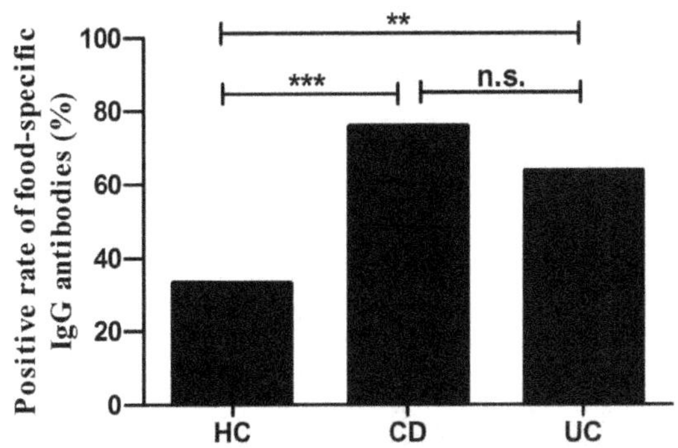


**Figure 1. Positive rate of food-specific IgG antibodies in Crohn's disease (CD), ulcerative colitis (UC) and healthy control (HC) groups.** Chi-square test, *** $P<0.001$, ** $P<0.005$, n.s. not significant.

Informed consent wasn't applied as the medical records and private information of all the subjects were anonymized and de-identified prior to analysis.

## Subjects

The study included a total of 112 patients with CD (n = 79) or UC (n = 33) in Ren Ji Hospital from June 2011 to December 2013. All patients met the diagnostic criteria for CD or UC according to the consensus on the diagnosis of IBD drawn up by European Crohn's and Colitis Organization (ECCO) [23,24] and were serologically tested of the food sIgG antibodies during their visit in hospital. In addition another 266 people, who came to our Health Care Centre to do checkups which contained the test as a routine item, were randomly chosen to represent the general population as healthy controls (HC).

## Data Collection

Medical records and clinical data of all the IBD patients were comprehensively reviewed and the general demographic data were summarized. The disease severity of CD or UC was based on Harvey-Bradshaw Index [25] or Modified Truelove-Witts Classi-

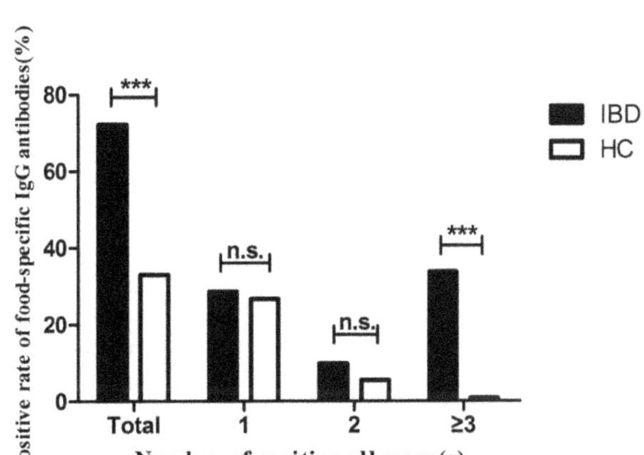


**Figure 2. Distribution of the number of positive allergen(s) with positive rate of food-specific IgG antibodies in patients with inflammatory bowel diseases (IBD) and healthy controls (HC).** Chi-square test, *** $P<0.001$, n.s. not significant.

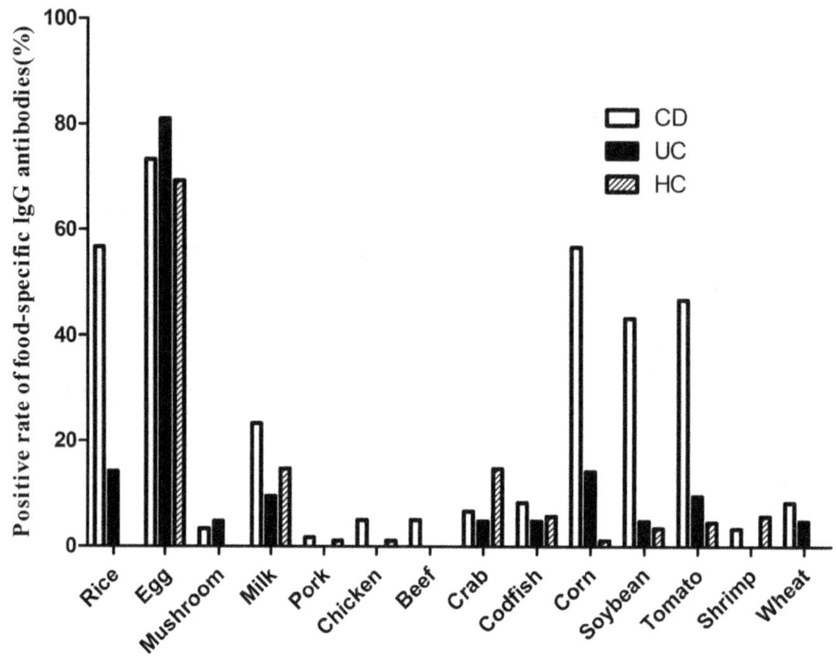


**Figure 3. Distribution of positive food allergens in Crohn's disease (CD), ulcerative colitis (UC) and healthy control (HC) groups.**

fication [26], respectively. The disease localization of both CD and UC was determined by Montreal Classification [27]. The complications that patients carried consisted of fistula, abdominal abscess, intestinal obstruction, perianal disease, hemorrhage of gastrointestinal tract and acute perforation. The simultaneous extraintestinal manifestations included oral ulcer, sacro-iliitis, rheumatoid arthritis, iritis, primary sclerotic cholangitis, hepatic adipose infiltration and cholelithiasis. Relevant laboratory findings contained peripheral white blood cell (WBC) counts, eosinophile granulocyte (EOS) counts, lymphocyte (LYM) counts, haemoglobin (Hb), serum albumin, erythrocyte sedimentation rate (ESR), high-sensitivity C-reactive protein (hs-CRP), serum total immunoglobulin (IgM, IgA and IgG) and anti double-stranded DNA antibodies (anti-dsDNA).

## Enzyme Linked Immunosorbent Assay (ELISA)

ELISA tests for the semi-quantitative analysis of serum IgG antibodies to 14 unique food allergens, including rice, egg, mushroom, milk, pork, chicken, beef, crab, codfish, corn, soybean, tomato, shrimp and wheat, were performed by the detection kit according to the operation manual (Biomerica, Inc. USA). The IgG concentration less than 50U/ml was considered negative (Grade 0). The values between 50–100U/ml, 100–200U/ml and more than 200U/ml were represented mild sensitivity (Grade +1), moderate sensitivity (Grade +2) and high sensitivity (Grade +3), respectively.

## Data Analysis

Statistics were performed with SPSS 19.0 (SPSS Inc. USA). Enumeration data were analyzed using chi-squared test, in which rates of multiple samples were compared by R×C contingency table analysis. Continuous numerical variables were expressed in the form of mean with 95% confidence interval (95% CI) and analyzed by Student's $t$ test. Regression analysis was utilized to identify the correlation/risk factors among variables. Two-tailed $P$-value$<0.05$ was regarded statistically significant.

# Results

## Demographic data of all subjects

The characteristic information of IBD patients and healthy controls were summarized in **Table 1**.

**Table 3.** Distribution of food specific IgG antibodies in different disease localizations.

| Localization | sIgG antibodies (+) | sIgG antibodies (−) |
|---|---|---|
| | (*n*, %) | (*n*, %) |
| Only small intestine (*N* = 40) | 33 (82.5) | 3 (17.5) |
| Only large intestine (*N* = 43) | 26 (60.5) | 17 (39.5) |
| Both small & large intestine (*N* = 29) | 22 (75.9) | 7 (24.1) |
| *P*-value | 0.072△ | |

△ Chi-square test (R×C contingency table analysis), not statistically significant ($P>0.05$).

**Table 4.** Distribution of food specific IgG antibodies at different IBD activity status.

| Disease status | sIgG antibodies (+) | Multiple positive (≥2) | High sensitivity |
|---|---|---|---|
| | *n* (%) | *n* (%) | *n* (%) |
| Remission (*N* = 7) | 6 (85.7) | 5 (71.4) | 3 (42.9) |
| Mild (*N* = 28) | 18 (64.3) | 7 (25) | 9 (32.1) |
| Moderate (*N* = 47) | 35 (74.5) | 23 (48.9) | 18 (38.3) |
| Severe (*N* = 30) | 22 (73.3) | 14 (46.7) | 14 (46.7) |
| *P*-value | 0.647$^{\triangle}$ | 0.079$^{\triangle}$ | 0.719$^{\triangle}$ |

$^{\triangle}$Chi-square test (R×C contingency table analysis), not statistically significant ($P>0.05$).

## Prevalence of serum IgG antibodies to 14 unique food allergens

Food specific IgG antibodies were detected positive in 75.9% (60/79) of CD patients, 63.6% (21/33) of UC patients and 33.1% (88/266) of HC (**Table 2**). The antibodies showed a significantly higher frequency in both CD and UC groups than in healthy controls (CD *vs* HC, $P = 0.000$; UC *vs* HC, $P = 0.001$) (**Figure 1**). However, there was no significant difference between CD and UC groups ($P = 0.184$). In general the total positive rate of all IBD patients was 72.3% (81/112), higher than the control group ($P = 0.000$). Among them 28.6% (32/112), 9.8% (11/112) and 33.9% (38/112) of subjects were respectively sensitive to one, two and more than two food allergens while the corresponding ratios of healthy controls were 26.7% (71/266), 5.6% (15/266) and 0.8% (2/266). There were more subjects who got intolerant to 3 or more antigens in IBD group than in HC group ($P = 0.000$) (**Figure 2**).

In the present study, the top five prevalent food allergens which caused positive sIgG antibodies in CD patients were egg (44/60, 73.3%), rice (34/60, 56.7%), corn (34/60, 56.7%), tomato (28/60, 46.7%) and soybean (26/60, 43.3%). Besides, the top five prevalent food allergens in UC group were egg (17/21, 81.0%), rice (3/21, 14.3%), corn (3/21, 14.3%), tomato (2/21, 9.5%) and milk (2/21, 9.5%). And healthy controls demonstrated the compositions of egg (61/88, 69.3%), milk (13/88, 14.8%), crab (13/88, 14.8%), codfish (5/88, 5.7%) and shrimp (5/88, 5.7%), which were similar to the results of a reported epidemiological survey in general population [28]. **Figure 3** showed the distribution of positive food allergens in CD, UC and HC groups.

## Association of food specific IgG antibodies with inflammatory segments

To analyze the association between food sIgG antibodies status and disease extent in gut, all 112 patients were divided into three subgroups according to endoscopic results (**Table 3**). The positive rate was found higher (82.5%) in patients with only small intestine involved but the statistical difference wasn't remarkable ($P = 0.072$).

## Relevance of food specific IgG antibodies with disease activity

We divided all 112 IBD patients into four subgroups according to clinical disease activity and compared the ratios of patients with positive IgG antibodies, multiple positive antibodies (≥2) and high sensitivity to at least one food allergen (**Table 4**). Although the

**Table 5.** Comparison of laboratory results in IBD patients with positive and negative food specific IgG antibodies.

| Laboratory results | sIgG antibodies (+) | sIgG antibodies (−) | *P*-value |
|---|---|---|---|
| | (N = 81) | (N = 31) | |
| WBC (×10$^9$/L) | 7.15(6.50–7.86) | 6.66(5.79–7.56) | 0.437 |
| EOS (×10$^9$/L) | 0.16(0.12–0.23) | 0.15(0.10–0.21) | 0.833 |
| LYM (×10$^9$/L) | 1.44(1.31–1.59) | 1.54(1.32–1.81) | 0.501 |
| Hb (g/L) | 114.31(109.52–119.06) | 114.23(104.84–122.58) | 0.986 |
| Albumin (g/L) | 36.19(34.82–37.72) | 35.98(33.67–38.28) | 0.889 |
| ESR (mm/h) | 28.07(23.01–33.58) | 21.35(15.65–27.61) | 0.160 |
| hs-CRP (mg/L) | 18.84(13.78–23.89) | 11.75(6.51–18.51) | 0.083 |
| IgM (g/L) | 1.22(0.99–1.49) | 0.79(0.60–1.03) | 0.045* |
| IgA (g/L) | 2.80(2.37–3.27) | 2.60(2.13–3.05) | 0.597 |
| IgG (g/L) | 12.90(11.94–13.94) | 10.92(9.50–12.48) | 0.041* |
| anti-dsDNA (IU/mL) | 3.31(2.85–3.75) | 3.56(2.72–4.61) | 0.609 |

Statistics were expressed as mean with 95% confidence interval.
Normal range: white blood cell (WBC), 3.69–9.16×10$^9$/L; eosinophile granulocyte (EOS), 0.02–0.50×10$^9$/L; lymphocyte (LYM), 0.8–4.0×10$^9$/L; haemoglobin (Hb), 113–172 g/L; albumin, 35–55 g/L; erythrocyte sedimentation rate (ESR) 0–20 mm/h; high-sensitivity C-reactive protein (hs-CRP), 0–3 mg/L; immunoglobulin M (IgM) 0.4–2.3 g/L; IgA, 0.7–4.0 g/L; IgG, 7–16 g/L; anti double-stranded DNA antibodies (anti-dsDNA), 0–7.0 IU/mL
Student's *t* test, *$P<0.05$.

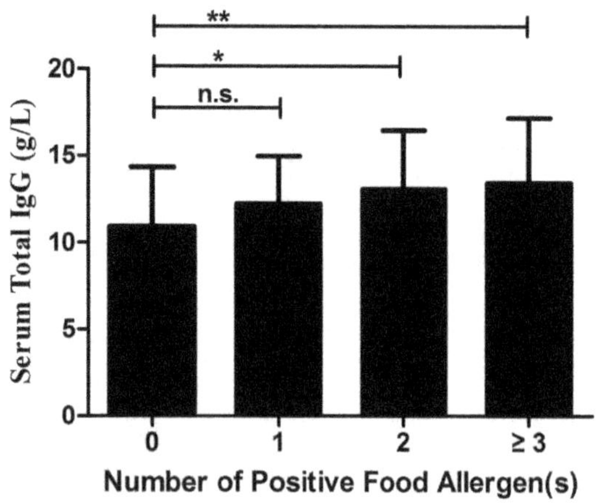


**Figure 4. Serum total IgG values in inflammatory bowel disease patients with multiple positive food allergens.** Statistics were shown as mean ± standard deviation. Chi-square test, * $P<0.05$; ** $P<0.005$, n.s. not significant.

general antibodies and multi-antibodies were found more common in remission group (85.7% and 71.4%) while the patients who were highly sensitive to specific food allergens seemed to be severer (46.7%), there was no significant differences among the four subgroups.

To further analyze the possible association with several laboratory values related to disease activity, IBD patients were classified into positive and negative IgG antibodies subgroups (**Table 5**). We did find a notable difference in general serum IgM ($P = 0.045$) and IgG ($P = 0.041$) levels between the two groups. Mean values of WBC, ESR and hs-CRP in the positive patients were recognized higher compared with the other group although no marked differences were found. The rest lab findings of the two groups were resembled.

Considering the relative levels of total IgG in relation to antigen specific IgG, we then divided all the IBD patients into 4 groups according to the number of positive allergen(s) (0, 1, 2, ≥3) and compared the difference of serum general IgG values among the groups (**Figure 4**). The mean values of each group were 10.92 (9.50–12.48) g/L, 12.24 (11.31–13.32) g/L, 13.08 (11.31–14.97) g/L and 13.42 (12.24–14.58) g/L, respectively. Patients with multiple positive allergens (≥2) were found with significant higher total IgG levels than sIgG-negative patients ($P = 0.044$, $P = 0.003$, respectively).

### Predictors for the occurrence of food specific IgG antibodies

To further identify the predictive factors, we utilized binary logistic regression analyses of several demographic and clinical parameters. The independent variables contained disease type (CD/UC), gender, age, complication, extraintestinal manifestation and intestinal surgery (**Table 6**). Only age was found as a predisposing as well as protective factor against the development of serum food-related IgG antibodies ($P = 0.002$).

## Discussion

In the present study, we have demonstrated that IgG antibodies against food specific allergens are distinctly elevated in IBD patients compared with healthy controls. This serologic antibody investigation is served as an aid in the diagnosis and management of food intolerance in clinical activities [29]. Food intolerance can be defined as a series of unpleasant symptoms including eructation, abdominal pain, diarrhea, fatigue, headache and palpitation after the intake of particular food products [29]. It is usually caused by enzyme deficiency as well as pharmacological effects of vasoactive amines present in foods. When certain food can't be fully digested, bodies may produce specific IgG antibodies which would form immune complexes with food particles and lead to excessive protective immune responses [30]. Food intolerance is not so similar to food allergy as the latter mainly occurs through the classically immediate IgE-mediated antibody responses and the obvious symptoms can be detected by most patients [31]. Meanwhile, IgG-mediated reaction characteristically acts as a particular delayed-type hypersensitivity response after the exposure to antigens and sometimes the symptoms are too occult for patients to recognize [22]. Some investigators considered them to be physiological since that the food sIgG antibodies can appear in healthy individuals [32], which was also proved in our data. However, several studies including our results have shown the higher prevalence of sIgG antibodies to food in IBD patients or animal models in contrast to normal controls [19,33], which arouse the attention to the relevance between IBD and food intolerance. Van Den Bogaerde *et al.* used colonoscopic allergen provocation test to determine the gut mucosal response to food antigens in Crohn's disease [34]. This intuitionistic study provided both *in vivo* and *in vitro* evidence that CD patients were more sensitive to exogenous food antigens than healthy people and the reactions were gut specific.

Food sIgG antibodies were discovered frequent in IBD patients with small intestine involved in the present research, which resembled the result of a study on the correlation of lactose malabsorption and disease segments [35]. Mishkin *et al.* demon-

**Table 6.** Correlation of food specific IgG antibodies with demographic and clinical parameters.

| Parameters | Odds ratio | 95% CI | *P*-value |
|---|---|---|---|
| Disease type (CD vs. UC) | 1.167 | 0.389–3.498 | 0.783 |
| Gender | 0.758 | 0.306–1.879 | 0.549 |
| Age | 0.945 | 0.912–0.979 | 0.002** |
| Complication | 2.269 | 0.719–7.157 | 0.162 |
| Extraintestinal manifestation | 1.302 | 0.438–3.868 | 0.635 |
| Intestinal surgery | 1.613 | 0.329–7.905 | 0.556 |

95% CI: 95% confidence interval; CD: Crohn's disease; UC: ulcerative colitis.
Binary logistic regression, $^{**}P<0.005$.

strated that CD of the proximal small bowel (duodenum, jejunum), terminal ileum, terminal ileum plus colon and colon alone were related with lactose malabsorption of 100%, 68.1%, 54.5% and 43.5%, respectively. Regression analysis of our data indicated age as a protective factor of food intolerance in IBD patients, which is opposite to the result of a cross sectional epidemiological study in other area of China [28]. We assume the difference might be associated with age structure of onset as inflammatory bowel diseases, especially Crohn's disease, tend to occur in younger people based on our clinical observation.

A survey demonstrated that 15.6% IBD patients believed diet could initiate the disease while 57.8% were convinced certain foods could play a role in causing relapses [36]. In our study, we found food sIgG antibodies were more frequent in patients who were during remission. Meanwhile, the patients who were highly sensitive to food allergens tended to be serious in disease activity and mean levels of ESR and hs-CRP were detected higher in sIgG-positive patients. Although the results didn't show statistical significance, they did provide us with a tendency. We consider the few remission cases (only 7) contributed to the above conflicting results.

The increased serum IgM values tested in sIgG-positive patients may indicate recent infection. Besides, we also found a higher level of serum total IgG antibodies in patients with positive allergens, especially with multiple ones in the study. The general increase on IgG levels may be an important reason for the increased amount of sIgG antibodies against food epitopes. It has been reported that mast cells can respond not only to IgE antibodies but also to IgG antibodies [37]. In addition IgG antibodies in food allergy may even influence allergen-IgE complex formation and bind to B cells, which is quite opposite the traditional concept that IgG antibodies are supposed to inhibit these processes [38]. Therefore IgG antibodies probably serve as mediation effects rather than inhibition in hypersensitivity reaction caused by food intolerance. Serum sIgG antibodies to non-food related antigens are mostly studied within inhaled antigens in respiratory allergic disorders such as asthma. Wang *et al.* investigated the relevance between asthma morbidity and sIgE/sIgG levels to inhaled allergen exposure [39]. They concluded that sIgE levels could serve as markers of asthma however sIgG was not that important as predictor or modifier. Due to the rich diversity of food and non-food allergens, we believe that the immune reactions can be very distinct for different allergens and the mechanisms of how sIgG functions may be complicated and needs further study.

How IBD and food intolerance interact with each other remains controversial. Disruption of epithelial tight junctions causes hyperpermeability in the gut of IBD patients and allows the antigen presenting cells (dendritic cells) to directly encounter food antigens in lamina propria to activate Th/B cells, thus resulting in high levels of sIgG antibodies [40]. Simultaneously this defect may also exacerbate inflammatory conditions. In another respect, lack of certain enzyme may lead to incomplete digestion of food and the remaining polypeptides then stimulate the secretion of sIgG antibodies as well as inflammatory cytokines, thereby bringing impairments to normal intestines [41]. The definite mechanism still remains unclear.

Although we used several methods to improve our study, there were still some limitations to the present results. The small quantity of cases may bring about the first shortcoming. The sample size needs to be enlarged to see the exact trend. We didn't contain the follow-up data of whether or not the IBD patients eliminated the food based on the presence of sIgG antibodies and whether the subsequent diet elimination had an effect on the diseases, which is also a limitation of our research. However, promising results have been reported in a randomized controlled trial [19]. Bentz *et al.* designed a double-blind, cross-over nutritional diet intervention according to circulating food sIgG antibodies with 40 CD patients and it did show therapeutic effects with regard to abdominal pain, stool frequency and general well-being. However, the investigators could not elucidate the exact mechanisms of the contribution of sIgG antibodies to disease activity. Anyway, we still consider serologic investigation of IgG antibodies to food antigens may bring benefits to dietary modification for IBD patients.

In conclusion, the prevalence of food specific IgG antibodies is remarkably higher in patients with inflammatory bowel diseases than healthy controls, and age may acts as a protective factor for their occurrence. Although the mechanisms of the interaction between food intolerance and IBD remain obscure, the sIgG antibodies may potentially show the clinical significance to indicate disease status and to ameliorate symptoms by guiding diets for patients.

## Acknowledgments

The authors would like to thank the Department of Clinical Laboratory at Ren Ji Hospital for assisting us to conduct the study.

## Author Contributions

Conceived and designed the experiments: CC QZ ZR. Performed the experiments: CC QZ. Analyzed the data: CC DZ AX SJ. Contributed reagents/materials/analysis tools: JS YQ DZ SJ. Wrote the paper: CC JS DZ ZR QZ.

## References


1. Bernstein CN (2001) Extraintestinal manifestations of inflammatory bowel disease. Curr Gastroenterol Rep 3: 477–483.
2. Vidal A, Gomez-Gil E, Sans M, Portella MJ, Salamero M, et al. (2008) Health-related quality of life in inflammatory bowel disease patients: the role of psychopathology and personality. Inflamm Bowel Dis 14: 977–983.
3. Macdonald TT, Monteleone G (2005) Immunity, inflammation, and allergy in the gut. Science 307: 1920–1925.
4. Goh K, Xiao SD (2009) Inflammatory bowel disease: a survey of the epidemiology in Asia. J Dig Dis 10: 1–6.
5. Magee EA, Edmond LM, Tasker SM, Kong SC, Curno R, et al. (2005) Associations between diet and disease activity in ulcerative colitis patients using a novel method of data analysis. Nutr J 4: 7.
6. Hou JK, Abraham B, El-Serag H (2011) Dietary intake and risk of developing inflammatory bowel disease: a systematic review of the literature. Am J Gastroenterol 106: 563–573.
7. Brunner B, Scheurer U, Seibold F (2007) Differences in yeast intolerance between patients with Crohn's disease and ulcerative colitis. Dis Colon Rectum 50: 83–88.
8. Haboubi NY, Jones S (2005) Influence of dietary factors on the clinical course of inflammatory bowel disease. Gut 54: 567.
9. Sakamoto N, Kono S, Wakai K, Fukuda Y, Satomi M, et al. (2005) Dietary risk factors for inflammatory bowel disease: a multicenter case-control study in Japan. Inflamm Bowel Dis 11: 154–163.
10. Jowett SL, Seal CJ, Pearce MS, Phillips E, Gregory W, et al. (2004) Influence of dietary factors on the clinical course of ulcerative colitis: a prospective cohort study. Gut 53: 1479–1484.
11. Sampson HA (2004) Update on food allergy. J Allergy Clin Immunol 113: 805–819; quiz 820.
12. David TJ (2000) Adverse reactions and intolerance to foods. Br Med Bull 56: 34–50.
13. Banai J (2009) Nutrition in inflammatory bowel disease. Orv Hetil 150: 839–845.
14. Binder JH, Gryboski JD, Thayer WR Jr, Spiro HM (1966) Intolerance to milk in ulcerative colitis. A preliminary report. Am J Dig Dis 11: 858–864.
15. Truelove SC (1961) Ulcerative colitis provoked by milk. Br Med J 1: 154–160.

16. Glassman MS, Newman LJ, Berezin S, Gryboski JD (1990) Cow's milk protein sensitivity during infancy in patients with inflammatory bowel disease. Am J Gastroenterol 85: 838–840.
17. Cashman KD, Shanahan F (2003) Is nutrition an aetiological factor for inflammatory bowel disease? Eur J Gastroenterol Hepatol 15: 607–613.
18. Atkinson W, Sheldon TA, Shaath N, Whorwell PJ (2004) Food elimination based on IgG antibodies in irritable bowel syndrome: a randomised controlled trial. Gut 53: 1459–1464.
19. Bentz S, Hausmann M, Piberger H, Kellermeier S, Paul S, et al. (2010) Clinical relevance of IgG antibodies against food antigens in Crohn's disease: a double-blind cross-over diet intervention study. Digestion 81: 252–264.
20. Zar S, Kumar D, Benson MJ (2001) Food hypersensitivity and irritable bowel syndrome. Aliment Pharmacol Ther 15: 439–449.
21. Mekkel G, Barta Z, Ress Z, Gyimesi E, Sipka S, et al. (2005) Increased IgE-type antibody response to food allergens in irritable bowel syndrome and inflammatory bowel diseases. Orv Hetil 146: 797–802.
22. Crowe SE, Perdue MH (1992) Gastrointestinal food hypersensitivity: basic mechanisms of pathophysiology. Gastroenterology 103: 1075–1095.
23. Stange EF, Travis SP, Vermeire S, Reinisch W, Geboes K, et al. (2008) European evidence-based Consensus on the diagnosis and management of ulcerative colitis: Definitions and diagnosis. J Crohns Colitis 2: 1–23.
24. Van Assche G, Dignass A, Panes J, Beaugerie L, Karagiannis J, et al. (2010) The second European evidence-based Consensus on the diagnosis and management of Crohn's disease: Definitions and diagnosis. J Crohns Colitis 4: 7–27.
25. Harvey RF, Bradshaw JM (1980) A simple index of Crohn's-disease activity. Lancet 1: 514.
26. Truelove SC, Witts LJ (1955) Cortisone in ulcerative colitis; final report on a therapeutic trial. Br Med J 2: 1041–1048.
27. Satsangi J, Silverberg MS, Vermeire S, Colombel JF (2006) The Montreal classification of inflammatory bowel disease: controversies, consensus, and implications. Gut 55: 749–753.
28. Sai XY, Zheng YS, Zhao JM, Zhao W (2011) A cross sectional survey on the prevalence of food intolerance and its determinants in Beijing, China. Chin J Epidemiol 32(3):302–05 (in Chinese).
29. Palmieri B, Esposito A, Capone S, Fistetto G, Iannitti T (2011) Food intolerance: reliability and characteristics of different diagnostic alternative tests. Minerva Gastroenterol Dietol 57: 1–10.
30. Ortolani C, Pastorello EA (2006) Food allergies and food intolerances. Best Pract Res Clin Gastroenterol 20: 467–483.
31. Wuthrich B (2009) Food allergy, food intolerance or functional disorder. Praxis (Bern 1994) 98: 375–387.
32. Husby S, Oxelius VA, Teisner B, Jensenius JC, Svehag SE (1985) Humoral immunity to dietary antigens in healthy adults. Occurrence, isotype and IgG subclass distribution of serum antibodies to protein antigens. Int Arch Allergy Appl Immunol 77: 416–422.
33. Foster AP, Knowles TG, Moore AH, Cousins PD, Day MJ, et al. (2003) Serum IgE and IgG responses to food antigens in normal and atopic dogs, and dogs with gastrointestinal disease. Vet Immunol Immunopathol 92: 113–124.
34. Van Den Bogaerde J, Cahill J, Emmanuel AV, Vaizey CJ, Talbot IC, et al. (2002) Gut mucosal response to food antigens in Crohn's disease. Aliment Pharmacol Ther 16: 1903–1915.
35. Mishkin B, Yalovsky M, Mishkin S (1997) Increased prevalence of lactose malabsorption in Crohn's disease patients at low risk for lactose malabsorption based on ethnic origin. Am J Gastroenterol 92: 1148–1153.
36. Zallot C, Quilliot D, Chevaux JB, Peyrin-Biroulet C, Gueant-Rodriguez RM, et al. (2013) Dietary beliefs and behavior among inflammatory bowel disease patients. Inflamm Bowel Dis 19: 66–72.
37. Malbec O, Daeron M (2007) The mast cell IgG receptors and their roles in tissue inflammation. Immunol Rev 217: 206–221.
38. Meulenbroek LA, de Jong RJ, den Hartog Jager CF, Monsuur HN, Wouters D, et al. (2013) IgG antibodies in food allergy influence allergen-antibody complex formation and binding to B cells: a role for complement receptors. J Immunol 191: 3526–3533.
39. Wang J, Visness CM, Calatroni A, Gergen PJ, Mitchell HE, et al. (2009) Effect of environmental allergen sensitization on asthma morbidity in inner-city asthmatic children. Clin Exp Allergy 39: 1381–1389.
40. Chahine BG, Bahna SL (2010) The role of the gut mucosal immunity in the development of tolerance against allergy to food. Curr Opin Allergy Clin Immunol 10: 220–225.
41. Isolauri E, Rautava S, Kalliomaki M (2004) Food allergy in irritable bowel syndrome: new facts and old fallacies. Gut 53: 1391–1393.

13

# Immunization with Hypoallergens of Shrimp Allergen Tropomyosin Inhibits Shrimp Tropomyosin Specific IgE Reactivity

**Christine Y. Y. Wai[1], Nicki Y. H. Leung[1], Marco H. K. Ho[2], Laurel J. Gershwin[3], Shang An Shu[4], Patrick S. C. Leung[4], Ka Hou Chu[1]***

**1** School of Life Sciences, The Chinese University of Hong Kong, Shatin, Hong Kong SAR, China, **2** Department of Pediatrics and Adolescent Medicine, The University of Hong Kong, Hong Kong SAR, China, **3** Department of Pathology, Microbiology and Immunology, School of Veterinary Medicine, University of California Davis, Davis, California, United States of America, **4** Division of Rheumatology/Allergy, School of Medicine, University of California Davis, Davis, California, United States of America

## Abstract

Designer proteins deprived of its IgE-binding reactivity are being sought as a regimen for allergen-specific immunotherapy. Although shrimp tropomyosin (Met e 1) has long been identified as the major shellfish allergen, no immunotherapy is currently available. In this study, we aim at identifying the Met e 1 IgE epitopes for construction of hypoallergens and to determine the IgE inhibitory capacity of the hypoallergens. IgE-binding epitopes were defined by three online computational models, ELISA and dot-blot using sera from shrimp allergy patients. Based on the epitope data, two hypoallergenic derivatives were constructed by site-directed mutagenesis (MEM49) and epitope deletion (MED171). Nine regions on Met e 1 were defined as the major IgE-binding epitopes. Both hypoallergens MEM49 and MED171 showed marked reduction in their *in vitro* reactivity towards IgE from shrimp allergy patients and Met e 1-sensitized mice, as well as considerable decrease in induction of mast cell degranulation as demonstrated in passive cutaneous anaphylaxis assay. Both hypoallergens were able to induce Met e 1-recognizing IgG antibodies in mice, specifically $IgG_{2a}$ antibodies, that strongly inhibited IgE from shrimp allergy subjects and Met e 1-sensitized mice from binding to Met e 1. These results indicate that the two designer hypoallergenic molecules MEM49 and MED171 exhibit desirable preclinical characteristics, including marked reduction in IgE reactivity and allergenicity, as well as ability to induce blocking IgG antibodies. This approach therefore offers promises for development of immunotherapeutic regimen for shrimp tropomyosin allergy.

**Editor:** Jacques Zimmer, Centre de Recherche Public de la Santé (CRP-Santé), Luxembourg

**Funding:** The work described in this paper was fully supported by a research grant from the Research Grants Council, Hong Kong Special Administrative Region, China (CUHK 463911). The funders had no role in study design, data collection and analysis, decision to publish, or preparation of the manuscript.

**Competing Interests:** The authors have declared that no competing interests exist.

* Email: kahouchu@cuhk.edu.hk

## Introduction

Food allergy is a type 1 hypersensitivity disorder that affects up to 10% of the general population [1] and frequently lead to anaphylaxis. Food-related acute allergic reactions account for up to 49% of all anaphylaxis-related emergency department (ED) visits [2–4] and for patients discharged from ED, 54% filled epinephrine autoinjection prescription within one year [5]. Among all food allergies, shellfish allergy is one of the most common types with a prevalence of 0.6% in the world population [6], and is particularly common in Asian countries [7]. Shellfish is also considered as one of the four most common food, which could provoke anaphylaxis [8]. With an emerging trend in both shellfish production and consumption, the increase in the prevalence of shellfish allergy is predictable [9]. Improved clinical management of this disorder is therefore needed, and comprehensive studies of the molecular characteristics of shellfish allergens and therapeutic regimens are eminent.

At the molecular level, the muscle protein tropomyosin was identified as the major shrimp ingestion-related allergen in *Metapenaeus* and *Penaeus* spp [10–12]. Biochemically, tropomyosin is a coiled-coiled secondary structure protein of 34–38 kDa and functions in contractile activities of muscle cells [13]. While shrimp allergy has long been a model for studying shellfish allergy, our laboratory has cloned and expressed tropomyosin from *Metapenaeus ensis* (Met e 1), which exhibits specific serological IgE reactivity with serum samples from shrimp allergy patients [11]. This study has facilitated the subsequent identification of tropomyosin as an allergen common in crustaceans and mollusks [14–18]. Greatly attributed to the high amino acid sequence homology among the crustaceans and mollusks tropomyosins (93.8% and 77.2%, respectively), as well as a 61.4% sequence homology between the arthropods and mollusks tropomyosins, this protein is believed to be the major cross-reactive shellfish pan-allergen [13,19]. Specifically, there are more than 99% sequence homology between the two most common reference shrimp allergens Met e 1 and the tropomyosin from *Penaeus aztecus*

(Pen a 1) [12]. Met e 1 and Pen a 1 are therefore ideal model allergens, to be engineered for shrimp allergy immunotherapy studies but also possibly at other tropomyosin-induced shellfish allergies.

Although food avoidance and epinephrine injection are currently the first-line treatments in patients with anaphylaxis, allergen-specific immunotherapy (SIT) is the major strategy for clinical management of allergy as it has the capacity to modify the course of the disease. However, conventional modalities for SIT using native allergens are constrained due to the potential risk of allergic side-effects during treatment. In this context, hypoallergen with low/no IgE reactivity is desirable for SIT. Notably, the nature of allergenic epitopes and hypoallergens might greatly affect the SIT outcome such as the induction and generation of blocking antibodies, shifting of the Th1/Th2 paradigm and induction of peripheral tolerance by recruitment of regulatory T cells [20–25]. Molecular characterization of allergens, exemplified by the identification of IgE-binding epitopes, is thus imperative for the design of safer immunotherapy regimens [26]. Ayuso et al. have applied the concept of a hypoallergenic mutant by introducing 12 point mutations into the eight IgE-binding epitopes [27] within the five allergenic regions of Pen a 1 [28]. Although this mutant showed a reduction of allergenic potency of 90–98% in humanized rat basophilic leukemia (RBL) release assay, maximal releases were similar between the mutant and wild-type Pen a 1. This result suggests that other significant allergenic epitopes may exist in addition to the eight allergenic sites reported, thus additional approaches are necessary to construct a hypoallergen of shellfish tropomyosin.

To circumvent this issue, we have chosen a two-pronged approach in designing shrimp tropomyosin hypoallergens. In this study, the first objective is to define the major IgE-binding epitopes of *Metapenaeus* tropomyosin Met e 1. The second objective of this study is to construct hypoallergenic derivatives of Met e 1 by introducing point mutations within the IgE-binding epitopes identified, or by deleting these epitopes. The IgE reactivity, allergenicity, immunogenicity and the inhibitory potential of the hypoallergen-induced antibodies towards IgE antibodies of subjects allergic to shrimp and Met e 1-sensitized mice [29] are characterized and compared to the wild type allergen Met e 1. Herein, we specifically used serum samples from children and adolescents allergic to shrimp in mapping the IgE-binding epitopes. Previous study reported greater epitope diversity among children allergic to shrimp than adult patients [30] and outgrown of shellfish allergy is rarely reported [31,32]. We therefore believe that the use of pediatric serum samples could resolve an epitope profile of Met e 1 that is comprehensive, clinically relevant and common among shrimp allergy patients in any age group. The hypoallergens constructed based on this epitope profile should also be applicable in immunotherapy targeting at both pediatric and adult patients.

## Materials and Methods

### Serum samples

Serum samples were obtained from 12 subjects (aged 3–17 years) with confirmed clinical history of allergic responses to shrimp and positive skin prick test (Table S1). Specific IgE reactivities to purified recombinant shrimp tropomyosin Pen a 1 and Met e 1 were characterized by ImmunoCAP and ELISA, respectively. None of the recruited subjects have other allergies. Serum samples (n = 8) obtained from healthy, non-atopic volunteers without Met e 1-specific IgE were used as a negative control.

### Ethics statement

A written consent was obtained from the parents of the children enrolled in the study (Institutional Review Board of the University of Hong Kong/Hospital Authority Hong Kong West Cluster, Ref. No. UW10-115). The use and storage of human sera were approved by the Joint Chinese University of Hong Kong - New Territories East Cluster Clinical Research Ethics Committee with a written informed consent (CREC Ref. No. CRE-2010-514). All animal protocols were approved by the Animal Experimentation Ethics Committee, The Chinese University of Hong Kong (ref No. 11/006/GRF and 463911), in accordance with the Department of Health (Hong Kong) guidelines in Care and Use of Animals. All experiments were performed under licenses granted from the Government of Hong Kong Special Administrative Region.

### Identification of allergenic epitopes

There were three independent methods used to predict the immunodominant allergenic epitopes including 1) computational prediction of IgE binding epitopes, 2) ELISA against overlapping peptides that span the entire Met e 1 sequence, and 3) dot-immunoblotting of overlapping peptides against the entire Met e 1 sequence. 18 overlapping peptides spanning the full-length (274 amino-acids) Met e 1 were commercially synthesized (GenScript). Each peptide had 20 amino acids (except for peptide 18 that contains 19 amino acids) with five amino acids overlapping with the adjacent peptides at the N-terminus. Individual peptides were dissolved in distilled water, aliquoted and stored at −20°C until required.

1) Three computational models from the Immune Epitope Database (IEDB) Analysis Resource were employed to predict the major linear IgE-binding epitopes of Met e 1, including Bepipred Antibody Epitope Prediction, Kolaskar & Tongaonkar Antigenicity model and Emini Surface Accessibility Prediction. Bepipred Antibody Epitope Prediction predicts the location of IgE-binding epitopes based on the hidden Markov model and propensity scale method [33]. The Kolaskar & Tongaonkar Antigenicity model is based on the physiochemical properties of amino acid residues [34]. Emini Surface Accessibility Prediction is based on the calculation of the surface accessibility scale [35].
2) For peptide ELISA, 3 μg of each peptide were coated on 96-well plates (Nunc, maxisorp) in 0.05 M carbonate buffer overnight. After blocking with 1% BSA/PBS for 1.5 h, the plates were incubated with individual serum samples (150 dilution) at room temperature for 2 h. Thereafter, the plates were incubated with biotinylated goat anti-human IgE (Vector) in 11000 dilution for 45 min followed by incubation with Avidin D, Peroxidase labeled antibody (Vector) in 11000 dilution for 30 min. The plates were then developed with TMB substrate reagent set (BD Biosciences) for 15 min and the reaction was terminated by 2 N $H_2SO_4$. Absorbance was measured at 450 nm using an ELISA plate reader (Bio-Rad). All absorbance values were background-corrected, in which the background absorbance was the OD value of Met e 1-coated wells incubated with secondary and tertiary antibodies only. All the above procedures were performed at room temperature. The plates were washed with PBS/0.5% Tween-20 (PBST) three times and PBS once between each step and all dilutions were made in 1% BSA/PBS.
3) For dot-immunoblotting, 3 μg of each peptide (3 μL) were spotted onto a 0.2 μm nitrocellulose membrane (Bio-Rad). The membrane was allowed to air-dry and thereafter fixed

with 2.5% glutaraldehyde/PBS for 10 min [36]. The membrane was incubated with diluted serum (150 dilution) overnight at 4°C after a 2-h blocking in 3% skim milk/TBS. The membrane was incubated with mouse monoclonal anti-human IgE-alkaline phosphatase antibody (Sigma Aldrich) at 12000 dilution for 1 h at room temperature followed by signal development with NBT/BCIP (Roche). All dilutions were made with 3% skim milk/TBS and all washing steps were performed with TBST) once and TBS three times with shaking.

## Design of hypoallergenic shrimp tropomyosins

With the high structural flexibility and spontaneous unfolding property of tropomyosin [37], we believe that the possibility of having only one single amino acid per epitope that is crucial for IgE binding is unlikely. Restricted homologous substitution may not be sufficient to result in tropomyosin variants with greatly reduced IgE reactivity. Therefore, the amino acid sequence of Met e 1 was compared to the non-allergenic fish tropomyosins of four species *Salmo salar* (Atlantic salmon; GenBank accession number NP_001117128.1), *Epinephelus coioides* (orange-spotted grouper; ADG29138.1), *Siniperca chuatsi* (Mandarin fish; AEK21799.1) and *Thunnus thynnus* (Atlantic bluefin tuna; BAD01050.1) (Fig. S1). All nine identified IgE-binding regions in Met e 1 were converted into the homologous sequence of fish tropomyosins and 49 point mutations in total were introduced to construct the mutation mutant MEM49 (Fig. 1A & B). To construct the deletion mutant, all nine IgE-binding epitopes were deleted (Fig. 1B). This mutant, named MED171, contained only 171 amino acid residues. The amino acid sequences of MEM49 and MED171 were reverse translated using MEGA 5.0 and the encoding sequences of the two mutants were synthesized commercially by GenScript. Synthetic genes of each of the mutants were cloned into pET30(a)+ (Novagen) expression vector via *EcoRV* and *HindIII* restriction sites. The sequences and reading frame of MEM49 and MED171 in the plasmid were confirmed by dideoxynucleotide sequencing.

## Preparation of recombinant wild type and mutant shrimp tropomyosin

cDNA coding for the full length shrimp tropomyosin Met e 1 and the encoding sequences of MEM49 and MED171 were cloned into His-tag expression vector pET30(a)+ (Novagen) and expressed in *Escherichia coli* BL21 (DE3) (Invitrogen) by culturing in MagicMedia (Invitrogen) at 37°C overnight. His-tagged recombinant Met e 1 (rMet e 1), MEM49 and MED171 were purified using the HisPur Cobalt Spin Column (Thermo Scientific) according to the manufacturer's instructions. Protein concentration was determined by BCA assay (Sigma Aldrich) while the purity was determined by Sodium dodecyl sulfate-polyacrylamide gel electrophoresis (SDS-PAGE) and Coomassie blue staining.

## Mice sensitization and immunization

3–4 weeks old female Balb/c mice were acquired from the Laboratory Animal Services Centre, The Chinese University of Hong Kong. All animals were maintained on a shrimp-free diet and housed in pathogen-free conditions. To induce Met e 1 hypersensitivity in mice, sensitization was performed as described previously by intragastric administration of 0.1 mg of recombinant tropomyosin plus cholera toxin on days 0, 12, 19 and 26 and challenged on day 33 [29]. Mice fed with phosphate-buffered saline plus cholera toxin were included as controls. Blood samples were collected 4 h after the challenge for antibody analysis.

For immunization experiments, 5–6 weeks old female Balb/c mice were intraperitoneally immunized three times on days 0, 7 and 14 with 0.1 mg purified rMet e 1, MEM49 or MED171 adsorbed to 1 mg $Al(OH)_3$. Blood was collected 4 h after the last injection for the determination of antibody levels.

## Direct ELISA

To examine the IgE reactivity to rMet e 1, MEM49 or MED171, 96-well ELISA plates were coated with 5 μg/mL of either rMet e 1, MEM49 or MED171 in 0.05 M carbonate buffer overnight at 4°C, blocked with 1% BSA/PBS for 2 h and incubated with serum samples from shrimp allergy subjects or Met e 1-sensitized mice (110 dilution) overnight at 4°C. After washing, plates were incubated with biotinylated anti-human (Vector) or anti-mouse IgE antibodies (BD Pharmigen) and Avidin D, Peroxidase labeled antibody (Vector), each at 11000 dilution at room temperature for 1 h and 30 min, respectively. The plates were then developed with TMB substrate reagent set (BD Biosciences) for 15 min and the reaction was terminated by 2 N $H_2SO_4$.

To determine the reactivity of IgG and $IgG_{2a}$ antibodies raised in rMet e 1, MEM49 and MED171 immunized mice, sera in serial dilutions (1400 to 125600) were incubated in the rMet e 1, MEM49 or MED171 coated plates (5 μg/mL) for 2 h at room temperature. The plates were then incubated with goat anti-mouse IgG or anti-mouse $IgG_{2a}$ (Southern Biotech) in 12000 dilution for 45 min followed by incubation with Avidin D, Peroxidase labeled antibody (Vector) in 11000 dilution for 30 min. The plates were then developed with TMB substrate reagent set (BD Biosciences) for 5 min and the reaction was terminated by 2 N $H_2SO_4$.

## Passive cutaneous anaphylaxis

Passive cutaneous anaphylaxis was performed to determine the *in vivo* allergenicity of MEM49 and MED171. Backs of naïve Balb/c mice were shaved, followed by intradermal injection of Met e 1-specific IgE-containing sera (undiluted sera in a total volume of 100 μL) under isoflurane narcosis. Two hours later, mice were injected intravenously with a mixture of 100 μL of 0.5% Evan's blue dye (Sigma Aldrich) and 0.1 mg rMet e 1, MEM49 or MED171. Thirty minutes after dye-rMet e 1 administration, mice were sacrificed by cervical dislocation and skins of their backs were immediately inverted for the measurement of blue region diameters.

## Competitive inhibition ELISA

Competitive inhibition ELISA was performed to evaluate the blocking capacity of hypoallergen-induced blocking antibodies. Briefly, rMet e 1 was used to coat 96-well plates (5 μg/mL) overnight at 4°C and blocked with 1% BSA/PBS for 2 h. Plates were then washed and blocked with 100 μL of 110 diluted sera from mice immunized MEM49, or MED171 overnight at 4°C. Thereafter, 100 μL of sera from shrimp allergy patients or Met e 1-sensitized mice at a predetermined dilution (110–120 dilution) were added and incubated at room temperature for 2 h. The wells were then washed and followed by the addition of biotinylated anti-human or anti-mouse IgE antibodies, HRP-Avidin D and developed as described above. The blocking ability of the induced IgG antibodies was determined using the equation $[(OD_{no\ inhibitor} - OD_{inhibitor})/OD_{no\ inhibitor}] \times 100\%$ and expressed as percentage inhibition.

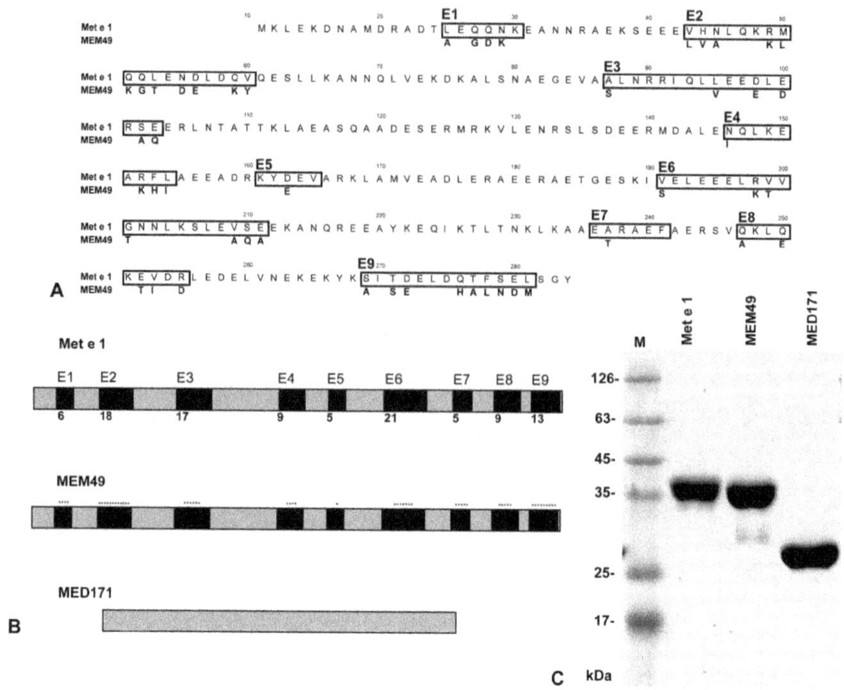


**Figure 1. Design of two hypoallergenic mutants.** MEM49 was constructed by substitution of 49 different amino acid residues within the nine Met e 1 epitopes to the homologous fish tropomyosin sequence. MED171 was constructed by deletion of epitopes E1 to E9 of Met e1. (**A**) Location of the IgE-binding epitopes in tropomyosin. The IgE epitopes designated as E1–E9 are shown in boxes and the location of the 49 amino acid residues in Met e 1 that are converted in MEM49 are also shown as one letter amino acid code. (**B**) Schematic representation of Met e 1, MEM49 and MED171. Epitopes E1 to E9 in Met e 1 are represented as black boxes and the number of amino acids in each epitope is indicated. Amino acid residue changes in MEM49 are shown as *. MED171 is a truncated peptide with the epitopes E1–E9 deleted. (**C**) SDS-PAGE of Met e 1, MEM49 and MED171 after Coomassie Blue staining. Note the 35 kDa molecular weight of Met e 1 and MEM49 and the expected smaller size of MED171 compared to Met e 1.

### Statistical analysis

Data were presented as mean ± SEM. The statistical comparison was determined by one-way analysis of variance (ANOVA) followed by the Student-Newman-Keuls test using SigmaStat 3.1. The difference was considered statistically significant at $p<0.05$.

## Results

### IgE-binding epitopes of Met e 1 and hypoallergen design

By ELISA, sera from patients with shrimp allergy (n = 12) had significantly higher IgE reactivity against five peptides (P3, P5, P10, P13 and P16) when compared with other peptides ($p<0.05$) (Fig. 2A). None of the sera from control subjects (n = 8) showed IgE-binding activity towards these or other peptides (data not shown).

Allergenic regions on Met e 1 were also defined based on the intensity of peptide spots and the frequency of recognition in dot-immunoblotting (Fig. 2B). A peptide with >50% recognition (6 out of 12 patients) or an epitope score (calculated by the summation of the IgE reactivity score (strong reactivity: 3; median: 2; low: 1)) higher than the mean intensity score (8.83, calculated by adding all epitope scores and dividing by 18 peptides) was defined as a major IgE-binding epitope. Based on these criteria, eight peptides (P1, P3, P10, P11, P15, P16, P17 and P18) were identified as the major Met e 1-specific IgE-binding sequences. The discrepancy in epitopes determined by ELISA and dot-immunoblotting (Fig. 2C) was apparently due to assay sensitivity and peptide presentation on different materials in the two assays.

Three online immunoinformatics models were applied to define the IgE epitopes. (Fig. 2C & Fig. S2). Seven epitopes, with six to 16 amino acid residues in length, were identified using Emini Surface Accessibility Prediction based on the surface probability score (Fig. S2A). Ten allergenic regions, between six to 19 amino acid residues in length, were defined under the Kolaskar & Tongaonkar Antigenicity model based on the antigenic propensity score (Fig. S2B). Using Bepipred Antibody Epitope Prediction, 15 regions from one to 28 amino acid residues in length were recognized as IgE-binding epitopes (Fig. S2C). In comparing the predictions by these three models, Emini Surface Accessibility Prediction and Bepipred Antibody Epitope Prediction yielded very similar epitope results (>85% similarity, calculated as the degree of overlapping amino acid residues), while the prediction by Kolaskar & Tongaonkar Antigenicity deviated from those of the other two models. Only six regions resulted in consensus between Emini Surface Accessibility Prediction and Kolaskar & Tongaonkar Antigenicity, but with a low degree of overlap ranging between 14% and 37%.

Data obtained by ELISA and dot-immunoblotting, as well as from the three predictions models, were combined and equally weighted for defining the major IgE-binding epitopes (Fig. 2C). Logically, sequences that are determined as IgE reactive both experimentally and by modeling studies are more likely to represent IgE-binding epitopes in the native protein. Therefore, only regions that were suggested as IgE reactive by at least one of the experimental assays, and at least two other of the above assays or models, were considered as major epitopes [38]. Altogether, nine major IgE-binding epitopes of Met e 1 ranging from five to twenty-one amino acid residues in length were identified, namely

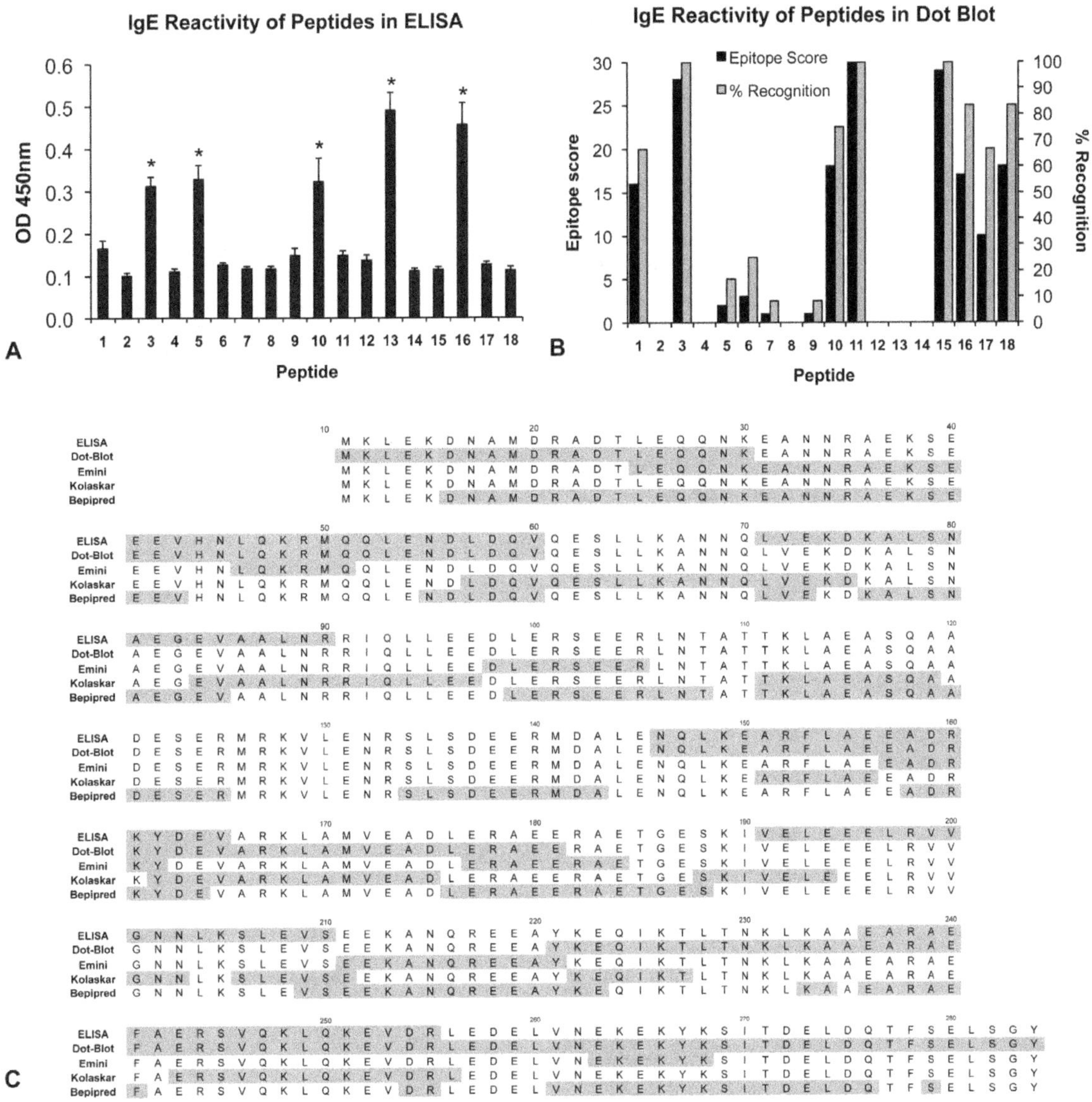

**Figure 2. Determination of Met e 1 IgE-binding epitopes.** Epitopes were determined by ELISA, dot-immunoblotting and three prediction models Emini Surface Accessibility Prediction Kolaskar & Tongaonkar Antigenicity model and Bepipred Antibody Epitope Prediction. (**A**) Histogram of the IgE binding reactivity against the Met e 1 peptides as determined by ELISA. (**B**) Histogram of IgE binding reactivity against the Met e1 peptides as determined by dot-immunoblotting. (**C**) Alignment of Met e 1 IgE-binding epitope sequences as determined by ELISA, dot-immunoblotting and each of the three prediction models.

E1–E9, with positions at Met e $1^{25-30}$, Met e $1^{43-60}$, Met e $1^{87-103}$, Met e $1^{146-154}$ Met e $1^{161-165}$, Met e $1^{191-211}$, Met e $1^{236-241}$, Met e $1^{247-255}$ and Met e $1^{269-281}$, respectively (Fig. 1A). Based on these epitopes, we constructed two tropomyosin mutants, by site-directed mutagenesis (MEM49) and epitope deletion (MED171). The locations of the IgE epitopes and their corresponding amino acid changes in mutants MEM49 and MED171 are shown in Fig. 1A and B. Approximately 4 mg of purified soluble recombinant proteins of MEM49 and MED171 could be obtained from 1 liter of *E.coli* culture. SDS-PAGE analysis of purified recombinant proteins of the mutation mutant MEM49 and the deletion mutant MED171 showed a 35-kDa MEM49 band and a 27-kDa MED171 band, compared to a 35 kDa rMet e 1 band (Fig. 1C).

## Immunoreactivity of tropomyosin mutants

Sera from 8/8 shrimp allergy patients and Met e 1-sensitized mice showed a marked decrease in IgE reactivity to MEM49 and MED171 (Fig. 3). Reactivity of MEM49 and MED171 towards patient IgE decreased by an average of 71.4% and 77.4% relative to Met e 1, respectively (Fig. 3A & B), while that to mouse IgE decreased by an average of 90.5% and 97.6%, respectively (Fig. 3C & D). Notably, the IgE-binding reactivity of MED171 was significantly lower than that of MEM49 ($p<0.05$) when tested with mouse sera. In addition to *in vitro* reduction in IgE reactivity, both MEM49 and MED171 did not trigger mast cell degranulation in passive cutaneous anaphylaxis assays. In contrast to a > 2.5 cm blue region induced by intradermal injection of Met e 1-specific IgE and intravenous injection of Met e 1 with Evan's blue dye, no Evan's blue dye extravasation could be induced by intravenous injection of either hypoallergens (Fig. 3E). More importantly, none of the MEM49- or MED171-immunized mice produced Met e 1-recognizing IgE antibodies (OD 0.071±0.001 and 0.092±0.003, respectively) and hypoallergen-specific IgE antibodies, comparing to an IgE level of OD 0.405±0.056 upon Met e 1 immunization (Table 1). These clearly demonstrated that both MEM49 and MED171 had marked reduction in their *in vivo* allergenicity.

## Hypoallergen-immunized mice produced Met e 1-specific IgG antibodies and inhibited IgE binding to Met e 1

Mice immunized with either rMet e 1, MEM49 or MED171 produced robust IgG antibodies that recognized rMet e 1 with OD 1.778±0.037, 0.571±0.082 and 1.089±0.085, respectively (Table 1). Moreover, IgG antibodies induced by MED171 exhibited better rMet e 1 recognition when compared to those induced by MEM49 at all tested dilutions (Fig. 4A). It is noteworthy that only the hypoallergens MEM49 and MED171, but not Met e 1, could induce the production of Met e 1-specific $IgG_{2a}$ antibodies (Fig. 4B). We further examined if the sera IgG antibodies from hypoallergen-immunized mice were able to block Met e 1-specific IgE from binding to rMet e 1 by competitive inhibition ELISA. Serological IgG from MEM49 and MED171 were able to inhibit 46.2±3.41% and 45.9±3.54% of IgE from shrimp allergy patients from binding to Met e 1, respectively (Fig. 4C). MEM49- and MED171-IgG could better inhibit mouse IgE binding to Met e 1 with average of 82.5±3.24% and 87.6±2.84%, respectively (Fig. 4D).

## Discussion

Knowledge of the IgE-binding epitopes of allergens is fundamental for designing hypoallergenic derivatives, which are regarded as one of the best candidates applicable in SIT. Successful SIT using hypoallergens has been well demonstrated in mouse models of respiratory allergies [39–42] as well as in clinical trials on birch pollen allergy patients [43–45]. The fish parvalbumin mutant Mut-CD/EF that displays a 95% reduction in IgE reactivity and ability to induce blocking IgG antibodies might represent the only best-known hypoallergen among all the most common food allergens [46]. Meanwhile, hypoallergens of the major shellfish allergen tropomyosin that could be translated into specific immunotherapy are unavailable.

Although several shrimp allergens including arginine kinase [47,48], sacroplasmic calcium-binding protein [49,50], myosin light chain [51,52] and troponin C [51] have been identified and registered by the IUIS-allergen database, tropomyosin is reactive to >80% patients allergic to shrimp and is regarded as the major shrimp and shellfish cross-reactive allergen [10,11]. Herein, we have defined the IgE-binding epitopes of the shrimp tropomyosin Met e 1 by ELISA, dot-immunoblotting and three online models as prediction tool represents an emerging strategy in epitope mapping studies among food and drug allergies [38,53,54]. Using this combination, we aimed to achieve higher accuracy, including a lower chance of missing important epitopes, more complete recovery and a higher resolution of epitopes. Using this approach, nine major IgE-binding Met e 1 epitopes were identified. These epitopes range from five to twenty one amino acid residues in length, with some of these allergenic regions longer than the IgE-binding epitopes of other allergens [53,55–57]. This variation may be due to the relatively simple coiled-coiled secondary structure of tropomyosin and/or the high flexibility of this molecule [37], possibly resulting in the higher proportion of surface-exposing IgE-binding sequences. The discovery that six IgE-binding epitopes

**Table 1.** Immunoreactivity of mutants as hypoallergen vaccines in mouse.

| Group | Met e 1 | | | | MEM49 | | | | MED171 | | | |
|---|---|---|---|---|---|---|---|---|---|---|---|---|
| | IgE | | IgG | | IgE | | IgG | | IgE | | IgG | |
| | no. of mice reacted | OD | no. of mice reacted | OD | no. of mice reacted | OD | no. of mice reacted | OD | no. of mice reacted | OD | no. of mice reacted | OD |
| **Immunized with rMet e 1** | 6 | 0.405±0.056 | 6 | 1.778 ±0.037 | 0 | 0.038 ±0.008 | 6 | 1.733 ±0.054 | 0 | 0.08 ±0.002 | 6 | 0.754 ±0.087 |
| **Immunized with MEM49** | 0 | 0.071 ±0.01 | 6 | 0.571 ±0.082 | 0 | 0.081 ±0.002 | 6 | 1.852 ±0.319 | 0 | 0.069 ±0.006 | 6 | 0.283 ±0.015 |
| **Immunized with MED171** | 0 | 0.092 ±0.003 | 6 | 1.089 ±0.085 | 0 | 0.069 ±0.009 | 6 | 0.857 ±0.073 | 0 | 0.089 ±0.005 | 6 | 1.121 ±0.098 |

Balb/c mice (n = 6 in each group) were immunized with rMet e 1, MEM49 or MED171 and their serological IgE and IgG reactivity were analyzed. Note that IgE is only induced in the rMet e 1-immunized mice and IgG to Met e 1, MEM49 and MED171 are cross-reactive.

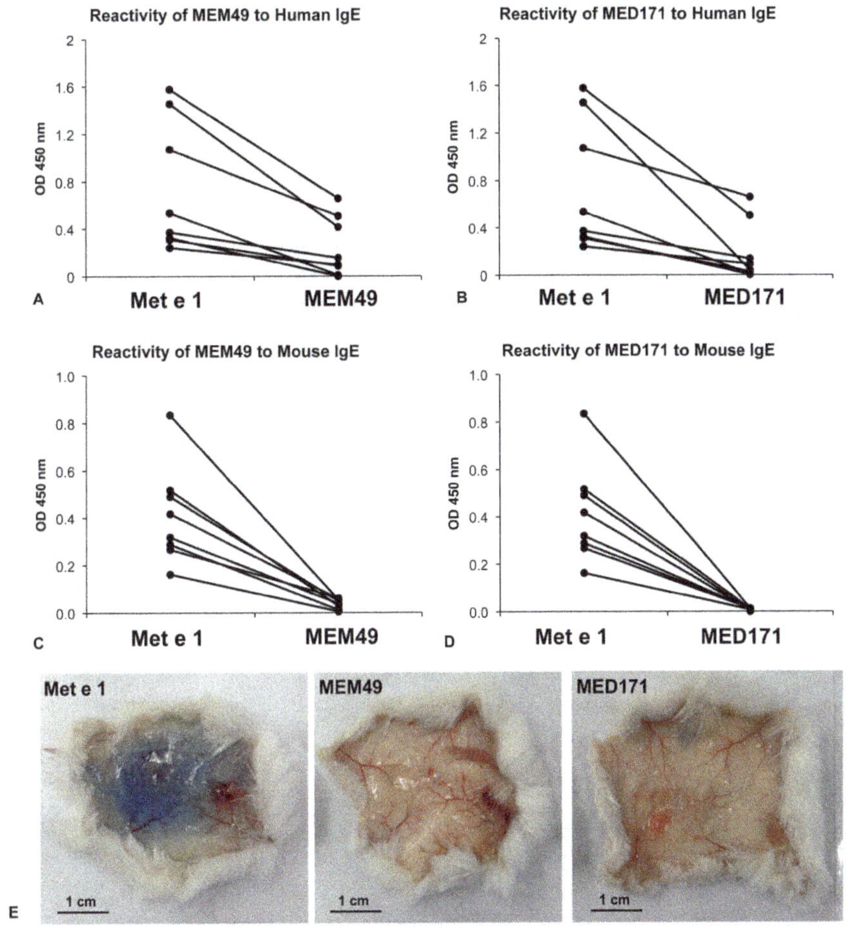


**Figure 3. *In vitro* and *in vivo* IgE reactivity and allergenicity of the hypoallergens.** Reactivity of (**A**) MEM49 and (**B**) MED171 to IgE from shrimp allergy patients (n = 8) and reactivity of (**C**) MEM49 and (**D**) MED171 to IgE of Met e 1-sensitized mice (n = 8) in ELISA. (**E**) *In vivo* IgE reactivity and allergenicity of Met e 1, MEM49 and MED171 as determined by PCA assay. Note that the *in vitro* and *in vivo* IgE reactivity and allergenicity of MEM49 and MED171 are significantly lower than those of Met e 1, as shown by the significantly lower absorbance value at 450 nm and absence of Evan's blue dye extravasation.

identified in our work overlap with those previously reported for Pen a 1 [27,28] is not surprising because the two proteins only have one amino acid difference at residue 69. The three Met e 1 IgE epitopes (E1, E5 and E7) newly identified in this study (Fig. 2A) may partly account for the limited success of a Pen a 1 hypoallergen in reducing allergenicity to shrimp tropomyosin [27]. Incidentally, serum samples from adults were used in the Pen a 1 study while serum samples from children and adolescents were used in determining the IgE-binding epitopes of Met e 1. The presumed greater epitope diversity in children with shrimp allergy than adults [30] may account for the additional epitopes revealed in the present study. Interestingly, some of the Met e 1 epitopes predicted by Bepipred Antibody Epitope Prediction are only one to five amino acid residues apart. Although this model was designed for continuous B cell epitope prediction, a recent study suggests that the results are similar to the predicted discontinuous B cell epitopes [58]. Hence, the epitopes predicted by this model may possibly represent the discontinuous epitopes of Met e 1, although more sophisticated experiments such as crystal structure resolution of allergen/IgE complex could be conducted to confirm the identity of the discontinuous epitopes of Met e 1. Nevertheless, the identification of previously unidentified IgE-binding epitopes in our study as compared to the study on Pen a 1 may be partly explained by the characterization of both linear and discontinuous IgE-binding epitopes here.

In the immunotherapy of allergy, a major goal is to reduce IgE-mediated side-effects during the course of immunotherapy. The two major strategies to reduce IgE reactivity include mutating the amino acid residues involved in IgE-binding, and disrupting the three-dimensional structure of the allergen [59]. Based on our IgE-epitope data, we constructed two hypoallergenic derivatives of Met e 1.

First, hypoallergen MEM49 was constructed by replacing 49 amino acid residues within the nine Met e 1 IgE-binding epitopes with the homologous tropomyosin sequences of fish. Tropomyosin sequences of more than ten fish species are available on GenBank. Herein, we have chosen tropomyosin sequences from four common edible fish species, *Salmo salar*, *Epinephelus coioides*, *Siniperca chuatsi* and *Thunnus thynnus* for comparison. To our knowledge, these fish tropomyosins have not been documented as ingestion-related allergens (however, see Liu et al. which shows that tilapia tropomyosin may be related to autoimmune diseases [60]) and are thus valid candidates for such a homologous conversion. The advantage of homologous substitution is that MEM49 would retain its natural conformation and thereby ensuring a strong allergen-specific IgG response [61]. On the other

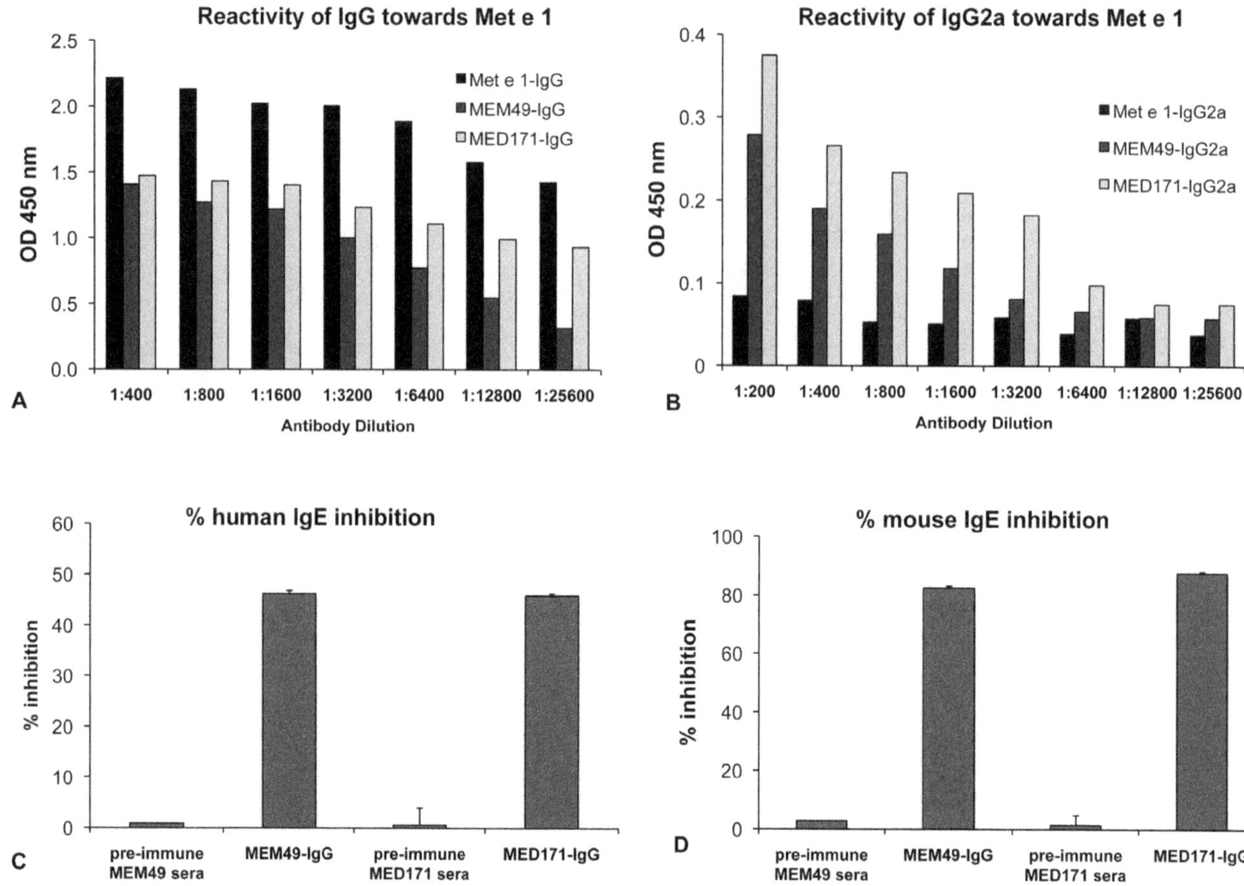


**Figure 4. Immuno-reactivity of hypoallergens and inhibitory potential of the induced IgG antibodies.** Reactivity of the rMet e 1-, MEM49- and MED171-induced (**A**) IgG and (**B**) $IgG_{2a}$ antibodies towards the wild type allergen rMet e 1. Note that specific $IgG_{2a}$ could only be induced by the hypoallergens. Inhibitory potential of the induced IgG towards Met e 1-specific IgE from (**C**) shrimp allergy subjects (n = 8) and (**D**) Met e 1-sensitized mice (n = 8) determined by competitive inhibition ELISA. Percentage inhibition was calculated by $[(OD_{no\ inhibitor} - OD_{inhibitor})/OD_{no\ inhibitor}] \times 100\%$. Note that the MEM49- and MED171-induced IgG antibodies could significantly inhibit IgE of shrimp allergy patients and Met e 1-sensitized mice from binding to Met e 1.

hand, we believe that with the high structural flexibility of tropomyosin and its spontaneous unfolding property [37], the possibility of having only one single critical amino acid per epitope that is responsible for IgE binding is unlikely. Therefore, restricted homologous substitution may not be sufficient to significantly reduce the IgE-binding reactivity of the variant. Hence, all the identified IgE-binding regions in Met e 1 were converted into the homologous sequence of fish tropomyosins.

The second hypoallergen MED171 was designed by deleting all IgE-binding epitopes, which results in a smaller-sized truncated tropomyosin variant of only 171 amino acid residues. With the disruption of all epitopes and possibly its structural flexibility as in tropomyosin, IgE reactivity and allergenicity of MED171 should be more significantly abolished. From our data, both variant showed significant reduction in their *in vitro* reactivity towards Met e 1-specific IgE from patients and sensitized mice. Both of them also lost their *in vivo* allergenicity in inducing mast cell degranulation or IgE synthesis. Direct ELISA also demonstrated that the IgE reactivity of MED171 is significantly lower than MEM49 when tested with sera from Met e 1-sensitized mice (2.4% IgE reactivity retained comparing to 9.5% in MEM49), which matches with our initial expectation.

We noted that most of the human shrimp tropomyosin $CD4^+$ T cell epitopes mapped by Ravkov et al. [62] remain intact in both hypoallergens and therefore, both MEM49 and MED171 should retain their immunogenicity in inducing IgG antibodies. This is supported by our data that a robust Met e 1-specific IgG response was induced by MEM49 and MED171. Notably, we specifically detected the production of $IgG_{2a}$ antibodies in mice immunized with MEM49 or MED171, but not with the wild type allergen Met e 1. The Th1-driven allergen-specific $IgG_{2a}$ antibody in mouse and $IgG_4$ antibody in human induced during SIT are considered to be blocking antibodies and correlate well with clinical improvements [63–71]. The fast-acting blocking IgG antibodies provides protection possibly through the formation of IgG/FcγRIIb complex on mast cells that down-regulates IgE receptor FcεRI signaling and mast cell degranulation [70,72], sequestration of the circulating allergen by the induced IgGs [73], and/or IgE internalization facilitated by the formation of IgG/FcγRIIb immune complex [74]. In fact, our study provides evidence that a MEM49- or MED171-based treatment may bring forth this beneficial effect, because we found that both hypoallergens were able to induce strong Met e 1-specific $IgG_{2a}$ responses even a pro-Th2 adjuvant was used during immunization. Such production of specific $IgG_{2a}$ and absence of Met e 1-specific IgE might correspond to the Th1-driving potential of the two hypoallergens. Most importantly, these antibodies were able to significantly block IgE of both shrimp allergy subjects and Met e 1-sensitized mice from binding to Met e 1. Such inhibitory and Th1-inducing potential are beneficial and it is likely that a MEM49- or MED171-based vaccine will modulate shrimp tropomyosin-induced allergic responses.

To our knowledge, this is the first study providing experimental evidence of a shellfish allergen-specific IgG blocking antibodies induced by hypoallergens. Our results demonstrate significant decrease in the *in vivo* and *in vitro* IgE reactivity and allergenicity of the two designer shrimp tropomyosin hypoallergens MEM49 and MED171 when compared to the wild type allergen Met e 1 and more importantly, robust IgG antibodies' responses with inhibitory potential to Met e 1-specific IgE antibodies of shrimp allergy subjects and Met e 1-sensitized mice. Finally, this work signifies an important discovery that could potentiate the development of prophylactic and/or therapeutic therapies in shellfish allergy.

## Supporting Information

**Figure S1** Comparison of the tropomyosin sequences for the construction of hypoallergen MEM49. Tropomyosin sequence of Met e 1 was compared to that of four fish species *Salmo salar* (Atlantic salmon), *Epinephelus coioides* (orange-spotted grouper), *Siniperca chuatsi* (Mandarin fish) and *Thunnus thynns* (Atlantic bluefin tuna). Amino acid deviations within each IgE-binding epitope (framed) were identified and subsequently mutated into the homologous sequence of fish tropomyosins (bold letters shaded in gray) for the construction of hypoallergen MEM49.
(TIF)

**Figure S2** Computational prediction of tropomyosin IgE-binding epitopes. **(A)** Surface probability score of each amino acid residue of Met e 1 in Emini Surface Accessbility Prediction. **(B)** Antigenic propensity score of each amino acid residue of Met e 1 in Kolaskar & Tongaonkar Antigenicity. **(C)** Epitope score of each amino acid residue of Met e 1 in Bepipred Linear Epitope Prediction.
(TIF)

**Table S1** Clinical characteristics and shrimp tropomyosin-specific IgE of the shrimp allergy patients included in this study. 12 patients 3–17 years old with documented history of shrimp allergy were recruited in this study for mapping the major IgE-binding epitopes of Met e 1 and characterizing the IgE reactivity of the hypoallergens.
(DOCX)

## Acknowledgments

The authors thank K.C. Cheung and Y.F. Lam for their technical assistance and D. Wilmshurst (The Chinese University of Hong Kong) for editorial comments on this manuscript.

## Author Contributions

Conceived and designed the experiments: CYYW PSCL KHC. Performed the experiments: CYYW NYHL. Analyzed the data: CYYW SAS MHKH PSCL KHC. Contributed reagents/materials/analysis tools: MHKH. Contributed to the writing of the manuscript: CYYW PSCL SAS LJG KHC.

## References

1. Chafen JJ, Newberry SJ, Riedl MA, Bravata DM, Maglione M, et al. (2010) Diagnosing and managing common food allergies: a systematic review. JAMA 303: 1848–1856.
2. Clark S, Espinola J, Rudders SA, Banerji A, Camargo CA Jr (2011) Frequency of US emergency department visits for food-related acute allergic reactions. J Allergy Clin Immunol 127: 682–683.
3. Harduar-Morano L, Simon MR, Watkins S, Blackmore C (2011) A population-based epidemiologic study of emergency department visits for anaphylaxis in Florida. J Allergy Clin Immunol 128: 594–600.
4. Nowak RM, Macias CG (2014) Anaphylaxis on the other front line: perspectives from the emergency department. Am J Med 127: S34–44.
5. Landsman-Blumberg PB, Wei W, Douglas D, Smith DM, Clark S, et al. (2013) Food-induced anaphylaxis among commercially insured US adults: Patient concordance with postdischarge care guidelines. J Allergy Clin Immunol Pract 1: 595–601 e591.
6. Sicherer SH (2011) Epidemiology of food allergy. J Allergy Clin Immunol 127: 594–602.
7. Ho MH, Lee SL, Wong WH, Ip P, Lau YL (2012) Prevalence of self-reported food allergy in Hong Kong children and teens–a population survey. Asian Pac J Allergy Immunol 30: 275–284.
8. Lopata AL, O'Hehir RE, Lehrer SB (2010) Shellfish allergy. Clin Exp Allergy 40: 850–858.
9. Hajeb P, Selamat J (2012) A contemporary review of seafood allergy. Clin Rev Allergy Immunol 42: 365–385.
10. Shanti KN, Martin BM, Nagpal S, Metcalfe DD, Rao PVS (1993) Identification of tropomyosin as the major shrimp allergen and characterization of its IgE-binding epitopes. J Immunol 151: 5354–5363.
11. Leung PSC, Chu KH, Chow WK, Ansari A, Bandea CI, et al. (1994) Cloning, expression, and primary structure of *Metapenaeus ensis* tropomyosin, the major heat-stable shrimp allergen. J Allergy Clin Immunol 94: 882–890.
12. Daul CB, Slattery M, Reese G, Lehrer SB (1994) Identification of the major brown shrimp (Penaeus aztecus) allergen as the muscle protein tropomyosin. Int Arch Allergy Immunol 105: 49–55.
13. Leung NY, Wai CY, Shu S, Wang J, Kenny TP, et al. (2014) Current immunological and molecular biological perspectives on seafood allergy: a comprehensive review. Clin Rev Allergy Immunol 46: 180–197.
14. Chu KH, Wong SH, Leung PSC (2000) Tropomyosin is the major mollusk allergen: reverse transcriptase polymerase chain reaction, expression and IgE reactivity. Mar Biotechnol (NY) 2: 499–509.
15. Leung PSC, Chen YC, Mykles DL, Chow WK, Li CP, et al. (1998) Molecular identification of the lobster muscle protein tropomyosin as a seafood allergen. Mol Mar Biol Biotechnol 7: 12–20.
16. Leung PSC, Chen YC, Gershwin ME, Wong SH, Kwan HS, et al. (1998) Identification and molecular characterization of *Charybdis feriatus* tropomyosin, the major crab allergen. J Allergy Clin Immunol 102: 847–852.
17. Leung PSC, Chow WK, Duffey S, Kwan HS, Gershwin ME, et al. (1996) IgE reactivity against a cross-reactive allergen in crustacea and mollusca: evidence for tropomyosin as the common allergen. J Allergy Clin Immunol 98: 954–961.
18. Leung PSC, Chu KH (2001) cDNA cloning and molecular identification of the major oyster allergen from the Pacific oyster *Crassostrea gigas*. Clin Exp Allergy 31: 1287–1294.
19. Reese G, Ayuso R, Lehrer SB (1999) Tropomyosin: an invertebrate pan-allergen. Int Arch Allergy Immunol 119: 247–258.
20. Gieras A, Cejka P, Blatt K, Focke-Tejkl M, Linhart B, et al. (2011) Mapping of conformational IgE epitopes with peptide-specific monoclonal antibodies reveals simultaneous binding of different IgE antibodies to a surface patch on the major birch pollen allergen, Bet v 1. J Immunol 186: 5333–5344.
21. Vickery BP, Lin J, Kulis M, Fu Z, Steele PH, et al. (2013) Peanut oral immunotherapy modifies IgE and IgG4 responses to major peanut allergens. J Allergy Clin Immunol 131: 128–134.
22. Smarr CB, Bryce PJ, Miller SD (2013) Antigen-specific tolerance in immunotherapy of Th2-associated allergic diseases. Crit Rev Immunol 33: 389–414.
23. Jutel M, Van de Veen W, Agache I, Azkur KA, Akdis M, et al. (2013) Mechanisms of allergen-specific immunotherapy and novel ways for vaccine development. Allergol Int 62: 425–433.
24. Dall'Antonia F, Gieras A, Devanaboyina SC, Valenta R, Keller W (2011) Prediction of IgE-binding epitopes by means of allergen surface comparison and correlation to cross-reactivity. J Allergy Clin Immunol 128: 872–879.
25. Hecker J, Diethers A, Schulz D, Sabri A, Plum M, et al. (2012) An IgE epitope of Bet v 1 and fagales PR10 proteins as defined by a human monoclonal IgE. Allergy 67: 1530–1537.
26. Wai CYY, Leung NYH, Chu KH, Leung PSC (2012) From molecule studies of allergens to development of immunotherapy of allergies. J Aller Ther 3: 1000124.
27. Reese G, Viebranz J, Leong-Kee SM, Plante M, Lauer I, et al. (2005) Reduced allergenic potency of VR9-1, a mutant of the major shrimp allergen Pen a 1 (tropomyosin). J Immunol 175: 8354–8364.
28. Ayuso R, Lehrer SB, Reese G (2002) Identification of continuous, allergenic regions of the major shrimp allergen Pen a 1 (tropomyosin). Int Arch Allergy Immunol 127: 27–37.
29. Leung PSC, Lee YS, Tang CY, Kung WY, Chuang YH, et al. (2008) Induction of shrimp tropomyosin-specific hypersensitivity in mice. Int Arch Allergy Immunol 147: 305–314.

30. Ayuso R, Sanchez-Garcia S, Lin J, Fu ZY, Ibanez MD, et al. (2010) Greater epitope recognition of shrimp allergens by children than by adults suggests that shrimp sensitization decreases with age. J Allergy Clin Immunol 125: 1286–1293.
31. Boyce JA, Assa'ad A, Burks AW, Jones SM, Sampson HA, et al. (2010) Guidelines for the Diagnosis and Management of Food Allergy in the United States: Summary of the NIAID-Sponsored Expert Panel Report. J Allergy Clin Immunol 126: 1105–1118.
32. Tsabouri S, Triga M, Makris M, Kalogeromitros D, Church MK, et al. (2012) Fish and shellfish allergy in children: review of a persistent food allergy. Pediatr Allergy Immunol 23: 608–615.
33. Larsen JE, Lund O, Nielsen M (2006) Improved method for predicting linear B-cell epitopes. Immunome Res 2: 2.
34. Kolaskar AS, Tongaonkar PC (1990) A semi-empirical method for prediction of antigenic determinants on protein antigens. FEBS Lett 276: 172–174.
35. Emini EA, Hughes JV, Perlow DS, Boger J (1985) Induction of Hepatitis-a virus-neutralizing antibody by a virus-specific synthetic peptide. Journal of Virology 55: 836–839.
36. Li KW, Geraerts WP, van Elk R, Joosse J (1988) Fixation increases sensitivity of India ink staining of proteins and peptides on nitrocellulose paper. Anal Biochem 174: 97–100.
37. Nitanai Y, Minakata S, Maeda K, Oda N, Maeda Y (2007) Crystal structures of tropomyosin: Flexible coiled-coil. Regulatory Mechanisms of Striated Muscle Contraction 592: 137–151.
38. Sun X, Shan X, Yan Z, Zhang Y, Guan L (2013) Prediction and characterization of the linear IgE epitopes for the major soybean allergen beta-conglycinin using immunoinformatics tools. Food Chem Toxicol 56: 254–260.
39. Bauer R, Scheiblhofer S, Kern K, Gruber C, Stepanoska T, et al. (2006) Generation of hypoallergenic DNA vaccines by forced ubiquitination: preventive and therapeutic effects in a mouse model of allergy. J Allergy Clin Immunol 118: 269–276.
40. Saarne T, Neimert-Andersson T, Gronlund H, Jutel M, Gafvelin G, et al. (2011) Treatment with a Fel d 1 hypoallergen reduces allergic responses in a mouse model for cat allergy. Allergy 66: 255–263.
41. Wiedermann U, Herz U, Vrtala S, Neuhaus-Steinmetz U, Renz H, et al. (2001) Mucosal tolerance induction with hypoallergenic molecules in a murine model of allergic asthma. Int Arch Allergy Immunol 124: 391–394.
42. Linhart B, Valenta R (2012) Mechanisms underlying allergy vaccination with recombinant hypoallergenic allergen derivatives. Vaccine 30: 4328–4335.
43. Purohit A, Niederberger V, Kronqvist M, Horak F, Gronneberg R, et al. (2008) Clinical effects of immunotherapy with genetically modified recombinant birch pollen Bet v 1 derivatives. Clin Exp Allergy 38: 1514–1525.
44. van Hage-Hamsten M, Johansson E, Roquet A, Peterson C, Andersson M, et al. (2002) Nasal challenges with recombinant derivatives of the major birch pollen allergen Bet v 1 induce fewer symptoms and lower mediator release than rBet v 1 wild-type in patients with allergic rhinitis. Clin Exp Allergy 32: 1448–1453.
45. Niederberger V, Horak F, Vrtala S, Spitzauer S, Krauth MT, et al. (2004) Vaccination with genetically engineered allergens prevents progression of allergic disease. Proc Natl Acad Sci U S A 101 Suppl 2: 14677–14682.
46. Swoboda I, Bugajska-Schretter A, Linhart B, Verdino P, Keller W, et al. (2007) A recombinant hypoallergenic parvalbumin mutant for immunotherapy of IgE-mediated fish allergy. J Immunol 178: 6290–6296.
47. Garcia-Orozco KD, Aispuro-Hernandez E, Yepiz-Plascencia G, Calderon-de-la-Barca AM, Sotelo-Mundo RR (2007) Molecular characterization of arginine kinase, an allergen from the shrimp Litopenaeus vannamei. Int Arch Allergy Immunol 144: 23–28.
48. Yu CJ, Lin YF, Chiang BL, Chow LP (2003) Proteomics and immunological analysis of a novel shrimp allergen, Pen m 2. J Immunol 170: 445–453.
49. Ayuso R, Grishina G, Ibanez MD, Blanco C, Carrillo T, et al. (2009) Sarcoplasmic calcium-binding protein is an EF-hand-type protein identified as a new shrimp allergen. J Allergy Clin Immunol 124: 114–120.
50. Shiomi K, Sato Y, Hamamoto S, Mita H, Shimakura K (2008) Sarcoplasmic calcium-binding protein: identification as a new allergen of the black tiger shrimp Penaeus monodon. Int Arch Allergy Immunol 146: 91–98.
51. Bauermeister K, Wangorsch A, Garoffo LP, Reuter A, Conti A, et al. (2011) Generation of a comprehensive panel of crustacean allergens from the North Sea Shrimp Crangon crangon. Mol Immunol 48: 1983–1992.
52. Ayuso R, Grishina G, Bardina L, Carrillo T, Blanco C, et al. (2008) Myosin light chain is a novel shrimp allergen, Lit v 3. J Allergy Clin Immunol 122: 795–802.
53. Chen JC, Chiu LL, Lee KL, Huang WN, Chuang JG, et al. (2012) Identification of critical amino acids in an immunodominant IgE epitope of Pen c 13, a major allergen from *Penicillium citrinum*. PLoS One 7: e34627.
54. Zheng LN, Lin H, Pawar R, Li ZX, Li MH (2011) Mapping IgE binding epitopes of major shrimp (*Penaeus monodon*) allergen with immunoinformatics tools. Food Chem Toxicol 49: 2954–2960.
55. Mine Y, Rupa P (2003) Fine mapping and structural analysis of immunodominant IgE allergenic epitopes in chicken egg ovalbumin. Protein Eng 16: 747–752.
56. Rabjohn P, Helm EM, Stanley JS, West CM, Sampson HA, et al. (1999) Molecular cloning and epitope analysis of the peanut allergen Ara h 3. J Clin Invest 103: 535–542.
57. Yuan HC, Wu KG, Chen CJ, Su SN, Shen HD, et al. (2012) Mapping of IgE and IgG4 antibody-binding epitopes in Cyn d 1, the major allergen of Bermuda grass pollen. Int Arch Allergy Immunol 157: 125–135.
58. Bergmann-Leitner ES, Chaudhury S, Steers NJ, Sabato M, Delvecchio V, et al. (2013) Computational and experimental validation of B and T-cell epitopes of the *in vivo* immune response to a novel malarial antigen. PLoS One 8: e71610.
59. Valenta R, Ferreira F, Focke-Tejkl M, Linhart B, Niederberger V, et al. (2010) From allergen genes to allergy vaccines. Annu Rev Immunol 28: 211–241.
60. Liu R, Holck AL, Yang E, Liu C, Xue W (2013) Tropomyosin from tilapia (Oreochromis mossambicus) as an allergen. Clin Exp Allergy 43: 365–377.
61. Cromwell O, Hafner D, Nandy A (2011) Recombinant allergens for specific immunotherapy. J Allergy Clin Immunol 127: 865–872.
62. Ravkov EV, Pavlov IY, Martins TB, Gleich GJ, Wagner LA, et al. (2013) Identification and validation of shrimp-tropomyosin specific CD4 T cell epitopes. Hum Immunol 74: 1542–1549.
63. James LK, Shamji MH, Walker SM, Wilson DR, Wachholz PA, et al. (2011) Long-term tolerance after allergen immunotherapy is accompanied by selective persistence of blocking antibodies. J Allergy Clin Immunol 127: 509–516.
64. Subbarayal B, Schiller D, Mobs C, de Jong NW, Ebner C, et al. (2013) Kinetics, cross-reactivity, and specificity of Bet v 1-specific IgG4 antibodies induced by immunotherapy with birch pollen. Allergy 68: 1377–1386.
65. van Neerven RJ, Wikborg T, Lund G, Jacobsen B, Brinch-Nielsen A, et al. (1999) Blocking antibodies induced by specific allergy vaccination prevent the activation of CD4+ T cells by inhibiting serum-IgE-facilitated allergen presentation. J Immunol 163: 2944–2952.
66. Wachholz PA, Soni NK, Till SJ, Durham SR (2003) Inhibition of allergen-IgE binding to B cells by IgG antibodies after grass pollen immunotherapy. J Allergy Clin Immunol 112: 915–922.
67. Worm M, Lee HH, Kleine-Tebbe J, Hafner RP, Laidler P, et al. (2011) Development and preliminary clinical evaluation of a peptide immunotherapy vaccine for cat allergy. J Allergy Clin Immunol 127: 89–97, 97 e81–14.
68. Li XM, Srivastava K, Grishin A, Huang CK, Schofield B, et al. (2003) Persistent protective effect of heat-killed Escherichia coli producing "engineered," recombinant peanut proteins in a murine model of peanut allergy. J Allergy Clin Immunol 112: 159–167.
69. Rupa P, Mine Y (2012) Oral immunotherapy with immunodominant T-cell epitope peptides alleviates allergic reactions in a Balb/c mouse model of egg allergy. Allergy 67: 74–82.
70. Strait RT, Morris SC, Finkelman FD (2006) IgG-blocking antibodies inhibit IgE-mediated anaphylaxis in vivo through both antigen interception and Fc gamma RIIb cross-linking. J Clin Invest 116: 833–841.
71. Walgraffe D, Matteotti C, el Bakkoury M, Garcia L, Marchand C, et al. (2009) A hypoallergenic variant of Der p 1 as a candidate for mite allergy vaccines. J Allergy Clin Immunol 123: 1150–1156.
72. Daeron M, Malbec O, Latour S, Arock M, Fridman WH (1995) Regulation of high-affinity IgE receptor-mediated mast cell activation by murine low-affinity IgG receptors. J Clin Invest 95: 577–585.
73. Schmitz N, Dietmeier K, Bauer M, Maudrich M, Utzinger S, et al. (2009) Displaying Fel d1 on virus-like particles prevents reactogenicity despite greatly enhanced immunogenicity: a novel therapy for cat allergy. J Exp Med 206: 1941–1955.
74. Uermösi C, Zabel F, Manolova V, Bauer M, Beerli RR, et al. (2014) IgG-mediated down-regulation of IgE bound to mast cells: a potential novel mechanism of allergen-specific desensitization. Allergy 69: 338–347.

# 14

# Biochemical, Biophysical and IgE-Epitope Characterization of the Wheat Food Allergen, Tri a 37

**Sandra Pahr[1,2], Regina Selb[3], Milena Weber[1], Margarete Focke-Tejkl[1], Gerhard Hofer[4], Andela Dordić[4], Walter Keller[4], Nikolaos G. Papadopoulos[5], Stavroula Giavi[5], Mika Mäkelä[6], Anna Pelkonen[6], Verena Niederberger[3], Susanne Vrtala[1,2], Rudolf Valenta[1]***

**1** Division of Immunopathology, Department of Pathophysiology and Allergy Research, Center of Pathophysiology, Infectiology and Immunology, Medical University of Vienna, Vienna, Austria, **2** Christian Doppler Laboratory for the Development of Allergen Chips, Medical University of Vienna, Vienna, Austria, **3** Department of ENT, Medical University of Vienna, Vienna, Austria, **4** Institute of Molecular Biosciences, Karl-Franzens University Graz, Graz, Austria, **5** Allergy Department, 2nd Pediatric Clinic, University of Athens, Athens, Greece, **6** Skin and Allergy Hospital, Helsinki University Central Hospital, Helsinki, Finland

## Abstract

Wheat is an important staple food and potent allergen source. Recently, we isolated a cDNA coding for wheat alpha-purothionin which is recognized by wheat food allergic patients at risk for severe wheat-induced allergy. The purpose of the present study was the biochemical, biophysical and IgE epitope characterization of recombinant alpha-purothionin. Synthetic genes coding for alpha-purothionin were expressed in a prokaryotic system using *Escherichia coli* and in a eukaryotic expression system based on baculovirus-infected Sf9-insect cells. Recombinant proteins were purified and characterized by SDS-PAGE, mass spectrometry, circular dichroism, chemical cross-linking and size exclusion chromatography. Five overlapping peptid were synthesized for epitope mapping. Alpha-purothionin-specific rabbit antibodies were raised to perform IgE-inhibition experiments and to study the resistance to digestion. The IgE reactivity of the proteins and peptides from ten wheat food allergic patients was studied in non-denaturing RAST-based binding assays. Alpha-purothionin was expressed in the prokaryotic (EcTri a 37) and in the eukaryotic system (BvTri a 37) as a soluble and monomeric protein. However, circular dichroism analysis revealed that EcTri a 37 was unfolded whereas BvTri a 37 was a folded protein. Both proteins showed comparable IgE-reactivity and the epitope mapping revealed the presence of sequential IgE epitopes in the N-terminal basic thionin domain (peptide1:KSCCRSTLGRNCYNLCRARGAQKLCAGVCR) and in the C-terminal acidic extension domain (peptide3:KGFPKLALESNSDEPDTIEYCNLGCRSSVC, peptide4:CNLGCRSSVCDYMV-NAAADDEEMKLYVEN). Natural Tri a 37 was digested under gastric conditions but resistant to duodenal digestion. Immunization with EcTri a 37 induced IgG antibodies which recognized similar epitopes as IgE antibodies from allergic patients and inhibited allergic patients' IgE binding. Reactivity to Tri a 37 does not require a folded protein and the presence of sequential IgE epitopes indicates that sensitization to alpha-purothionin occurs via the gut. Both allergens can be used for *in-vitro* diagnosis of wheat food allergy. The induction of blocking IgG antibodies suggests the usefulness for immunotherapy.

**Editor:** Simon Patrick Hogan, Cincinnati Children's Hospital Medical Center, University of Cincinnati College of Medicine, United States of America

**Funding:** This study was supported by research grants from Phadia-Thermo Fisher, Uppsala, Sweden, the Christian Doppler Research Association, Austria, project F4605 of the Austrian Science Fund (FWF) and in part by the European Commission's Seventh Framework program under grant agreement no. 261357. The funders had no role in study design, data collection and analysis, decision to publish, or preparation of the manuscript.

**Competing Interests:** Rudolf Valenta has served as a consultant for Phadia/Thermofisher, Uppsala, Sweden and has received research grants from this company. The other authors have no conflict of interest to declare.

* Email: rudolf.valenta@meduniwien.ac.at

## Introduction

Wheat is one of the most important components of our daily nutrition. It contains several essential dietary constituents such as carbohydrates, fats, dietary fibers, minerals, proteins, vitamins and water. [1] However, wheat also belongs to the most important allergy-eliciting foods causing local manifestations as well as severe systemic reactions. [2] In fact, in a population of wheat food allergic children more than 50% had experienced anaphylaxis upon wheat ingestion [3] and wheat has been reported as one of the major food allergen sources involved in food-induced anaphylaxis in a study analysing 1000 patients with food allergy. [4] However, only a few allergen molecules have been identified to be involved in severe allergy to wheat. Among the known wheat food allergens, $\omega_5$-gliadin (Tri a 19) [5], $\alpha/\beta$-gliadins (Tri a 21) [6] and HMW glutenin (Tri a 26) [7] have been described as markers for wheat-dependent exercise-induced anaphylaxis. Furthermore, LTP (lipid transfer protein; Tri a 14) [8] was reported to play an important role in the development of wheat-induced anaphylaxis.

Very recently we identified a novel wheat food allergen, alpha purothionin, which according to the allergen nomenclature system was designated Tri a 37. In 20% of wheat food allergic patients we found IgE reactivity to Tri a 37 which was associated with a four-fold increased risk of experiencing severe wheat-induced anaphylaxis. [9]

The latter finding suggested that Tri a 37 may be a true wheat food allergen (class I food allergen). [9] Class I food allergens usually contain sequential epitopes and sensitization occurs mainly via the gastrointestinal tract. [10,11] The wheat allergens $\omega_5$-gliadin, the HMW glutenins [7,12] as well as allergens from other food allergen sources, such as egg (ovomucoid) [13] and cow's milk (alpha-, beta-casein) are examples for class I food allergens. [14]

Here we report the recombinant expression of Tri a 37 in a prokaryotic system using *Escherichia coli* cells (EcTri a 37) and in an eukaryotic system (baculovirus infected insect cells - BvTri a 37) which yielded an unfolded and a folded form of Tri a 37 and thus allowed us to study the potential relevance of conformational IgE epitopes. Both allergens were characterized regarding biochemical and biophysical properties. A detailed IgE epitope mapping of Tri a 37 was performed with synthetic peptides spanning the complete Tri a 37 sequence. Furthermore, we raised a rabbit antiserum against Tri a 37 to study the natural Tri a 37 under conditions of gastric and duodenal digestion in wheat extract and performed IgE-inhibition experiments to investigate the protective activity of IgG antibodies induced by immunization with Tri a 37.

## Materials and Methods

### Recombinant production of EcTri a 37

The cDNA coding for the mature Tri a 37 with a 3′ sequence coding for a hexahistidine tag was produced as synthetic gene with codons optimized for expression in *E.coli* and subcloned into the pET17b expression vector (ATG-biosynthetics, Merzhausen, Germany). The recombinant allergen was then expressed in *E.coli* BL21 (DE3) cells and purified by nickel affinity chromatography from the inclusion body fraction (Quiagen, Hilden, Germany). [15] The purified recombinant allergen EcTri a 37 was eluted from the column in 8 M urea, 100 mM $NaH_2PO_4$, 10 mM Tris, pH 4.6, then dialyzed step-wise against 10 mM $NaH_2PO_4$ buffer pH 4.0 in which it remained soluble up to 2 mg/ml and could be stored at −20°C. Specific rabbit antibodies against alpha purothionin were raised by immunization of a New Zealand white rabbit with purified EcTri a 37 (200 µg per injection) using once Freund's complete adjuvant and twice Freund's incomplete adjuvant. (Charles River, Kisslegg, Germany). Pre-immune serum was obtained from the rabbit before immunization.

### Recombinant production of BvTri a 37

**Subcloning of Tri a 37 and production of recombinant bacmid DNA.** The cDNA (364 bp) coding for Tri a 37 (accession number AFQ60540.1) containing an additional 3′ sequence coding for a hexahistidine tag was produced as synthetic gene and subcloned into the BamHI/SmaI sites of pUC57 (GenScript, NJ, USA) with codons optimized for insect cell expression. This cDNA was then cloned into the BamHI/SmaI sites of the pTM1 vector harbouring the baculoviral polyhedrin promoter sequence. [16] The plasmid containing the Tri a 37 insert was transformed into XL-1 Blue competent cells (Agilent technologies, Santa Clara, USA) and selected for ampicillin and tetracycline. The correct insertion of the cDNA was confirmed by restriction analysis of plasmid mini-prep DNA (Promega, Madison, Wisconsin, USA) with BamHI/SmaI and by sequence analysis (VBC Biotech, Vienna, Austria). Following the manual instructions (Version A, 15 December 2008) of the Bac-to-Bac TOPO Expression System (Life Technologies, Carlsbad, CA, USA), the recombinant donor plasmid containing the proper DNA sequence was transformed into competent DH10Bac *E.coli* cells, which allow the transposition of the DNA of interest into a baculoviral bacmid. Using blue/white selection and screening for resistance to kanamycin, tetracycline (ROTH, Karlsruhe, Germany) and gentamicin (Life Technologies, Carlsbad, CA, USA) colonies containing the Tri a 37 insert within the bacmid DNA were identified. The presence of the correct recombinant bacmid DNA containing the Tri a 37 gene was confirmed by PCR analysis. A white colony was inoculated in 100 µl water and heated for 5 min at 95°C. PCR analysis was performed using M13 primers (VBC Genomics) and GoTaq DNA polymerase (Promega, Madison, Wisconsin, USA). After midi-prep (Promega) of a positive overnight culture, occurrence of the correct DNA insert was again confirmed by PCR.

**Production of recombinant baculovirus, determination of viral titer.** Recombinant baculovirus was produced using the Bac-to-Bac insect cell expression system (Life Technologies). The recombinant bacmid DNA containing the Tri a 37 DNA was transfected into Sf9 insect cells (Life Technologies) in order to produce recombinant baculovirus. Sf9 insect cells were grown in Sf-900 II SFM media (Life Technologies) supplemented with 10 µg/ml gentamicin (Life Technologies), 2.5% Fetal Bovine Serum (Life Technologies) and maintained in the log phase ($3\times10^5$–$3\times10^6$ cells/ml) at 27°C for the entire experiment. For transfection, a total of $2\times10^6$ Sf9 insect cells in 2 ml media per well were seeded in a 6-well-plate and incubated for 30 min at 27°C for cell attachment. After replacing the medium containing gentamicin and fetal bovine serum with medium, 100 µl transfection cocktail consisting of 6 µl transfection reagent (FuGENE HD Transfection Reagent, Promega, Madison), 2 µg recombinant bacmid DNA, $H_2O$ ad 100 ◦l were added to each well. After 7hrs, the medium was removed, replaced with fresh medium containing gentamicin and FBS and incubated for 72hrs at 27°C. Baculoviral stock (P1 viral stock) was collected from the supernatant after centrifugation at 750 xrpm for 5 min at room temperature and stored at 4°C in the dark until use. To determine the viral titre, a plaque assay was performed seeding 2 ml of Sf9 cells ($1\times10^6$ Sf9 cells/well) in 6-well-plates for 1 hour. After removing medium from the cells, attached insect cells were infected with 1 ml/well of serial viral dilutions (P1: $10^4$, $10^5$, $10^6$; P2 and P3: $10^5$, $10^6$, $10^7$, $10^8$), using 1xDPBS (Life Technologies, Carlsbad, CA, USA), for 1 hour at room temperature. The supernatant was removed and infected insect cells were covered with 2 ml of Sf-900 medium 1.3X (Life Technologies) containing 1% low-melting agarose and 10 µg/ml of gentamicin. Plates were kept, without moving, for 1 hour at room temperature allowing the agarose mixture to solidify. After wrapping the plate in moisturized paper, the plate was covered with aluminium foil and incubated for 5–7 days at 27°C. Plaques were stained with 2 ml of neutral red solution (Sigma Aldrich, Munich, Germany), diluted 1:10 in 1xPBS for 2 hours at room temperature. After removal of the staining solution, plaques became visible and were counted. For further amplification of P1 stock to generate a high-titer P2 stock, the following formula was used: inoculum required (ml) = [MOI (pfu/cell) x number of cells]/titer of viral stock (pfu/ml). Ten ml of cells ($2\times10^6$ cells/ml → $2\times10^7$ cells) were infected with 2 ml of P1 stock ($1\times10^6$ pfu/ml) to obtain a MOI (multiplicity of infection: number of virus particles per cell) of 0.1. The viral titer of P2 stock was again determined by plaque assay and stored as described above for P1 viral stock.

In optimization experiments, several conditions (MOI 1, 2, 3, 4; durations of expression 24hrs, 48hrs, 72hrs, 96hrs) were tested to optimize the protocol. Samples were taken, centrifuged at 10,000 rpm for 2 min, sample buffer was added to the supernatants and stored at 4°C. All collected samples were subjected to

14% SDS-PAGE, blotted onto nitrocellulose and tested with Tri a 37-specific rabbit antibodies to detect the level of BvTri a 37 expression.

**Expression of BvTri a 37.** For expression of BvTri a 37, 200 ml of $2\times10^6$ cells/ml Sf9 cells present in fresh Sf-900 II SFM medium (+Gm, -FBS) were infected with the viral P2 stock to reach MOI = 1 for 96hrs while shaking at 80 rpm/min at 27°C in the dark. After centrifugation at 750 xrpm for 15 min, PMSF (10 µg/ml) were added to secreted protein-containing supernatants. For protein purification under native conditions, using nickel affinity chromatography (Qiagen), supernatants were dialyzed against lysis buffer (50 mM $NaH_2PO_4$, 300 mM NaCl, 1 mM Imidazole, pH 8.0) o/N, and incubated with pre-equilibrated nickel agarose in a batch procedure o/N. The agarose batch was filled into column, washed with wash buffer (50 mM $NaH_2PO_4$, 300 mM NaCl, 20 mM Imidazole, pH 8.0) and eluted with elution buffer (50 mM $NaH_2PO_4$, 300 mM NaCl, 250 mM Imidazole, PH 8.0). BvTri a 37-containing fractions were pooled and dialyzed against 10 mM $NaH_2PO_4$ pH 8.0 and stored at −20°C.

## Characterization of recombinant proteins

The protein concentrations of both recombinant allergens were determined in parallel by BCA assay (Pierce, Rockford, IL) and purity was assessed by Coomassie Blue-stained 14% SDS–PAGE. The protein was analysed under reducing and non-reducing conditions. [17] Nitrocellulose-blotted, recombinant EcTri a 37 and BvTri a 37 (2 µg each) were tested with serum (dilution 1:10) from a wheat food allergic patient (Patient 1, Table 1) and buffer as a control. Bound IgE antibodies were detected with $^{125}$I-labeled anti-human IgE antibodies (Demeditec Diagnostics, Kiel, Germany) and visualized by autoradiography. Aqueous wheat seed extract (20 µg) was blotted and probed with Tri a 37-specific rabbit antibodies and for control purposes with the corresponding pre-immune serum (dilution 1:10.000). Bound IgG antibodies were detected with $^{125}$I-labeled goat anti-rabbit IgG antibodies (Perkin Elmer, Boston, USA) and visualized by autoradiography. The identity of the recombinant proteins was confirmed by mass spectrometry (Bruker, Billerica, MA). [18] Mass spectrometry, size exclusion chromatography and circular dichroism measurement (CD) were performed as previously described. [18] For the chemical crosslinking of oligomers in solution 2 ng of EcTri a 37 or BvTri a 37 were incubated in a total volume of 15 µl with 0.01–0.2% v/v glutaraldehyde for 15 minutes at room temperature. To generate samples in a reduced condition 10 mM DTT was added 10 minutes prior to the glutaraldehyde. The reaction was stopped by adding 2 µl of a 1 M glycine solution. The resulting products were assessed by 18% SDS-PAGE and by size exclusion chromatography. [18]

Tri a 37 was analyzed using the Expasy ProtScale accessibility program for the presence of surface-exposed areas. [19]

## Sera from wheat allergic patients used for testing the IgE reactivity of the allergens

Sera were obtained from European wheat food allergic patients (Austria n = 1; Finland: n = 3; Greece: n = 6; total: n = 10) aged 3–41 years (mean age 12 years). Patients were diagnosed on the basis of a case history demonstrating that allergic symptoms (airway symptoms, gastrointestinal symptoms, skin symptoms, systemic anaphylaxis) were unambiguously related to the ingestion of wheat or wheat-containing products. A grading of symptoms and definition of anaphylaxis was performed according to the international position paper and recommendations for the definition of anaphylaxis (Table 1). [20] In six of the patients,

**Table 1.** Demographic, clinical and serological characterization of wheat food-allergic patients.

| Patient | Age | Sex | Wheat-induced Symptoms | Wheat-induced anaphylaxis | Total IgE (kU/L) | Wheat-specific IgE (kUA/L) | Wheat SPT Mean wheal diameter (mm) | Wheat challenge | omega-5-gliadin (kUA/L) | Tri a 36 | Reaction after |
|---|---|---|---|---|---|---|---|---|---|---|---|
| 1 | 41 | F | AS, GIS | yes | 252 | 180 | pos | n.d. | 9.66 | + | wheat-containing products |
| 2 | 5 | M | SS | no | 7559 | 45.2 | 6 | open (pos) | 2.37 | + | open challenge |
| 3 | 14 | M | AS, SS | yes | 636 | >200 | 8 | open (pos) | n.d. | + | bread |
| 4 | 3 | M | GIS, SS | yes | 165 | 11.7 | 8 | n.d. | 0.22 | + | pasta soup, baby cereals |
| 5 | 10 | M | AS, GIS | yes | 802 | 456 | 7 | n.d. | 20.3 | + | cereals |
| 6 | 11 | M | GIS | no | 1642 | 519 | 12 | open (pos) | 3.33 | + | open challenge |
| 7 | 22 | M | GIS | no | n.d. | 47 | 6 | open (pos) | 0.46 | + | open challenge |
| 8 | 4 | F | AS, SS, GIS | yes | 483 | 66.3 | 4.5 | open (pos) | 4.56 | + | open challenge |
| 9 | 6 | F | AS, SS | yes | 74 | 7.57 | 6 | open (pos) | 0.04 | + | open challenge |
| 10 | 3 | F | SS | no | 59.4 | 3.1 | 3 | n.d. | 0.01 | - | wheat soup |

Abbreviations: kU/L: kilounit per liter, kUA/L: kilounit antigen per liter, AS: airway symptoms, GIS: gastrointestinal symptoms, SS: skin symptoms, n.d.: not done, SPT: skin prick test.

open food challenge was performed and positive challenge results were obtained. Skin prick tests with wheat seed extract were performed and positive in each of the wheat allergic patients. For each patient IgE-mediated sensitization to wheat was confirmed by measurements of allergen-specific IgE (CAP-FEIA, Thermofisher, Uppsala, Sweden). Patients were further characterized for their reactivity to the two major wheat food allergens omega-5-gliadin (Tri a 19) and LMW glutenin (Tri a 36). [21]

### Ethical Considerations

Serum samples were obtained in the course of routine allergy diagnosis with permission of the Helsinki University Hospital Review Board/Section for Pediatrics (Dnro 374/E7/2004), Regional Committee of Ethics of the Kopodistrian University of Athens (289/2007) and the Ethics Committee of the Medical University of Vienna (565/2007). Written informed consent was obtained from adult patients and in case of children, from their parents. A retrospective analysis of allergen-specific IgE antibodies was performed with anonymized serum samples with permission of the Ethics Committee of the Medical University of Vienna.

### Determination of IgE-reactivity by dot-blotting

IgE-reactivity of EcTri a 37, BvTri a 37 and five peptides (P1–P5) was tested by by non-denaturing, RAST-based IgE dot blotting. [15] For dot blotting, aliquots of aqueous wheat seed extract (2 µg/dot), HSA (0.5 µg/dot), recombinant EcTri a 37, BvTri a 37 and peptides (0.5 µg/dot) were dotted onto nitrocellulose strips (Schleicher & Schuell, Dassel, Germany). Strips were incubated with 1:10 diluted sera of allergic patients sera (1–10) or with 1:10,000 diluted EcTri a 37-specific rabbit antibodies. As a control, serum of a non-atopic individual (N), rabbit pre-immune serum or buffer (B) alone were included. Bound IgE antibodies were detected with $^{125}$I-labeled anti-human IgE antibodies (Demeditec Diagnostics, Kiel, Germany), bound rabbit antibodies with $^{125}$I-labeled anti-rabbit IgG antibodies (Perkin Elmer, Waltham, USA) and visualized by autoradiography. [22]

### Synthesis, characterization and antibody reactivity of Tri a 37 peptides

Five 10aa- overlapping peptides spanning the Tri a 37 sequence (Table 2; accession number AFQ60540.1) were synthesized (Microwave peptide synthesizer liberty CEM GmbH, Germany) using a Fmoc (9-fluorenylmethoxycarbonyl)-strategy with HBTU [2-(1H-Benzotriazol-1-yl)1,1,3,3 tetramethyluronium hexafluorophosphat] activation as described by Focke *et al.* [23] Table 2 shows the amino acid sequences of Tri a 37-derived peptides. Four of the five peptides had a length of 30 amino acids whereas peptide 4 was synthesized without C-terminal cysteine and hence only 29 aa long. After purification by HPLC to a purity >90%, the identities of the peptides were confirmed by mass spectrometry.

### Inhibition of allergic patients' IgE-binding to EcTri a 37 by rabbit IgG antibodies as determined by ELISA inhibition assay

ELISA plates (Nunc-Immuno Plate, Maxisorp, Thermofisher Scientific, Denmark) were coated with EcTri a 37 diluted in PBS (c = 2 µg/ml) overnight at 4°C. After washing plates twice with PBST and blocking with blocking buffer (PBST, 1% [w/v] BSA) for 2 hours at room temperature, plates were incubated overnight at 4°C with rabbit anti-EcTri a 37 immune-serum or the corresponding pre-immune serum which had been diluted 1:50 in PBST, 0.5% (w/v) BSA. After washing, plates were incubated with 1:10 diluted sera from wheat food allergic patients (Table 1; Patients 1, 3, 4) overnight at 4°C and bound human IgE antibodies were detected with horseradish peroxisase (HRP)-coupled goat anti-human IgE antibodies (KPL, Gaithersburg, MD) diluted 1:2,500 in PBST, 0.5% (w/v) BSA. The color reaction was induced by addition of 1.7 mM 2,2′-azino-di-[3-ethyl-benzthiezolin-sulfonet] (Sigma-Aldrich) in 60 mM citric acid, 77 mM $Na_2HPO_4 \cdot 2H_2O$ and 3 mM $H_2O_2$.OD measurements were performed after 30 minutes in an ELISA reader (Spectra Max PLUS 384, Molecular Devices, Germany) at 405 nm-490 nm. The percentage of inhibition of IgE binding was calculated as follows: 100-(ODimmune/ODpre)x100, where ODimmune and ODpre represent the extinction coefficients after pre incubation with the immune serum or with the pre-immune serum, respectively.

### *In-vitro* digestion assays

Gastric and duodenal *in-vitro* digestion assay with wheat seed extract was performed as described. [24,25] Aliquots containing 10 µg undigested or digested extract were loaded on SDS-PAGE and blotted onto nitrocellulose membranes. Membranes were incubated either with rabbit Abs raised against EcTri a 37 or the corresponding pre-immune serum. Bound rabbit Abs were detected with $^{125}$I-labeled anti-rabbit IgG Abs (Perkin Elmer, Waltham, USA) and visualized by autoradiography.

## Results

### Expression of recombinant Tri a 37 proteins as unfolded and folded protein

rTri a 37 expressed in a prokaryotic system using *E.coli* cells was designated EcTri a 37, however rTri a 37 expressed in baculovirus-infected insect cells was termed BvTri a 37. Both recombinant proteins were purified by Nickel affinity chromatography and showed a similar migration behaviour in Coomassie Blue-stained SDS-PAGE under reducing conditions where they appeared as bands of approximately 18kDa which differs from their calculated molecular weights (EcTri a 37 including N-terminal methionine and C-terminal hexahistine-tag: 12.757 Da; BvTri a 37 including a D and P residue at the N-terminus and a C-terminal hexahistidine-tag: 12.838 Da) and may be explained by the high content of positively charged amino acids (Figure 1A). Under non-reducing conditions, BvTri a 37 appeared as single band of approximately 14 kDa whereas EcTri a 37 showed an additional second band of approximately 18 kDa but no high molecular weight aggregates were visible in both protein preparations (Figure 1A). Using serum IgE from a wheat food allergic patient, monomeric EcTri a 37 and BvTri a 37 were detected at approximately 18 kDa by immunoblotting. Tri a 37-specific rabbit antibodies reacted with natural, monomeric Tri a 37 at 15 kDa in a nitrocellulose-blotted aqueous wheat seed extract (Figure 1B).

MALDI-ToF analysis of EcTri a 37 resulted in a mass peak of 12.742 Da corresponding to the predicted molecular weight of the monomeric protein including methionine and a hexahistidine-tag. (Figure 1C, left). Three BvTri a 37 preparations were analyzed by MALDI-ToF. For one preparation the molecular weight determined by mass spectrometry (i.e., 11.837 Da) was smaller than the calculated mass (Figure 1B, right) whereas for the two other preparations the measured masses were 12.829 Da and 12.913 Da, respectively, which fitted the calculated mass (i.e., 12.838 Da). The smaller mass of the first preparation was most likely was due to N-terminal proteolytic degradation because the His-tag was intact as shown by immunoblotting with an anti-His-tag antibody (data not shown). Chemical cross-linking experiments

**Table 2.** Characterization of Tri a 37-derived peptides and of the two Tri a 37 domains.

| Peptides | Sequence | Molecular weight | Isoelectric point |
|---|---|---|---|
| P1 | KSCCRSTLGRNCYNLCRARGAQKLCAGVCR | 3291.91 | 9.69 |
| P2 | AQKLCAGVCRCKISSGLSCPKGFPKLALES | 3095.75 | 9.21 |
| P3 | KGFPKLALESNSDEPDTIEYCNLGCRSSVC | 3276.66 | 4.51 |
| P4 | CNLGCRSSVCDYMVNAAADDEEMKLYVEN | 3243.62 | 4.02 |
| P5 | EEMKLYVENCADACVSFCNGDAGLPSLDAY | 3228.58 | 3.71 |
| | | **Thionin domain (45 aa)** | **C-terminal acidic extension domain (65 aa)** |
| | **basic aa** | 22.20% | 3.10% |
| | **acidic aa** | 0% | 22% |
| | **pI** | 9.75 | 3.35 |
| | **hydrophobic aa** | 18% | 22% |
| | **hydrophilic aa** | 60% | 48% |

and size exclusion experiments showed that both, EcTri a 37 and BvTri a 37, occurred as monomeric proteins (data not shown).

The far-UV CD spectrum of EcTri a 37 indicated that the recombinant protein was unfolded which is characterized by minimum at approximately 205 nm. By contrast, BvTri a 37 appeared as folded protein showing a CD spectrum typical for a predominant α-fold with two minima at 208 and 222 nm and a maximum at approximately 190 nm (Figure 1D).

## Unfolded EcTri a 37 and folded BvTri a 37 show comparable IgE-reactivity

The IgE-reactivity of both recombinant allergens EcTri a 37 and BvTri a 37 was tested in non-denaturing, RAST-based IgE-dot blot experiments with sera from 10 patients with confirmed wheat-induced food allergy (Figure 2A; Table 1). Both allergens showed very similar and specific IgE-binding capacity when tested with the sera from the five wheat allergic patients who were sensitized to Tri a 37 (patients #1–5) but not with sera from wheat allergic patients who were not sensitized to Tri a 37 (patients #6–10). Also Tri a 37-specific rabbit antibodies reacted with both recombinant allergens in a comparable manner (Figure 2A). Allergic patients' sera, but not serum from a non-allergic subject or buffer displayed IgE reactivity to wheat extract. Likewise, wheat extract was recognized by the rabbit anti-Tri a 37 antibodies but not by the pre-immune serum or buffer. The negative control protein HSA showed no reactivity (Figure 2A).

## Tri a 37 contains sequential IgE epitopes in the N- as well as C- terminal domain

In order to study the IgE epitopes of Tri a 37 in more detail, we tested the sera from the wheat allergic patients also for IgE reactivity with synthetic Tri a 37 peptides (Figure 2B). Five overlapping peptides spanning the Tri a 37 sequence were synthesized and purified (Figure 3, Table 2). With the exception of peptide 4 which was 29 amino acids long, the synthesized peptides were 30 amino acids long with overlaps of ten amino acids (Figure 3A). The molecular weights of the peptides range from 3095 to 3291 Dalton. Three of the synthesized peptides were from the original IgE-reactive recombinant fragment whereas peptides 1 and 2 also included portions of the N-terminal thionin domain which is rich in basic amino acids and has a pI of 9.75 whereas the C-terminal acidic extension domain is acidic (pI 3.53) (Figure 3A; Table 2). Hence, the isoelectric points of the individual peptides ranged from 3.71 to 9.69 depending on the domain from which they originated (Table 2). Peptides 1, 3 and 4 from both domains were recognized by IgE antibodies from Tri a 37-sensitized patients and also by Tri a 37-specific rabbit antibodies. Peptides 2 and 5 did not react with IgE from the tested patients and also not with rabbit IgG antibodies raised by immunization with rTri a 37 (Figure 2B). According to the prediction of surface-exposed portions of Tri a 37, the IgE-reactive peptides were derived from surface-exposed regions (e.g., peptides 3 and 4) but included also less surface-exposed areas (i.e., peptide 1) (Figure 3B).

## IgG antibodies induced by immunization with EcTri a 37 recognize similar epitopes as allergic patients IgE and inhibit allergic patients' IgE binding to Tri a 37

EcTri a 37- specific rabbit IgG antibodies were then used to investigate their ability to inhibit wheat food allergic patients' IgE binding (Table 1; Patient 1, 3, 4) to the allergen in ELISA competition experiments. In patients 3 and 4 who showed the strongest IgE binding to Tri a 37, rabbit anti-Tri a 37 antibodies caused a 64% and 73% inhibition of IgE binding respectively whereas the inhibition in patient 1 who showed low levels of Tri a 37-specific IgE was 39% (Figure 4).

## Natural Tri a 37 in wheat extracts is digested under gastric digestion conditions

Figure 5 shows nitrocellulose-blotted wheat extracts which were subjected to gastric and duodenal digestion and then probed with rabbit anti-Tri a 37 antibodies. Undigested Tri a 37 was detected at 15 kDa whereas one minute of gastric digestion led to the loss of the signal. Under duodenal digestion conditions, Tri a 37 could be detected even after 45 minutes at 15 kDa and an additional smaller IgG binding band at 10 kDa became visible after 10 minutes of digestion (Figure 5).

## Discussion

Here we showed that IgE recognition of Tri a 37, a wheat food allergen which is associated with severe wheat-induced anaphy-

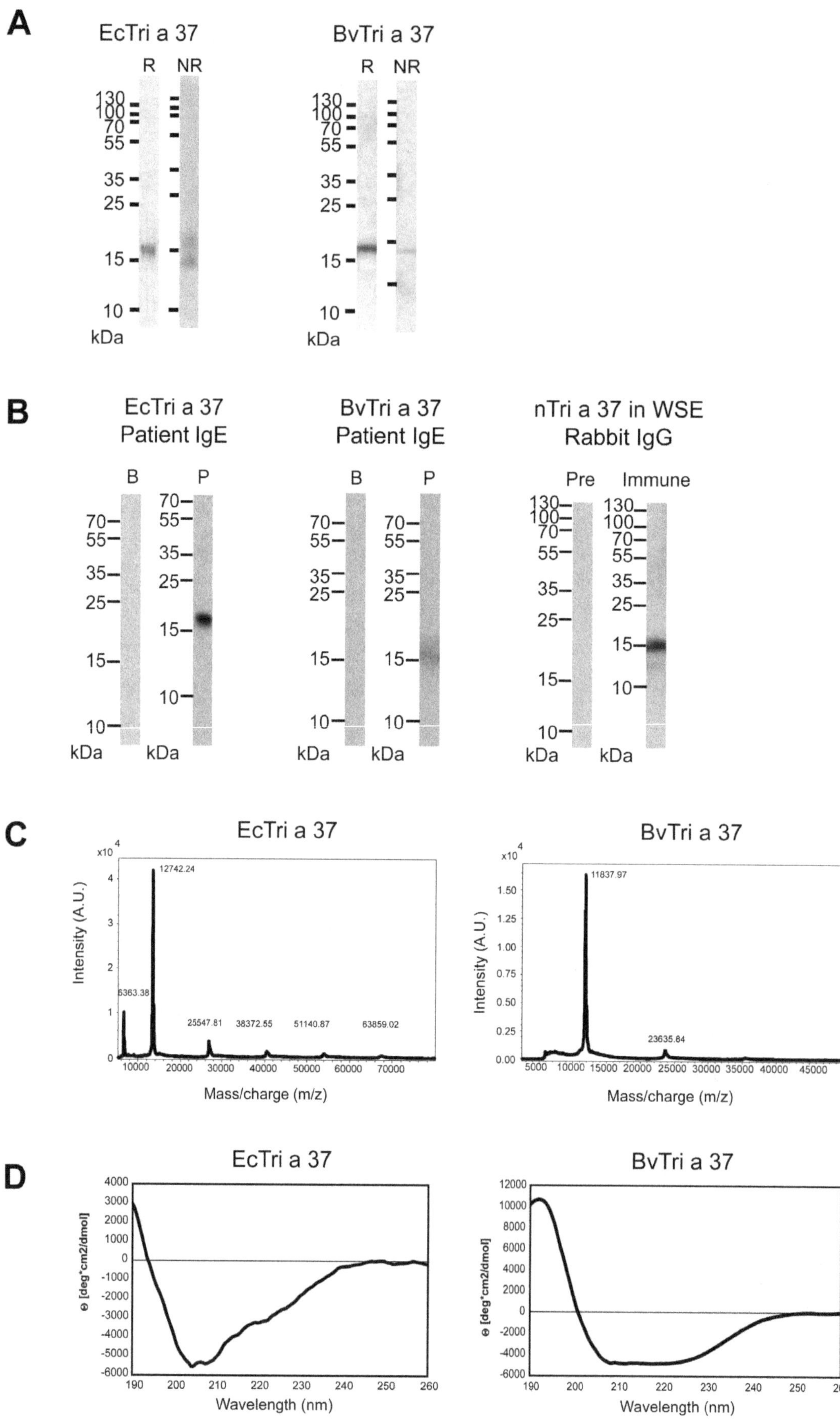
A
EcTri a 37
R NR
BvTri a 37
R NR
kDa
B
EcTri a 37
Patient IgE
B P
BvTri a 37
Patient IgE
B P
nTri a 37 in WSE
Rabbit IgG
Pre Immune
kDa
C
EcTri a 37
Intensity (A.U.)
Mass/charge (m/z)
BvTri a 37
Intensity (A.U.)
Mass/charge (m/z)
D
EcTri a 37
Wavelength (nm)
BvTri a 37
Wavelength (nm)

**Figure 1. Characterization of purified Tri a 37 expressed in *E.coli* cells (EcTri a 37) and in baculovirus-infected insect cells (BvTri a 37) as well as detection of natural Tri a 37 in wheat seed extract.** (**A**) Coomassie brilliant blue-stained SDS-PAGE under reducing (lane R) and under non-reducing (lane NR) conditions. A protein molecular weight marker (kDa) is shown on the left side. (**B**) Detection of IgE-reactivitiy to Western-blotted EcTri a 37 and BvTri a 37, using serum from a wheat food allergic patient (P) and buffer (B) as a control. Western-blotted wheat seed extract was tested with Tri a 37-specific rabbit antibodies (Immune) or the corresponding pre-immune serum (Pre). Bound human IgE and rabbit IgG antibodies were detected with $^{125}$Iodine-labeled antibodies and visualized by autoradiography. Molecular weights are indicated in kilo Dalton (kDa). (**C**) Mass spectrometry of recombinant EcTri a 37 and BvTri a 37. The mass/charge ratios are shown on the *x*-axes, and the intensities are displayed on the *y*-axes as percentages of the most intensive signals obtained in the investigated mass range. (**D**) Circular dichroism analysis of recombinant EcTri a 37 and BvTri a 37. The spectra are expressed as mean residue ellipticities (θ) (*y*-axes) at given wavelengths (*x*-axes).

laxis does not require conformational epitopes. Using two different expression systems, an unfolded variant of rTri a 37 (i.e., EcTri a 37) was produced by prokaryotic expression and a folded form was obtained by expression in baculovirus-infected insect cells (i.e., BvTri a 37). The differences in fold between the two recombinant proteins were not due to differences in glycosylation because Tri a 37 does not contain any glycosylation sites. However, Tri a 37 contains 14 cystein residues of which 8 are known to form 4 disulphide bridges in a correctly folded N-terminal thionin domain for which the three-dimensional structure was obtained by x-ray crystallography and nuclear magnetic resonance analysis. [26,27] Interestingly, both, the folded as well as the unfolded Tri a 37 occurred as monomeric proteins in SDS-PAGE under non-reducing conditions and when analyzed by size exclusion chromatography indicating that in both proteins the 14 cysteins were mainly engaged in the formation of intra-molecular but did not form inter-molecular disulphide bonds. The presence and lack of structural fold in the two proteins therefore may be attributed to correct versus partly incorrect formation of intra-molecular disulphide bonds. Comparable IgE binding capacity of EcTri a 37 and BvTri a 37 in non-denaturing, RAST-based IgE binding assay revealed that wheat food allergic patients' IgE recognition does not require structural fold of Tri a 37. A more detailed analysis of IgE epitopes was performed with 5 synthetic peptides spanning the complete Tri a 37 sequence which had an overlap of 9–10 amino acids. Using these synthetic peptides, sequential IgE binding sites were found at the N-terminal thionin domain and the C-terminal extension domain. Not all Tri a 37-reactive sera reacted also with peptides which may be due to the fact that certain IgE-reactive areas were not covered by the peptides due to limited overlap or length. Nevertheless, our data demonstrate that IgE recognition of Tri a 37 thus does not require fold and is directed against sequential epitopes which is typical for class I food allergens which sensitize mainly via the gut such as other wheat food-, milk, egg and peanut allergens. When we digested natural wheat extract containing Tri a 37, we found that the allergen was digested under conditions of gastric digestion whereas it was stable under conditions of duodenal digestion. This finding fits to the observation that Tri a 37 contains sequential epitopes which are represented by peptides. IgE recognition of sequential epitopes might thus be explained by sensitization to proteolytic fragments of Tri a 37. In this context it is tempting to speculate that sensitization to Tri a 37 and symptoms caused by Tri a 37 may be modulated by conditions affecting gastric digestion such as pathologies of the gastrointestinal tract and low acidic conditions

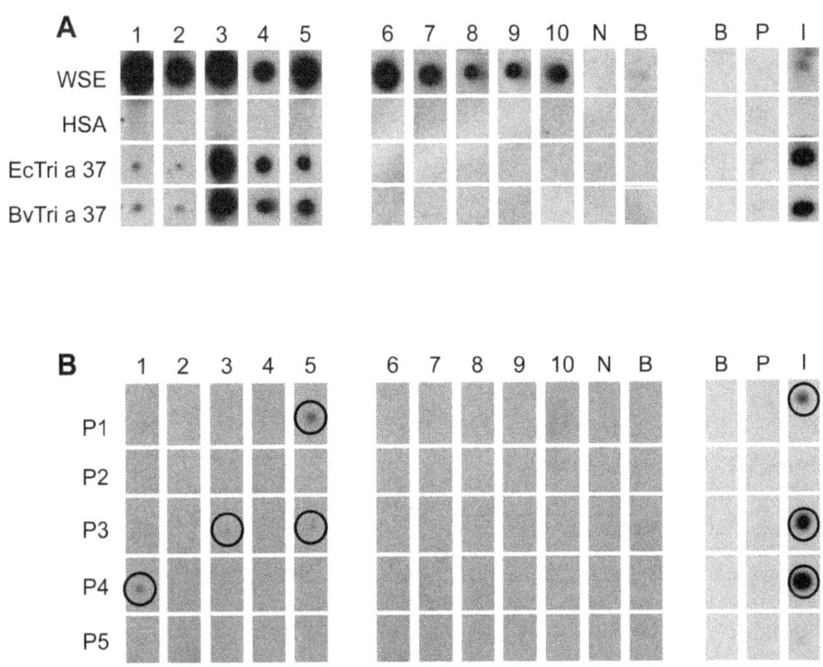


**Figure 2. Antibody-recognition of EcTri a 37, BvTri a 37 and Tri a 37 peptides.** (**A**) Nitrocellulose-dotted wheat seed extract (WSE), human serum albumin (HSA), EcTri a 37 and BvTri a 37 were tested with sera from ten wheat food allergic patients (1–10), with serum from a non-allergic individual (N), buffer alone (B), with Tri a 37-specific rabbit antibodies (I), the corresponding rabbit pre-immune serum (P) and buffer control (B). (**B**) Testing of Tri a 37 peptides (P1–P5) as in (A).

**A**

**Thionin domain** **C-terminal acidic extension domain**

| | |
|---|---|
| Tri a 37 | KSCCRSTLGRNCYNLCRARGAQKLCAGVCRCKISSGLSCPKGFPKLALESNSDEPDTIEYCNLGCRSSVCDYMVNAAADDEEMKLYVENCADACVSFCNGDAGLPSLDAY |
| P1 (AA 1-30) | KSCCRSTLGRNCYNLCRARGAQKLCAGVCR |
| P2 (AA 21-50) | AQKLCAGVCRCKISSGLSCPKGFPKLALES |
| P3 (AA 41-70) | KGFPKLALESNSDEPDTIEYCNLGCRSSVC |
| P4 (AA 61-90) | CNLGCRSSVCDYMVNAAADDEEMKLYVEN |
| P5 (AA 81-110) | EEMKLYVENCADACVSFCNGDAGLPSLDAY |

**Tri a 37**

| | |
|---|---|
| **AA 1-46** | **Thionin domain** |
| **AA 47-110** | **C-terminal acidic extension domain** |
| underlined | IgE -reactive cDNA clone |
| boxed | cysteins |
| red | basic AAs (H/K/R) |
| blue | acidic AAs (D/E) |

**B** **ProtScale (% accessible residues)**

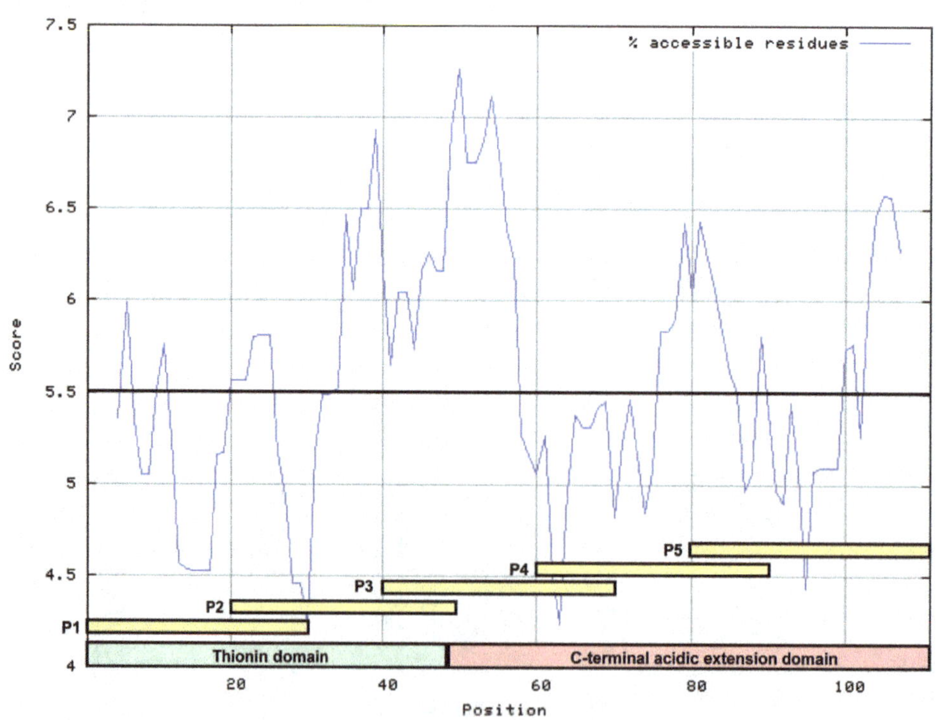


**Figure 3. Localization of synthetic peptides in the Tri a 37 sequence and surface accessibility prediction.** (**A**) Amino acid sequence of Tri a 37 showing the N- and C-terminal domain and the originally isolated IgE-reactive fragment (underlined). Cysteins are boxed, basic and acidic amino acids are coloured in red and blue, respectively. Synthetic Tri a 37 peptides P1–P5 are indicated. (**B**) Surface accessibility plot of the Tri a 37 amino acid sequence. The numbers of the amino acids, the thionin domain (green), the C-terminal acidic extension domain (pink), the synthetic peptides (yellow) are indicated on the x-axis. The calculated accessibility of the residues is indicated on the y-axis. Scores above 5.5 (bold horizontal line) represent regions of high surface accessibility.

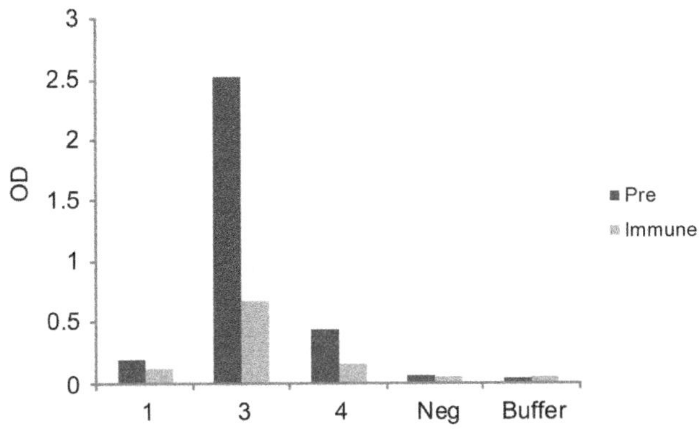


**Figure 4. Inhibition of allergic patients' IgE binding to Tri a 37 by rabbit anti-Tri a 37 antibodies.** Tri a 37 was tested for IgE reactivity with sera from three Tri a 37-allergic patients (1, 3, 4), serum from a non-allergic individual or buffer after pre-incubation with rabbit anti-Tri a 37 antibodies (Immune) or the rabbits pre-immune serum (Pre). Shown are the optical density (O.D.) levels corresponding to bound IgE.

which may occur in in children or elderly persons or as consequence of antacid medication. [28,29]

Currently several approaches of allergen-specific immunotherapy are pursued for food allergies, among them oral, sublingual and epicutaneous immunotherapy with natural food allergens [30] and also injection immunotherapy approaches using recombinant food allergens. [31] In this context, we investigated the ability of rabbit IgG antibodies which were induced by immunization with recombinant Tri a 37, to inhibit allergic patients IgE binding to Tri a 37. In fact, we found that Tri a 37-specific IgG inhibited allergic patients IgE binding to Tri a 37 indicating that it may be possible to perform injection immunotherapy with recombinant Tri a 37 with the goal to induce blocking IgG antibodies which are known to play a major role in immunotherapy.

In conclusion we showed that IgE epitopes of Tri a 37 are of the non-conformational type, including sequential epitopes and that rTri a 37 expressed in *E.coli* as well as insect cells can be used for the serological detection of Tri a 37-specific IgE in diagnostic tests. Furthermore, it may be possible to use rTri a 37 for immunotherapy in sensitized individuals.

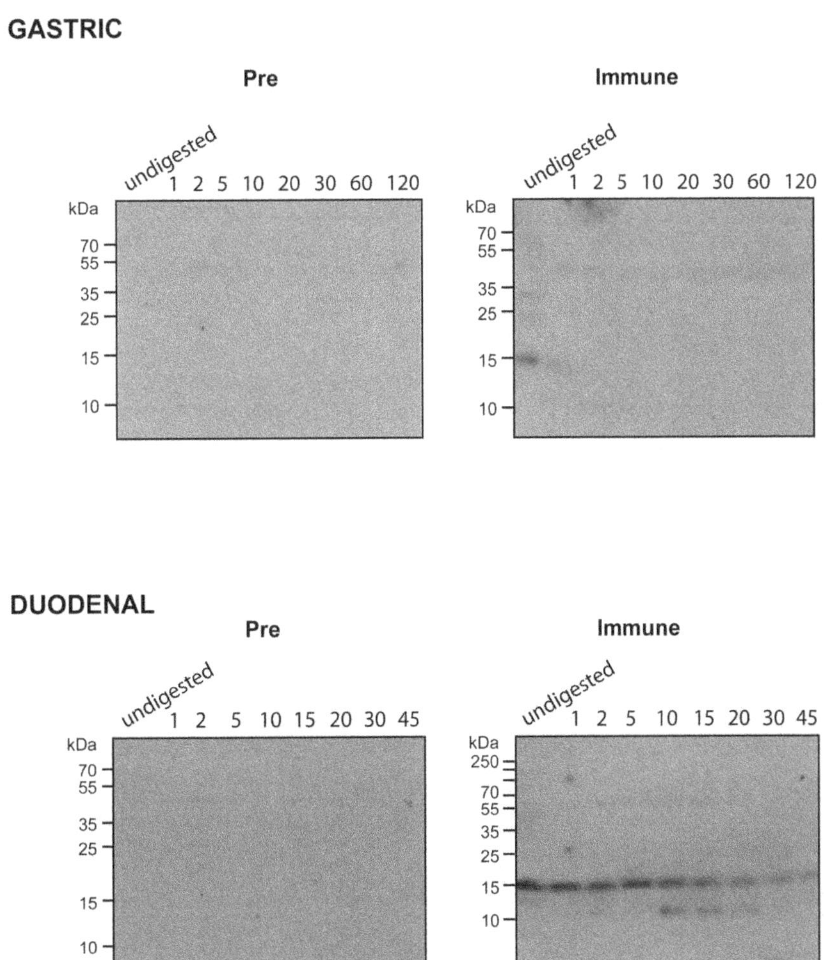


**Figure 5. Effects of gastric and duodenal digestion on natural Tri a 37.** Undigested wheat seed extract (undigested) or after different times of gastric (top panel) or duodenal digestion (lower panel) was subjected to SDS-PAGE and blotted to nitrocellulose. Nitrocelluloses were then tested with rabbit anti-Tri a 37 antibodies (Immune) and the corresponding pre-immune serum (Pre). Bound IgG antibodies were detected with $^{125}$I-labeled anti-rabbit IgG antibodies and visualized by autoradiography.

## Author Contributions

Conceived and designed the experiments: SP RV. Performed the experiments: SP MW MFT GH AD. Analyzed the data: SP RV WK VN SV. Contributed reagents/materials/analysis tools: RS NGP SG MM AP. Wrote the paper: SP RV.

## References


1. Cordain L (1999) Cereal grains: humanity's double-edged sword. World Rev Nutr Diet **84**: p. 19–73.
2. Helm RM, Burks AW (2008) Food allergens. Clin Allergy Immunol **21**: p. 219–35.
3. Pourpak Z, Mansouri M, Mesdaghi M, Kazemnejad A, Farhoudi A (2004) Wheat allergy: clinical and laboratory findings. Int Arch Allergy Immunol **133**(2): p. 168–73.
4. Asero R, Antonicelli L, Arena A, Bommarito L, Caruso B (2009) Causes of food-induced anaphylaxis in Italian adults: a multi-centre study. Int Arch Allergy Immunol **150**(3): p. 271–7.
5. Matsuo H, Kohno K, Morita E (2005) Molecular cloning, recombinant expression and IgE-binding epitope of omega-5 gliadin, a major allergen in wheat-dependent exercise-induced anaphylaxis. FEBS J **272**(17): p. 4431–8.
6. Hofmann SC, Fischer J, Eriksson C, Bengtsson GO, Biedermann T, et al. (2012) IgE detection to alpha/beta/gamma-gliadin and its clinical relevance in wheat-dependent exercise-induced anaphylaxis. Allergy **67**(11): p. 1457–60.
7. Matsuo H, Kohno K, Niihara H, Morita E (2005) Specific IgE determination to epitope peptides of omega-5 gliadin and high molecular weight glutenin subunit is a useful tool for diagnosis of wheat-dependent exercise-induced anaphylaxis. J Immunol **175**(12): p. 8116–22.
8. Palacin A, Bartra J, Muñoz R, Diaz-Perales A, Valero A, et al. (2010) Anaphylaxis to wheat flour-derived foodstuffs and the lipid transfer protein syndrome: a potential role of wheat lipid transfer protein Tri a 14. Int Arch Allergy Immunol **152**(2): p. 178–83.
9. Pahr S, Constantin C, Papadopoulos NG, Giavi S, Mäkelä M, et al. (2013) alpha-Purothionin, a new wheat allergen associated with severe allergy. J Allergy Clin Immunol : **132**(4): 1000—3. e1–4.
10. Reese G, Ayuso R, Leong-Kee SM, Plante MJ, Lehrer SB (2001) Characterization and identification of allergen epitopes: recombinant peptide libraries and synthetic, overlapping peptides. J Chromatogr B Biomed Sci Appl **756**(1–2): p. 157-63.
11. Nowak-Wegrzyn A (2007) Food allergy to proteins. Nestle Nutr Inst Workshop Ser **59**: p. 17–31; discussion 31—6.
12. Battais F, Mothes T, Moneret-Vautrin DA, Pineau F, Kanny G, et al. (2005) Identification of IgE-binding epitopes on gliadins for patients with food allergy to wheat. Allergy **60**(6): p. 815–21.
13. Roth-Walter F, Starkl P, Zuberbier T, Hummel K, Nöbauer K, et al. (2013) Glutathione exposes sequential IgE-epitopes in ovomucoid relevant in persistent egg allergy. Mol Nutr Food Res **57**(3): p. 536–44.
14. Vila L, Beyer K, Järvinen KM, Chatchatee P, Bardina L, et al. (2001) Role of conformational and linear epitopes in the achievement of tolerance in cow's milk allergy. Clin Exp Allergy, 2001. **31**(10): p. 1599–606.
15. Pahr S, Constantin C, Mari A, Scheiblhofer S, Thalhamer J, et al. (2012) Molecular characterization of wheat allergens specifically recognized by patients suffering from wheat-induced respiratory allergy. Clin Exp Allergy **42**(4): p. 597–609.
16. Marlovits TC, Zechmeister T, Schwihla H, Ronacher B, Blaas D (1998) Recombinant soluble low-density lipoprotein receptor fragment inhibits common cold infection. J Mol Recognit **11**(1–6): p. 49-51.
17. Chen KW, Blatt K, Thomas WR, Swoboda I, Valent P, et al. (2012) Hypoallergenic Der p 1/Der p 2 combination vaccines for immunotherapy of house dust mite allergy. J Allergy Clin Immunol **130**(2): p. 435–43 e4
18. Campana R, Vrtala S, Maderegger B, Dall'Antonia Y, Zafred D, et al. (2011) Altered IgE epitope presentation: A model for hypoallergenic activity revealed for Bet v 1 trimer. Mol Immunol **48**(4): p. 431–41.
19. Janin J (1979) Surface and inside volumes in globular proteins. Nature **277**(5696): p. 491–2.
20. Sampson HA, Muñoz-Furlong A, Campbell RL, Adkinson NF Jr, Bock SA, et al. (2006) Second symposium on the definition and management of anaphylaxis: summary report—second National Institute of Allergy and Infectious Disease/Food Allergy and Anaphylaxis Network symposium. Annals of emergency medicine **47**(4): p. 373–80.
21. Baar A, Pahr S, Constantin C, Giavi S, Manoussaki A, et al. (2014) Specific IgE reactivity to Tri a 36 in children with wheat food allergy. J Allergy Clin Immunol **133**(2): p. 585–7.
22. Valenta R, Duchene M, Ebner C, Valent P, Sillaber C, et al. (1992) Profilins constitute a novel family of functional plant pan-allergens. J Exp Med **175**(2): p. 377–85.
23. Focke M, Mahler V, Ball T, Sperr WR, Majlesi Y, et al. (2001) Nonanaphylactic synthetic peptides derived from B cell epitopes of the major grass pollen allergen, Phl p 1, for allergy vaccination. FASEB J **15**(11): p. 2042–4.
24. Baar A, Pahr S, Constantin C, Scheiblhofer S, Thalhamer J, et al. (2012) Molecular and immunological characterization of Tri a 36, a low molecular weight glutenin, as a novel major wheat food allergen. J Immunol **189**(6): p. 3018–25.
25. Vieths S, Reindl J, Müller U, Hoffmann A, Haustein D (1999) Digestibility of peanut and hazelnut allergens investigated by a simple in vitro procedure. Eur Food Res Technol **209**(6): p. 379–388.
26. Teeter MM, Ma XQ, Rao U, Whitlow M (1990) Crystal structure of a protein-toxin alpha 1-purothionin at 2.5A and a comparison with predicted models. Proteins **8**(2): p. 118–32.
27. Clore GM, Nilges M, Sukumaran DK, Brünger AT, Karplus M, et al. (1986) The three-dimensional structure of alpha1-purothionin in solution: combined use of nuclear magnetic resonance, distance geometry and restrained molecular dynamics. EMBO J **5**(10): p. 2729–35.
28. Untersmayr E, Jensen-Jarolim E (2008) The role of protein digestibility and antacids on food allergy outcomes. J Allergy Clin Immunol **121**(6): p. 1301–8; quiz 1309–10.
29. Untersmayr E, Schöll I, Swoboda I, Beil WJ, Förster-Waldl E, et al. (2003) Antacid medication inhibits digestion of dietary proteins and causes food allergy: a fish allergy model in BALB/c mice. J Allergy Clin Immunol **112**(3): p. 616–23.
30. Jones SM, Burks AW, Dupont C (2014) State of the art on food allergen immunotherapy: Oral, sublingual, and epicutaneous. J Allergy Clin Immunol **133**(2): p. 318–23.
31. Zuidmeer-Jongejan L, Fernandez-Rivas M, Poulsen LK, Neubauer A, Asturias J, et al. (2012) FAST: towards safe and effective subcutaneous immunotherapy of persistent life-threatening food allergies. Clin Transl Allergy **2**(1): p. 5.

# 15

# Enlarging the Toolbox for Allergen Epitope Definition with an Allergen-Type Model Protein

Hanna Berkner[1]*, Christian Seutter von Loetzen[1]*, Maximilian Hartl[1], Stefanie Randow[2], Michaela Gubesch[2], Lothar Vogel[2], Felix Husslik[2], Andreas Reuter[2], Jonas Lidholm[3], Barbara Ballmer-Weber[4], Stefan Vieths[2], Paul Rösch[1], Dirk Schiller[2]*

1 Department of Biopolymers, University of Bayreuth, Bayreuth, Bavaria, Germany, 2 Division of Allergology, Paul-Ehrlich-Institut, Langen, Hesse, Germany, 3 ImmunoDiagnostics Division, Thermo Fisher Scientific Inc., Uppsala, Uppsala län, Sweden, 4 Department of Dermatology, Allergy Unit, University Hospital Zürich, Zürich, Zürich, Switzerland

## Abstract

***Background:*** Birch pollen-allergic subjects produce polyclonal cross-reactive IgE antibodies that mediate pollen-associated food allergies. The major allergen Bet v 1 and its homologs in plant foods bind IgE in their native protein conformation. Information on location, number and clinical relevance of IgE epitopes is limited. We addressed the use of an allergen-related protein model to identify amino acids critical for IgE binding of PR-10 allergens.

***Method:*** Norcoclaurine synthase (NCS) from meadow rue is structurally homologous to Bet v 1 but does not bind Bet v 1-reactive IgE. NCS was used as the template for epitope grafting. NCS variants were tested with sera from 70 birch pollen allergic subjects and with monoclonal antibody BV16 reported to compete with IgE binding to Bet v 1.

***Results:*** We generated an NCS variant ($\Delta$29NCS$_{N57/I58E/D60N/V63P/D68K}$) harboring an IgE epitope of Bet v 1. Bet v 1-type protein folding of the NCS variant was evaluated by $^{1}$H-$^{15}$N-HSQC NMR spectroscopy. BV16 bound the NCS variant and 71% (50/70 sera) of our study population showed significant IgE binding. We observed IgE and BV16 cross-reactivity to the epitope presented by the NCS variant in a subgroup of Bet v 1-related allergens. Moreover BV16 blocked IgE binding to the NCS variant. Antibody cross-reactivity depended on a defined orientation of amino acids within the Bet v 1-type conformation.

***Conclusion:*** Our system allows the evaluation of patient-specific epitope profiles and will facilitate both the identification of clinically relevant epitopes as biomarkers and the monitoring of therapeutic outcomes to improve diagnosis, prognosis, and therapy of allergies caused by PR-10 proteins.

**Editor:** Nick Gay, University of Cambridge, United Kingdom

**Funding:** The authors have no support or funding to report.

**Competing Interests:** Hanna Berkner and Jonas Lidholm are employees of Thermo Fisher Scientific. The other authors declare no conflict of interest.

* Email: Dirk.Schiller@pei.de

These authors contributed equally to this work.

## Introduction

Millions of patients with allergies to tree pollen are sensitized (produce IgE antibodies) to the major allergen of birch (*Betula verrucosa*) pollen, Bet v 1 [1]. Bet v 1-binding IgE cross-reacts with Bet v 1-homologous proteins from plant foods, leading to allergy to such foods in a majority of birch pollen-allergic subjects [2]. Despite all efforts so far, a complete IgE epitope profile of Bet v 1 or of a Bet v 1-related allergen is still lacking, although knowledge of clinically relevant IgE binding determinants would benefit diagnosis, therapy, and current understanding of the sometimes puzzling clinical phenomena of pollen-related food allergies. Structural information on IgE epitopes of Bet v 1 and Bet v 1-like allergens in foods is limited. To date only IgE epitopes of allergens Art v 1 (pollen), Phl p 2 (grass), and β-lactoglobulin (milk) were determined from X-ray crystallography and NMR spectroscopy of IgE-allergen complexes [3–5]. Conformational IgE epitopes of allergens from the PR10-protein family, however, are unknown. Allergen variants carrying substitutions of either individual or multiple residues to either attenuate or induce IgE antibody binding (epitope grafting) identified individual residues crucial for IgE recognition by Bet v 1 [6–10] and Bet v 1-type allergens from apple [11,12], cherry [13,14], and celeriac [15]. In addition, monoclonal antibodies have been used to localize potential IgE epitopes of Bet v 1 and related allergens [10,16–19]. The only structural information on an epitope of Bet v 1 to date was obtained from X-ray crystallography of a complex between the monoclonal Bet v 1-specific mouse IgG BV16 and the major isoform of Bet v 1, Bet v 1 a [20]. Binding of BV16 to Bet v 1 reduces serum IgE interactions, indicating competition of IgE and monoclonal IgG for an overlapping binding site of Bet v 1 [21,22].

IgE-allergen interactions are usually analyzed with polyclonal serum IgE, making it difficult to differentiate individual IgE interaction sites. Engineering of recombinant allergen variants often changes the native protein conformation which is essential for IgE interaction. Thus we suggest to use a non-IgE binding protein with allergen-like conformation as a scaffold that can be modulated on the individual amino acid level to stepwise induce IgE recognition capabilities. For this purpose we recently cloned, expressed, purified, and characterized the enzyme norcoclaurine synthase (NCS) from the meadow rue *Thalictrum flavum* as a recombinant protein variant Δ29NCS [23,24]. As Bet v 1, NCS is a member of the pathogenesis-related protein family (PR-10) sharing the typical Bet v 1 protein fold [25], but has no known allergenic properties. NCS is thus an ideal protein model candidate to study epitopes of PR-10 allergens.

Here we aimed at establishing a recombinant model protein system to specifically analyze epitopes of PR-10 allergens. For this purpose we used the truncated variant Δ29NCS. To study the impact of individual amino acids in IgE binding within NCS we generated variants of Δ29NCS, analyzed their IgE antibody binding with sera of birch pollen allergic subjects and determined the cross-reactivity of suspected IgE epitopes grafted onto NCS.

## Methods

### Patients

Sixty-nine patients with a convincing history of pollinosis to early flowering tree pollen and specific IgE levels>0.35 $kU_A/L$ to birch pollen measured by ImmunoCAP (Thermo Fisher Scientific, Uppsala, Sweden) were included as serum donors. Patients were recruited at the Allergy Unit, Department of Dermatology, University Hospital Zürich, Switzerland, at the Hospital Borkum Riff, Borkum, Germany, and at the Paul-Ehrlich-Institut, Langen, Germany. Study participants provided written informed consent. Ethics approval by the local ethics committee 'Kantonale Ethikkomission Zürich, Switzerland' of the University Hospital in Zürich, Switzerland and the local ethics committee 'Ethik-Kommission, Fachbereich Medizin der Johann Wolfgang Goethe-Universität, Frankfurt am Main, Germany' of the University Hospital in Frankfurt included consent form and consent procedure. Sera 52–69 were published elsewhere [26]. Serum 70 was purchased from DLab Diagnose GmbH, Hamburg, Germany. Serum from one non-allergic subject was used as negative control for the specific IgE measurements. The positive serum pool (IgE>0.35 $kU_A/L$ against Δ29NCS_5x) comprised sera 11, 14, 20–23, 32, 42, 47, and 70. The negative serum pool (IgE< 0.35 $kU_A/L$ against Δ29NCS_5x) comprised sera 4, 12, 18, 29–31, 33, 40, 43, and 46.

### Determination of specific IgE

Specific IgE levels to recombinant proteins were determined by ImmunoCAP in Phadia 100 and 250 instruments (Thermo Fisher Scientific, Uppsala, Sweden) according to the manufacturer's instructions. In the case of Bet v 1, Api g 1.01 and Cor a 1.04, commercial ImmunoCAP tests were used, whereas for Pru av 1, Dau c 1.01, NCS and its variants, experimental ImmunoCAPs were manufactured by coupling the recombinant allergens individually to the solid phase, as described elsewhere [27,28].

### Cloning, expression and purification of Δ29NCS, Bet v 1 variants, and Bet v 1-related allergens

Mutations leading to the amino acid exchanges/insertion in $\Delta29NCS_{N57/I58E/D60N/V63P}$, $\Delta29NCS_{N57/I58E/D60N/V63P/D68K}$, and Bet v $1_{N43A/E45S/N47A/K55A}$ were sequentially introduced into pET29b-Δ29NCS [23] and pET15b-Bet v 1, respectively, with the QuickChange kit from Stratagene (Heidelberg, Germany). All protein variants were expressed and purified via their $His_6$-tag as described [23] with minor changes. To yield higher amounts of soluble protein, the synthesis of the protein variants was induced by the addition of 1 mM IPTG at 25°C followed by incubation overnight. A synthetic gene encoding soy allergen Gly m 4 was cloned into pET15b and purified as described above for Bet v 1. The following Bet v 1-related allergens were expressed and purified as described: Pru av 1 (cherry) [29], Dau c 1 (carrot) [26], and Cor a 1.04 (hazelnut) [30]. rApi g 1.01 (celeriac) was purchased from Biomay, Vienna, Austria.

### Circular dichroism

Far UV circular dichroism (CD) spectra of the Δ29NCS variants were acquired at 293 K using a Jasco J-810 spectropolarimeter (Japan Spectroscopic, Gross-Umstadt, Germany) at a band width of 1 nm and a sensitivity of 100 mdeg in a 0.2 cm cell. All proteins were analyzed at a concentration of 2.5 μM in 5 mM sodium phosphate, pH 7.0. Each measurement comprised the average of 10 repeated scans between 260 and 190 nm.

### NMR spectroscopy

NMR samples were prepared by dissolving lyophilized $^{15}N$-labeled protein in 20 mM sodium phosphate, pH 7.0, 1 mM DTT, 0.04% sodium azide and 10% $D_2O$. $^1H$-$^{15}N$-HSQC spectra were recorded on a Bruker Avance 700 MHz spectrometer at 298 K. NMR data were processed using in-house software and were visualized with NMR view [31].

### Modelling of NCS variants

Structure predictions of $\Delta29NCS_{N57/I58E/D60N/V63P}$, $\Delta29NCS_{N57/I58E/D60N/V63P/D68K}$, and Bet v $1_{N43I/E45S/N47D/K55A}$ were performed by using the Phyre server [32]. The calculated models were based on the structures of wild type NCS [25] (pdb 2VNE) and Bet v 1a [33] (pdb 1BV1), respectively, with a confidence of 100% and a sequence coverage of at least 85%.

### Binding of monoclonal antibody BV16 to Bet v 1 and related allergens

Nunc Maxisorp plates (Fisher Scientific, Schwerte, Germany) were coated overnight at room temperature with 250 ng/100 μl proteins (Δ29NCS_5x; Δ29NCS; Dau c 1; Pru av 1; Bet v 1; Gly m 4; Cor a 1), with 50 ng/100 μl Api g 1, and with 25 ng/100 μl Bet v 1 and Bet v 1_4x in phosphate-buffered saline (PBS). After blocking with PBS containing 2% BSA a dilution series of the murine monoclonal anti-Bet v 1 antibody BV16 [34] was added for 1 h at room temperature in PBS containing 0.05% Tween 20 and 0.1% BSA. Allergen-specific IgG was detected with horseradish peroxidase-conjugated goat anti-mouse IgG antibody (A3673, SigmaAldrich, Taufkirchen, Germany) diluted 1:3000 in PBS containing 0.05% Tween 20 and 0.1% BSA as described for the IgE ELISA below.

### Inhibition IgE ELISA

For IgE-ELISA inhibition experiments, Nunc Maxisorp plates (Fisher Scientific, Schwerte, Germany) were coated overnight at room temperature with 300 ng/100 μl Δ29NCS_5x with 10 mM potassium phosphate-buffered saline (PBS). After blocking with PBS containing 2% BSA, plates were incubated with the human serum pool (dilution 1:10) and increasing concentrations ($3*10^{-5}$–3 µg/well) of recombinant inhibitors (Bet v 1, Bet v 1_4x, Dau c 1.01, Pru av 1, Gly m 4, Cor a 1.04, and Api g 1.01, respectively) for 3 hrs at room temperature with PBS containing 0.05% Tween 20 and 0.1% BSA. Allergen-specific IgE was detected with horseradish peroxidase-conjugated mouse anti-human IgE antibody (Clone B3102E8, Southern Biotech via Biozol, Eching, Germany) diluted 1:1000 with PBS containing 0.05% Tween 20 and 0.1% BSA. The substrate for horseradish peroxidase was 3,3′,5,5′-tetramethylbenzidine (Roth, Karlsruhe, Germany) and the reaction was stopped by addition of 25% $H_2SO_4$. The absorbance was measured at 450 nm.

For the IgE-ELISA inhibition experiment with monoclonal antibody, ascites fluid of Bet v 1-specific antibody BV16 [34] (diluted: 1:1000; 1:10000, and 1:100000 in PBS containing 0.05% Tween and 0.1% BSA) was pre-incubated with 9 ng/well Bet v 1 as inhibitor for 2 hrs at room temperature. As a negative control, dilution buffer alone was preincubated with Bet v 1. After blocking with PBS containing 2% BSA, rBet v 1 and serum pool IgE diluted 1:10 (final concentration) were incubated on the plate for 3 hrs at room temperature. Human IgE was detected as described below.

### Indirect ELISA for IgE binding to Bet v 1 variants

For IgE-ELISA experiments, Nunc Maxisorp plates (Nunc via Fisher Scientific, Schwerte, Germany) were coated overnight at room temperature with 25 ng/100 µl recombinant Bet v 1 and Bet v 1_4x, respectively with phosphate-buffered saline (PBS). Blocking and IgE detection was done as described for IgE ELISA above.

### SDS-PAGE and immunoblot analysis

SDS-PAGE was performed with 15% separating gels and 5% stacking gels using a discontinuous buffer system [35]. For immunoblot analysis, 0.5 µg/cm of recombinant protein Δ29NCS_5x was transferred onto 0.2 µm nitrocellulose membranes by semi-dry blotting at 0.8 mA/cm$^2$ for 1 h [36]. After blocking with Tris-buffered saline (TBS) containing 0.3% Tween 20 blots were cut into strips and incubated overnight at room temperature with 5 µl of human serum pool with or without increasing amounts of recombinant allergens as inhibitors (Δ29NCS_5x and Bet v 1, respectively) with TBS containing 0.05% Tween 20 (TBST 0.05%) and 0.1% BSA (TBST 0.05%–0.1% BSA). After incubation for 1 h with horseradish peroxidase labelled mouse anti-human IgE antibody (Clone B3102E8, Southern biotech via Biozol, Eching, Germany), diluted 1:100000 with TBST 0.05%–0.1% BSA, IgE-binding proteins were visualized by chemiluminescence (LumiGLO Reserve diluted 1:3, KPL via Medac, Wedel, Germany).

### Mediator release from humanized Rat Basophil Leukaemia (RBL) cells

The mediator release assay followed an established protocol [37]. Briefly, RBL cells expressing the α-chain of human FcεRI were sensitized overnight with the positive serum pool of human sera (diluted 1:20). After washing, cells were stimulated with serial dilutions of allergens. Degranulation was quantified by photometric measurement of β-hexosaminidase activity in the culture supernatants and was expressed as percent of the total cellular β-hexosaminidase content obtained by lysing the cells with Triton X-100 (Sigma-Aldrich, Steinheim, Germany) after correction for spontaneous release (sensitized cells without allergen).

### MS analysis of recombinant protein variants

The identity of recombinant proteins was confirmed by liquid chromatography mass spectrometry (LC-MS). Recombinant proteins were excised from Coomassie stained SDS-PAGE gels and analyzed as described elsewhere [38]. Differing from this, peptides were eluted with 25 mM $NH_4HCO_3$; 10% aceto nitrile (ACN) and the digestion was stopped by adding 5% formic acid. The peptides were analyzed by using a nano-ultra performance LC system coupled to a nano-ESI- MS (nano Acquity UPLC nanoESI Synapt-MS, Waters, Milford, US) with a 5 µm symmetry 180 µm×20 mm c18 pre-column and a 1.7 µm BEH 130 100 µm×100 mm c18 separation column. After 3 minutes of trapping (99% water at 5 µl/minute), a 30 minutes gradient (3–40% ACN at 500 nl/minute) was applied to separate peptides. MS was operated in V mode, acquiring MSE data and applying standard parameters. Data analysis was performed with protein lynx global server version 2.4 (Waters), searching an in house database consisting of the Uniprot database (as of May 2011, restricted to reviewed entries of eukaryotic organisms) and the amino acid sequences of the recombinant variants Δ29NCS, Δ29NCS_4x and Δ29NCS_5x. The identification of a protein was accepted at a false positive rate of less than 4%; peptide mass accuracy was 9 parts per million (ppm) or better.

### Miscellaneous

Amino acid sequence alignments were carried out with ClustalO [39]. 3D protein models were analyzed and illustrated using PyMol [40].

## Results

### Δ29NCS variants have Bet v 1-type tertiary structure

IgE antibody binding to PR-10 allergens depends on the presence of a native protein fold of the allergen. The crystal structure of recombinant norcoclaurine synthase (NCS, pdb 2VNE) revealed a conformation identical to that of Bet v 1, even though the sequence identity of these proteins is only 25% [25]. We recently optimized purification of a properly folded N-terminally truncated variant of NCS (Δ29NCS), which comprises the complete structurally corresponding amino acid sequence of Bet v 1 [23]. We generated two Δ29NCS variants harboring single amino acids of a Bet v 1 epitope for IgG that competes with IgE [20,22] (Figures 1 and 2A). In addition, Asp68 of NCS was exchanged for Lysine, a corresponding amino acid of Bet v 1 involved in IgE binding [22,41] and located directly adjacent to the epitope. Initially we tested whether the rΔ29NCS variants have the typical Bet v 1 conformation using circular dichroism (CD) and nuclear magnetic resonance (NMR) spectroscopy (Figure 2B, 2C and Figure S1). Both the CD and $^1H^{15}N$-HSQC NMR spectra of $\Delta29NCS_{N57/I58E/D60N/V63P}$ (Δ29NCS_4x) and $\Delta29NCS_{N57/I58E/D60N/V63P/D68K}$ (Δ29NCS_5x) indicated that the amino acid substitutions in the NCS variants did not change the proteins' secondary or tertiary structures and confirmed that the native protein conformation is maintained in the variants (Figure 2D).

### Δ29NCS variants selectively bind IgE from sera of birch pollen allergic subjects

To assess potential cross-reactive IgE binding to rΔ29NCS variants, 70 sera of birch pollen allergic subjects were analyzed for IgE binding to a range of PR-10 proteins using ImmunoCAP tests (Table 1). All sera had sIgE to Bet v 1 (from 0.69 to>100 $kU_A/L$) and a majority to the PR-10 food allergens Pru av 1.01 (cherry, < 0.35 to 58.2 $kU_A/L$), Cor a 1.04 (hazelnut, <0.35 to>100 $kU_A/$

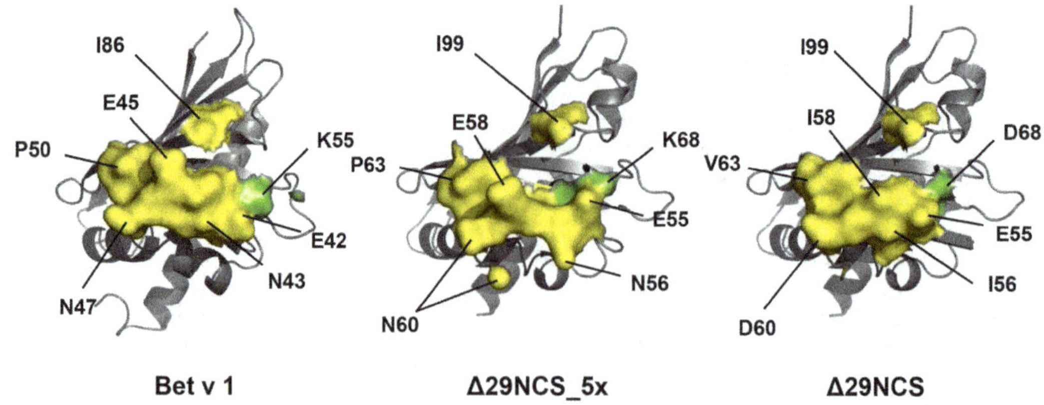


**Figure 1. Grafting of an epitope onto Δ29NCS.** Left panel: 13 of the 16 amino acids comprising the Bet v 1 epitope (Bet v $1_{E42/N43/I44/E45/G46/N47/G48/G49/P50/G51/T52/R70/D72/H76/I86/K97}$) of mouse monoclonal IgG antibody BV16 (yellow). Six amino acids of the epitope are labeled. Lys55 of Bet v 1 located adjacent to the epitope is highlighted (green). Middle panel: the corresponding 13 residues of the Bet v 1 epitope for BV16 and a lysine corresponding to K55 of Bet v 1 have been grafted onto Δ29NCS to generate Δ29NCS_4x (Δ29NCS $_{N57/I58E/D60N/V63P}$) (not shown) and Δ29NCS_5x (Δ29NCS $_{N57/I58E/D60N/V63P/D68K}$). Right panel: corresponding surface area of Δ29NCS. Protein models were based on the structures of NCS (pdb 2VNE) and Bet v 1a (pdb 1BV1), and modelled with a confidence of 100% and a sequence coverage of at least 85%.

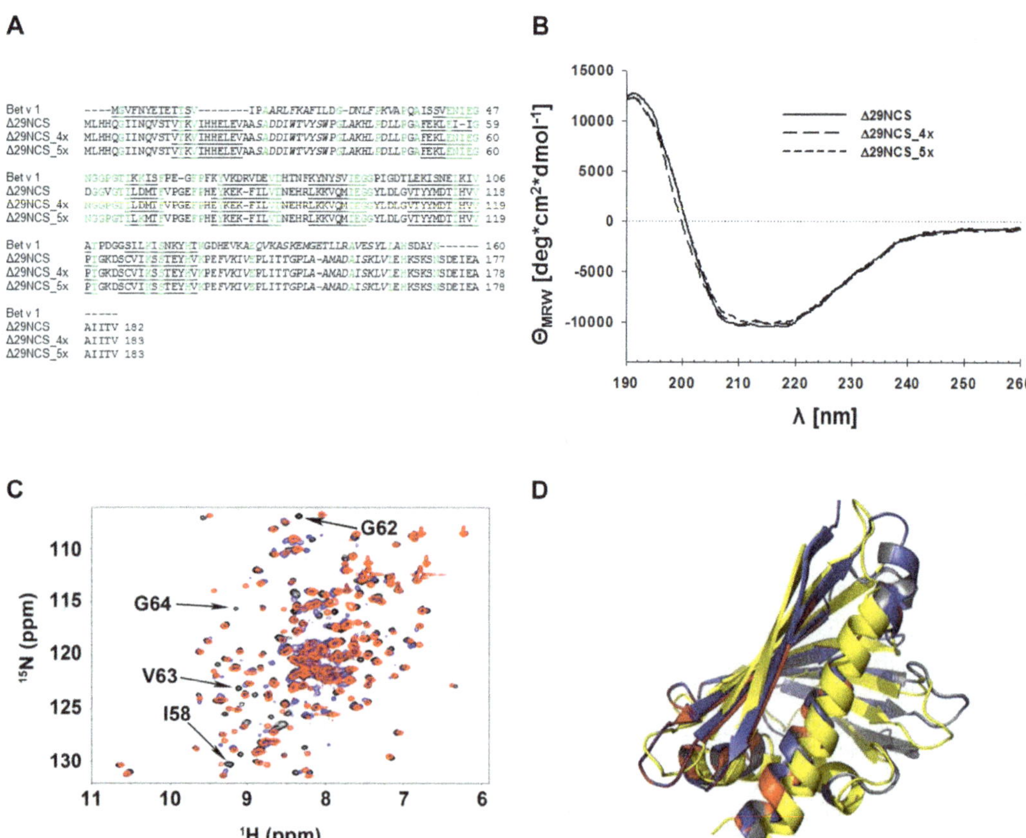


**Figure 2. Δ29NCS, Δ29NCS_4x, and Δ29NCS_5x structures are virtually identical to the Bet v 1 structure.** (A) Structural sequence alignment. β-strands (underlined), helices (italic), and amino acid identities (green) to Bet v 1 (pdb: 1BV1) are 23.8% (Δ29NCS), 26.8% (Δ29NCS_4x), and 27.5% (Δ29NCS_5x), respectively. (B) Circular dichroism of Δ29NCS variants. (C) Overlay of three $^{1}$H-$^{15}$N-HSQC spectra of Δ29NCS variants. Black arrows, signals numbered and named according to Δ29NCS. Black: Δ29NCS, blue: Δ29NCS_4x, red: Δ29NCS_5x. The arrows highlight signals of selected amino acids that are expected to differ between the three Δ29NCS variants. Labeling is according to Δ29NCS scheme. (D) Overlay of secondary structure topologies of Δ29NCS (grey), Δ29NCS_4x (blue), Δ29NCS_5x (red), and Bet v 1 (yellow).

**Table 1.** Human sera used in this study.

| Patient | Serological data: specific IgE ($kU_A/L$) and CAP classes (0–6) | | | | | | | | | | | | | | | |
|---|---|---|---|---|---|---|---|---|---|---|---|---|---|---|---|---|
| No. | rBet v 1 | | rPru av 1 | | rCor a 1.04 | | Dau c 1.01 | | rApi g 1.01 | | Δ29NCS | | Δ29NCS_4x N57/I58E/D60N/V63P | | Δ29NCS_5x N57/I58E/D60N/V63P/D68K | |
| 1 | 73.4 | 5 | 32.20 | 4 | 78.8 | 5 | 5.05 | 3 | 5.74 | 3 | 0.75 | 2 | 3.34 | 2 | 11.3 | 3 |
| 2 | 11.1 | 3 | 2.47 | 2 | 6.8 | 3 | <0.35 | 0 | <0.35 | 0 | <0.35 | 0 | 0.39 | 1 | 1.38 | 2 |
| 3 | 43.3 | 4 | 16.1 | 3 | 38.3 | 4 | 14.1 | 3 | 11.8 | 3 | <0.35 | 0 | <0.35 | 0 | 2.89 | 2 |
| 4 | 79.4 | 5 | 22.4 | 4 | >100 | 6 | 3.36 | 2 | 5.95 | 3 | <0.35 | 0 | <0.35 | 0 | <0.35 | 0 |
| 5 | 48.6 | 4 | 12.1 | 3 | 57.8 | 5 | 6.54 | 3 | 6.84 | 3 | <0.35 | 0 | 0.99 | 2 | 1.75 | 2 |
| 6 | 89.9 | 5 | 34.6 | 4 | >100 | 6 | 1.64 | 2 | 2.00 | 2 | <0.35 | 0 | <0.35 | 0 | 13.8 | 3 |
| 7 | 69.6 | 5 | 18.0 | 4 | 55.2 | 5 | 9.55 | 3 | 10.7 | 3 | <0.35 | 0 | 1.74 | 2 | 7.34 | 3 |
| 8 | >100 | 6 | 51.2 | 5 | 61.7 | 5 | 28.1 | 4 | 26.9 | 4 | 0.45 | 1 | 0.93 | 2 | 7.34 | 3 |
| 9 | >100 | 6 | 41.7 | 4 | 71.6 | 5 | 45.3 | 4 | 43.1 | 4 | <0.35 | 0 | <0.35 | 0 | 4.42 | 3 |
| 10 | 68.4 | 5 | 18.7 | 4 | 67.3 | 5 | <0.35 | 0 | 0.74 | 2 | <0.35 | 0 | <0.35 | 0 | 17.4 | 4 |
| 11 | >100 | 6 | 13.1 | 3 | 92.4 | 5 | 4.06 | 3 | 1.66 | 2 | <0.35 | 0 | <0.35 | 0 | 5.15 | 3 |
| 12 | 5.61 | 3 | 1.86 | 2 | 4.88 | 3 | <0.35 | 0 | 0.39 | 1 | <0.35 | 0 | <0.35 | 0 | <0.35 | 0 |
| 13 | 54.3 | 5 | 2.79 | 2 | 25.9 | 4 | 1.22 | 2 | 1.59 | 2 | <0.35 | 0 | <0.35 | 0 | 0.55 | 1 |
| 14 | 24.2 | 4 | 7.71 | 3 | 29.3 | 4 | <0.35 | 0 | 1.28 | 2 | <0.35 | 0 | 3.02 | 2 | 10.0 | 3 |
| 15 | 47.5 | 4 | 29.5 | 4 | 29.7 | 4 | 3.11 | 2 | 3.74 | 3 | <0.35 | 0 | 1.62 | 2 | 2.85 | 2 |
| 16 | 22.5 | 4 | 3.34 | 2 | 11.1 | 3 | <0.35 | 0 | 1.06 | 2 | <0.35 | 0 | 0.63 | 1 | 2.56 | 2 |
| 17 | 73.8 | 5 | 12.8 | 3 | 69.8 | 5 | 33.4 | 4 | 38.2 | 4 | <0.35 | 0 | <0.35 | 0 | 2.45 | 2 |
| 18 | 25.6 | 4 | 6.60 | 3 | 12.0 | 3 | 3.76 | 3 | 5.91 | 3 | <0.35 | 0 | <0.35 | 0 | <0.35 | 0 |
| 19 | 17.2 | 3 | 5.35 | 3 | 18.5 | 4 | 1.71 | 2 | 2.16 | 2 | <0.35 | 0 | 0.40 | 1 | 1.77 | 2 |
| 20 | 37.5 | 4 | 9.78 | 3 | 37.0 | 4 | 6.18 | 3 | 6.76 | 3 | <0.35 | 0 | 1.03 | 2 | 3.27 | 2 |
| 21 | 31.0 | 4 | 9.42 | 3 | 28.6 | 4 | 5.38 | 3 | 5.98 | 3 | <0.35 | 0 | 0.85 | 2 | 3.36 | 2 |
| 22 | 35.4 | 4 | 11.6 | 3 | 21.7 | 4 | <0.35 | 0 | 1.01 | 2 | <0.35 | 0 | <0.35 | 0 | 5.36 | 3 |
| 23 | 24.5 | 4 | 3.36 | 2 | 25.5 | 4 | 4.08 | 3 | 4.73 | 3 | <0.35 | 0 | 0.36 | 1 | 4.47 | 3 |
| 24 | 24.2 | 4 | 7.78 | 3 | 27.3 | 4 | 1.83 | 2 | 3.23 | 2 | <0.35 | 0 | <0.35 | 0 | 1.82 | 2 |
| 25 | 77.7 | 5 | 6.97 | 3 | 15.2 | 3 | 6.58 | 3 | 7.93 | 3 | <0.35 | 0 | <0.35 | 0 | 1.28 | 2 |
| 26 | 25.4 | 4 | 8.16 | 3 | 20.9 | 4 | 1.58 | 2 | 2.00 | 2 | <0.35 | 0 | <0.35 | 0 | 2.81 | 2 |
| 27 | 17.8 | 4 | 9.9 | 3 | 14.1 | 3 | <0.35 | 0 | <0.35 | 0 | <0.35 | 0 | 0.49 | 1 | 3.08 | 2 |
| 28 | 35.4 | 4 | 17.8 | 4 | 23.4 | 4 | 3.51 | 3 | 0.39 | 1 | <0.35 | 0 | 2.09 | 2 | 11.3 | 3 |
| 29 | 37.1 | 4 | 8.82 | 3 | 4.99 | 3 | 4.99 | 3 | 4.57 | 3 | <0.35 | 0 | <0.35 | 0 | <0.35 | 0 |
| 30 | 41.6 | 4 | 4.03 | 3 | 34.1 | 4 | 16.7 | 3 | 16.7 | 3 | <0.35 | 0 | <0.35 | 0 | <0.35 | 0 |
| 31 | 36.4 | 4 | 2.93 | 2 | 12.7 | 3 | 0.61 | 1 | 1.91 | 2 | <0.35 | 0 | <0.35 | 0 | <0.35 | 0 |
| 32 | 92.4 | 5 | 14.2 | 3 | 33.7 | 4 | 4.21 | 3 | 7.11 | 3 | <0.35 | 0 | 1.47 | 2 | 16.1 | 3 |
| 33 | 19.0 | 4 | 2.16 | 2 | 15.9 | 3 | 0.35 | 1 | 1.62 | 2 | <0.35 | 0 | <0.35 | 0 | <0.35 | 0 |

**Table 1.** Cont.

| Patient | Serological data: specific IgE ($kU_A/L$) and CAP classes (0–6) | | | | | | | | | | | | | | | |
|---|---|---|---|---|---|---|---|---|---|---|---|---|---|---|---|---|
| No. | rBet v 1 | | rPru av 1 | | rCor a 1.04 | | Dau c 1.01 | | rApi g 1.01 | | Δ29NCS | | Δ29NCS_4x N57/I58E/D60N/V63P | | Δ29NCS_5x N57/I58E/D60N/V63P/D68K | |
| 34 | 44.2 | 4 | 4.3 | 3 | 18.3 | 4 | 0.39 | 1 | <0.35 | 0 | <0.35 | 0 | 0.93 | 2 | 2.95 | 2 |
| 35 | >100 | 6 | 58.2 | 5 | 98.5 | 5 | 15.9 | 3 | 20.5 | 4 | <0.35 | 0 | <0.35 | 0 | 4.65 | 3 |
| 36 | 78.3 | 5 | 11.5 | 3 | 34.5 | 4 | 1.89 | 2 | 0.89 | 2 | 0.46 | 1 | <0.35 | 0 | 5.58 | 3 |
| 37 | 17.1 | 3 | 11.4 | 3 | 18.1 | 4 | 5.74 | 3 | 4.73 | 3 | <0.35 | 0 | 1.23 | 2 | 4.01 | 3 |
| 38 | 17.2 | 3 | 5.56 | 3 | 12.4 | 3 | 4.22 | 3 | 5.16 | 3 | <0.35 | 0 | <0.35 | 0 | 0.94 | 2 |
| 39 | 94.2 | 5 | 17.1 | 3 | 30.9 | 4 | 9.13 | 3 | 12.1 | 3 | 0.46 | 1 | 0.74 | 2 | 1.19 | 2 |
| 40 | 19.0 | 4 | 9.86 | 3 | 13.0 | 3 | 3.02 | 2 | 4.03 | 3 | <0.35 | 0 | <0.35 | 0 | <0.35 | 0 |
| 41 | 6.9 | 3 | 1.27 | 2 | 6.61 | 3 | <0.35 | 0 | <0.35 | 0 | <0.35 | 0 | <0.35 | 0 | 0.63 | 1 |
| 42 | 51.8 | 5 | 13.8 | 3 | 22.2 | 4 | 0.67 | 1 | 0.77 | 2 | <0.35 | 0 | 1.15 | 2 | 6.09 | 3 |
| 43 | 14.2 | 3 | 4.36 | 3 | 15.9 | 3 | 5.82 | 3 | 6.51 | 3 | <0.35 | 0 | <0.35 | 0 | <0.35 | 0 |
| 44 | 18.6 | 4 | 1.87 | 2 | 6.84 | 3 | <0.35 | 0 | <0.35 | 0 | <0.35 | 0 | <0.35 | 0 | <0.35 | 0 |
| 45 | 4.01 | 3 | 2.18 | 2 | 3.59 | 3 | <0.35 | 0 | <0.35 | 0 | <0.35 | 0 | <0.35 | 0 | <035 | 0 |
| 46 | 3.51 | 3 | <0,35 | 0 | 1.22 | 2 | <0.35 | 0 | <0.35 | 0 | <0.35 | 0 | <0.35 | 0 | <0.35 | 0 |
| 47 | 16.1 | 3 | 3.00 | 2 | 9.48 | 3 | 1.91 | 2 | 4.85 | 3 | <0.35 | 0 | 3.80 | 3 | 5.88 | 3 |
| 48 | 32.2 | 4 | 8.73 | 3 | 14.0 | 3 | 1.43 | 2 | 2.40 | 2 | <0.35 | 0 | <0.35 | 0 | 0.72 | 2 |
| 49 | 17.4 | 3 | 2.99 | 2 | 7.05 | 3 | 2.72 | 2 | 2.23 | 2 | <0.35 | 0 | <0.35 | 0 | 1.64 | 2 |
| 50 | 21.2 | 4 | 15.4 | 3 | 23.3 | 4 | <0.35 | 0 | <0.35 | 0 | <0.35 | 0 | <0.35 | 0 | <0.35 | 0 |
| 51 | 28.8 | 4 | 5.82 | 3 | 13.8 | 3 | 0.89 | 2 | 1.01 | 2 | <0.35 | 0 | <0.35 | 0 | 0.40 | 1 |
| 52 | 18.4 | 4 | 5.69 | 3 | 9.34 | 3 | 0.48 | 1 | 0.56 | 1 | <0.35 | 0 | <0.35 | 0 | <0.35 | 0 |
| 53 | 19.0 | 4 | 2.02 | 2 | 8.52 | 3 | 3.58 | 3 | 3.81 | 3 | <0.35 | 0 | 0.40 | 1 | 1.92 | 2 |
| 54 | 0.90 | 2 | <0.35 | 0 | 0.58 | 1 | <0.35 | 0 | <0.35 | 0 | <0.35 | 0 | <0.35 | 0 | <0.35 | 0 |
| 55 | 13.8 | 3 | 7.73 | 3 | 10.0 | 3 | 0.49 | 1 | 2.28 | 2 | <0.35 | 0 | 0.49 | 1 | 2.39 | 2 |
| 56 | 5.47 | 3 | 1.49 | 2 | 4.04 | 3 | <0.35 | 0 | <0.35 | 0 | <0.35 | 0 | <0.35 | 0 | <0.35 | 0 |
| 57 | 19.0 | 4 | 10.6 | 3 | 16.0 | 3 | 0.84 | 2 | 0.58 | 1 | <0.35 | 0 | 1.55 | 2 | 4.3 | 3 |
| 58 | 0.69 | 1 | 0.35 | 1 | <0.35 | 0 | <0.35 | 0 | <0.35 | 0 | <0.35 | 0 | <0.35 | 0 | <0.35 | 0 |
| 59 | 52.3 | 5 | 14.8 | 3 | 34.9 | 4 | 6.61 | 3 | 9.04 | 3 | <0.35 | 0 | <0.35 | 0 | 1.49 | 2 |
| 60 | 1.58 | 2 | 0.41 | 1 | 1.27 | 2 | <0.35 | 0 | <0.35 | 0 | <0.35 | 0 | <0.35 | 0 | <0.35 | 0 |
| 61 | 77.8 | 5 | 23.5 | 4 | 57.3 | 5 | 12.6 | 3 | 11.5 | 3 | <0.35 | 0 | 4.52 | 3 | 9.2 | 3 |
| 62 | 50.8 | 5 | 13.3 | 3 | 27.6 | 4 | 0.4 | 1 | 0.94 | 2 | <0.35 | 0 | <0.35 | 0 | <0.35 | 0 |
| 63 | 17.0 | 3 | 4.73 | 3 | 8.27 | 3 | <0.35 | 0 | <0.35 | 0 | <0.35 | 0 | <0.35 | 0 | 0.60 | 1 |
| 64 | 8.46 | 3 | 2.28 | 2 | 4.69 | 3 | 0.54 | 1 | <0.35 | 0 | <0.35 | 0 | <0.35 | 0 | <0.35 | 0 |
| 65 | 2.80 | 2 | 0.40 | 1 | 1.45 | 2 | 0.35 | 1 | <0.35 | 0 | <0.35 | 0 | <0.35 | 0 | <0.35 | 0 |
| 66 | 6.85 | 3 | 2.56 | 2 | 6.23 | 3 | 0.52 | 1 | 1.09 | 1 | <0.35 | 0 | <0.35 | 0 | 0.41 | 1 |

**Table 1.** Cont.

| Patient | Serological data: specific IgE ($kU_A$/L) and CAP classes (0–6) | | | | | | | | | | | | | | | |
|---|---|---|---|---|---|---|---|---|---|---|---|---|---|---|---|---|
| No. | rBet v 1 | | rPru av 1 | | rCor a 1.04 | | Dau c 1.01 | | rApi g 1.01 | | Δ29NCS | | Δ29NCS_4x N57/I58E/D60N/V63P | | Δ29NCS_5x N57/I58E/D60N/V63P/D68K | |
| 67 | 33.1 | 4 | 5.37 | 3 | 18.8 | 4 | 0.45 | 1 | 1.02 | 2 | <0.35 | 0 | <0.35 | 0 | 1.6 | 2 |
| 68 | 31.5 | 4 | 8.82 | 3 | 15.7 | 3 | 0.41 | 1 | 0.68 | 1 | <0,35 | 0 | 1.02 | 2 | 4.87 | 3 |
| 69 | 3.03 | 2 | <0.35 | 0 | 2.61 | 2 | <0.35 | 0 | <0.35 | 0 | <0.35 | 0 | <0.35 | 0 | <0.35 | 0 |
| 70* | 67 | - | n.d. | - | 33 | - | <0.3 | - | <0.3 | - | n.d. | - | n.d. | - | n.d. | - |
| 71** | <0.35 | 0 | <0.35 | 0 | <0.35 | 0 | <0.35 | 0 | <0.35 | 0 | <0.35 | 0 | <0.35 | 0 | <0.35 | 0 |

*sIgE determined by ISAC. **Non-allergic control. Sera 52–69 were published elsewhere [40].
Summary of specific Immunoglobulin E against recombinant Bet v 1 and Δ29NCS variants.

L), Dau c 1.01 (carrot, <0.35 to 98.5 $kU_A$/L), and Api g 1.01 (celeriac, <0.35 to 43.1 $kU_A$/L), respectively. In contrast, most of the sera (66/70, 94%) tested negative (<0.35 $kU_A$/L) to Δ29NCS, whereas 25/70 (36%) showed significant IgE binding (0.35 to 3.34 $kU_A$/L, $p < 0.0001$) to Δ29NCS_4x and 50/70 (71%) to Δ29NCS_5x (0.35 to 17.4 $kU_A$/L, $p < 0.0001$). Thus, gradual substitution of certain amino acids of the low-IgE binding protein Δ29NCS with those of Bet v 1 at the corresponding positions induced significant binding of serum IgE from subjects with birch pollinosis.

## Δ29NCS_5x presents an IgE epitope that cross-reacts with a subset of Bet v 1-homologous allergens

Since the majority of the patients' sera IgE bound Δ29NCS_5x, we asked whether this interaction was due to a Bet v 1-specific IgE epitope presented by the Δ29NCS variant. Therefore we used serum with sIgE to both Bet v 1 and Δ29NCS_5x and tested its IgE interaction with the Δ29NCS_5x variant in the presence of Bet v 1 (Figure 3). As expected, no IgE interaction of the serum pool with Δ29NCS was observed (Figure 3A). In contrast, IgE binding to Δ29NCS_5x was inhibited by Δ29NCS_5x itself and Bet v 1 in a dose-dependent manner, suggesting the presence of an IgE epitope shared by the two proteins.

Next, we asked whether the IgE epitope presented by Δ29NCS_5x is cross-reactive with PR-10 food allergens. Thus, we performed competitive IgE binding experiments (ELISA) with the PR-10 food allergens Cor a 1.04, Gly m 4, Dau c 1.01, Api g 1.01, and Pru av 1, respectively (Figure 3B). Bet v 1 as well as Cor a 1.04 and Gly m 4 competed for serum IgE binding to Δ29NCS_5x, whereas only very low inhibition of IgE binding to Δ29NCS_5x was observed with Api g 1, Pru av 1, and Dau c 1, respectively. We conclude that the IgE epitope offered by Δ29NCS_5x is not ubiquitous but specific for a subgroup of PR-10 allergens.

## The IgE cross-reactive epitope of Δ29NCS_5x overlaps with an IgG binding site

Δ29NCS harbors 47% and Δ29NCS_5x 76% of the structurally resolved IgG epitope (total of 16 amino acids) of Bet v 1, as defined earlier [20]. We therefore asked whether the IgE binding epitope of Δ29NCS_5x overlaps with the binding site of BV16 on Bet v 1. Thus, we tested serum IgE binding of immobilized Δ29NCS_5x in the presence of both Bet v 1 and increasing amounts of BV16 (Figure 3C). In the absence of BV16, IgE binding to Δ29NCS_5x was inhibited to 84% by Bet v 1. The observed Bet v 1-induced inhibition of IgE-Δ29NCS_5x interaction could, however, been abolished by the monoclonal antibody BV16 in a dose-dependent manner. This result suggests a structural overlap between the individual cross-reactive IgE epitope of Δ29NCS_5x and the Bet v 1-specific IgG epitope recognized by monoclonal antibody BV16. Furthermore, when we tested BV16 binding only Bet v 1, Gly m 4, Cor a 1.04, and Δ29NCS_5x interacted markedly with the monoclonal antibody, whereas Dau c 1.01, Api g 1.01 1, Pru av 1, and Δ29NCS did not (Figure 3D).

## Subtle structural differences define the IgE cross-reactivity pattern of Bet v 1-homologous allergens

The differential interaction of Δ29NCS_5x and Pr-10 allergens as above with both serum IgE and the Bet v 1-specific mouse monoclonal BV16 let us to hypothesize that Δ29NCS_5x displays an epitope shared only with Bet v 1, Cor a 1.04, and Gly m 4, but not with Dau c 1.01, Api g 1.01, and Pru av 1. Thus, we structurally aligned the epitope grafted onto Δ29NCS_5x and the corresponding surface areas of cross-reactive and non-cross-reactive Bet v 1-related proteins (Figure 4). Residue by residue comparison of the epitope revealed that N43, E45, N47, and K55 of Bet v 1 are shared with Δ29NCS_5x, Gly m 4, and Cor a 1.04, but not with Pru av 1, Api g 1.01, and Dau c 1.01, thus mirroring the IgE/IgG inhibition results (cf. Figure 3) and suggesting that they are critical determinants of IgE cross-reactivity and BV16 binding. To challenge this hypothesis we investigated the substitutional variant Bet v 1_4x (Bet v $1_{N43I/E45S/N47D/K55A}$). As for Δ29NCS_5x and Δ29NCS_4x, the amino acid substitutions did not alter the protein conformation according to CD and $^1H^{15}N$-HSQC NMR spectroscopy (Figure S2). Serum IgE binding to Bet v 1_4x was virtually identical to that of wild type Bet v 1 (Figure 5A). However, inhibition of IgE binding to Δ29NCS_5x was strongly reduced by Bet v 1_4x as compared to Bet v 1 (Figure 5B), and interaction of monoclonal BV16 with Bet v 1_4x was virtually abolished (Figure 5C). The capacity of Bet v 1_4x to induce mediator release in humanized rat basophil leukemia cells *via* allergen mediated cross-linking of receptor bound human IgE was only slightly reduced as compared to wild type Bet v 1, suggesting the presence of further IgE epitopes compensating for the loss of one IgE epitope in Bet v 1_4x (Figure 5D). As expected, the Δ29NCS variants did not induce mediator release due to the lack of a second IgE epitope needed for allergen-mediated IgE cross-linking. Since Bet v 1_4x could not compete with Δ29NCS_5x for binding to serum IgE, we conclude that we have identified an epitope in a subset of PR-10 allergens that binds cross-reactive IgE and IgG.

## Discussion

To analyze epitopes of allergens it is common to genetically engineer specific allergen variants and test their antibody binding capacity in comparison to the respective wild type allergen. A residual response, however, can be misleading if the epitope to be analyzed is conformational and proper binding of the antibody is dependent on the native fold of the allergen. In this case any observed compromised antibody-allergen interaction may well be due to an altered protein conformation of the allergen variant rather than due to the exchange of amino acids crucial for direct antibody binding. Furthermore, the analysis of epitopes in allergens is often hampered by the fact that the polyclonal serum antibody repertoire makes it technically challenging to measure and assign the functionality of single epitopes in the background of the overall multiple antibody binding to the allergen. As the

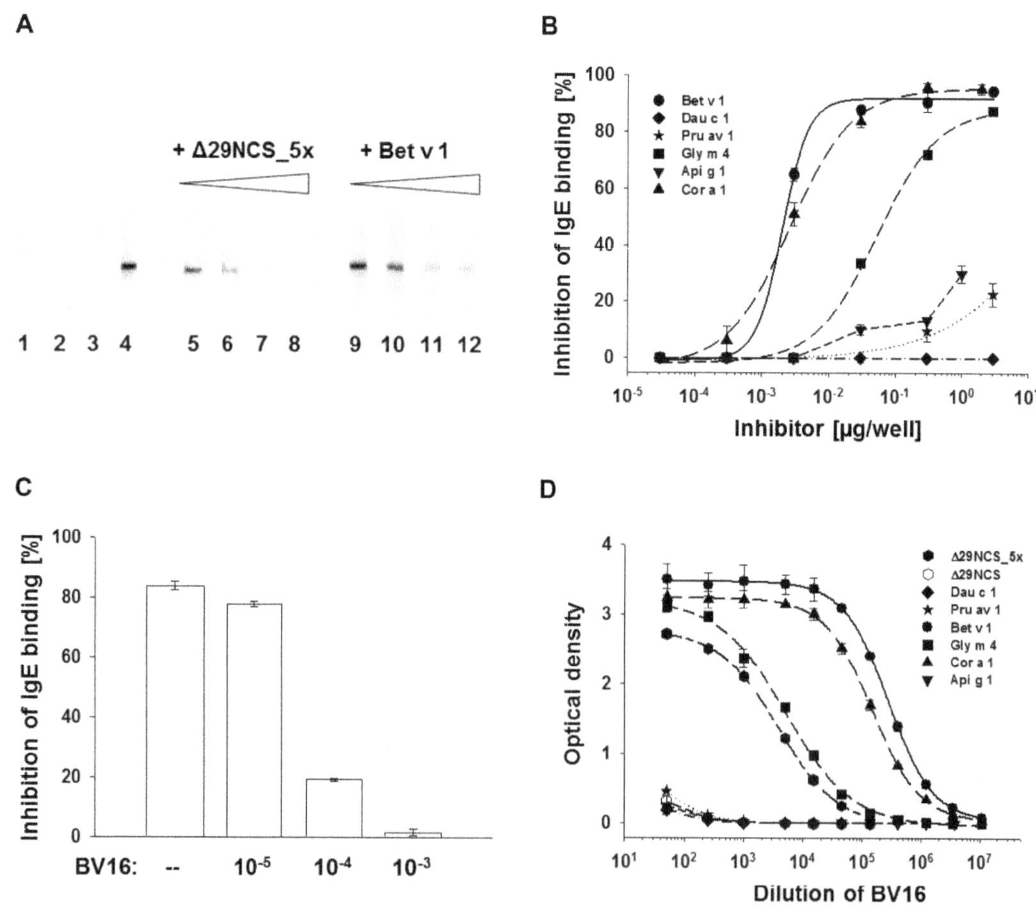


**Figure 3. Δ29NCS_5x presents a cross-reactive Ig epitope.** (A) Inhibition of IgE binding to Δ29NCS_5x. Binding of serum IgE to Δ29NCS (lane 3) and to Δ29NCS_5x (lane 4) in the presence of increasing amounts of inhibitors Δ29NCS_5x (lanes 5–8) or Bet v 1 (lanes 9–12). No serum (lane 1) and negative serum pool (lane 2) served as control. (B) Dose-dependent inhibition of IgE binding to surface-coated Δ29NCS_5x in the presence of increasing concentrations of PR-10 allergens in ELISA. (C) Inhibition of IgE binding to surface-coated Δ29NCS_5x in the presence of both Bet v 1 and serial dilutions of Bet v 1-binding monoclonal mouse IgG antibody BV16 (–: no BV16; $10^{-5}$ to $10^{-3}$: dilutions of BV16) in ELISA. (D) Binding of mouse monoclonal IgG antibody BV16 to surface-coated Bet v 1-related proteins. 250 ng of protein (50 ng of Api g 1) was coated and incubated with dilution series of the monoclonal BV16 in ELISA.

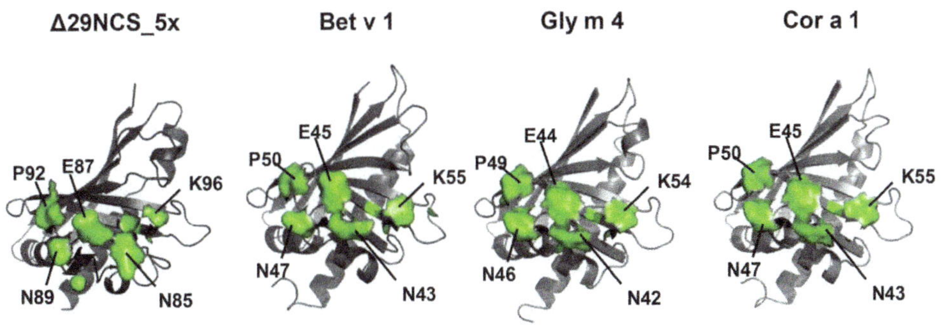


| Δ29NCS_5x | E84 | N85 | I86 | E87 | G88 | N89 | G90 | G91 | P92 | G93 | T94 | K96 | K111 | I113 | N117 | I127 | Y138 |
|---|---|---|---|---|---|---|---|---|---|---|---|---|---|---|---|---|---|
| Bet v 1 | E42 | N43 | I44 | E45 | G46 | N47 | G48 | G49 | P50 | G51 | T52 | K55 | R70 | D72 | H76 | I86 | K97 |
| Gly m 4 | E41 | N42 | V43 | E44 | G45 | N46 | G47 | G48 | P49 | G50 | T51 | K54 | K69 | E71 | E75 | V85 | K96 |
| Cor a 1 | E42 | N43 | I44 | E45 | G46 | N47 | G48 | G49 | P50 | G51 | T52 | K55 | K70 | E72 | H76 | I86 | K97 |

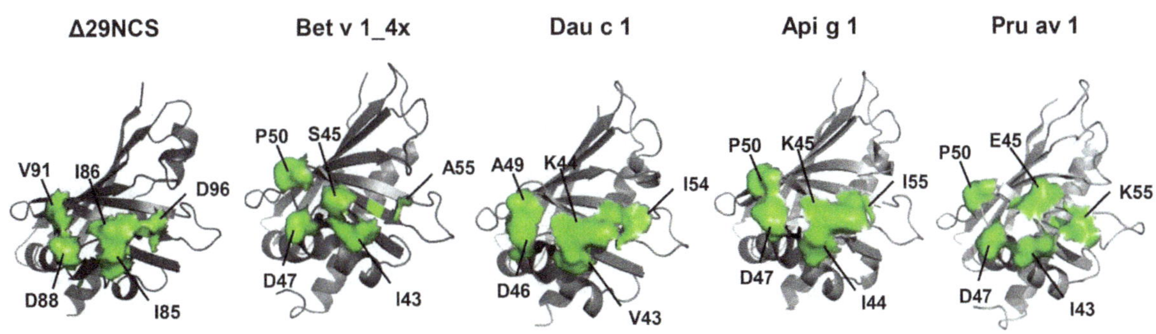


| Δ29NCS | E84 | I85 | I86 | --- | G87 | D88 | G89 | G90 | V91 | G92 | T93 | D96 | K111 | I113 | N117 | I127 | Y138 |
|---|---|---|---|---|---|---|---|---|---|---|---|---|---|---|---|---|---|
| Bet v 1_4x | E42 | I43 | I44 | S45 | G46 | D47 | G48 | G49 | P50 | G51 | T52 | A55 | R70 | D72 | H76 | I86 | K97 |
| Dau c 1 | E42 | --- | V43 | K44 | G45 | D46 | G47 | G48 | A49 | G50 | T51 | I54 | R69 | D71 | K75 | I85 | S96 |
| Api g 1 | E43 | --- | I44 | K45 | G46 | D47 | G48 | G49 | P50 | G51 | T52 | I55 | R70 | D72 | K76 | I86 | S97 |
| Pru av 1 | E42 | I43 | L44 | E45 | G46 | D47 | G48 | G49 | P50 | G51 | T52 | K55 | K70 | D72 | K76 | I86 | K97 |

**Figure 4. Structural alignment of the Bet v 1 epitope forBV16 and amino acids critical for Ig cross-reactivity in PR-10 allergens.** Upper panel: model structures of Δ29NCS_5x and PR-10 allergens showing IgE cross-reactivity with Δ29NCS_5x. The amino acids comprising the BV16-binding epitope and lysine 55 of Bet v 1 and the corresponding residues of Δ29NCS_5x, Gly m 4, and Cor a 1 are listed. Residues of the epitope and of position 55 of Bet v 1 that are critical for Ig cross-reaction are highlighted in green. Lower panel: model structures of Δ29NCS and allergens that do not show IgE cross-reactivity with Δ29NCS_5x. The amino acids corresponding to the epitope in the cross-reactive proteins are listed and highlighted in green.

majority of epitopes of inhalative allergens is thought to be conformational and the IgE repertoire of allergic patients to a specific allergen is polyclonal, we circumvented these issues by employing a model protein that i) does not interact with patients' IgE, ii) has a stable allergen-like protein fold, and iii) allows the analysis of individual antibody binding by amino acid substitutions.

Here we analyzed a non IgE-binding variant of the PR-10 enzyme Δ29NCS of the common meadow rue with Bet v 1-type protein structure [25]. We showed that amino acid insertion/substitution did not alter the Bet v 1-like protein fold of Δ29NCS, although it induced significant binding of IgE from sera of birch pollen allergic subjects. IgE that bound to the epitope presented by the model protein Δ29NCS_5x, cross-reacted with a subgroup of PR-10 allergens. As analyzed with a Bet v 1 variant with exchanged residues that mediate antibody binding to the epitope, the observed IgE cross-reaction depended on a subset of amino acids not ubiquitously present in PR-10 allergens. The functional IgE epitope identified in this study overlaps with the known binding site of the Bet v 1-specific murine monoclonal antibody BV16.

The native protein conformation of Bet v 1 and highly likely other PR-10 allergens is critical for IgE interaction since i) neither sequential IgE binding peptides of Bet v 1 nor IgE binding truncated variants of Bet v 1 have been described so far [42] ii) a folding variant of Bet v 1 with native primary structure, but permanently altered secondary structure has very low IgE reactivity [43]. iii) several Bet v 1 variants with amino acid substitutions that induced an altered protein conformation showed reduced binding of serum IgE [7,44]. Thus we thoroughly studied the secondary and tertiary structure of our model protein by CD and $^{1}H^{15}N$-HSQC NMR spectroscopy. The CD spectra of the Δ29NCS variants were virtually identical and typical for PR-10 proteins. Furthermore, the $^{1}H^{15}N$-HSQC spectra of the Δ29NCS variants were superimposable for the majority of resonances, and the spectra are in agreement with the notion of only minor local

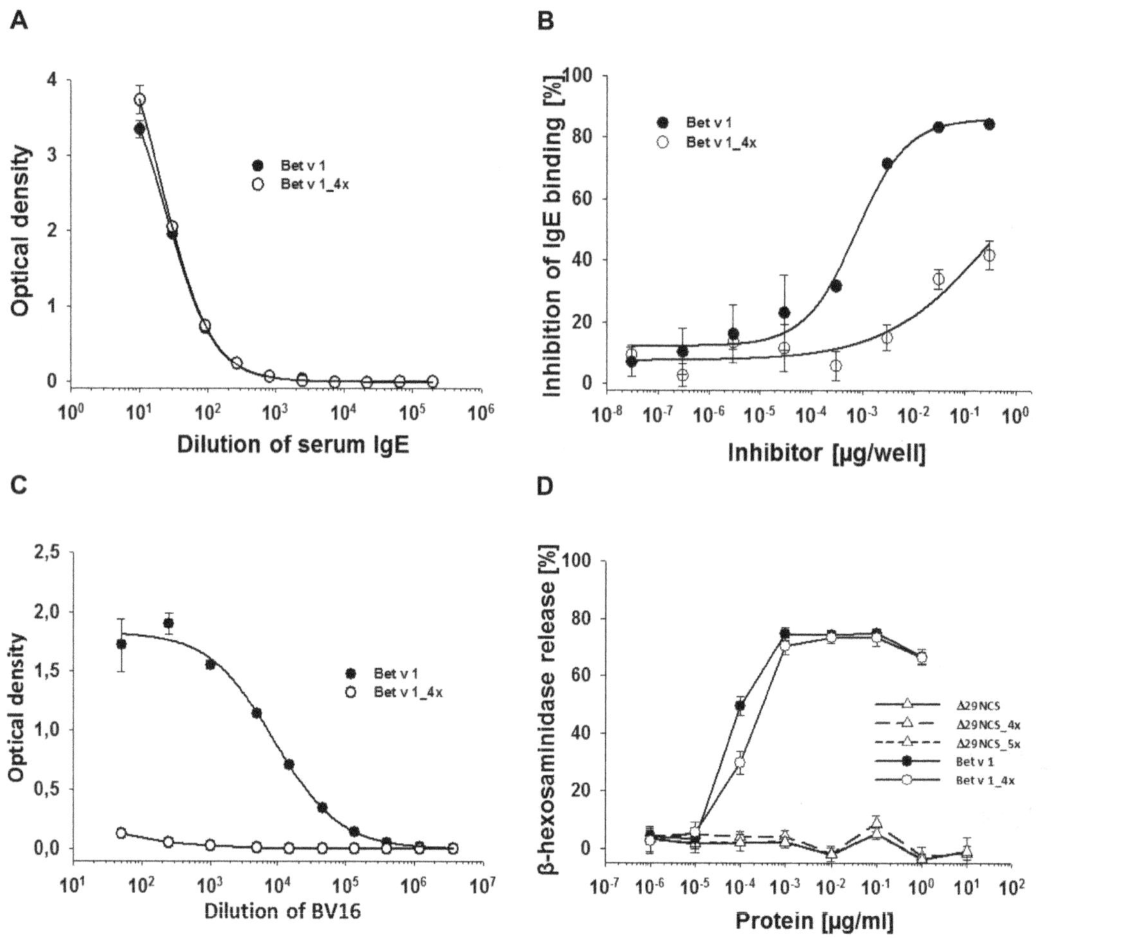


**Figure 5. Amino acids critical forIgE and IgG cross-reactivity in a subgroup of Bet v 1-related proteins.** (A) Binding of serial dilutions of pool serum IgE to surface-coated equimolar amounts of Bet v 1 and Bet v 1_4x (Bet v $1_{N43I/E45S/N47D/K55A}$) in ELISA. (B) Inhibition of IgE binding to surface-coated Δ29NCS_5x in the presence of either Bet v 1 or Bet v 1_4x in ELISA. (C) Binding of serial dilutions of monoclonal BV16 to surface-coated equimolar amounts of Bet v 1 and Bet v 1_4x in ELISA. (D) Mediator release induced by recombinant NCS and Bet v 1 variants. Humanized RBL cells were sensitized with a pool of human birch-specific sera. Cross-linking of membrane-bound human IgE by IgE-protein interaction and subsequent release of β-hexosaminidase was determined with serial dilutions of the proteins.

differences caused by the amino acid substitutions (cf. Figure 2C), but otherwise identical protein conformation of the Δ29NCS variants. Hence, the Δ29NCS variants have the typical PR-10 protein structure and fulfill the essential requirement for molecular epitope analysis.

When we tested the impact of specific amino acids on serum IgE binding, we found that amino acid substitutions in Δ29NCS with structurally corresponding residues of Bet v 1 induced a significant increase in IgE interaction of the model protein to up to four CAP classes (cf. Table 1). As the protein folds of the Δ29NCS variants were essentially identical, we concluded that the observed serological IgE interaction of the model protein was caused solely by the residues substituted. This hypothesis was further confirmed by the allergen variant Bet v $1_{N43I/E45S/N47D/K55A}$ (Bet v 1_4x) which showed only little competition for serum IgE binding to Δ29NCS_5x and did not bind the Bet v 1-reactive murine monoclonal antibody BV16. Interestingly, residue E45 of Bet v 1 has already been identified as being critical for both IgE and BV16 interaction [17,22]. Thus we confirmed the existence of a functional overlapping Bet v 1 epitope for human IgE and murine IgG, with the majority (71%) of our study population having serum IgE against the epitope displayed by Δ29NCS_5x.

Since Bet v 1-specific IgE cross-reacts with PR-10 food allergens [2], we analyzed whether the functional epitope presented by Δ29NCS_5x is also relevant for IgE cross-reactivity. Binding of patients' IgE to Δ29NCS_5x could be inhibited by Bet v 1, Gly m 4, and Cor a 1.04, respectively, suggesting that Δ29NCS_5x displays an epitope shared by these allergens. Interestingly, the PR-10 allergens Pru av 1, Dau c 1.01, and Api g 1.01 did not cross-react with the NCS variant. Since the observed IgE reactivity of the PR-10 allergens we studied correlated well with their binding to the monoclonal antibody BV16, we assumed subtle structural differences within the epitope between the allergens. A sequential/structural alignment of the BV16 epitope indeed revealed that five amino acids are identical and oriented in a similar fashion among the cross-reactive proteins, but not in the non-cross-reactive proteins. To confirm our hypothesis, we generated a corresponding Bet v 1 variant to address these sequential differences and found that the protein variant behaved like the non-cross-reactive Bet v 1-homologous allergens with regard to binding IgG (BV16) and competing with serum IgE for Δ29NCS_5x.

Whereas the structural epitope of an antigen usually spans a molecular surface area of about 400–1000 Å$^2$ and comprises

10–25 amino acids, only a small subset of these residues dominates the energetics of the antibody-antigen interaction and thus constitutes the functional (active) epitope [45,46]. Our model system is ideal for the analysis of functional epitopes, since even low-affinity and individual antibody binding might be detected due to the lack of multiple antibody binding sites in our model protein.

Some information on functional IgE epitopes of Bet v 1 and other PR-10 allergens has emerged in recent years. These studies analyzed the interaction of IgE with either native Bet v 1 isoforms or recombinant allergen variants [8,9,12–16,22,47]. Even though great care had been taken to ensure a Bet v 1-like conformation of the studied protein variants, they were inevitably targeted by a polyclonal IgE antibody response, making it difficult to define the importance and architecture of any single epitope structure. Moreover, bioinformatic approaches are emerging that use either peptide:IgE interaction or structure-based comparison of allergen surfaces to localize Ig epitopes [18,26,48–50]. We believe that our approach to induce measurable antibody interaction of allergen-like protein variants is ideal to identify individual residues critical for antibody interaction. However, the truncated version of NCS used in this study still carries N- and C-terminal extensions that might locally interfere with epitope analysis. Thus our future research aims to further optimize our model protein system and adapt it to the average number of amino acids of PR-10 allergens.

No mediator release in humanized rat basophil leukemia cells sensitized with sera of birch pollen allergic subjects has been observed with the Δ29NCS variants, indicating that no additional IgE epitope that would mediate IgE receptor cross-linking is displayed in the variants (cf. Figure 5D). In contrast, Bet v 1_4x induced full wild type-like mediator release indicating that the lack of one particular epitope is easily compensated by polyclonal serum IgE. Thus our allergen model system also allows the investigation of the role of epitopes of different affinities to IgE antibodies in the IgE-mediated activation of basophils and mast cells, a crucial step of Type I allergic reactions.

In summary, we have established a protein model system which enables the specific analysis of functional IgE and IgG epitopes and their homologies among PR-10 allergens. Upon single amino acid substitutions of the non-allergenic protein variant Δ29NCS, individual epitopes are identified in a residue-specific manner by detection of newly generated immunoglobulin interactions of the model protein. Our system allows the evaluation of patient-specific epitope profiles and will facilitate both the identification of clinically relevant epitopes as biomarkers and the monitoring of therapeutic outcomes to improve diagnosis, prognosis, and therapy of allergies caused by PR-10 proteins.

## Supporting Information

**Figure S1 $^{1}$H-$^{15}$N-HSQC spectra of different NCS variants.** Spectra of (**A**) 400 μM Δ29NCS (black) (**B**) 250 μM $\Delta29NCS_{N57/I58E/D60N/V63P}$ (Δ29NCS_4x) (blue), and (**C**) 400 μM $\Delta29NCS_{N57/I58E/D60N/V63P/D68K}$ (Δ29NCS_5x) (red). The proteins were measured in 20 mM sodium phosphate, pH 7.0, 1 mM DTT, 0.04% sodium azide and 10% $D_2O$ at a 700 MHz spectrometer at 298 K. Due to its solubility limit $\Delta29NCS_{N57/I58E/D60N/V63P}$ (Δ29NCS_4x) was measured at a lower protein concentration.
(TIF)

**Figure S2 Folding and structural integrities of Bet v 1 and Bet v 1_4x variant.** (A) Circular dichroism of Bet v 1 and Bet v 1_4x. (B) $^{1}$H-$^{15}$N-HSQC spectra of Bet v 1 variants. Overlay of the spectra of 100 μM Bet v 1 (petrol) and 100 μM Bet v 1_4x (purple). The proteins were measured in 20 mM sodium phosphate, pH 7.0, 1 mM DTT, 0.04% sodium azide and 10% $D_2O$ at a 700 MHz spectrometer at 298 K.
(TIF)

## Acknowledgments

We thank Rob Aalberse for initial discussion on the project, Ramona Heissmann for excellent technical assistance, Daniela Weigand and Iris Lauer for providing recombinant Dau c 1 and Cor a 1, respectively, Kay-Martin Hanschmann for statistical analysis of the data, and Thomas Holzhauser for critically reading the manuscript.

## Author Contributions

Conceived and designed the experiments: HB PR SV MH DS. Performed the experiments: HB MH CSvL SR MG LV. Analyzed the data: HB CSvL MH SR MG LV FH AR SV PR DS. Contributed reagents/materials/analysis tools: SV MG JL. Wrote the paper: MH DS. Recruitment of patients and clinical evaluation of data: BB-W.

## References


1. D'Amato G, Cecchi L, Bonini S, Nunes C, Annesi-Maesano I, et al. (2007) Allergenic pollen and pollen allergy in Europe. Allergy 62: 976–990.
2. Vieths S, Scheurer S, Ballmer-Weber B (2002) Current understanding of cross-reactivity of food allergens and pollen. Ann N Y Acad Sci. 964: 47–68.
3. Niemi M, Jylhä S, Laukkanen ML, Söderlund H, Mäkinen-Kiljunen S, et al. (2007) Molecular interactions between a recombinant IgE antibody and the beta-lactoglobulin allergen. Structure 15: 1413–1421.
4. Padavattan S, Flicker S, Schirmer T, Madritsch C, Randow S, et al. (2009) High-affinity IgE recognition of a conformational epitope of the major respiratory allergen Phl p 2 as revealed by X-ray crystallography. J Immunol 182: 2141–2151.
5. Razzera G, Gadermaier G, de Paula V, Almeida MS, Egger M, et al. (2010) Mapping the interactions between a major pollen allergen and human IgE antibodies. Structure 18: 1011–1021.
6. Ferreira F, Ebner C, Kramer B, Casari G, Briza P, et al. (1998) Modulation of IgE reactivity of allergens by site-directed mutagenesis: potential use of hypoallergenic variants for immunotherapy. FASEB J 12: 231–242.
7. Holm J, Gajhede M, Ferreras M, Henriksen A, Ipsen H, et al. (2004) Allergy vaccine engineering: epitope modulation of recombinant Bet v 1 reduces IgE binding but retains protein folding pattern for induction of protective blocking-antibody responses. J Immunol 173: 5258–5267.
8. Holm J, Ferreras M, Ipsen H, Würtzen PA, Gajhede M, et al. (2011) Epitope grafting, re-creating a conformational Bet v 1 antibody epitope on the surface of the homologous apple allergen Mal d 1. J Biol Chem 286: 17569–17578.
9. Klinglmayr E, Hauser M, Zimmermann F, Dissertori O, Lackner P, et al. (2009) Identification of B-cell epitopes of Bet v 1 involved in cross-reactivity with food allergens. Allergy 64: 647–651.
10. Hecker J, Diethers A, Schulz D, Sabri A, Plum M, et al. (2012) An IgE epitope of Bet v 1 and fagales PR10 proteins as defined by a human monoclonal IgE. Allergy 67: 1530–1537.
11. Son DY, Scheurer S, Hoffmann A, Haustein D, Vieths S (1999) Pollen-related food allergy: cloning and immunological analysis of isoforms and mutants of Mal d 1, the major apple allergen, and Bet v 1, the major birch pollen allergen. Eur J Nutr 38: 201–215.
12. Ma Y, Gadermaier G, Bohle B, Bolhaar S, Knulst A, et al. (2006) Mutational analysis of amino acid positions crucial for IgE-binding epitopes of the major apple (Malus domestica) allergen, Mal d 1. Int Arch Allergy Immunol 139: 53–62.
13. Scheurer S, Son DY, Boehm M, Karamloo F, Franke S, et al. (1999) Cross-reactivity and epitope analysis of Pru a 1, the major cherry allergen. Mol Immunol 36: 155–167.
14. Neudecker P, Lehmann K, Nerkamp J, Haase T, Wangorsch A, et al. (2003) Mutational epitope analysis of Pru av 1 and Api g 1, the major allergens of cherry (Prunus avium) and celery (Apium graveolens): correlating IgE reactivity with three-dimensional structure. Biochem J 376: 97–107.
15. Wangorsch A, Ballmer-Weber BK, Rosch P, Holzhauser T, Vieths S (2007) Mutational epitope analysis and cross-reactivity of two isoforms of Api g 1, the major celery allergen. Mol Immunol 44: 2518–2527.

16. Wiche R, Gubesch M, König H, Fötisch K, Hoffmann A, et al. (2005) Molecular basis of pollen-related food allergy: identification of a second cross-reactive IgE epitope on Pru av 1, the major cherry (Prunus avium) allergen. Biochem J 385: 319–327.
17. Schirmer T, Hoffmann-Sommergruber K, Susani M, Breiteneder H, Markovic-Housley Z (2005) Crystal structure of the major celery allergen Api g 1: molecular analysis of cross-reactivity. J Mol Biol 351: 1101–1109.
18. Gieras A, Cejka P, Blatt K, Focke-Tejkl M, Linhart B, et al. (2011) Mapping of conformational IgE epitopes with peptide-specific monoclonal antibodies reveals simultaneous binding of different IgE antibodies to a surface patch on the major birch pollen allergen, Bet v 1. J Immunol 186: 5333–5344.
19. Levin M, Davies AM, Liljekvist M, Carlsson F, Gould HJ, et al. (2014) Human IgE against the major allergen Bet v 1 - defining an epitope with limited cross-reactivity between different PR-10 family proteins. Clin Exp Allergy 44: 288–299.
20. Mirza O, Henriksen A, Ipsen H, Larsen JN, Wissenbach M, et al. (2000) Dominant epitopes and allergic cross-reactivity: complex formation between a Fab fragment of a monoclonal murine IgG antibody and the major allergen from birch pollen Bet v 1. J Immunol 165: 331–338.
21. Spangfort MD, Mirza O, Svensson LA, Larsen JN, Gajhede M et al. (1999) Crystallization and preliminary X-ray analysis of birch-pollen allergen Bet v 1 in complex with a murine monoclonal IgG Fab′ fragment. Acta Crystallogr D Biol Crystallogr 55: 2035–2036.
22. Spangfort MD, Mirza O, Ipsen H, Van Neerven RJ, Gajhede M, et al. (2003) Dominating IgE-binding epitope of Bet v 1, the major allergen of birch pollen, characterized by X-ray crystallography and site-directed mutagenesis. J Immunol 171: 3084–3090.
23. Berkner H, Engelhorn J, Liscombe DK, Schweimer K, Wöhrl BM, et al. (2007) High-yield expression and purification of isotopically labeled norcoclaurine synthase, a Bet v 1-homologous enzyme, from Thalictrum flavum for NMR studies. Protein Expr Purif 56: 197–204.
24. Berkner H, Schweimer K, Matecko I, Rosch P (2008) Conformation, catalytic site, and enzymatic mechanism of the PR10 allergen-related enzyme norcoclaurine synthase. Biochem J 413: 281–290.
25. Ilari A, Franceschini S, Bonamore A, Arenghi F, Botta B, et al. (2009) Structural basis of enzymatic (S)-norcoclaurine biosynthesis. J Biol Chem 284: 897–904.
26. Ballmer-Weber BK, Wangorsch A, Bohle B, Kaul S, Kündig T, et al. (2005) Component-resolved in vitro diagnosis in carrot allergy: does the use of recombinant carrot allergens improve the reliability of the diagnostic procedure? Clin Exp Allergy 35: 970–978.
27. Axen R, Drevin H, Kober A, Yman L (1988) A new laboratory system applied to allergy testing. N Engl Reg Allergy Proc 9: 503.
28. Marknell DeWitt A, Niederberger V, Lehtonen P, Spitzauer S, Sperr WR, et al. (2002) Molecular and immunological characterization of a novel timothy grass (Phleum pratense) pollen allergen, Phl p 11. Clin Exp Allergy 32: 1329–1340.
29. Scheurer S, Metzner K, Haustein D, Vieths S (1997) Molecular cloning, expression and characterization of Pru a 1, the major cherry allergen. Mol Immunol 34: 619–629.
30. Lauer I, Alessandri S, Pokoj S, Reuter A, Conti A, et al. (2008) Expression and characterization of three important panallergens from hazelnut. Mol Nutr Food Res 52 Suppl 2: S262–S271.
31. Johnson BA and Blevins RA (1994) NMR View: A computer program for the visualization and analysis of NMR data. J Biomol NMR 4: 603–614.
32. Kelley LA and Sternberg MJ (2009) Protein structure prediction on the Web: a case study using the Phyre server. Nat Protoc 4: 363–371.
33. Gajhede M, Osmark P, Poulsen FM, Ipsen H, Larsen JN, et al. (1996) X-ray and NMR structure of Bet v 1, the origin of birch pollen allergy. Nat Struct Biol 3: 1040–1045.
34. Larsen JN, Casals AB, From NB, Stroman P, Ipsen H (1993) Characterization of recombinant bet vI, the major pollen allergen of Betula verrucosa (white birch), produced by fed-batch fermentation. Int Arch Allergy Immunol 102: 249–258.
35. Laemmli UK (1970) Cleavage of structural proteins during the assembly of the head of bacteriophage T4. Nature 227: 680–685.
36. Kyhse-Andersen J (1984) Electroblotting of multiple gels: a simple apparatus without buffer tank for rapid transfer of proteins from polyacrylamide to nitrocellulose. *J Biochem Biophys Methods* 10: 203–209.
37. Vogel L, Luttkopf D, Hatahet L, Haustein D, Vieths S (2005) Development of a functional in vitro assay as a novel tool for the standardization of allergen extracts in the human system. Allergy 60: 1021–1028.
38. Albrecht M, Alessandri S, Conti A, Reuter A, Lauer I, et al. (2008) High level expression, purification and physico- and immunochemical characterisation of recombinant Pen a 1: a major allergen of shrimp. Mol Nutr Food Res 52 Suppl 2: S186–S195.
39. Sievers F, Wilm A, Dineen D, Gibson TJ, Karplus K, et al. (2011) Fast, scalable generation of high-quality protein multiple sequence alignments using Clustal Omega. Mol Syst Biol 7: 539.
40. DeLano WL (2002) The PyMOL Molecular Graphics System.
41. Subbarayal B, Schiller D, Möbs C, de Jong NW, Ebner C, et al. (2013) Kinetics, cross-reactivity, and specificity of Bet v 1-specific IgG4 antibodies induced by immunotherapy with birch pollen. Allergy 68: 1377–1386.
42. Lebecque S, Dolecek C, Laffer S, Visco V, Denépoux S, et al. (1997) Immunologic characterization of monoclonal antibodies that modulate human IgE binding to the major birch pollen allergen Bet v 1. J Allergy Clin Immunol 99: 374–384.
43. Kahlert H, Suck R, Weber B, Nandy A, Wald M, et al. (2008) Characterization of a hypoallergenic recombinant Bet v 1 variant as a candidate for allergen-specific immunotherapy. Int Arch Allergy Immunol 145: 193–206.
44. Wallner M, Hauser M, Himly M, Zaborsky N, Mutschlechner S, et al. (2011) Reshaping the Bet v 1 fold modulates T(H) polarization. J Allergy Clin Immunol 127: 1571–1578.
45. Dall′Acqua W, Goldman ER, Lin W, Teng C, Tsuchiya D, et al. (1998) A mutational analysis of binding interactions in an antigen-antibody protein-protein complex. Biochemistry 37: 7981–7991.
46. Jenkins JA, Griffiths-Jones S, Shewry PR, Breiteneder H, Mills EN (2005) Structural relatedness of plant food allergens with specific reference to cross-reactive allergens: an in silico analysis. J Allergy Clin Immunol 115: 163–170.
47. Ferreira F, Hirtenlehner K, Jilek A, Godnik-Cvar J, Breiteneder H, et al. (1996) Dissection of immunoglobulin E and T lymphocyte reactivity of isoforms of the major birch pollen allergen Bet v 1: potential use of hypoallergenic isoforms for immunotherapy. J Exp Med 183: 599–609.
48. Mittag D, Batori V, Neudecker P, Wiche R, Friis EP, et al. (2006) A novel approach for investigation of specific and cross-reactive IgE epitopes on Bet v 1 and homologous food allergens in individual patients. Mol Immunol 43: 268–278.
49. Dall′Antonia F, Gieras A, Devanaboyina SC, Valenta R, Keller W (2011) Prediction of IgE-binding epitopes by means of allergen surface comparison and correlation to cross-reactivity. J Allergy Clin Immunol 128: 872–879.
50. Jimenez-Lopez JC, Gachomo EW, Ariyo OA, Baba-Moussa L, Kotchoni SO (2012) Specific conformational epitope features of pathogenesis-related proteins mediating cross-reactivity between pollen and food allergens. Mol Biol Rep 39: 123–130.

# 16

# IgE Recognition Patterns of Profilin, PR-10, and Tropomyosin Panallergens Tested in 3,113 Allergic Patients by Allergen Microarray-Based Technology

**Enrico Scala, Claudia Alessandri, Paola Palazzo, Debora Pomponi, Marina Liso, Maria Livia Bernardi, Rosetta Ferrara, Danila Zennaro, Mario Santoro, Chiara Rasi, Adriano Mari***

Center for Molecular Allergology, IDI-IRCCS, Rome, Italy

## Abstract

***Background:*** IgE recognition of panallergens having highly conserved sequence regions, structure, and function and shared by inhalant and food allergen sources is often observed.

***Methods:*** We evaluated the IgE recognition profile of profilins (Bet v 2, Cyn d 12, Hel a 2, Hev b 8, Mer a 1, Ole e 2, Par j 3, Phl p 12, Pho d 2), PR-10 proteins (Aln g 1, Api g 1, Bet v 1.0101, Bet v 1.0401, Cor a 1, Dau c 1 and Mal d 1.0108) and tropomyosins (Ani s 3, Der p 10, Hel as 1, Pen i 1, Pen m 1, Per a 7) using the Immuno-Solid phase Allergen Chip (ISAC) microarray system. The three panallergen groups were well represented among the allergenic molecules immobilized on the ISAC. Moreover, they are distributed in several taxonomical allergenic sources, either close or distant, and have a route of exposure being either inhalation or ingestion.

***Results:*** 3,113 individuals (49.9% female) were selected on the basis of their reactivity to profilins, PR-10 or tropomyosins. 1,521 (48.8%) patients were reactive to profilins (77.6% Mer a 1 $IgE^{+}$), 1,420 (45.6%) to PR-10 (92.5% Bet v 1 $IgE^{+}$) and 632 (20.3%) to tropomyosins (68% Der p 10 $IgE^{+}$). A significant direct relationship between different representative molecules within each group of panallergens was found. 2,688 patients (86.4%) recognized only one out of the three distinct groups of molecules as confirmed also by hierarchical clustering analysis.

***Conclusions:*** Unless exposed to most of the allergens in the same or related allergenic sources, a preferential IgE response to distinct panallergens has been recorded. Allergen microarray IgE testing increases our knowledge of the IgE immune response and related epidemiological features within and between homologous molecules better describing the patients' immunological phenotypes.

**Editor:** Dennis W. Metzger, Albany Medical College, United States of America

**Funding:** The study has been funded by the Italian Ministry of Health, Current Research Program 2006-2008. Extensive IgE testing carried out routinely by the ISAC microarray system has been made possible by using the reimbursement system established by the Regional Public Health Care Service for laboratory IgE detection. The funders had no role in study design, data collection and analysis, decision to publish, or preparation of the manuscript.

**Competing Interests:** The authors have declared that no competing interests exist.

* E-mail: adriano.mari@idi.it

## Introduction

The prevalence of allergic diseases has dramatically increased in last decades, mostly in developed countries [1,2]. Comprehensive and reliable allergy diagnostic testing are needed, also for therapeutic decision making [3]. In vitro diagnosis of allergic sensitizations is based on the measurement of specific IgE in sera of allergic patients [4]. Most of the currently available singleplex in vitro assays measure the IgE reactivity to extracts obtained from raw material derived from several organisms or their tissues. No information about the number of molecules involved or about the molecular profile associated with a given clinical manifestation is currently provided by extract-based testing.

A major problem is represented by the possibility that positive results, employing extracts, could be caused by IgE recognition of homologous molecules instead of molecules that represent the genuine marker of sensitization to a given biological source [5]. In the past 10 years the production of highly purified natural or recombinant allergens together with the recent advances in microarray technology provided the background for the development of a multiplexed assay as efficient means to test IgE sensitization to hundreds of allergenic molecules simultaneously in large populations [6–8].

Adverse reactions after the ingestion of animal- or plant-derived foods caused by IgE cross-reactive molecules shared by inhalant and food allergen sources are often seen in clinical practice [9]. These molecules are commonly defined as "pan-allergens" and represent families of homologous and structurally related proteins belonging to different biological sources (i.e. profilins, PR-10 molecules, tropomyosins) [10–12]. As the three molecule groups considered in the present study have different distributions in nature, namely profilins are ubiquitous eukaryotic proteins, found in both animal and plant sources, tropomyosins are highly conserved eukaryotic proteins, but are not found in plants, and

**Table 1.** List, characteristics, and Allergome reference code for the three panallergen groups, ranked by prevalence of IgE reactivity among and within groups.

| Panallergens | | | | IgE Reactive Patients | | | |
|---|---|---|---|---|---|---|---|
| **Allergen** | **Common name** | **Allergome Code** | **Molecule Sequence Identity°** | **N.** | **%** | **N.** | **%** |
| **Mer a 1** | *Profilin* | 476 | 100 | 1,521 | 48.8 | 1181 | 77.6 |
| **Hev b 8** | | 397 | 81 | | | 1019 | 67.0 |
| **Bet v 2** | | 127 | 84 | | | 986 | 64.8 |
| **Ole e 2*** | | 490 | 85 | | | 977 | 64.2 |
| **Hel a 2** | | 377 | 75 | | | 889 | 58.4 |
| **Pho d 2** | | 571 | 80 | | | 876 | 57.6 |
| **Cyn d 12** | | 279 | 76 | | | 857 | 56.3 |
| **Par j 3** | | 510 | 78 | | | 688 | 45.2 |
| **Phl p 12** | | 553 | 82 | | | 551 | 36.2 |
| **Bet v 1** | *PR-10* | 89 | 100 | 1,420 | 45.6 | 1314 | 92.5 |
| **Cor a 1** | | 232 | 83 | | | 960 | 67.6 |
| **Aln g 1** | | 7 | 81 | | | 741 | 52.2 |
| **Mal d 1** | | 464 | 65 | | | 696 | 49.0 |
| **Api g 1** | | 40 | 41 | | | 163 | 11.5 |
| **Dau c 1** | | 287 | 39 | | | 59 | 4.2 |
| **Der p 10** | *Tropomyosin* | 311 | 100 | 632 | 20.3 | 430 | 68.0 |
| **Pen i 1*** | | 527 | ≈80# | | | 326 | 51.6 |
| **Pen m 1*** | | 872 | 80 | | | 313 | 49.5 |
| **Ani s 3** | | 37 | 73 | | | 313 | 49.5 |
| **Hel as 1** | | 378 | 64 | | | 309 | 48.9 |
| **Per a 7** | | 542 | 79 | | | 272 | 43.0 |

*Natural purified molecules, all others are *E.coli*-produced recombinants. Biochemical, immunological and clinical details on each allergen are available at www.allergome.org.
°Generated using AllergomeAligner (www.allergome.org) assuming the first ranked IgE reactive allergen as reference sequence (= 100%).
#Complete Pen i 1 sequence is not available. From peptide fragment matching and IgE reactivity it is assumed to be close to Pen m 1.

PR-10 proteins are not found in animals, the "panallergen" definition has been herein used to identify allergenic molecules belonging to distant genera/orders rather than because they span across kingdoms. Profilins are actin-binding proteins having a molecular weight between 12–15 kDa, and present in the cell cytoplasm. They have been described as allergens in pollen sources and plant-derived food. Up to now 100 profilins have been described as allergenic, 55 of them in pollen from distant taxonomical species. PR-10 belong to the pathogenesis-related protein groups. They are molecules having a molecular weight of 16–18 kDa, produced in response to biotic and abiotic stresses, and described as allergens in pollen and plant-derived foods. Fifty three PR-10 have been described up to now, 17 from pollen of the *Fagales* order, whereas homologous from foods, like apple, carrot, celery, kiwi, are from quite distant taxonomical species. Tropomyosins are animal structural muscle proteins with a molecular weight of about 35 kDa. Tropomyosins are well described food allergens from crustaceans, but homologous allergens are found in arthropods not commonly used as food, like mites and cockroaches, causing allergic diseases by the inhalation route. Up to now 93 tropomyosins have been described as allergenic, 77 from shellfishes. All data on panallergens have been retrieved from Allergome (www.allergome.org), accessed April 30, 2011. This web-based platform can be used for more detailed and up to date descriptions of each allergen reported in the present study.

The aim of our study was to bring a further and more in deep insight into the distribution of the IgE reactivity to three panallergen groups (profilins, PR-10 and tropomyosins) in 3,113 individuals with a history of food allergy, rhinitis, asthma or atopic dermatitis, either looking at the reciprocal IgE positivity of each group compared to the others, or within each of the three panallergen groups. The study population is from Italy, extracted from a reported study [7], and being exposed and sensitized to the three groups of molecules. We selected these three groups of panallergens because they are well represented among the allergenic molecules immobilized on the available microarray version, and because they are distributed in several taxonomical allergenic sources, either close or distant, and having a route of exposure being either inhalation or ingestion. Thus, these three molecule groups have the highest probability to get in contact with the human immune system, though variable exposure levels could occur, largely depending on inhalant allergen seasonality, spatial (geographical) distributions, or frequency and amount of ingested food items.

## Methods

### Ethics Statement

The study was approved by the Institutional Review Board of Istituto Dermopatico dell'Immacolata – IDI-IRCCS, Rome, Italy

(n. 106-CE-2005). The Institutional Review Board approved that the study is based on the oral informed consent for blood sampling obtained from patients or caregivers during the allergy consult, as IgE detection by microarray testing was part of the routine procedures in each patient diagnostic work-up. All patients, being informed by the specialist performing demographic and clinical data collection and suggesting them the IgE testing as reported in the present study, approved the study itself.

## Study population

Data herein reported have been extracted and further analyzed from the total of 23,077 subjects previously reported by us [7]. Briefly, unselected consecutive subjects, 61.2% female; age range between 1 and 98 years old, referred for a history of food allergy, rhinitis, asthma, atopic dermatitis, latex allergy, acute or chronic urticaria to the Center for Molecular Allergology (IDI-IRCCS, Rome, Italy) from March 2006 to December 2007 [7]. Demographical (age and gender) and clinical (respiratory and food ingestion-related symptoms) data were recorded for all patients at history taking by means of the InterAll software for clinical data recording (InterAll version 3.0, Allergy Data Laboratories s.c., Latina, Italy) [13].

Three thousand, one hundred and thirteen individuals (49.9% female; age range between 2 and 96 years old) were selected on the basis of their IgE reactivity detected using the Immuno-Solid phase Allergen Chip (ISAC) system (VBC-Genomics, Vienna, Austria). Candidates had to be IgE positive to at least one allergen of the following group of panallergens: profilins (Bet v 2, Cyn d 12, Hel a 2, Hev b 8, Mer a 1, Ole e 2, Par j 3, Phl p 12, Pho d 2); PR-10 (Aln g 1, Api g 1, Bet v 1.0101, Bet v 1.0401, Cor a 1, Dau c 1 and Mal d 1.0108); tropomyosins (Ani s 3, Der p 10, Hel as 1, Pen i 1, Pen m 1, Per a 7). Selected subjects thus acted as our study group.

## Purified natural and recombinant allergens

Table 1 reports the characteristics of the recombinant and natural allergenic molecules listed above and used for the IgE microarray testing in this study. All the molecules studied were recombinant allergens expressed in *Escherichia coli*, with the exception of Ole e 2, Pen m 1, Pen i 1, which were naturally purified preparations. Table 1 displays the Allergome code (Allergen ID) for each molecule. Further details on single molecule characteristics are available via the Allergome web site (www.allergome.org) [13].

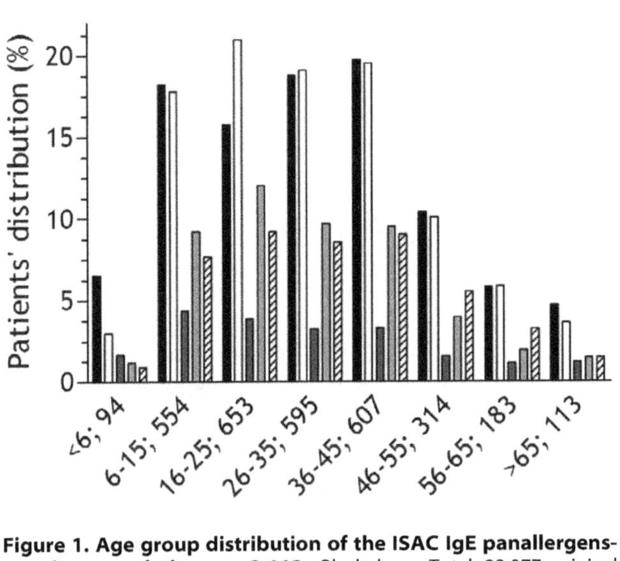


**Figure 1. Age group distribution of the ISAC IgE panallergens-reactive population; n = 3,113.** Black bars: Total 23,077 original allergic population; White Bars: Total 3,113 panallergens allergic population; Dark grey bars: PR-10; Hatched bars: Profilin; Light grey bars: Tropomyosin.

## Proteomic Allergen Microarray IgE Testing

**IgE microarray assay.** Glass microscopy slides, each bearing four reaction sites bearing immobilized allergens, as provided by the manufacturer (VBC-Genomics), were washed for 60 min in TBS-T buffer (150 mM sodium chloride, 10 mM Tris base, and 0.5% Tween 20, pH 8.0), rinsed with deionised water, and dried. Slides were placed into a humid chamber and 20 µl of undiluted serum from each patient was applied to the reaction site. After incubation with patient's sera for 120 min at R.T., slides were rinsed and washed for 15 min in TBS-T, for 5 min in deionised water and dried. To detect bound IgE antibodies, allergen chips were incubated for 60 min at room temperature with 20 µl of an Alexa Fluor 546 fluorescence-labeled (Alexa Fluor 546 protein labeling kit, Molecular Probes, Leiden, Netherlands) anti-human IgE antibody (Pharmingen, San Diego, CA) diluted 1:1000 in TBS-T containing 5% milk powder. Afterwards, slides were washed twice for 10 min with TBS-T, rinsed with deionised water, dried, and stored in the dark until scanning.

**Image and data acquisition, and quantification of IgE.** Images were acquired by scanning allergen chips with a ScanArray Gx Microarray Analysis System (Perkin Elmer Life and Analytical Sciences, Shelton, CT) with two different laser power settings. In the first scan, 70% of the laser power (50 db) was employed to obtain the highest possible signal intensities with acceptable background noise. In a second scanning step, laser power was reduced to 35 db in order to prevent saturated signals (65.535). Both images of each spot were analyzed using the ScanArray Express 3.0 software (PerkinElmer). Captured images saved as a TIFF file were imported into the ISAC software (VBC-Genomics) which specifically process the raw fluorescence value expressed as fluorescence index of each spot. From the three fluorescence values obtained for each allergen on triplicate spots, the mean value was calculated and used for further analysis. IgE values were expressed as $kU_A/l$ by interpolating the mean fluorescence value with a previously established reference curve [14–16]. At the end of each run data were exported to the InterAll software by a real-time connectivity, and saved in the patient's record where demographical and clinical data were saved earlier by the allergy specialist.

Though several ISAC biochips with different number of spotted allergens have been used during the study timeframe (ISAC79, ISAC81, ISAC86), we analyzed results from the 23 homologous molecules immobilized on all of them. For comparative purposes we used results available the same microarray testing for Phl p 1, Par j 2, and Der p 1, all considered genuine markers of sensitization to grass and parietaria pollen, and to house dust mite, respectively. The only route of exposure for all the selected genuine allergens is inhalation.

## Clustering analysis and Statistical evaluation

To verify the molecule IgE recognition profiles, we took advantage of the Genesis software version 1.7.2, originally developed for cluster analysis of genomics data [17]. The software has been adapted to be applied to proteomics of specific IgE detected by means of the ISAC molecule-based microarray.

Relatedness of IgE recognition profiles was tested by applying unsupervised Eisen's hierarchical cluster methods [18] to the data set, encompassing allergenic molecules across all samples and

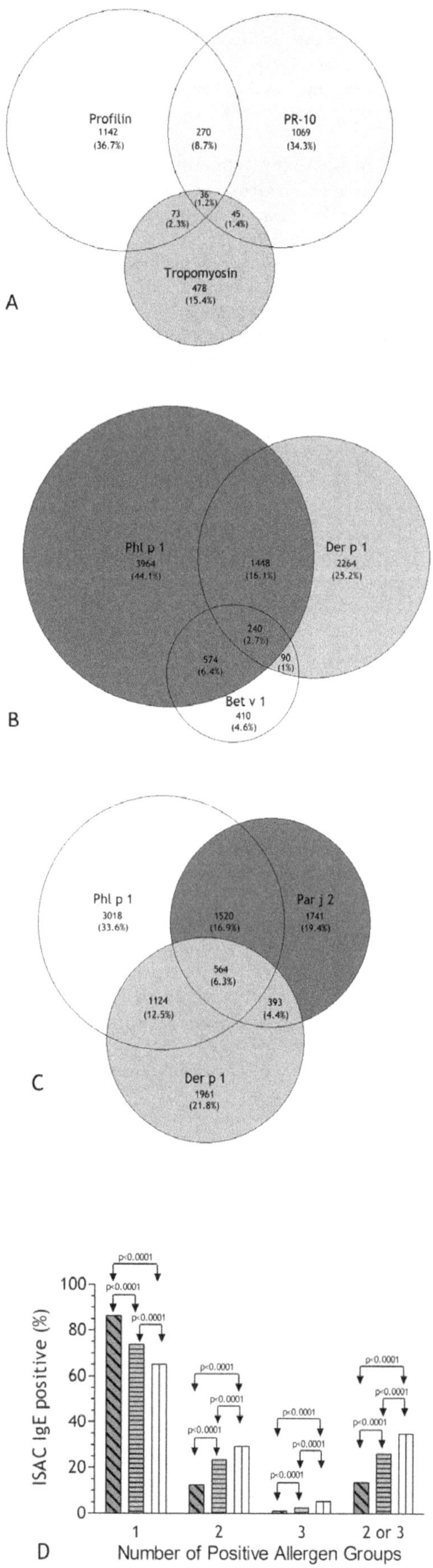


**Figure 2. Venn diagram comparative representations of the IgE reactivity distributions.** Panel A: Venn diagram of IgE reactivity distributions of the three panallergen groups, profilins, PR-10, and tropomyosin (n = 3,113); Panel B: Venn diagram of IgE reactivity distributions of genuine inhalant allergens Phl p 1, Der p 1, and including Bet v 1 when considered as a marker of genuine pollen sensitization; Panel C: Venn diagram of IgE reactivity distributions of exclusive genuine inhalant allergens Phl p 1, Der p 1, and Par j 2; Panel D: Statistical comparative evaluations of concurrent IgE reactivity to 1, 2, 3, or 2 and 3 groups in Venn diagrams shown in panel A (dark grey hatched bars), panel B (light grey horizontal line bars), panel C (white vertical line bars).

using as agglomeration rule the average linkage clustering as implemented in the Genesis software [17]. Unsupervised clustering involved the sorting of both homologous allergenic molecules and IgE recognition values. The IgE recognition tree was computed on the basis of a full data set and the distance between samples were computed by using Pearson correlation as similarity measures. Molecular allergens with a similar pattern of IgE recognition were grouped as hierarchical clusters and presented as heat-maps [7]. Each square in the heat-map represent the presence (red) or the absence (black) of IgE recognition of any given tested allergens for each tested subject. The red color intensity of every single square in the heat-map is directly associated with the measured IgE concentration. Interpretation of the heat-map generated by the software can be done either visually, where clustering IgE positive allergens tends to give more homogeneous red areas, or by taking into consideration the higher or lower level of dendrograms on allergen side of the graph.

Data collected in the InterAll database were also analyzed using the SPSS/PC + statistical package (SPSS, version 15, Chicago, IL). The levels of the variables of interest in the serum (IgE) from allergic patients were summarized showing the mean ± SD, in order to provide the most easily interpretable summary measure. However, differences between the levels of these variables were also tested using the nonparametric Mann–Whitney U-test. The degree of relationship between the quantitative variables studied was analyzed using Pearson Correlation test (r). Chi-square test has been used for prevalence comparisons. Statistical significance cut-off level has been set for $p<0.01$.

## Results

### Descriptive statistics

A total of 3,113 subjects (49.9% female), showing an IgE reactivity to at least one molecule belonging to profilin, PR-10, and tropomyosin allergen groups, represented our study group. The median age was 30.8±17.04 years, but male subjects were significantly younger (28.3±17.5 *vs* 30.4±16.1, Mann-Whitney Rank Sum Test $p<0.0001$). No major differences were recorded comparing to the median age of the entire studied population (30.8±18.3 years), whilst the gender distribution was different when compared to the original general population (55.2% female) from which our study group was extracted.

As shown in Table 1, profilin reactive individuals represented the largest group of patients, whilst tropomyosin reactive patients were the smaller one. Interestingly, PR-10 reactive individuals were prevalently female (Pearson $\chi^2$ test 4.8 $p=0.027$), whereas the opposite was observed in the case of tropomyosin reactivity ($\chi^2$ test 5.36 $p<0.021$). A slight, not significant, prevalence of male population (51.4%) was observed in profilin reactive patients, as well. Unless profilin sequence identity were above 75%, IgE recognition ranked between 76.6% and 36.2%. A broader

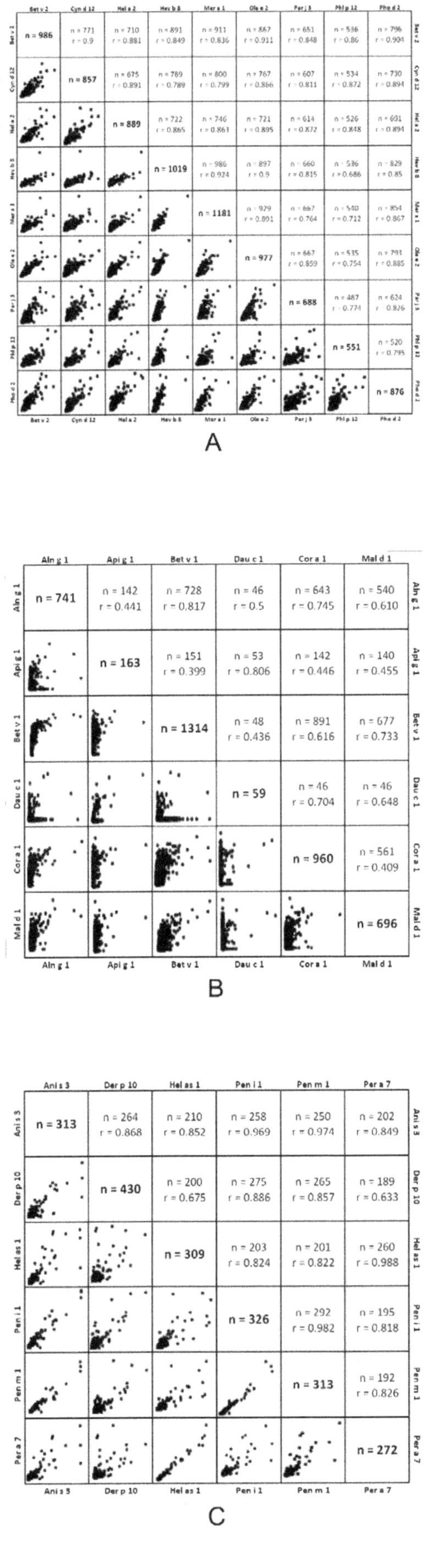

**Figure 3. Bivariate analysis of reciprocal relationships of IgE to profilin, PR-10, and tropomyosin panallergens.** The number of IgE reactive subjects and the Pearson coefficient are shown for paired allergens within the three panallergen groups. Pearson r values are reported below. Data were statistically significant in all cases (p<0.001). Panel A: Profilins; Panel B: PR-10; Panel C: Tropomyosins.

sequence identity was recorded within PR-10 molecules, having Dau c 1 (39%) the lowest sequence identity value. IgE prevalence was the broadest as well, ranging between 92.5% and 4.2%. Tropomyosins behaved as profilins, having the lowest sequence identity above 64%, but IgE prevalence ranged between 68% and 43%.

The panallergens IgE-positive cohort has been divided in eight consecutive age groups (Figure 1). Patients younger than 5 years old mainly recognized tropomyosin molecules, whilst the IgE profilin-reactive population was more prevalent between patients aged 6 to 45 years old. The prevalence of IgE reactivity to PR-10 molecules was the top ranked in patients older than 46.

Two thousand, six hundred and eighty-eight patients (86.4%) recognized just one out of the three distinct groups of panallergens, with a preferential recognition behavior (Figure 2, Panel A). Four hundred and twenty-four (13.6%) individuals had IgE to more than one panallergen group, but, among them, only 36 individuals (1.2%) recognized molecules belonging to all the three panallergen groups (Figure 2, Panel A). Among patients having IgE recognizing more than one panallergen group, 270 individuals (8.7%) had IgE to PR-10 and profilin molecules, 73 (2.3%) to tropomyosin and profilin, and 45 (1.4%) to tropomyosin and PR-10 panallergens (Figure 2, Panel A). To verify whether such distribution was related to any bias present in the patient recruitment phase or was related to any specific allergen sensitization process, data available for genuine allergen IgE testing were analyzed as reported in Figure 2 panel B and C. Concurrent sensitization to 2 or 3 genuine allergens was recorded with a statistically significant difference when compared to the distribution recorded for panallergens.

## Bivariate Correlation within Panallergen Groups

The association among the different molecules studied without distinction between independent and dependent variables was analyzed using the Pearson Correlation test. As shown in Figure 3, a significant direct relationship of IgE recognition of profilin, PR-10, and tropomyosin molecules, respectively, was recorded (p<0.001). Every single molecule belonging to a given group of panallergens, therefore, showed similar behavior of IgE recognition. In the case of PR-10 molecules, regardless the presence of a significant association between all molecules, the Pearson correlation coefficients analysis revealed a strong relationship (Pearson Correlation from 0.70 to 1) between Bet v 1, Aln g 1 and Cor a 1 from one side and between Api g 1 and Dau c 1 from the other, thus suggesting the presence of a distinct patterns of IgE recognition between PR-10 molecules belonging to inhalant and food allergens, respectively.

In the case of profilin and tropomyosin molecules, all the Pearson correlation coefficient resulted to be higher than 0.70, thus confirming a strong structural and immunological relationship between the tested molecules.

## Cluster analysis

Supervised two-way hierarchical clustering analysis, sorting for both allergenic molecules and IgE recognition values, generated distinct clusters of IgE recognition of profilin, PR-10, and

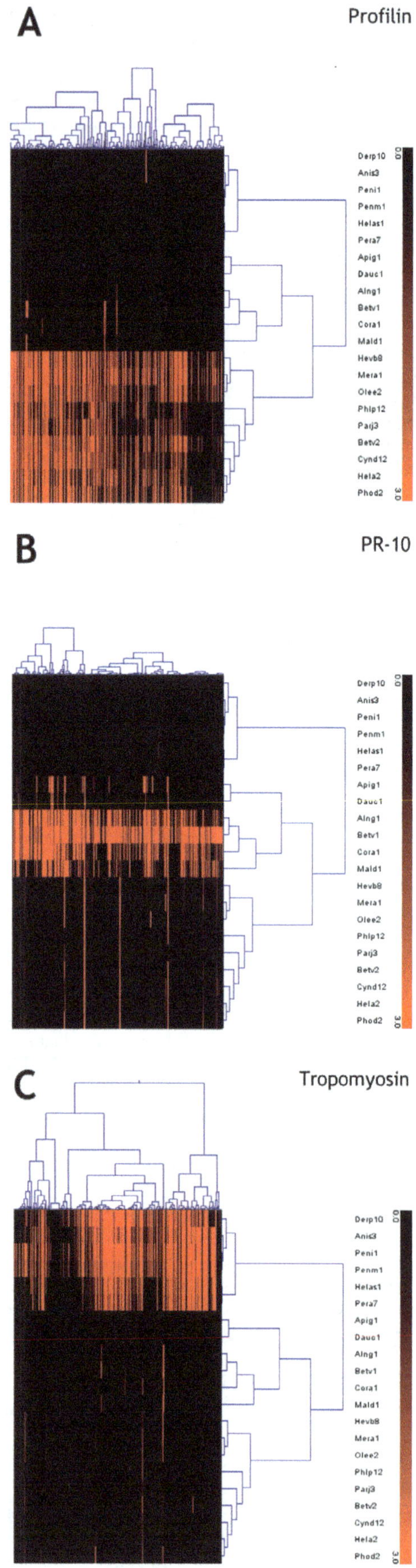


**Figure 4. Supervised two-way hierarchical clustering analysis of panallergen IgE values.** Subjects had at least one IgE-positive result to the panallergens under study. Allergens are reported on the y-axis, subjects on the x-axis. Black to dark red scale corresponds to IgE values from negative to strongly positive. Further explanations are in the 'Methods' section. Panel A: Profilins; Panel B: PR-10; Panel C: Tropomyosins.

tropomyosin molecules, as shown in Figure 4. The IgE recognition of these three distinct groups of molecules was exclusive in 86.4% of cases, as already mentioned, and also the clustering analysis confirmed the high level of exclusivity of IgE recognition of the three panallergens herein evaluated. Plant derived panallergens (PR-10 and profilin molecules) generated a larger cluster of reactivity distinct from the one generated by tropomyosin molecules. In the case of PR-10 molecules, two distinct clusters of IgE reactivity (between Api g 1 and Dau c 1 the first and between Bet v 1, Cor a 1 and Aln g 1 the second) were recorded. Also in the case of tropomyosin IgE reactivity, we observed two distinct clusters of reactivity: one shaped by Hel as 1 and Per a 7, the other by Ani s 3, Der p 10, Pen i 1 and Pen m 1, respectively.

## Discussion

In the present study we perform an in deep analysis of the prevalence of IgE reactivity to panallergens in a large cohort of allergic patients, evaluated by means of a microarray IgE detection system. We studied three groups of molecules belonging to different biological sources and tissues (profilin, PR-10, and tropomyosin), involved at the same time in respiratory and food allergy. Such allergens have been reported as representative examples of IgE "cross reactivity" between otherwise unrelated organisms [19–26].

We found that panallergen IgE recognition is exclusive in a large part of our Italian cohort. More than 86% of patients produce specific IgE to a group of panallergens but not to the others. As a result, in the vast majority of cases, the multiple reactivity to inhalant or food allergenic sources was caused by the sensitization to at least one representative molecule of a single panallergen group. Similarly, tropomyosin reactive individuals did not raise an IgE response to other panallergens, as also shown by the hierarchical clustering analysis (Figure 4). Comparatively we showed that when allergenic molecules sensitizing allergic patients by the inhalation route are considered a significant number of concurrent sensitization is recorded. Such number is higher when the exclusive inhalation route of sensitization and the following exposure is considered.

The use of the same approach, originally designed for genomic evaluation, in the epidemiological assessment of IgE reactivity to panallergens, might help in the management of large amount of data generated by serial proteomic evaluation of hundreds of molecules at the same time, in the same group of patients [7]. In this way, it is possible to identify subsets of patients having a similar IgE recognition profile. At the same time, it's also possible to confirm that molecules belonging to a given group of panallergen generate distinct clusters, as a result of the IgE recognition of the same group of molecules, at the same time by the same group of patients. Presumably, all the tropomyosin sensitized patients are also exposed to pollen and food PR-10 and profilins, but the vast majority of the cases did not recognize the other panallergens. If such behavior is more stringent when the IgE reactivity to tropomyosin is compared to the IgE recognition of the plant-derived molecules, the same finding is less obvious when we analyzed the latter groups of panallergens. Given that the possible role of HLA association in the mechanism of IgE response is not fully understood, further investigations of the immune mechanisms at the level of allergen-specific T cells and TCR-MHC/peptide interactions, could identify the MHC restriction elements capable of determine the preferential recognition of a given panallergen group instead of another. In absence of a genetically driven mechanism and in the light of IgE recognition of conformational epitopes, new hypotheses should be made to explain our findings.

Furthermore, as in the case of profilin IgE sensitization, molecules not commonly found in the environment such as Hev b 8, hardly found in latex gloves [27], or Mer a 1, *Mercurialis annua* pollen is rarely found in the atmosphere [28], turned out to be the most frequently recognized by patients' IgE, most likely primarily sensitized by other profilins. Such findings would suggest to carefully considering a molecule as the primary sensitizer merely on the basis of its higher or more frequent IgE reactivity. In the specific cases, latex and *Mercurialis* profilins could act just as the best "profilin" reagents for specific IgE detection among the many profilins already identified. Better conclusions on this issue could be drawn when some profilins, like Cuc m 2, the muskmelon profilin, commonly causing patients' reported symptoms [29], will be available for testing. Such observation can apply also to PR-10, as far as patients in the geographical area under consideration are not exposed to birch pollen [30], whereas IgE recognition of tested tropomyosins does not seem to suggest any leading role in either a molecule as sensitizer or just as the best reagent to detect group-related specific IgE. As in part already reported for the studied panallergens and other allergenic groups [31–33], in the case of profilin and PR-10, IgE co-recognition of allergens seems not to be as obvious as it should be from their sequence homology and structure similarity.

Discovering that the production of IgE is preferentially addressed to a panallergen rather than another is relevant also considering the different clinical phenotypes that these molecules could determine. Clinical reactions of panallergens, in fact, might range from very mild symptoms in the case of profilin reactivity [34,35], to mild or sometimes severe symptoms if PR-10 molecules are involved [36,37], to often severe reactions when IgE reactivity is directed to other panallergens, such as lipid transfer proteins [38,39]. The preferential IgE recognition of the panallergens would ease the clinical approach to patients sensitized to one or another group.

Another topic addressed by our study is represented by the possibility to evaluate the IgE reactivity to several representative molecules within each group of panallergens by means of the microarray [40]. In fact, the IgE epitope recognition of homologous molecules, within a given group of panallergens, could be the result of the somatic hyper-mutation and affinity maturation after the initial IgE recognition of the primary sensitizer as determined by the patient's different environmental exposure [41,42]. As shown in Figure 3, a significant relationship within every single group of molecules was clearly shown, as the consequence of an IgE co-recognition of all the homologous molecules belonging to the given panallergen group [43]. At the same time, different clusters of patients could be identified on the basis of the diversity of IgE recognition within every single group of panallergen (Figure 4). For instance, in the case of PR-10, two distinct subsets of patient could be identified: those IgE reactive to pollen-derived molecules (Bet v 1, Cor a 1 or Aln g 1) and those also reactive to food-derived PR-10 molecules (Dau c 1, Api g 1 or Mal d 1) (Figure 4). Similarly, in the case of tropomyosin reactivity, two distinct subsets of patients could be identified, the first reactive to Hel as 1 and Per a 7, and the other reactive to all the other tropomyosins. As a consequence, the presence of distinct representatives of a given group of panallergen represents an added value of the microarrayed system for the evaluation of IgE reactivity: it gives higher consistency to obtain more reliable results and could add further information on the hypothetical sensitizer in a given group of patients (Figure 3 and 4). All findings reported from using different analytical approaches require further evaluation using wet lab experimental studies using the same microarray-based technique, as already reported for another panallergen group, namely the lipid transfer proteins [44–46].

Overall, allergy diagnosis based on allergenic molecules is crucial for a correct evaluation of patients sensitized to panallergens. Molecular analysis represent the only way to establish the presence of new profiles represented by profilin, tropomyosin or PR-10 reactivity, conditions that are addressed to a preferential recognition of one panallergen, in the vast majority of cases, as suggested by our observations.

In conclusion, protein microarray techniques applied in allergy diagnosis allow the identification of several IgE reactivity patterns and possibly could lead to a better knowledge of the relationship between basic immunological mechanisms and clinical symptoms. We would put much emphasis on the opportunity that micro-technologies give us to broad our allergy testing and, at the same time, get detailed and in deep views of unselected patient's IgE immune recognition [7].

## Acknowledgments

We are grateful to Mr. Mauro Helmer-Citterich and Ms. Chiara Rafaiani who routinely performed the ISAC test during the time period the study has been carried out, Giorgio Perotti helping in setting the figures in the correct format, and to Dr. Silvia Monti for her timely and generous support to the work of each of us. We also thank allergists who transiently collaborate to the study.

The use of the InterAll allergy *e*-record has been kindly granted for free by Allergy Data Laboratories s.c. (Latina, Italy).

## Author Contributions

Conceived and designed the experiments: AM ES. Performed the experiments: ES CA MLB RF DZ AM PP DP ML. Analyzed the data: ES MS CR. Contributed reagents/materials/analysis tools: AM. Wrote the paper: ES CA AM.

## References

1. Simpson CR, Newton J, Hippisley-Cox J, Sheikh A (2008) Incidence and prevalence of multiple allergic disorders recorded in a national primary care database. J R Soc Med 101: 558–63.
2. Gupta R, Sheikh A, Strachan DP, Anderson HR (2004) Burden of allergic disease in the UK: secondary analyses of national databases. Clin Exp Allergy 34: 520–6.
3. Valenta R, Twaroch T, Swoboda I (2007) Component-resolved diagnosis to optimize allergen-specific immunotherapy in the Mediterranean area. J Investig Allergol Clin Immunol 17(Suppl 1): 36–40.
4. Grall F, Caroff J, Corson M, Morin JF, Clavier J (1977) Correlations between specific IgE cutaneous tests and the clinical diagnosis of allergies in asthma and respiratory equivalents. Rev Fr Allergol Immunol Clin 17: 7–12.
5. Mari A (2001) Multiple pollen sensitization: a molecular approach to the diagnosis. Int Arch Allergy Immunol 125: 57–65.
6. Hiller R, Laffer S, Harwanegg C, Huber M, Schmidt WM, et al. (2002) Microarrayed allergen molecules: diagnostic gatekeepers for allergy treatment. FASEB J 16: 414–6.
7. Scala E, Alessandri C, Bernardi ML, Ferrara R, Palazzo P, et al. (2010) Cross-sectional survey on immunoglobulin E reactivity in 23 077 subjects using an allergenic molecule-based microarray detection system. Clin Exp Allergy 40: 911–21.
8. Mari A, Alessandri C, Bernardi ML, Ferrara R, Scala E, et al. (2010) Microarrayed Allergen Molecules for the Diagnosis of Allergic Diseases. Curr Allergy Asthma Rep 10: 357–64.

9. Lidholm A, Ballmer-Weber BK, Mari A, Vieths S (2006) Component-resolved diagnostics in food allergy. Curr Opin Allergy Clin Immunol 6: 234–40.
10. Radauer C, Bublin M, Wagner S, Mari A, Breiteneder H (2008) Allergens are distributed into few protein families and possess a restricted number of biochemical functions. J Allergy Clin Immunol 121: 847–52.
11. Chapman MD (2008) Allergen nomenclature. Clin Allergy Immunol 21: 47–58.
12. Chapman MD, Pomes A, Breiteneder H, Ferreira F (2007) Nomenclature and structural biology of allergens. J Allergy Clin Immunol 119: 414–20.
13. Mari A, Rasi C, Palazzo P, Scala E (2009) Allergen databases: current status and perspectives. Curr Allergy Asthma Rep 9: 376–83.
14. Harwanegg C, Hiller R (2006) Protein microarrays for the diagnosis of allergic diseases: state-of-the-art and future development. Eur Ann Allergy Clin Immunol 38: 232–6.
15. Harwanegg C, Laffer S, Hiller R, Mueller MW, Kraft D, et al. (2003) Microarrayed recombinant allergens for diagnosis of allergy. Clin Exp Allergy 33: 7–13.
16. Jahn-Schmid B, Harwanegg C, Hiller R, Bohle B, Ebner C, et al. (2003) Allergen microarray: comparison of microarray using recombinant allergens with conventional diagnostic methods to detect allergen-specific serum immunoglobulin E. Clin Exp Allergy 33: 1443–9.
17. Sturn A, Quackenbush J, Trajanoski Z (2002) Genesis: cluster analysis of microarray data. Bioinformatics 18: 207–8.
18. Eisen MB, Spellman PT, Brown PO, Botstein D (1998) Cluster analysis and display of genome-wide expression patterns. Proc Natl Acad Sci U S A 95: 14863–8.
19. Lombardero M, Garcia-Selles FJ, Polo F, Jimeno L, Chamorro MJ, et al. (2004) Prevalence of sensitization to Artemisia allergens Art v 1, Art v 3 and Art v 60 kDa. Cross-reactivity among Art v 3 and other relevant lipid-transfer protein allergens. Clin Exp Allergy 34: 1415–21.
20. Gamboa PM, Caceres O, Antepara I, Sanchez-Monge R, Ahrazem O, et al. (2007) Two different profiles of peach allergy in the north of Spain. Allergy 62: 408–14.
21. Moneret-Vautrin DA (2005) Cross reactivity of food allergens and its clinical relevance. Bull Acad Natl Med 189: 1491–501.
22. Klinglmayr E, Hauser M, Zimmermann F, Dissertori O, Lackner P, et al. (2009) Identification of B-cell epitopes of Bet v 1 involved in cross-reactivity with food allergens. Allergy 64: 647–51.
23. Vieths S, Scheurer S, Ballmer-Weber B (2002) Current Understanding of Cross-Reactivity of Food Allergens and Pollen. Ann N Y Acad Sci 964: 47–68.
24. Lehrer SB, Reese G (1998) Cross-reactivity between cockroach allergens and arthropod, nematode and mammalian allergens. Rev Fr Allergol Immunol Clin 38: 846–8.
25. Carrapatoso I, Rodrigues F, Geraldes L, Faria E, Todo-Bom A, et al. (2008) Clinical and immunological patterns in patients with shrimp hypersensitivity and Dermatophagoides pteronyssinus cross-reactivity. Rev Port Imunoalergol 16: 449–66.
26. Leung PS, Chow WK, Duffey S, Kwan HS, Gershwin ME, et al. (1996) IgE reactivity against a cross-reactive allergen in crustacea and mollusca: evidence for tropomyosin as the common allergen. J Allergy Clin Immunol 98: 954–61.
27. Yeang HY, Hamilton RG, Bernstein DI, Arif SAM, Chow K-S, et al. (2006) Allergen concentration in natural rubber latex. Clin Exp Allergy 36: 1078–86.
28. Ariano R, Panzani RC, Falagiani P, Chiapella M, Augeri G (1993) Respiratory allergy to the pollen of Mercurialis annua (Euphorbiaceae). Ann Allergy 70: 249–54.
29. Cuesta-Herranz J, Barber D, Blanco C, Cistero-Bahima A, Crespo JF, et al. (2010) Differences among Pollen-Allergic Patients with and without Plant Food Allergy. Int Arch Allergy Immunol 153: 182–92.
30. Mari A, Wallner M, Ferreira F (2003) Fagales pollen sensitization in a birch-free area: a respiratory cohort survey using Fagales pollen extracts and birch recombinant allergens (rBet v 1, rBet v 2, rBet v 4). Clin Exp Allergy 33: 1419–28.
31. D'Avino R, Bernardi ML, Wallner M, Palazzo P, Camardella L, et al. (2011) Kiwifruit Act d 11 is the first member of the ripening-related protein family identified as an allergen. Allergy 66: 870–7.
32. Radauer C, Willerroider M, Fuchs H, Hoffmann-Sommergruber K, Thalhamer J, et al. (2006) Cross-reactive and species-specific immunoglobulin E epitopes of plant profilins: an experimental and structure-based analysis. Clin Exp Allergy 36: 920–9.
33. Radauer C, Adhami F, Furtler I, Wagner S, Allwardt D, et al. (2011) Latex-allergic patients sensitized to the major allergen hevein and hevein-like domains of class I chitinases show no increased frequency of latex-associated plant food allergy. Mol Immunol 48: 600–9.
34. van Ree R, Akkerdaas J, van Leeuwen WA, Fernandez-Rivas M, Asero R, et al. (2000) New Perspectives for the diagnosis of food allergy. Allergy Clin Immunol Int 12: 7–12.
35. Ebo D, Hagendorens M, Bridts C, De Clerck L, Stevens W (2004) Sensitization to cross-reactive carbohydrate determinants and the ubiquitous protein profilin: mimickers of allergy. Clin Exp Allergy 34: 137–44.
36. Wensing M, Akkerdaas JH, van Leeuwen WA, Stapel SO, Bruijnzeel-Koomen CA, et al. (2002) IgE to Bet v 1 and profilin: Cross-reactivity patterns and clinical relevance. J Allergy Clin Immunol 110: 435–42.
37. Kleine-Tebbe J, Vogel L, Crowell DN, Haustein UF, Vieths S (2002) Severe oral allergy syndrome and anaphylactic reactions caused by a Bet v 1- related PR-10 protein in soybean, SAM22. J Allergy Clin Immunol 110: 797–804.
38. Pastorello EA, Robino A (2004) Clinical role of lipid transfer proteins in food allergy. Mol Nutr Food Res 48: 356–62.
39. Wagner S, Breiteneder H (2002) The latex-fruit syndrome. Biochem Soc Trans 30: 935–40.
40. Harwanegg C, Hiller R (2004) Protein microarrays in diagnosing IgE-mediated diseases: spotting allergy at the molecular level. Expert Rev Mol Diagn 4: 539–48.
41. Erazo A, Kutchukhidze N, Leung M, Christ AP, Urban JF Jr., et al. (2007) Unique Maturation Program of the IgE Response In Vivo. Immunity 26: 191–203.
42. Kerzel S, Rogosch T, Struecker B, Maier RF, Zemlin M (2010) IgE Transcripts in the Circulation of Allergic Children Reflect a Classical Antigen-Driven B Cell Response and Not a Superantigen-Like Activation. J Immunol 185: 2253–60.
43. Mari A, Scala E, Ronconi AM, Carabella G (2005) Sequence Homology and IgE Co-Recognition of Allergenic Molecules: Comparative results obtained using the Allergome O-Ring Graphical Representation. Allergy Clin Immunol Int 17(Suppl 1): 205.
44. Ciardiello MA, Palazzo P, Bernardi ML, Carratore V, Giangrieco I, et al. (2010) Biochemical, immunological and clinical characterization of a cross-reactive nonspecific lipid transfer protein 1 from mulberry. Allergy 65: 597–605.
45. Gadermaier G, Harrer A, Girbl T, Palazzo P, Himly M, et al. (2009) Isoform identification and characterization of Art v 3, the lipid-transfer protein of mugwort pollen. Mol Immunol 46: 1919–24.
46. Krause S, Reese G, Randow S, Zennaro D, Quaratino D, et al. (2009) Lipid transfer protein (Ara h 9) as a new peanut allergen relevant for a Mediterranean allergic population. J Allergy Clin Immunol 124: 771–8.e5.

# 17

# Thioredoxin from the Indianmeal Moth *Plodia interpunctella*: Cloning and Test of the Allergenic Potential in Mice

**Elisabeth Hoflehner[1], Marina Binder[1], Wolfgang Hemmer[2], Vera Mahler[3], Raphael C. Panzani[4], Reinhart Jarisch[2], Ursula Wiedermann[1], Michael Duchêne[1]***

**1** Institute of Specific Prophylaxis and Tropical Medicine, Center for Pathophysiology, Infectiology and Immunology, Medical University of Vienna, Vienna, Austria, **2** Floridsdorfer Allergiezentrum, Vienna, Austria, **3** Department of Dermatology, University of Erlangen-Nuremberg, Erlangen, Germany, **4** Centre de recherche en allergologie, Marseille, France

## Abstract

***Background/Objective:*** The Indianmeal moth *Plodia interpunctella* is a highly prevalent food pest in human dwellings, and has been shown to contain a number of allergens. So far, only one of these, the arginine kinase (Plo i 1) has been identified.

***Objective:*** The aim of this study was to identify further allergens and characterise these in comparison to Plo i 1.

***Method:*** A cDNA library from whole adult *P. interpunctella* was screened with the serum of a patient with indoor allergy and IgE to moths, and thioredoxin was identified as an IgE-binding protein. Recombinant thioredoxin was generated in *E. coli*, and tested together with Plo i 1 and whole moth extracts in IgE immunoblots against a large panel of indoor allergic patients' sera. BALB/c mice were immunised with recombinant thioredoxin and Plo i 1, and antibody production, mediator release from RBL cells, T-cell proliferation and cytokine production were measured.

***Result:*** For the first time a thioredoxin from an animal species was identified as allergen. About 8% of the sera from patients with IgE against moth extracts reacted with recombinant *P. interpunctella* thioredoxin, compared to 25% reacting with recombinant Plo i 1. In immunised BALB/c mice, the recombinant allergens both induced classical Th2-biased immune responses such as induction IgE and IgG1 antibodies, upregulation of IL-5 and IL-4 and basophil degranulation.

***Conclusion:*** Thioredoxin from moths like Plo i 1 acts like a classical Type I allergen as do the thioredoxins from wheat or corn. This clearly supports the pan-allergen nature of thioredoxin. The designation Plo i 2 is suggested for the new *P. interpunctella* allergen.

**Editor:** Jean Kanellopoulos, University Paris Sud, France

**Funding:** This study was supported by Grant 8643 from the "Jubiläumsstiftung der Österreichischen Nationalbank", and by Grant H-1760/2006 from the "Hochschuljubiläumsstiftung der Stadt Wien", Vienna, Austria. The funders had no role in study design, data collection and analysis, decision to publish, or preparation of the manuscript.

**Competing Interests:** The authors have declared that no competing interests exist.

* E-mail: michael.duchene@meduniwien.ac.at

These authors contributed equally to this work.

## Introduction

Arthropods represent more than three quarters of all animal species, and get into contact with humans in multiple ways. Arthropod antigens can cause Type I allergies with various manifestations, such as the acute and life-threatening insect venom allergies [1], perennial rhinitis, dermatitis and bronchial asthma caused by house dust mites [2] or cockroaches [3,4], as well as oral symptoms caused by seafood [5].

Although moths like cockroaches are typical and widespread household pests, there is much less research on Type I allergy against moth proteins. Historically, that moths cause inhalant allergies had been reported as early as 1928 by Vaughan [6]. In the following decades, there have been occasional case reports on bronchial asthma caused by moths, such as by the clothes moth *Tineola bisselliella* in an infested home [7] or the wax moth *Galleria mellonella* in a company producing fish bait [8]. More recently, IgE immunoblots of clothes moth [9] or silkworm moth [10] demonstrated specific IgE against moth antigens.

The Indianmeal moth *Plodia interpunctella* is a common household and stored product pest. Its larvae feed on dry foodstuffs such as grains, nuts, dried fruit, or chocolate. This pest had been suspected early to be a possible source of allergens in mills [11]. The first *P. interpunctella* allergen to be identified on the molecular level (Plo i 1) was an arginine kinase [12]. Arginine kinase (EC 2.7.3.3) phosphorylates arginine, whereas the related creatine kinase (EC 2.7.3.2) acts on creatine. Both enzymes thus help to store metabolic energy, where creatine kinase is typically found in vertebrates and arginine kinase is found in lower species such as arthropods and some protozoa [13]. The arthropod arginine kinases exhibit IgE cross-reactivity [12], and several further arginine kinases have been identified as allergens, *e.g.* from shrimp [14,15] and mite [16].

IgE immunoblots of *P. interpunctella* whole larval extracts were positive in 51% when probed with sera from indoor allergic patients [12]. In this study we extend this work using extracts from adult moths. IgE screening of a cDNA library of the imago stage of *P. interpunctella* revealed a further allergen, a thioredoxin.

Thioredoxins are ubiquitous redox-active proteins found in eukaryotes and prokaryotes. They activate proteins by reduction of cysteine disulphide bonds [17,18]. Thioredoxins have been identified as allergens in wheat and maize [19] as well as fungi such as *Malassezia* spp. [20]. In human allergic bronchopulmonary aspergillosis, IgE cross-reactivity of fungal and human thioredoxin was found to result in IgE autoreactivity [21]. Recently, wheat flour thioredoxin was identified as an allergen in patients with baker's asthma [22].

In this study, the allergenic potential of thioredoxin as a new arthropod allergen was examined in comparison to Plo i 1 by IgE immunoblotting and in a mouse immunisation model.

## Materials and Methods

### Ethics statement and patient characteristics

The study was approved by the ethics committee of the Medical University of Vienna and the Vienna General Hospital (application EK Nr. 322/2008). The anonymised sera to be tested in immunoblots (n = 156, of which n = 154 were allergic patients'sera and n = 2 nonallergic control sera) are displayed in detail in Table 1.

The diagnosis of Type I allergy was based on case history and symptoms (rhinitis/conjunctivitis, allergic asthma), skin prick testing as well as CAP-RAST (Pharmacia, Uppsala, Sweden) testing using a panel of extracts from indoor (house dust mite, cat dander) and outdoor (birch pollen, grass pollen) allergen sources. The cDNA library from adult *P. interpunctella* was screened with the serum from an indoor-allergic patient with IgE reactivity to Indianmeal moths.

### Construction of a *P. interpunctella* cDNA library from imagines

*P. interpunctella* larvae were left to hide for metamorphosis in a roll of cardboard with vertical holes. When the moths emerged, they were immediately frozen in liquid nitrogen. Four hundred moths (around 3.2 g) were homogenised in 30 ml of TRIzol reagent (Life Technologies, Frederick, MD), and about 10 mg of total RNA were extracted. Poly(A)$^+$ RNA was prepared using the Poly(A)Ttract system (Promega, Madison, WI, USA) with a yield of 4.9 µg from 4 mg of total RNA. The cDNA library prepared with the Uni-ZAP system (Stratagene, La Jolla, CA, USA) [23] contained $1.25\times10^6$ clones.

### IgE screening of the λZAP cDNA library

λZAP phages ($2.8\times10^5$) from the primary library were plated on *Escherichia coli* XL1-Blue (Stratagene). Synthesis of recombinant proteins was induced by adding nitrocellulose filters (Schleicher & Schuell, Dassel, Germany) soaked in 10 mM isopropylthio β-D-galactoside (IPTG). The filters were blocked, and probed with a 1/10 dilution of a serum which contained IgE against several moth proteins. IgE bound to recombinant moth proteins was detected by $^{125}$I-labeled anti-IgE antibodies (Pharmacia) followed by autoradiography. Further rounds of screening were then performed to obtain single phage clones.

The cDNA-containing plasmids were obtained from the isolated phages by *in vivo* excision [23]. Twenty two cDNAs were sequenced using Thermosequenase (Amersham Pharmacia Biotech, Piscataway, NJ, USA) and IRD800-labeled primers on a LI-COR sequencer (LI-COR, Lincoln, NE, USA). The deduced protein sequences were compared with the SwissProt database using the FastA program [24]. Nucleotide sequences were aligned with the ClustalW program [25].

### Expression of *P. interpunctella* thioredoxin in *E. coli*

The oligodeoxynucleotide primers ExTrxF 5′-GGG ACT TC**C ATA TG**T CGA TCC ACA TCA AAG ACG TTG AGG AC-3′ and ExTrxR 5′-TCC G**CT CGA G**TT AAT GAT GGT GAT GAT GAT GCT TGA GTT TCA AAA TGG TGG ACC G-3′ were used for PCR to amplify the *P. interpunctella* thioredoxin coding sequence from the cDNA template (clone 1). The primers contain *Nde*I and *Xho*I restriction sites (bold) for cloning into the expression plasmid pET-17b (Novagen, Merck, Darmstadt, Germany) plus a hexahistidine-encoding sequence (underlined) for recombinant protein purification.

The recombinant pET-17b plasmid was transformed into *E. coli* BL21-CodonPlus (DE3) (Stratagene). The cultures were grown to an $OD_{600}$ of 0.75, recombinant protein production was induced by addition of 1 mM IPTG and shaking overnight at 18°C.

**Table 1.** Demographics and symptoms of the groups of patients' sera examined in this study.

| Symptomatic Type I allergy against | Abbre-viation in Fig. 1 | Number of patients | Age range | Mean age | Female: male ratio | RC [%] | Asthma [%] | AD [%] |
|---|---|---|---|---|---|---|---|---|
| House dust mites but not animal dander | M | 69 | 1–64 | 21.3 | 31 : 38 | 77 | 38 | 6 |
| House dust mites and animal dander | M+D | 43 | 9–61 | 30.0 | 16 : 27 | 74 | 49 | 12 |
| Animal dander but not house dust mites | D−M | 20 | 3–56 | 27.7 | 10 : 10 | 60 | 65 | 0 |
| Seafood | SF | 22 | 17–76 | 38.5 | 7 : 15 | 50 | 36 | 0 |
| Nonallergic controls | NC | 2 | 37–49 | 44.0 | 1 : 1 | 0 | 0 | 0 |
| Total allergy patients | | 154 | 1–76 | 27.0 | 64 : 90 | 70 | 44 | 6 |
| Total individuals | | 156 | 1–76 | 27.2 | 65 : 91 | | | |

The sera were from Floridsdorfer Allergiezentrum, Vienna, Austria. The last three colums give the percentage of patients reporting rhinitis and/or conjuctivitis (RC), asthma or asthma-like symptoms ("asthma"), or atopic dermatitis (AD).

Harvesting of cells, lysis and purification of recombinant thioredoxin via metal chelate affinity chromatography under native conditions were performed according to the supplier's protocol (Qiagen, Hilden, Germany). Recombinant *P. interpunctella* arginine kinase (Plo i 1) was produced as described [12].

## IgE-immunoblots of moth extracts and the recombinant allergens

Whole extracts from imagines of the Mediterranean flour moth (*Ephestia kuehniella*), a species closely related to *P. interpunctella* but considerably larger, were obtained by grinding of 150 moths with liquid nitrogen in a mortar. Fifteen ml of 1× reducing gel loading buffer were added, samples were denatured for 10 min at 95°C, and debris was removed by centrifugation. The whole extracts or, respectively, the purified recombinant allergens (arginine kinase (Plo i 1) and moth thioredoxin) were separated on preparative 12.5% SDS - polyacrylamide gels with an approximate protein concentration of 20 μg/cm (extracts) or 10 μg/cm (of each purified recombinant protein) as estimated by Coomassie blue-stained test gels. Proteins were blotted onto nitrocellulose membranes (Schleicher & Schuell), and 5 mm strips were cut after the transfer. The strips were blocked 2×5 min and 1×30 min at room temperature with buffer G (42 mM $Na_2HPO_4$, 6.4 mM $NaH_2PO_4$, 0.5% (v/v) Tween 20, 0.5% (w/v) bovine serum albumin, 0.05% (w/v) $NaN_3$, pH 7.5), and incubated with a 1/10 dilution of patients' sera in buffer G overnight at 4°C. After washing 2×5 min and 1×30 min in buffer G, bound IgE was detected by overnight incubation at room temperature with $^{125}$I-labeled anti-IgE antibodies (IBL, Hamburg, Germany), washing as above, and autoradiography at −80°C.

## Ethics statement on animal treatment and sampling

The animal study was performed according to institutional guidelines for animal use and care. The study was approved under the number GZ BMBWK-66.009/0246-BrGT/2005 by the Austrian Federal Ministry of Science and Research.

Female BALB/c mice (n = 5 per group, aged 7 weeks) were purchased from the Research Institute for Laboratory Animal Breeding (Himberg, Austria). Sensitisation was performed by four subcutaneous (s.c.) injections (day 0, 14, 28, 42) of 1 μg, 5 μg or 25 μg of Plo i 1 (arginine kinase) or Plo i 2 (thioredoxin) adsorbed to aluminium hydroxide ($Al(OH)_3$; Serva, Heidelberg, Germany). Control mice were sham-treated with PBS. Blood samples were taken before treatment (day 0), and 7 days after the last immunisation (day 49) by tail bleeding. At sacrifice cell suspensions from spleens were prepared as described [26].

## Allergen-specific antibody levels in mouse sera

Microtiter plates (Nunc, Roskilde, Denmark) were coated with 5 μg/ml of the recombinant allergens Plo i 1 or Plo i 2, respectively, and incubated with sera. Serum samples were diluted 1/500 for IgG2a, 1/1000 for IgG1 and 1/10 for IgE. Rat anti-mouse IgG2a, IgG1 and IgE antibodies (1/500, Pharmingen, San Diego, CA) were used, followed by peroxidase-conjugated mouse anti-rat IgG antibodies (1/2000, Jackson Immuno Lab, West Grove, PA) [26]. Data are shown as optical density (OD) after subtraction of baseline levels from pre-immune sera.

## Rat basophil leukaemia cell mediator release assay (RBL assay)

Sera were incubated with RBL-2H3 cells (cell line from rat basophilic leukemia, available from ATCC, No. CRL-2256) at dilutions of 1/10. IgE-dependent degranulation of RBL cells was induced by adding 0.03 μg of each allergen (Plo i 1 or Plo i 2) diluted in 100 μl Tyrode's buffer. Supernatants were analysed for ß-hexosaminidase activity as described previously [27]. Data are reported as percen-tages of total ß-hexosaminidase released after addition of 1% Triton X-100 and are shown after subtraction of baseline release levels obtained with pre-immune sera.

## Lymphocyte proliferation and cytokine production

Proliferation of splenocytes ($2\times10^5$ cells/well) after stimulation with the recombinant allergens Plo i 1 or, respectively, Plo i 2 (2 μg/well) was measured as described previously [27]. The ratio of the mean proliferation after antigen stimulation (counts per minute [cpm]) and medium control values [cpm], *i.e.* the stimulation index [SI], was calculated.

Levels of IL-4, IL-5 and IFN-γ were measured in spleen cell cultures ($5\times10^6$ cells/well) incubated for 48 hours with Plo i 1 or Plo i 2 (10 μg/well) [26]. Cytokine levels were measured with mouse ELISA kits (Endogen, Woburn, MA) and were shown in pg/ml after subtraction of baseline levels of unstimulated cultures.

## Statistics

Data are expressed as means ± SEMs. For statistical analysis p values$<$0.05 were defined significant. Pair-wise comparison of allergen- sensitised versus sham-treated control groups was performed by using the non-parametric Kruskal–Wallis test, followed by ad hoc post analysis.

# Results

## Prevalence of IgE binding to moth extracts in sera from indoor-allergic patients

Previously we had shown that 51% of unselected patients with indoor allergies had serum IgE antibodies against *P. interpunctella* larval extracts. In the present study we tested 154 anonymised type I allergic patients' sera and two non-allergic control sera from Vienna (see Table 1). These comprised the following groups of patients: patients with indoor allergies to house dust mite (n = 69), to house dust mite and animal dander (n = 43), to animal dander but not house dust mite (n = 20), in addition seafood allergic patients (n = 22), and two non-allergic control sera.

Extracts from whole *E. kuehniella* moths, flour moths closely related to *P. interpunctella*, but yielding significantly more extract per animal, were used to prepare immunoblot strips. These strips were used to probe all the sera for IgE antibodies against moth antigens. The results are shown in Fig. 1 (top parts). A low IgE reactivity, which we interpret as weak binding of the moth antigens to the secondary antibody, was observed in the sera from nonallergic individuals (NC) and the buffer controls (BC) and is always taken into account. In the indoor allergic patient groups, 48% the sera reacted significantly with moth allergens contained in the whole extract, similar to the 51% found previously for *P. interpunctella* larval antigens [12]. This varied from 43% in the group of indoor allergic patients with mite allergy only (M) to 53% in the patients with allergies to mites and animal dander (M+D). In the group with indoor allergy to animal dander but not to mites (D−M), 50% reacted with moth allergens. Although the frequency of IgE recognition did not vary so much between the groups, a striking difference was observed in the quantity of moth specific IgE. In a number of the mite allergic and moth IgE-positive patients, and even more in the mite and dander allergic and moth IgE-positive patients, very high moth specific IgE levels were observed. None of the 20 patients tested negative for mites (D−M) showed such a high level of reactivity. The binding of IgE to moth antigens was highest, however, in the group of seafood allergic patients (SF), in

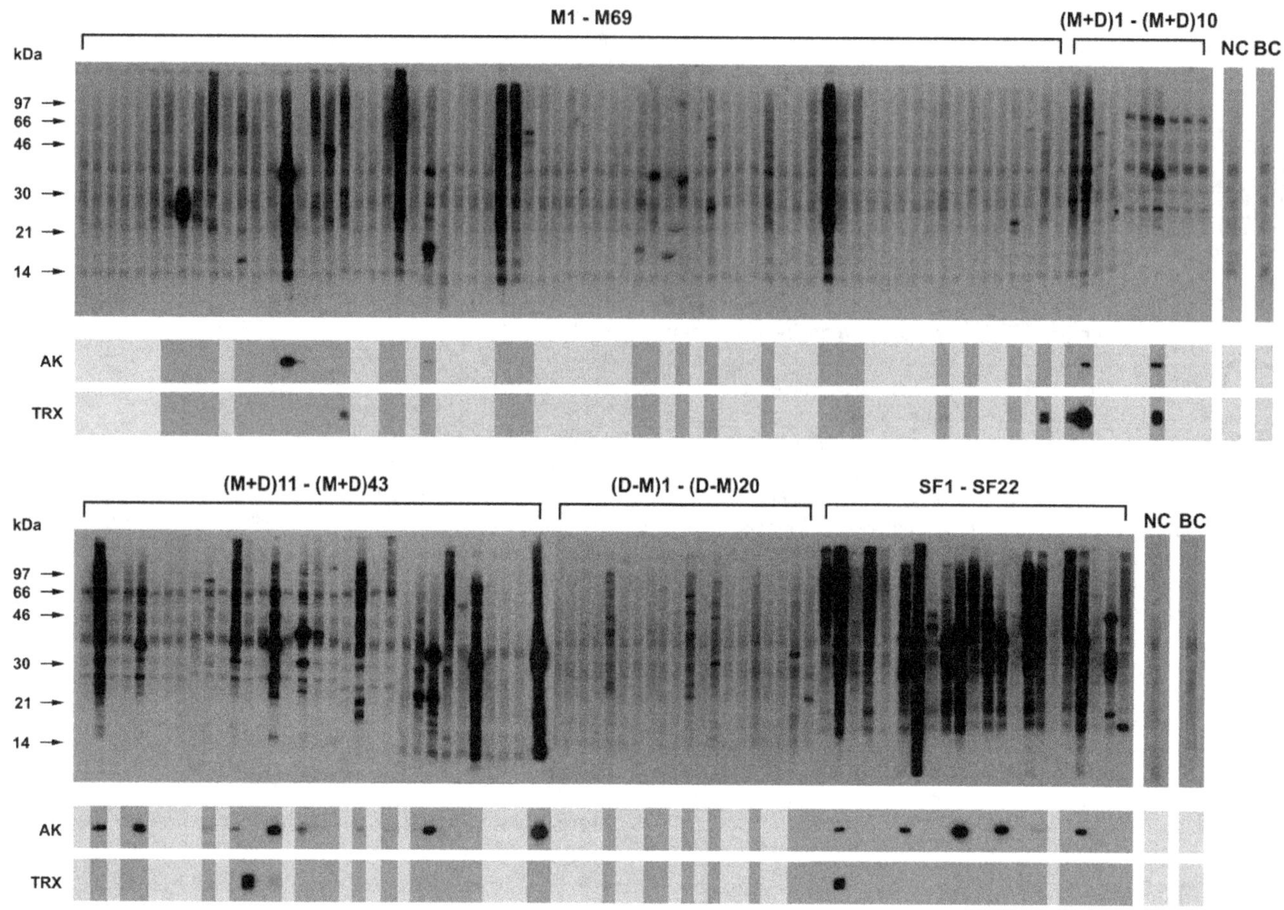


**Figure 1. IgE immunoblots with patients' sera.** Top panels: extracts from whole mediterranean flour moths (*E. kuehniella*) were separated by polyacrylamide electrophoresis, blotted onto nitrocellulose, and probed with the sera from various groups of patients with indoor allergy or seafood allergy as well as from control individuals. The indoor allergic patient groups were: M, housedust mite allergic patients (n = 69), M+D, patients allergic to mites and animal dander (n = 43), D−M, patients with allergy to animal dander but not to mites (n = 20). Patients SF, seafood allergic patients (n = 22), NC, nonallergic control individuals (n = 2), BC, buffer control without serum, only secondary anti-IgE antibody. Molecular weights [kDa] are indicated at the left side. Bottom panels, the recombinant *P. interpunctella* 40 kDa arginine kinase (AK) and 12 kDa thioredoxin (TRX) were probed with those patients' sera containing IgE to *E. kuehniella*, and only the parts of the strips containing the two recombinant allergens are shown.

relative numbers, 95% of the sera were positive, and 55% of these sera contained very high levels of levels of IgE binding to moth antigens.

Taken together, immunoreactive bands of various molecular weights were observed on the blots and in order to identify more moth allergens, a moth cDNA library was constructed and screened.

## Cloning of *P. interpunctella* thioredoxin as an IgE-binding protein from adult moths

As described above, a λZAP cDNA library from *P. interpunctella* imagines was probed with the serum from a patient with indoor allergies and IgE binding to several moth antigens. The primary screen gave 40 strong and 10 weak positive signals. After reprobing, 22 single cDNA clones were obtained and sequenced. Twenty of these encoded a *P. interpunctella* protein with significant sequence similarity to thioredoxins. Three of the 20 clones contained single base insertions and deletions resulting in truncation of the open reading frame. The other 17 clones comprised the identical open reading frame encoding a protein of 11.7 kDa. The 3′-untranslated region of 689 bp between the stop codon and the poly-A tail was rather long. Minor differences were obtained in this region, but these did not allow to group the cDNAs into possible isoforms. The complete sequence of clone 1 was submitted to the EMBL/GenBank/DDBJ databases (accession number FR681573).

The BlastP search clearly identified the protein as thioredoxin. Fig. 2 shows *P. interpunctella* thioredoxin (Pi) aligned with selected other thioredoxins. The most closely related sequence with 83% amino acid identity was from the domestic silkworm *Bombyx mori* (Bm). The thioredoxin from the more distantly related arthropod *Litopenaeus vannamei* (Lv) and human thioredoxin (Hs) were 58% and 46% identical, respectively, to *P. interpunctella* thioredoxin. The allergenic fungal thioredoxin (2J23_A) Mala s 13 from *Malassezia sympodialis* (Ms) and wheat (*Triticum aestivum*) thioredoxin Tri a 25 (Ta) (CAB96931) were 46% and 41% identical. All the sequences contained the active site consensus WCGPC with the two redox-active cysteines.

We obtained only two other IgE-positive cDNAs from the same screen not coding for thioredoxin. The delicate extraction of RNA from adult moth material, a possible advantage of λZAP phage expressing thioredoxin leading to a preponderance in the composition of the plated library, or a peculiarity of the patient's serum used for screening may contribute to this finding. We did

```
Pi                    MSIHIKDVEDLTARLTEA  GDKLVVIDFMATWCGPCKIIGPKL 42
Bm                    -------SD--KT--A--  G----------------M----- 42
Lv                    -VYQV--Q--S-KQ-N--  GN-------Y--------M-A--- 42
Hs                    -VKQ-ESKTAFQEA-DA-  G-----V--S--------M-K-FF 42
Ms     MRGSHHHHHHLVPRG-VQVISSY-QFKQV-G    G--V-----W--------M---VF 55
Ta   MAASAATATAAAVGAGEV-SVHSL-QW-MQIE--NAAK-------T-S-----R-MA-IF 60

Pi   DEIA AEMADSIVVVKVDVDECEDIATEYSINTMPTFVFVKNGKPVEQFSGANVEKLRST 101
Bm   ---- ---S-----------------S--N--S-----------KLDE------D--KT- 101
Lv   E-LS QS-S- V-FL-----------QDNQ-AC----L-M---QKLDSL-----D--LEL 100
Hs   HSLS EKYSN VIFLE----D-Q-V-S-CEVKC----Q-F-K-QK-GE-----K---EA- 100
Ms   EK-SDTPAG-KVGFY------QSQ--Q-VG-RA------F---QKIDTVV--DPS--QAA 115
Ta   ADL-  KKFPAA-FL------LKS--EQF-VEA----L-M-E-DVKDRVV--IK-E-TNK 118

Pi   ILKLK   106
Bm   ---H-   106
Lv   VE-N-   105
Hs   -NE-V   105
Ms   -TQHSA  121
Ta   VGLHAAQ 125
```

**Figure 2. Comparison of thioredoxin sequences.** The deduced amino acid sequence of *P. interpunctella* thioredoxin Plo i 2 (Pi) was aligned with *Bombyx mori* thioredoxin (ABM92269) (Bm) with 83% identity. The other arthropod thioredoxin from the shrimp *Litopenaeus vannamei* (ACA60746) (Lv) was 58% identical, and human thioredoxin (NP_003320) (Hs) shared 47% amino acid identity with Pi. The allergenic fungal thioredoxin (2J23_A) Mala s 13 from *Malassezia sympodialis* (Ms) and wheat (*Triticum aestivum*) thioredoxin Tri a 25 (Ta) (CAB96931) were 46% and 41% identical, respectively with Plo i 2. The residues equal to Plo i 2 are marked with dashes. The important thioredoxin consensus sequence WCGPC with the two active site cysteines was found in all the sequences (bold type).

not investigate this matter in more detail and focused on the characterisation of thioredoxin as a novel allergen from moths.

## Prevalence of IgE binding to recombinant *P. interpunctella* thioredoxin and arginine kinase (Plo i 1) in sera from indoor-allergic patients

Recombinant thioredoxin (11.7 kDa) and arginine kinase, Plo i 1, (39.9 kDa) [12] from *P. interpunctella* were separated together under denaturing and reducing conditions in SDS-PAGE, blotted onto nitrocellulose, and strips were probed with the sera that had shown positive reactivity with the whole moth extracts. The signals from the recombinant allergens arginine kinase Plo i 1 and thioredoxin are displayed in Fig. 1 as two blocks AK (40 kDa) and TRX (12 kDa) mounted below the whole moth extract strips.

Counting only the clearly positive signals, seven patients' sera had IgE towards *P. interpunctella* thioredoxin, six in the various indoor allergic groups and one in the seafood allergic group, but none in mite negative group. This corresponds to 8% of all moth extract positive patients, 5% of all allergic patients of this study. Again the strongest signals were observed in patients with concomitant mite allergy or concomitant mite and dander allergy, and in the seafood allergic patients. Due to this small but significant number of sera with IgE to moth thioredoxin, we proposed to name this allergen Plo i 2, and it is now available in the IUIS allergen nomenclature database as Plo i 2.0101.

In contrast to the Plo i 1 homolog, we noted the absence of 12 kDa bands of the natural thioredoxin in the blots from the whole moth extracts. This could have several causes, for example, the concentration of thioredoxin could simply be low, or as the immunoblots for whole moth extracts were not optimised for small proteins, some thioredoxin might have been lost during blotting. Alternatively, thioredoxin still bound covalently to its interaction partners [17,18] could migrate at higher molecular weights. Finally, the patients' IgE could possibly recognise *P. interpunctella* thioredoxin better than the *E. kuehniella* homolog. To investigate this cross-reactivity, we performed an inhibition experiment as

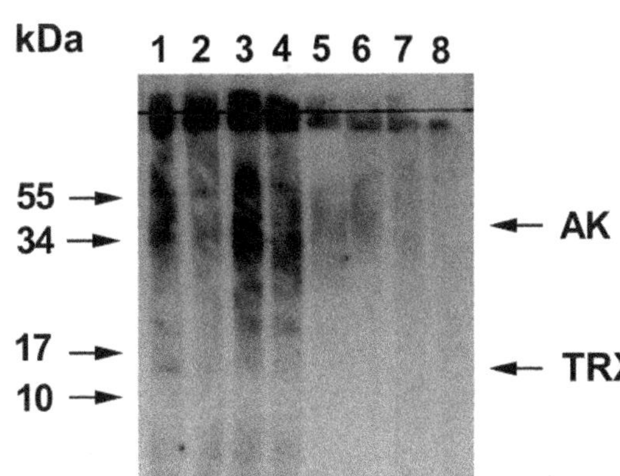


**Figure 3. Immunoblot inhibition experiment.** Extracts from *E. kuehniella* were separated by polyacrylamide electrophoresis, blotted onto nitrocellulose, and strips were probed with serum samples preincubated with or without 10 μg of recombinant allergen overnight. Lane 1, thioredoxin (Plo i 2) positive serum; lane 2, same serum preincubated with recombinant *P. interpunctella* thioredoxin; lane 3, arginine kinase (Plo i 1) positive serum; lane 4, same serum preincubated with recombinant Plo i 1; lane 5, nonallergic control serum, lane 6, same serum preincubated with Plo i 2; lane 7, same serum preincubated with Plo i 1; lane 8, buffer control. Molecular weights [kDa] are indicated at the left side, the positions of thioredoxin (TRX) and arginine kinase (AK) at the right side.

done previously [12] (Fig. 3). Two 1 ml samples of a 1:10 dilution of a thioredoxin positive serum in buffer G (see Materials and Methods) were preincubated with or without 10 µg of recombinant *P. interpunctella* thioredoxin overnight at 4°C, and then used to probe strips of blotted *E. kuehniella* antigens as described above (Fig. 3, lanes 1, 2). Similarly an inhibition was carried out with a Plo i 1 positive serum and recombinant Plo i 1 (Fig. 3, lanes 3, 4) or a nonallergic control serum (Fig. 3, lanes 5–7), here lane 5 shows the uninhibited serum, lane 6 was preincubated with recombinant thioredoxin and lane 7 with recombinant arginine kinase. Lane 8 represents the buffer control. One important result of the experiment was that the 12 kDa thioredoxin band only appeared after the blot was exposed for 14 days instead of two days. This shows that the extracts contained only a low concentration of thioredoxin and explain the absence of signals in the previous blots. With the help of specific antibodies against recombinant Plo i 2, it should be possible to better quantify the allergen in the extracts and to check if it forms covalent adducts of larger molecular weight with its interaction partners.

The main result of the inhibition experiment was that recombinant Plo i 2 was able to block the binding of the patient's IgE to the *E. kuehniella* thioredoxin (Fig. 3, lane 2) as well as recombinant Plo i 1 blocked the binding to *E. kuehiella* arginine kinase (Fig. 3, lane 4). So the allergens from the closely related moths are cross-reactive.

The immunoblot experiment with the recombinant arginine kinase (Fig. 1, lower panels) showed that 21 of all the patients with IgE to moth extracts (25%) had specific IgE to Plo i 1, and again

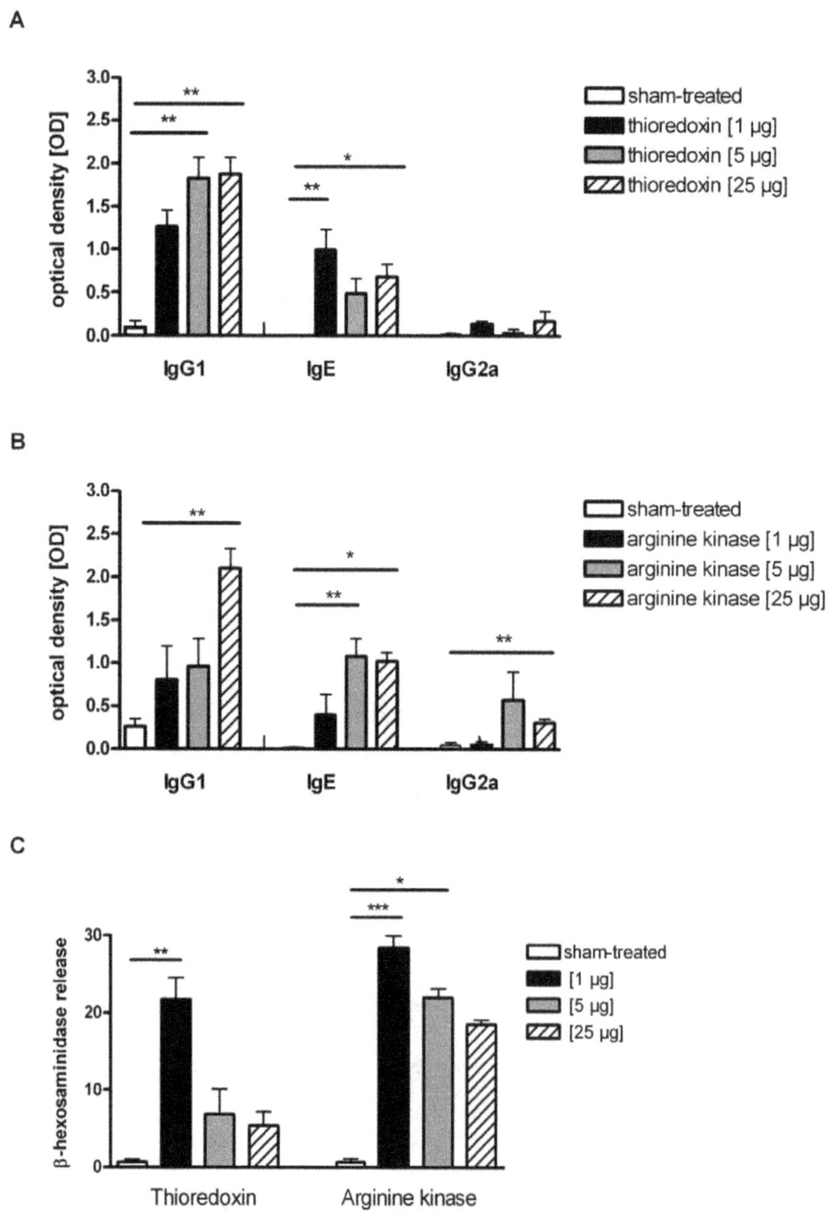


**Figure 4. Antibody levels in mouse sera.** (A), thioredoxin, (B), arginine kinase-specific antibody responses in sera after immunisation with three different antigen concentrations (1 µg, 5 µg, 25 µg) measured by ELISA; (C), IgE-mediated basophil degranulation in sera, β- hexosaminidase release from thioredoxin- and arginine kinase-sensitised mice, treated with 1 µg (black bars), 5 µg (grey bars) or 25 µg (striped bars), compared to sham-treated controls (white bars). *p<0.05, **p<0.01, ***p<0.005.

the groups with mite, mite and dander, and seafood allergies had the highest prevalence and displayed the strongest signals, no Plo i 1 positive reactions were detected in any mite negative patient. The prevalence of IgE to Plo i 1 is the same as the 25% frequency of recognition of Plo i 1 in moth larval extract positive patients observed previously [12].

## Antibody production in sensitised mice

To investigate the immunogenicity of thioredoxin (Plo i 2) and arginine kinase (Plo i 1) we sensitised mice four times subcutaneously with three different concentrations of the recombinant allergens (1 μg, 5 μg, 25 μg). Treatment with thioredoxin induced strong Th2 responses with increased IgG1 levels for all three concentrations, whereas treatment with 5 μg and 25 μg showed significantly increased antibody levels in comparison to sham-treated mice. IgE antibody production in thioredoxin-treated mice was significantly upregulated after sensitisation with the lowest concentration of 1 μg and with the highest concentration of 25 μg allergen, respectively, compared to controls. The typical Th1-associated IgG2a was only enhanced in mice, treated with 1 μg and 25 μg thioredoxin (Fig. 4A).

Arginine kinase-specific IgG1 was induced with all three concentrations, but only treatment with 25 μg showed a significantly increased antibody production, compared to controls. Whereas arginine kinase-specific IgE was significantly induced with a concentration of 5 μg as well as 25 μg, in comparison to sham-treated mice, IgG2a production was significantly increased in 25 μg- arginine kinase-treated mice (Fig. 4B).

For thioredoxin, IgE-dependent basophil degranulation was induced with all three concentrations, significantly increased only in 1 μg-sensitised group in comparison to controls. Similarly, immunisation with 1 μg and 5 μg arginine kinase induced significantly high IgE-depended basophil degranulation compared to controls (Fig. 4C).

## Cytokine production in sensitised mice

Both arginine kinase and thioredoxin induced strong cellular responses with high IL-5 and IL-4 levels in restimulated spleen cell cultures, while IFN-γ was induced only by arginine kinase. Th2 cytokine production in splenocytes of thioredoxin-treated mice showed significantly induced IL-5 levels in 1 μg-sensitised groups, compared to sham-treated mice. Thioredoxin-specific IL-4 was increased in all treated groups, in comparison to controls. Thioredoxin did not induce IFN-γ (Fig. 5A). Arginine kinase showed similar high IL-5 levels for all three sensitisation concentrations like thioredoxin. In particular, application of 5 μg arginine kinase showed the highest IL-5 and IL-4 production. Sensitisation with 5 μg or 25 μg arginine kinase induced significantly increased IL-4 levels compared to sham-treated group. Moreover, a low production of IFN-γ was measured in arginine kinase-treated mice, which reached significant IFN-γ levels in 1 μg and 5 μg treated mice compared to controls (Fig. 5B).

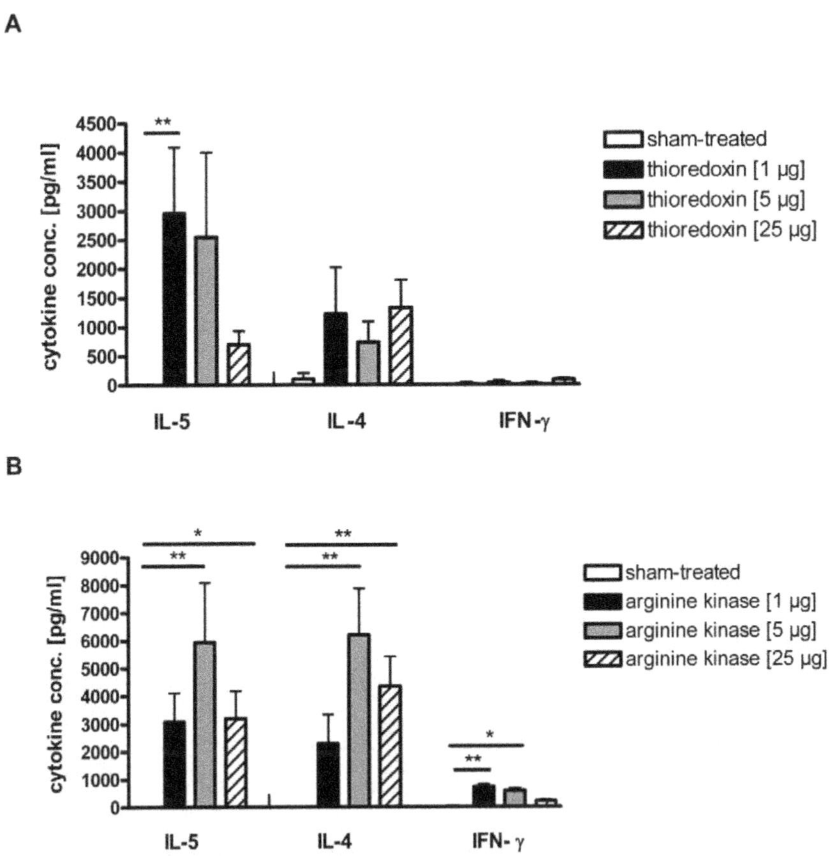


**Figure 5. Cellular immune responses.** IL-5, IL-4 and IFN-γ levels in supernatants of restimulated spleen cell cultures of mice, treated with 1 μg (black bars), 5 μg (grey bars) or 25 μg (striped bars) of (A), thioredoxin or (B), arginine kinase, or sham-treated (white bars). Groups were compared to sham-treated controls. *p<0.05, **p<0.01.

### Proliferative response of stimulated lymphocytes

Thioredoxin restimulated splenocytes showed an increased proliferation response (SI: 4) for all 3 treatment groups. Immunisation with 25 µg thioredoxin provoked a significantly induced proliferation compared to sham-treated mice.

Arginine kinase-sensitised mice showed cellular responses only in the group with 1 µg treatment concentration, not with 5 µg or 25 µg, in comparison to controls (Fig. 6).

## Discussion

The IgE immunoblot experiments probing indoor allergic patients' sera with extracts from adult moths confirmed previous results on larval extracts [12] and showed IgE positivity in 48% of the sera of indoor allergic patients, therefore moths have to be considered a relevant source of allergens.

The complex and only partially resolved immunoblot band patterns show that there are numerous moth IgE antigens. Although many patients without mite allergy have IgE against moth components, the *in vitro* reactivity is weaker than in mite positive patients. As some of these individuals may bind to cross-reactive carbohydrate determinants (CCDs) in the moth extracts, we do not know at this time how much mite-independent moth allergy could exist. Certainly, the allergens cross-reactive between moth and mite may contribute to this enhanced IgE reactivity. An additional phenomenon is that the mite and animal dander allergic patients together with the seafood allergic patients show the highest levels of IgE binding to moths. It appears as if these polysensitised patients show a stronger atopic predisposition and higher IgE levels. So far we do not know what is the contribution of moth allergens in the sensitisation of these patients.

IgE screening of a *P. interpunctella* cDNA library produced a number of immunopositive clones mostly encoding thioredoxin. Testing the moth positive sera against recombinant thioredoxin gave a positive reaction in 5% of all examined allergic patients, 8% of moth positive patients, whereas recombinant Plo i 1 tested positive in 14% of all sera, 25% of moth positive sera. The data show that thioredoxin (now named Plo i 2) is a minor allergen, however, the majority of those with positive reactivity showed a high level of thioredoxin-specific IgE. The prevalence of thioredoxin reactivity was highest in the group of indoor allergic patients reacting with mites and animal dander.

Recombinant thioredoxin like arginine kinase induced a Th2-biased immune response with significantly enhanced IgE and IgG1 antibody levels at the humoral site as well as a marked upregulation of IL-5 and IL-4 cytokines on the cellular site. Moreover, significantly enhanced IgE-mediated basophil degranulation with even 1 µg allergen confirmed the clinical relevant Th2-biased immune response of thioredoxin as well.

Thioredoxin is a truly ubiquitous protein with pleiotropic activities found both in eukaryotes and prokaryotes. It had been identified as an allergen in wheat and maize [19], in fungi [20,21], and in this study for the first time in a representative from the

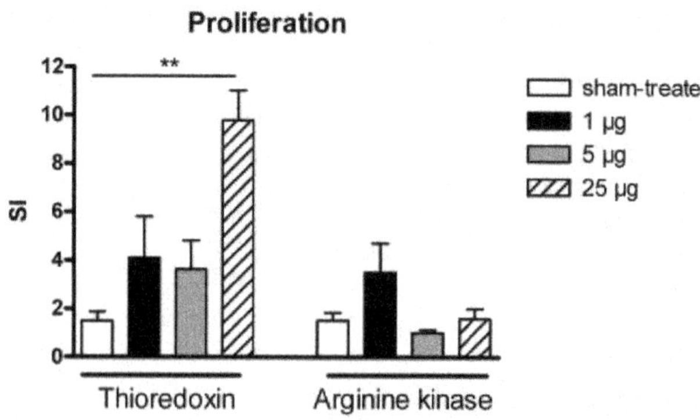


**Figure 6. In vitro splenocyte stimulation.** Stimulation index [SI] of thioredoxin or arginine kinase restimulated spleen cell cultures of mice, treated with 1 µg (black bars), 5 µg (grey bars) or 25 µg (striped bars) antigen, compared to sham-treated controls (white bars). $^{**}p<0.01$.

animal kingdom strengthening its denomination as a member of a novel pan-allergen family [20] like the profilins [28].

Finally, we have noted that under certain conditions thioredoxins may also diminish the allergic response [29]. Treatment of commercial wheat allergen extract with reduced wheat thioredoxin, thioredoxin reductase, and NADPH reduced its allergenic potency, measured in a dog skin test model [30]. Similarly, thioredoxin reduced the allergenicity of β-lactoglobulin, the major bovine milk allergen [31]. In comparison to wild-type mice, transgenic mice overexpressing human thioredoxin showed a diminished mast cell histamine release in response to 2,4-dinitrophenylated bovine serum albumin [32]. Apoptosis can be induced in human bronchial epithelial cells by house dust mite-stimulated eosinophils. This effect is weaker when the epithelial cells overexpress human thioredoxin [33]. Further studies will have to show whether moth thioredoxin might also have any moderating activity on allergic responses similar to those reported for wheat and human thioredoxins.

## Acknowledgments

We thank Sabine Prozell and Matthias Schöller (Biologische Beratung, Berlin, Germany) for the *P. interpunctella* moths and Cornel Adler (Federal Biological Research Centre for Agriculture and Forestry, Berlin) for the *E. kuehniella* moths. Furthermore we thank Gerlinde Hofstetter (Department of Pathophysiology and Allergy Research, Medical University of Vienna) for help with the radioactive part of the immunoblot inhibition experiment.

## Author Contributions

Conceived and designed the experiments: EH MB UW MD. Performed the experiments: EH MB. Analyzed the data: EH MB WH VM RP RJ UW MD. Contributed reagents/materials/analysis tools: WH VM RP RJ. Wrote the paper: EH MD. Wrote applications for the ethics committees: UW MD.

## References

1. Hoffman DR (2008) Structural biology of allergens from stinging and biting insects. Curr Opin Allergy Clin Immunol 8: 338–342.
2. Thomas WR, Hales BJ, Smith WA (2010) House dust mite allergens in asthma and allergy. Trends Mol Med 16: 321–328.
3. Arruda LK, Vailes LD, Benjamin DC, Chapman MD (1995) Molecular cloning of German cockroach (*Blattella germanica*) allergens. Int Arch Allergy Immunol 107: 295–297.
4. Van Wijnen JH, Verhoeff AP, Mulder-Folkerts DK, Brachel HJ, Schou C (1997) Cockroach allergen in house dust. Allergy 52: 460–464.
5. Chu KH, Tang CY, Wu A, Leung PS (2005) Seafood allergy: lessons from clinical symptoms, immunological mechanisms and molecular biology. Adv Biochem Eng Biotechnol 97: 205–235.
6. Vaughan WT (1928) Some causes for failure in the specific treatment of allergy. J Lab Clin Med 13: 955–963.
7. Urbach E, Gottlieb PM (1941) Asthma from insect emanations. J Allergy 12: 485–495.
8. Stevenson DD, Mathews KP (1967) Occupational asthma following inhalation of moth particles. J Allergy 39: 274–283.

9. Baldo BA, Panzani RC (1988) Detection of IgE antibodies to a wide range of insect species in subjects with suspected inhalant allergies to insects. Int Arch Allergy Appl Immunol 85: 278–287.
10. Komase Y, Sakata M, Azuma T, Tanaka A, Nakagawa T (1997) IgE antibodies against midge and moth found in Japanese asthmatic subjects and comparison of allergenicity between these insects. Allergy 52: 75–81.
11. Wittich FW (1940) The nature of various mill dust allergens. J Lancet 418–421.
12. Binder M, Mahler V, Hayek B, Sperr WR, Schöller M, et al. (2001) Molecular and immunological characterization of arginine kinase from the Indianmeal moth, *Plodia interpunctella*, a novel cross-reactive invertebrate pan-allergen. J Immunol 167: 5470–5477.
13. Uda K, Fujimoto N, Akiyama Y, Mizuta K, Tanaka K, et al. (2006) Evolution of the arginine kinase gene family. Comp Biochem Physiol Part D Genomics Proteomics 1: 209–218.
14. Yu CJ, Lin YF, Chiang BL, Chow LP (2003) Proteomics and immunological analysis of a novel shrimp allergen, Pen m 2. J Immunol 170: 445–453.
15. Lopata AL, O'Hehir RE, Lehrer SB (2010) Shellfish allergy. Clin Exp Allergy 40: 850–858.
16. Hales BJ, Laing IA, Pearce LJ, Hazell LA, Mills KL, et al. (2007) Distinctive immunoglobulin E anti-house dust allergen-binding specificities in a tropical Australian Aboriginal community. Clin Exp Allergy 37: 1357–1363.
17. Fu C, Wu C, Liu T, Ago T, Zhai P, et al. (2009) Elucidation of thioredoxin target protein networks in mouse. Mol Cell Proteomics 8: 1674–1687.
18. Montrichard F, Alkhalfioui F, Yano H, Vensel WH, Hurkman WJ, et al. (2009) Thioredoxin targets in plants: the first 30 years. J Proteomics 72: 452–474.
19. Weichel M, Glaser AG, Ballmer-Weber BK, Schmid-Grendelmeier P, Crameri R (2006) Wheat and maize thioredoxins: a novel cross-reactive cereal allergen family related to baker's asthma. J Allergy Clin Immunol 117: 676–681.
20. Limacher A, Glaser AG, Meier C, Schmid-Grendelmeier P, Zeller S, et al. (2007) Cross-reactivity and 1.4-Å crystal structure of *Malassezia sympodialis* thioredoxin (Mala s 13), a member of a new pan-allergen family. J Immunol 178: 389–396.
21. Glaser AG, Menz G, Kirsch AI, Zeller S, Crameri R, et al. (2008) Auto- and cross-reactivity to thioredoxin allergens in allergic bronchopulmonary aspergillosis. Allergy 63: 1617–1623.
22. Sander I, Rozynek P, Rihs HP, van Kampen V, Chew FT, et al. (2011) Multiple wheat flour allergens and cross-reactive carbohydrate determinants bind IgE in baker's asthma. Allergy 66: 1208–1215.
23. Short JM, Fernandez JM, Sorge JA, Huse WD (1988) Lambda ZAP: a bacteriophage lambda expression vector with in vivo excision properties. Nucleic Acids Res 16: 7583–7600.
24. Pearson WR, Lipman DJ (1988) Improved tools for biological sequence comparison. Proc Natl Acad Sci U S A 85: 2444–2448.
25. Larkin MA, Blackshields G, Brown NP, Chenna R, McGettigan PA, et al. (2007) ClustalW and ClustalX version 2. Bioinformatics 23: 2947–2948.
26. Wiedermann U, Jahn-Schmid B, Bohle B, Repa A, Renz H, et al. (1999) Suppression of antigen-specific T- and B-cell responses by intranasal or oral administration of recombinant Bet v 1, the major birch pollen allergen, in a murine model of type I allergy. J Allergy Clin Immunol 103: 1202–1210.
27. Hufnagl K, Wagner B, Winkler B, Baier K, Hochreiter R, et al. (2003) Induction of mucosal tolerance with recombinant Hev b 1 and recombinant Hev b 3 for prevention of latex allergy in BALB/c mice. Clin Exp Immunol 133: 170–176.
28. Valenta R, Duchêne M, Ebner C, Valent P, Sillaber C, et al. (1992) Profilins constitute a novel family of functional plant pan-allergens. J Exp Med 175: 377–385.
29. Buchanan BB (2007) Thioredoxin and food allergy. J Allergy Clin Immunol 119: 513–514.
30. Buchanan BB, Adamidi C, Lozano RM, Yee BC, Momma M, et al. (1997) Thioredoxin-linked mitigation of allergic responses to wheat. Proc Natl Acad Sci U S A 94: 5372–5377.
31. Del Val G, Yee BC, Lozano RM, Buchanan BB, Ermel RW, et al. (1999) Thioredoxin treatment increases digestibility and lowers allergenicity of milk. J Allergy Clin Immunol 103: 690–697.
32. Son A, Nakamura H, Kondo N, Matsuo Y, Liu W, et al. (2006) Redox regulation of mast cell histamine release in thioredoxin-1 (TRX) transgenic mice. Cell Res 16: 230–239.
33. Chuang CY, Chang CH, Huang YL (2009) Thioredoxin mediates remodeling factors of human bronchial epithelial cells upon interaction with house dust mite-stimulated eosinophils. Inhal Toxicol 21: 153–167.

18

# Dietary Resveratrol Prevents the Development of Food Allergy in Mice

**Yui Okada[1,2], Kyoko Oh-oka[1], Yuki Nakamura[1], Kayoko Ishimaru[1], Shuji Matsuoka[3], Ko Okumura[4], Hideoki Ogawa[4], Masashi Hisamoto[2], Tohru Okuda[2], Atsuhito Nakao[1,4]***

**1** Department of Immunology, University of Yamanashi Faculty of Medicine Chuo, Yamanashi, Japan, **2** The Institute of Enology and Viticulture, University of Yamanashi, Koufu, Yamanashi, Japan, **3** Deparment of Pathology, Juntendo University School of Medicine, Bunkyo-ku, Tokyo, Japan, **4** Atopy Research Center, Juntendo University School of Medicine, Bunkyo-ku, Tokyo, Japan

## Abstract

***Background:*** Resveratrol is a bioactive polyphenol enriched in red wine that exhibits many beneficial health effects via multiple mechanisms. However, it is unclear whether resveratrol is beneficial for the prevention of food allergy. This study investigated whether resveratrol inhibited the development of food allergy by using a mouse model of the disease.

***Methodology/Principal Findings:*** Mice fed standard diet or standard diet plus resveratrol were sensitized by intragastric administration of ovalbumin (OVA) and mucosal adjuvant cholera toxin (CT). Several manifestations of food allergy were then compared between the mice. The effects of resveratrol on T cells or dendritic cells were also examined by using splenocytes from OVA-specific T cell-receptor (TCR) transgenic DO11.10 mice or mouse bone marrow-derived dendritic cells (BMDCs) *in vitro*. We found that mice fed resveratrol showed reduced OVA-specific serum IgE production, anaphylactic reaction, and OVA-induced IL-13 and IFN-ã production from the mesenteric lymph nodes (MLNs) and spleens in comparison to the control mice, following oral sensitization with OVA plus CT. In addition, resveratrol inhibited OVA plus CT-induced IL-4, IL-13, and IFN-ã production in splenocytes from DO11.10 mice associated with inhibition of GATA-3 and T-bet expression. Furthermore, resveratrol suppressed the OVA plus CT-induced CD25 expression and IL-2 production in DO11.10 mice-splenocytes in association with decreases in CD80 and CD86 expression levels. Finally, resveratrol suppressed CT-induced cAMP elevation in association with decreases in CD80 and CD86 expression levels in BMDCs.

***Conclusions/Significance:*** Ingestion of resveratrol prevented the development of a food allergy model in mice. Given the *in vitro* findings, resveratrol might do so by inhibiting DC maturation and subsequent early T cell activation and differentiation via downregulation of CT-induced cAMP activation in mice. These results suggest that resveratrol may have potential for prophylaxis against food allergy.

**Editor:** Stefan Bereswill, Charité-University Medicine Berlin, Germany

**Funding:** This work was supported by grants from the Ministry of Education, Culture, Sports, Science, and Technology, Japan (H23). The funders had no role in study design, data collection and analysis, decision to publish, or preparation of the manuscript.

**Competing Interests:** The authors have declared that no competing interests exist.

* E-mail: anakao@yamanashi.ac.jp

## Introduction

Food allergy is defined as an immune-mediated pathological reaction toward food antigens, which is a major health concern and epidemic in developed countries [1–3]. Generally, the mucosal immune system in the intestine is hyporesponsive to innocuous food antigens (termed "oral tolerance") due to different T cell events, such as anergy, clonal deletion, and the induction of regulatory T cells [4]. In contrast, mucosal sensitization to a food antigen occurs in patients with food allergy (a breakdown of the natural oral tolerance), which results in the antigen (allergen)-specific IgE production although the mechanisms are poorly understood [5,6]. The development of new approaches to prevent the disease is of significant importance for public health because allergen avoidance is currently the only way available for prevention of food allergy [7].

Resveratrol (*trans*-3, 4¢, 5, -trihydroxystilbene) is a polyphenolic compound that is abundant in grapes and red wine and functions as a phytoalexin that protects against fungus infections in plants [8,9]. Resveratrol has a wide range of biological and pharmacological activities in animal disease models and human health and diseases, including anti-inflammatory, anti-oxidative, and anti-carcinogenic properties via multiple molecular mechanisms [10]. Recently, resveratrol is of great interest since this reagent is reported to improve health and survival of mice on a high-calorie diet without apparent toxicity [11]. However, in spite of these extensive studies on the roles of resveratrol in human health and diseases, it remains unclear whether resveratrol is also beneficial for food allergy.

The primary aim of this study was to investigate whether ingestion of resveratrol inhibits mucosal sensitization to a food antigen, thereby suppressing the hallmark manifestations of food allergy such as antigen-specific IgE production, anaphylactic reaction, and Th2 cytokine production. For this purpose, we examined the effects of dietary resveratrol on a mouse model of food allergy induced by oral administration of ovalbumin (OVA) with mucosal adjuvant cholera toxin (CT) [12].

## Results

### Resveratrol Inhibits CT-driven Mucosal Sensitization to OVA in Mice

The mice were fed the standard diet or standard diet plus resveratrol (22.4 mg/kg diet, 0.01% resveratrol) for 5 weeks. The mice were orally administered 50 mg of OVA with 10 μg of CT 4 times a week for 4 weeks, beginning 1 week after the start of resveratrol administration (**Figure 1A**) and then were sacrificed at 5 weeks for the analysis as was noted below. The feeding dose was determined based on a study showing improved longevity of mice by chronic dietary resveratrol ingestion without toxicity [11].

Mice fed the standard diet showed the induction of serum OVA-specific IgE production following oral sensitization with OVA plus CT (**Figure 1B**) as previously described [12]. In contrast, the mice fed a standard diet plus resveratrol showed a decrease in OVA-specific IgE production after oral sensitization (**Figure 1B**). Consistent with the findings of the serum IgE levels, resveratrol-fed mice sensitized with OVA plus CT showed a smaller drop in the extent of rectal temperatures than the control mice sensitized with OVA plus CT, upon intraperitoneal OVA challenge (**Figure 1C**). In addition, OVA-specific IL-13 and IFN-ã productions from splenocytes and mesenteric lymph nodes (MLN)-derived cells were decreased in resveratrol-fed mice in comparison to those in control mice, following sensitization with OVA plus CT (**Figure 1D**). The frequencies of apoptotic cells in splenocytes and MLN cells freshly isolated from the mice fed standard diet and the mice fed the standard diet plus resveratrol were comparable based on propidium iodide (PI) and Annexin V staining (**Figure S1 A and B**). In addition, the frequencies of apoptotic cells in splenocytes and MLN cells from the mice fed standard diet and the mice fed the standard diet plus resveratrol were comparable following *in vitro* OVA re-stimulation based on PI and Annexin V staining (**Figure S1 C**). These data suggested that dietary resveratrol did not affect the cellular viability in spleen and MLN cells in mice. There were no significant changes in body weights and food or water intake in resveratrol-fed mice in comparison to those in control mice (data not shown). These results suggest that resveratrol inhibited CT-driven mucosal sensitization to OVA in mice without apparent toxicity in association with inhibition of OVA-specific both Th1 and Th2 differentiation.

### Resveratrol Inhibits OVA Plus CT-induced Th1 and Th2 Differentiation *in vitro*

The effects of resveratrol on OVA plus CT-stimulated spleen cells from OVA-specific TCR transgenic DO11.10 mice were examined to investigate how resveratrol inhibited CT-driven mucosal sensitization to OVA *in vivo* [13], hoping to mimic the effects of resveratrol *in vitro*. It is not possible to exactly measure the concentrations of resveratrol in the target tissues in mice (e.g. gut-associated lymphoid tissue: GALT); therefore, this study used the concentrations of resveratrol that can be attained by red wine intake (~10 μM) in humans [9] for the *in vitro* studies.

DO11.10 mice-splenocytes stimulated with OVA plus CT showed increased IFN-ã, IL-4, and IL-13 production in association with robust increases in mRNA levels of T-bet and GATA3, master transcriptional regulators of Th1 and Th2 differentiation, respectively (**Figure 2A and B**). The addition of 10 or 30 μM resveratrol inhibited those responses (**Figure 2A and B**). In contrast, we found that mRNA expression levels of Foxp3, a master regulator of regulatory T cells (Tregs) were not affected by the resveratrol treatment (**Figure 2A**). In addition, the treatment of DO11.10 mice-splenocytes with 10 or 30 μM resveratrol did not affect the cell viability based on trypan blue dye exclusion (**Figure S2**) and WST assay (**Figure 2C**), suggesting that the inhibition of Th1/Th2 differentiation by resveratrol was not due to a reduced cell viability by resveratrol. These results indicated that resveratrol inhibited OVA plus CT-induced both Th1 and Th2 differentiation *in vitro* as well as *in vivo*.

### Resveratrol Inhibits Early T Cell Activation Associated with Decrease of Co-stimulatory Molecule Expression in Antigen-presenting Cells (APCs)

The *in vitro* results suggest that resveratrol may inhibit OVA plus CT-induced T cell responses at the level of early T cell activation, thereby suppressing subsequent Th1 and Th2 cell differentiation. Therefore, the effects of resveratrol on early T cell activation markers, surface CD25 expression and IL-2 production, were examined by using DO11.10 mice-splenocytes *in vitro*.

DO11.10 mice-derived splenocytes stimulated with OVA plus CT showed increased surface expression levels of CD25 in OVA-specific $CD4^+$ T cells that were identified by staining with the anti-clonotypic antibody KJ1–26 (**Figure 3A and B**). Treatment of the cells with resveratrol (10 and 30 μM) decreased the frequency of $CD25^+$ KJ1–$26^+$ cells (**Figure 3A and B**). In addition, DO11.10 mice-derived splenocytes stimulated with OVA plus CT showed increased IL-2 production in the culture supernatants, which were inhibited by the addition of 30 μM resveratrol (**Figure 3C**). Furthermore, OVA plus CT-induced mRNA expression of co-stimulatory molecules CD80 and CD86 were decreased by resveratrol in DO11.10 mice-splenocytes (**Figure 3D**). These data suggest that resveratrol inhibited OVA plus CT-induced early T cell activation by decreasing the expression levels of co-stimulatory molecules in antigen presenting cells (APCs), most likely in DCs.

### Resveratrol Inhibits CT-induced cAMP Elevation in BMDCs

The adjuvant activity of CT is attributed, at least in part, to up-regulation of co-stimulatory molecules in APCs [14,15]. It is thought that CT-induced intracellular cAMP elevation is involved in the up-regulation of co-stimulatory molecules in APCs and licenses them for Th2 priming [16–18]. Therefore, the effects of resveratrol on cAMP elevation induced by CT in bone marrow-derived dendritic cells (BMDCs) were examined.

CT or prostaglandin E2 (PGE2) (as a positive control) induced cAMP elevation in BMDCs (**Figure 4A**) as reported previously [16]. Resveratrol (10 and 30 μM) inhibited CT-induced cAMP elevation in BMDCs (**Figure 4A**). In addition, OVA plus CT-induced surface CD80 and CD86 expression levels in BMDCs were decreased by 10 and 30 μM resveratrol as indicated by mean fluorescence intensity (**Figure 4B**). The treatment of BMDCs with 10 or 30 μM resveratrol did not affect the cell viability based on a WST assay (data not shown). These results suggest that resveratrol inhibits CT-induced cAMP elevation in BMDCs in association with decreases in the expression levels of co-stimulatory molecules.

### Dietary Resveratrol Protects Mice Against a Lethal dose of CT

We thought that, if resveratrol inhibits the adjuvant activity (e.g. cAMP elevation) of a low-dose of CT as described above, resveratrol might also protect mice against the toxic effects of

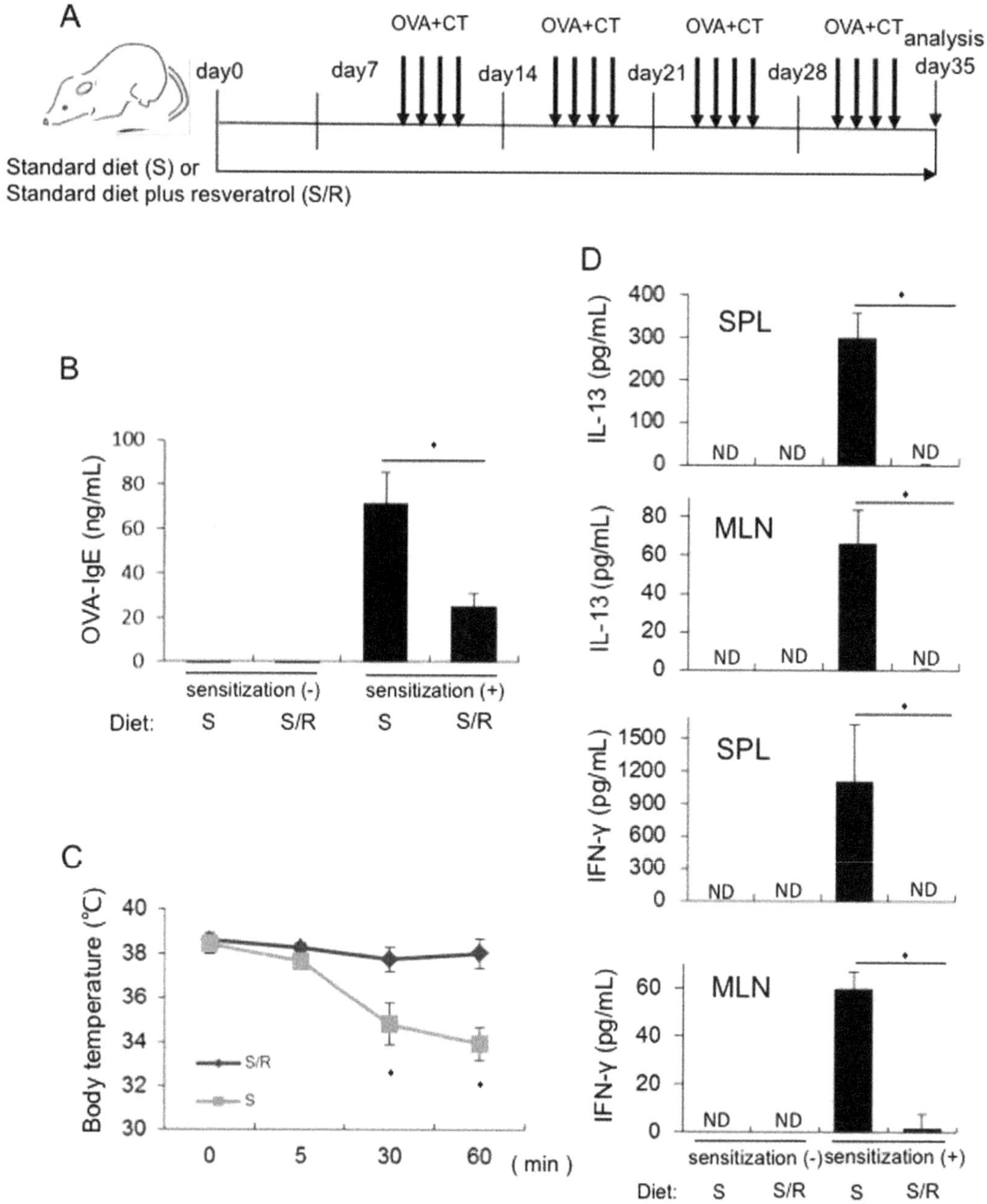


**Figure 1. Resveratrol inhibits CT-driven mucosal sensitization to OVA in mice.** Mice were fed the standard diet or standard diet plus resveratrol (22.4 mg/kg diet, 0.01% resveratrol) for 5 weeks (day 0–35). The mice were orally administered 50 mg of OVA with 10 µg of CT 1 week after the start of resveratrol feeding and 4 times a week for 4 weeks and sacrificed at the 5 weeks (on day 35) for the analysis below. A. Experimental protocol. B. Serum samples were collected on day 35 from the standard diet-fed and standard diet plus resveratrol-fed mice with or without OVA plus CT sensitization. OVA-specific serum IgE concentrations were measured by ELISA (n = 7 per group). C. The standard diet-fed and standard diet plus resveratrol-fed mice sensitized with OVA plus CT were challenged intraperitoneally with OVA on day 35 and rectal temperatures were measured with a digital thermometer at 0, 5, 30, and 60 minutes after the challenge (n = 10 per group). D. Splenocytes (SPL) and mesenteric lymph node (MLN) cells were obtained on day 35 from the standard diet-fed and standard diet plus resveratrol-fed mice with or without OVA plus CT sensitization and the cells were re-stimulated *in vitro* with OVA for 3 days (n = 5 per group). The culture supernatants were then collected and IL-13 and IFN-ã concentrations were measured by ELISA. (S: standard diet-fed mice, S/R: standard diet plus resveratrol-fed mice) Values represent the mean ± SD. *P<0.05 in comparison to the corresponding controls. Representative results from 2 independent experiments with same results are shown.

a high-dose of CT. Thus, we orally administered a high-dose of CT that causes severe toxicity to naïve mice fed with or without resveratrol.

One hundred percent of the mice fed the standard diet died by day 5 after a single challenge of 150 µg CT as previously described [19]. In contrast, 80% of the mice fed a standard diet plus resveratrol survived after the single challenge of CT (**Figure 5**).

These results suggest that dietary resveratrol protects mice against a lethal toxicity of CT at a high-dose, which may be related with the inhibitory effects of resveratrol on CT activity.

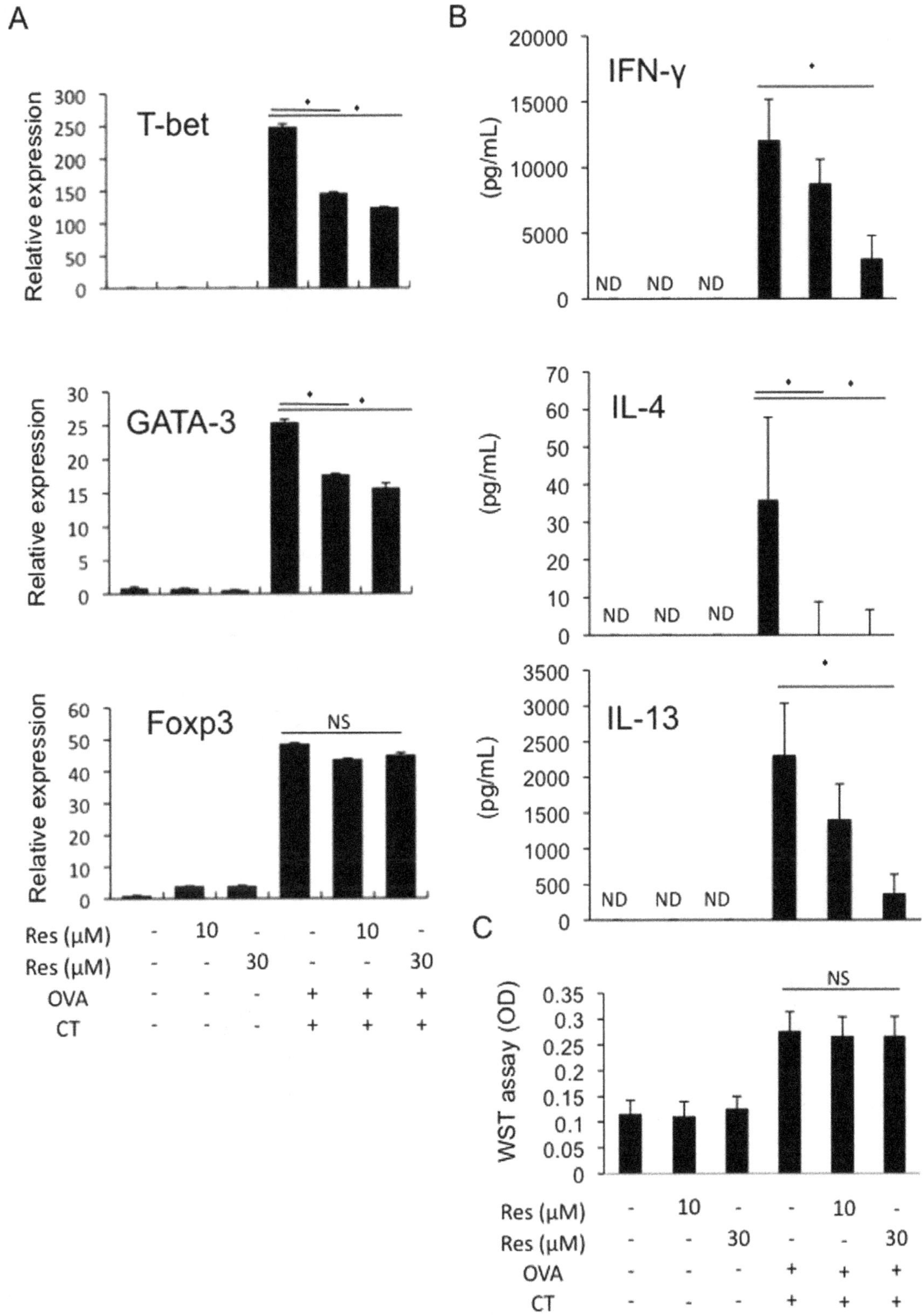


**Figure 2. Resveratrol inhibits OVA plus CT-induced Th1/2 cell differentiation *in vitro*.** DO11.10 mice-derived splenocytes were unstimulated or stimulated with 300 μg/ml OVA plus 12 pM CT and were cultured in the presence or absence of 10 or 30 μM resveratrol for the indicated times. Then the analysis described below was performed. A. After 3 day-culture, RNA samples were extracted from the cells and the cDNA samples were synthesized using reverse transcriptase system. Quantitative real-time PCR analysis was then done for T-bet, GATA3, and Foxp3 mRNAs. Relative expression levels are shown (n = 3 per group). B. After 3 day-culture, the supernatants were collected and IFN-ã, IL-4, and IL-13 concentrations were measured by ELISA (n = 9 per group). C. After 3 day-culture, the cells were subjected to a WST assay for evaluation of the cell viability (n = 4 per group). Values represent the mean ± SD. *P<0.05 in comparison to the corresponding controls. (ND: non-detected).

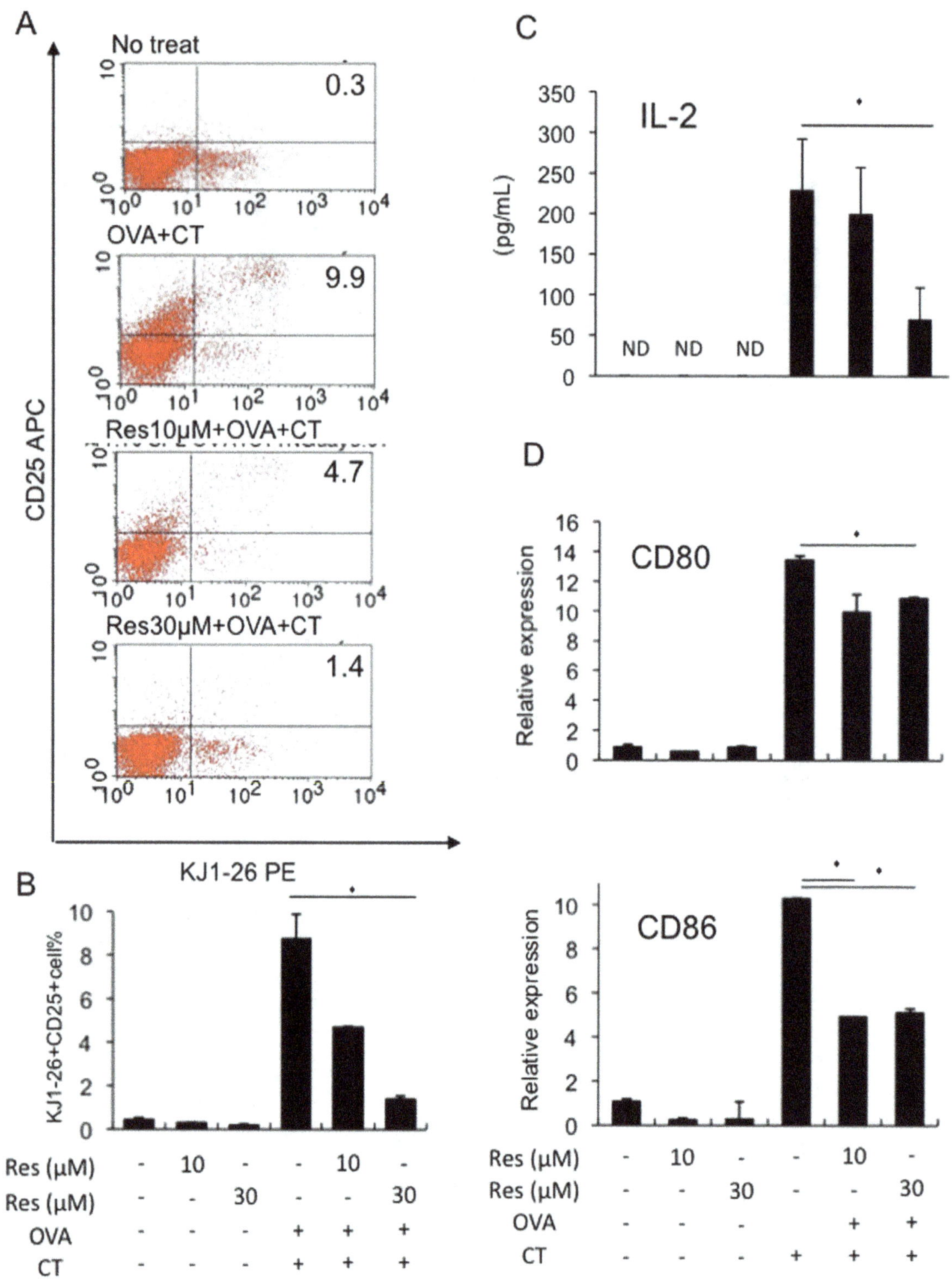


**Figure 3. Resveratrol inhibits early T cell activation and co-stimulatory molecule expression in APCs *in vitro*.** DO11.10 mice-derived splenocytes were un-stimulated (no treat) or stimulated with 300 μg/ml OVA plus 12 pM CT and were cultured in the presence or absence of 10 or 30 μM resveratrol for 1 day. Then the analysis described below was performed. A. After 1 day-culture, whole splenocytes were stained with PE-conjugated anti-KJ1-26 and APC-conjugated anti-CD25 antibody. Representative FACS plots are shown. Numbers indicate the proportion of the KJ1-$26^{+}$ $CD25^{+}$ cells. B. Quantitative analysis of A (n = 3 per group). C. After 1 day-culture, the supernatants were collected and IL-2 concentrations were measured by ELISA (n = 9 per group). D. After 1 day-culture, RNA samples were extracted from the splenocytes and the cDNA samples were synthesized using reverse transcriptase system. Quantitative real-time PCR analysis was then performed to assess CD80 and CD86 mRNA levels. Relative expression levels are shown (n = 3 per group). Values represent the mean ± SD. *P<0.05 in comparison to the corresponding controls. (ND: non-detected).

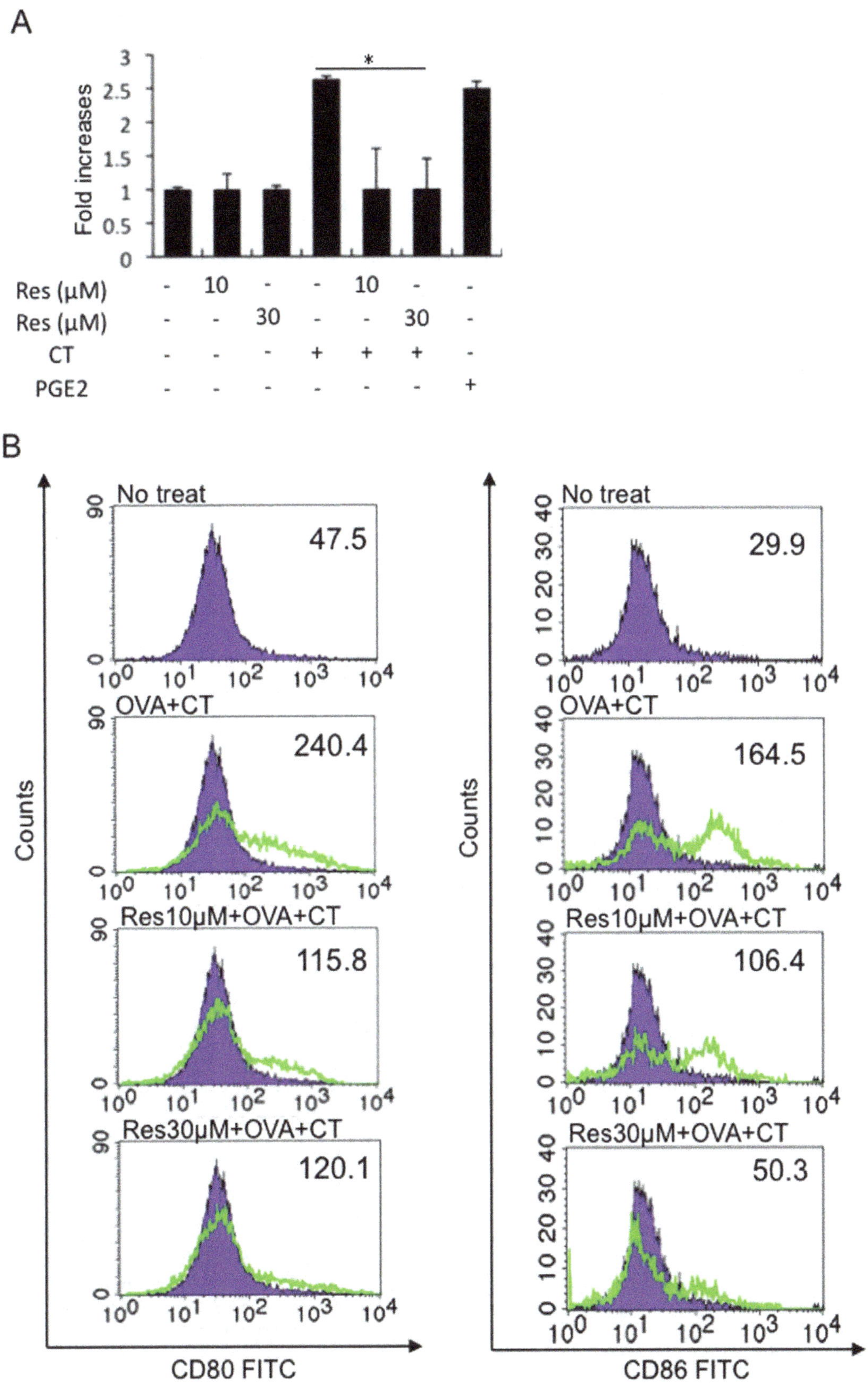


**Figure 4. Resveratrol inhibits CT-induced cAMP elevation in BMDCs.** A. Cultured BMDCs were un-stimulated or stimulated with 12 pM CT in the presence or absence of 10 or 30 μM resveratrol for 1 hour or 10 nM PGE2 (as a positive control) and intracellular cAMP levels were measured using a cAMP EIA kit. Relative changes in intracellular cAMP levels are indicated. Values represent the mean ± SD (n = 3 per group). B. Cultured

BMDCs were un-stimulated (no treat) or stimulated with 300 µg/ml OVA plus 12 pM CT and were cultured in the presence or absence of 10 or 30 µM resveratrol for 3 days. The cells were then stained with APC-conjugated anti-CD11c and FITC-conjugated anti-CD80 or CD86 antibody and were subjected to FACS analysis. A representative histogram regarding surface CD80 and CD86 expression levels on CD11c gated cells is shown. Numbers indicate the mean fluorescence intensity (MFI) of CD80 and CD86-stained cells. The filled histogram indicates un-stimulated (no treat) BMDCs for comparison. Representative results from 3 independent experiments with similar results are shown.

## Discussion

This study demonstrated that ingestion of resveratrol prevented CT-driven mucosal sensitization to OVA in mice without apparent toxic effects. The *in vitro* experiments showed that resveratrol was able to inhibit CT-induced cAMP elevation and maturation of DC and abrogated T cell activation and subsequent Th1/Th2 differentiation. The adjuvant activity of CT is largely attributed to its ability to induce co-stimulatory molecules in APCs via cAMP elevation [14,15,18]. Therefore, the current data suggest that resveratrol suppression of CT adjuvant activity is likely to be a key event associated with the inhibition of CT-induced mucosal sensitization to OVA *in vivo*. The findings that dietary resveratrol protected mice against a lethal dose of CT may support the hypothesis.

As stated above, the *in vivo* effects of resveratrol might be attributed to suppression of CT-induced DC maturation, which could occur in the gut-associated lymphoid tissue (GALT). However, the precise mechanisms by which resveratrol inhibits OVA-induced immune responses *in vivo* remain to be determined because resveratrol has a wide range of biological and pharmacological activities via multiple molecular mechanisms [10] and the bioavailability of resveratrol in mice (and also in humans) remains a major consideration [20]. In particular, further investigation should determine if it is possible to achieve the concentrations (10–30 µM) of resveratrol (that were used in the current *in vitro* studies) in the gut local environment in the resveratrol-fed mice.

Resveratrol treatment decreased OVA plus CT-induced co-stimulatory molecule expression levels in DO11.10 mice-splenocytes and in BMDCs. In consistent with this study, Sharma et al. previously reported that resveratrol at 20 µM suppressed the expression of co-stimulatory molecules (e.g. CD80) in LPS-stimulated mouse peritoneal macrophages *in vitro*, although the molecular mechanism was not addressed [21].

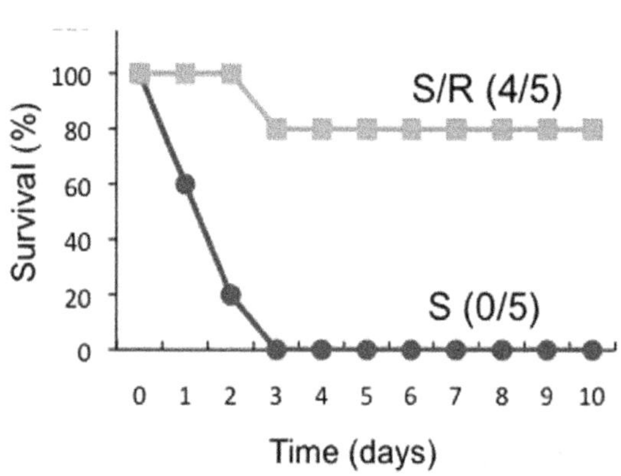


**Figure 5. Dietary resveratrol protects mice against a lethal dose of CT.** Survival of 8-week-old C57BL/6 mice orally challenged with CT at a dose of 150 µg monitored until day 10 after challenge (n = 5 per group). Representative results from 2 independent experiments with similar results are shown. (S: standard diet-fed mice, S/R: standard diet plus resveratrol-fed mice).

How resveratrol inhibits CT-induced cAMP elevation in BMDCs remains to be determined. Recently, Morinaga et al. reported that resveratrol inhibited CT-induced cAMP accumulation in Vero cells [22]. They suggested that resveratrol suppressed the CT activity indirectly by suppressing the internalization of CT or directly by interacting with CT and inhibiting its enzymatic activity to activate adenylate cyclase. These mechanisms might also occur in DC in this study.

Masilamani et al. and Zuercher et al. reported that dietary soybean isoflavons or polyphenol-enriched apple extract protected against CT-driven mucosal sensitization to peanut or OVA in mice, respectively [23,24]. Masilamani et al. also showed that soybean isoflavons inhibited CT-induced DC maturation and subsequent T cell activation [23], which is similar to the current findings in case of resveratrol. Therefore, dietary polyphenols present in vegetables and fruits might have the general potential to prevent food allergy and other allergic diseases [20]. The current study identifies resveratrol as a new dietary polyphenol having such an anti-allergic activity and shows that CT adjuvant activity is likely to be an important target of resveratrol in the context of a food allergy model.

In summary, this study suggests that dietary resveratrol can prevent mucosal sensitization to food antigens without apparent toxic effects. Resveratrol has beneficial properties in animal disease models and human health and, as such, many clinical trials are on going with relative safety [10,25]. The current results provide additional evidence that this remarkable natural substance may also be beneficial for prophylaxis against food allergy, where unmet preventive/therapeutic needs are greatest in allergic diseases.

## Methods

### Mice

Female 4–6 weeks Balb/c were purchased from Japan SLC (Tokyo, Japan) and DO11.10 transgenic mice [13] with Balb/c genetic backgrounds were bred under specific pathogen-free conditions. Susceptibility of mice to a lethal dose of CT was tested using 8 week-old C57BL/6 mice (Japan SLC, Tokyo, Japan). All animal experiments were approved by the Institutional Review Board of the University of Yamanashi.

### Dietary Resveratrol

The mice were maintained on a standard mouse diet for 2 weeks prior to the start of the experiment. All mice were housed 4–5 per cage with free access to food and water for 24 hours, under a 12:12 light/dark cycle. Mice were fed the standard diet or resveratrol (>99%, Sigma-Aldrich, St Louis, MO)-mixed standard diet (22.4 mg/kg diet, 0.01% resveratrol) for 5 weeks as previously described [11]. The diet was provided in cages for no more than 1 week. Food intake and body weight were measured on a weekly basis for the duration of the study.

### Mucosal Sensitization

The mice were orally sensitized with ovalbumin (OVA) at 1 week after the start of resveratrol feeding as previously described [12] with some modifications. Briefly, mice were administered

50 mg of OVA (Sigma-Aldrich, St Louis, MO) with 10 µg of CT (List Biologicals, Campbell, CA) in a final volume of 200 µl by using a mouse feeding needle 4 times a week for 4 weeks.

## Serum IgE Levels

Serum levels of OVA-specific IgE levels were determined using the mouse OVA-specific IgE ELISA kit at week 5 (DS Pharma Biomedical, Ohsaka, Japan), according to the manufacturers' instructions.

## Measurement of Anaphylaxis

All mice received a bolus i.p. challenge with OVA (100 µg) at week 5. Anaphylaxis was assessed in challenged mice by measuring changes in rectal temperature with a digital thermometer (Shibaura Electronics, Tokyo, Japan) at 0, 5, 30, 60 minutes after the challenge as previously described [26].

## Antigen-recall Response

The splenocytes and mesenteric lymph node (MLN) cells were obtained from the mice at week 5 and were cultured ($2\times10^6$ cells/well) for 72 hours in the presence of 300 µg/ml OVA. In the absence of OVA, IL-13 and IFN-ã production in the culture supernatants was not detected (data not shown).

## *In vitro* Cell Culture

Bone marrow-derived dendritic cells were generated from the femoral bone marrow cells of female mice as previously described [27]. DO11.10 mice derived-splenocytes or BMDCs were cultured in RPMI1640 (Sigma-Aldrich, St Louis, MO) containing 10% FCS and antibiotics. For experiments, the cells ($1\times10^6$ cells/well) were stimulated with 300 µg/ml OVA and 12 pM CT and were cultured for the indicated times. Resveratrol (10 and 30 µM) dissolved in DMSO or DMSO alone was added to the culture 30 minutes before the OVA plus CT stimulation. For some experiments, BMDCs were stimulated with 12 pM CT alone.

## Quantitative Real-time PCR

Total RNA was extracted from the cells using RNAeasy Mini kit (QUAGEN Inc., Valencia, CA). cDNA was then synthesized from 4 µg of total RNA using Reverse Transcriptase System (Applied Biosystems, Foster City, CA). Quantitative real-time PCR with specific primers and probes for mouse T-bet, GATA3, Foxp3, CD80, CD86, and GAPDH (Applied Biosystems, Foster City, CA) was then performed using the AB7300 real-time PCR system (Applied Biosystems) as previously described [28].

## ELISA

The amounts of IL-2, IL-4, IL-13, and IFN-ã in the culture supernatants were determined by using the mouse IL-2, IL-4, IL-13, and IFN-ã ELISA kits (eBioscience, San Diego, CA).

## Cell Viability Assay

The cells ($1\times10^5$ cells/well) were cultured with or without the indicated stimulations for 72 hours in a U-bottom 96-well microtiter plate. Cell viability was then determined by trypan blue dye exclusion and a WST assay using the Tetra Color ONE kit (Seikagaku Corporation, Tokyo, Japan) according to the manufacturer's instructions. To detect apoptotic cells, the spleen cells or MLN cells ($1\times10^6$) isolated from the mice were incubated with 5 µl FITC-conjugated Annexin V and 5 µl PI (BD Pharmingen, San Diego, CA, USA) in 500 µl PBS for 15 minutes. After washing with PBS, the cells were subjected to FACS analysis. For some experiments, the cells isolated from the mice were re-stimulated with 300 µg/ml OVA *in vitro* for 48 hours and stained with PI and Annexin V and subjected to FACS analysis.

## FACS

PE-conjugated anti-mouse KJ1–26, FITC-conjugated anti-mouse CD80 and CD86, and APC-conjugated anti-mouse CD11c antibody were purchased from BD PharMingen (San Diego, CA). APC-conjugated anti-mouse CD25 antibody were purchased from eBioscience Inc. (San Diego, CA). The cellular staining was analyzed on a FACSCalibur (BD Biosciences, San Diego, CA) using the CellQuest program (BD Biosciences). Before staining, Fc receptors were blocked with anti-CD16/32 antibody (2.4G2; BD Biosciences). Negative controls consisted of isotype-matched directly conjugated, nonspecific antibodies (BD Biosciences).

## cAMP Assay

cAMP was quantified using a cAMP EIA kit (Cayman Chemical Company, Ann Arbor, MI). Resveratrol (10 and 30 µM) was added to BMDCs ($5\times10^5$ cells/well) grown in 24-well plates and incubated at 37°C for 30 minutes before addition of 12 pM CT or 10 nM prostaglandin E2 (PGE2) (Tokyo Chemical Industry Co., Ltd., Tokyo, Japan) as a positive control and further incubation for 1 hour. The medium was then aspirated and 0.3 ml of 2% triton (Sigma-Aldrich, St Louis, MO) in EIA buffer (company supplied) was added. The cells were incubated for 10 min at room temperature and sedimented by centrifugation and the supernatant was used for assay following the manufacturer's instructions.

## Oral Administration of a Lethal Dose of CT to Mice

Mice were deprived of food for 2 hours and were deprived of water for another 2 hours and then were given a solution of sodium bicarbonate to neutralize stomach acidity before oral administration of CT as previously described [19]. Then 30 minutes later, mice were mildly sedated by anesthesia and given oral challenge with 150 µg CT in 10 mM Tris, pH7.5; they were monitored daily after the challenge if they were allowed to die after the lethal dose.

## Data Analysis

The statistical analysis was performed using un-paired Student's *t*-test. A value of $P<0.05$ was considered to be significant.

# Supporting Information

**Figure S1 The frequencies of apoptotic cells in splenocytes and mesenteric lymph node cells isolated from standard diet- or standard diet plus resveratrol-fed mice.** The splenocytes and mesenteric lymph node (MLN) cells were freshly isolated from the mice fed standard diet or fed the standard diet plus resveratrol at 5 weeks (day 35). A. B. The cells were immediately stained with propidium iodide (PI) and Annexin V and subjected to FACS analysis. Representative plots (left panels) and the quantitative data (right panels) of the splenocytes (SPL) (A) and MLN cells (B). C. The cells were stimulated with 300 µg/ml OVA *in vitro* for 2 days and were stained with PI and Annexin V and subjected to FACS analysis. The quantitative data of the splenocytes (SPL) and MLN cells are shown. Values represent the mean ± SD (A, B, n = 4 per group, C, n = 3 per group). (S: standard diet-fed mice, S/R: standard diet plus resveratrol-fed mice).
(TIF)

**Figure S2 The frequencies of viable cells in DO11.10 splenocytes stimulated in the presence or absence of resveratrol.** The splenocytes isolated from DO11.10 mice were stimulated with 300 μg/ml OVA +12 pM CT in the presence or absence of 10 or 30 μM resveratrol for 72 hours. The cells were then stained with trypan blue solution. Trypan blue exclusion rates relative to those in control group (OVA + CT stimulation) are shown. Values represent the mean ± SD (n = 4 per group).
(TIF)

## Acknowledgments

The authors thank Drs. Ryusukek Nakagawa and Naomi Shimokawa for their technical assistance and Ms. Yuko Ohnuma and Mutuko Hara for their valuable general assistance.

## Author Contributions

Conceived and designed the experiments: YO TO AN. Performed the experiments: YO K. Oh-oka YN KI. Analyzed the data: YO K. Oh-oka YN KI. Contributed reagents/materials/analysis tools: SM K. Okumura HO MH TO. Wrote the paper: YO AN.

## References

1. Crespo JF, Rodriguez J (2003) Food allergy in adult food. Allergy 58: 98–113.
2. Lack G (2008) Clinical practice. Food allergy. N Engl J Med 359: 1252–1260.
3. Wang J, Sampson HA (2011) Food allergy. J Clin Invest 121: 827–835.
4. Weiner HL, da Cunha AP, Quintana F, Wu H (2011) Oral tolerance. Immunol Rev 241: 241–259.
5. Burks AW, Laubach S, Jones SM (2008) Oral tolerance, food allergy, and immunotherapy: implications for future treatment. J Allergy Clin Immunol 121: 1344–1350.
6. Brandtzaeg P (2010) Food allergy: separating the science from the mythology. Nat Rev Gastroenterol Hepatol 7: 380–400.
7. Hamelmann E, Beyer K, Gruber C, Lau S, Matricardi PM, et al. (2008) Primary prevention of allergy: avoiding risk or providing protection? Clin Exp Allergy 38: 233–245.
8. German JB, Walzem RL (2000) The health benefits of wine. Annu Rev Nutr 20: 561–593.
9. Soleas GJ, Diamandis EP, Goldberg DM (2001) The world of resveratrol. Adv Exp Med Biol 492: 159–182.
10. Baur JA, Sinclair DA (2006) Therapeutic potential of resveratrol: the in vivo evidence. Nat Rev Drug Discov 5: 493–506.
11. Baur JA, Pearson KJ, Price NL, Jamieson HA, Lerin C, et al. (2006) Resveratrol improves health and survival of mice on a high-calorie diet. Nature 444: 337–342.
12. Li XM, Schofield BH, Huang CK, Kleiner GI, Sampson HA (1999) A murine model of IgE-mediated cow's milk hypersensitivity. J Allergy Clin Immunol 103: 206–214.
13. Murphy KM, Heimberger AB, Loh DY (1990) Induction by antigen of intrathymic apoptosis of $CD4^{+}CD8^{+}$TCRlow thymocytes in vivo. Science 250: 1720–1723.
14. Gagliardi MC, Sallusto F, Marinaro M, Langenkamp A, Lanzavecchia A, et al. (2000) Cholera toxin induces maturation of human dendritic cells and licences them for Th2 priming. Eur J Immunol 30: 2394–2403.
15. Blázquez AB, Berin MC (2008) Gastrointestinal dendritic cells promote Th2 skewing via OX40L. J Immunol 180: 4441–4450.
16. Bagley KC, Abdelwahab SF, Tuskan RG, Fouts TR, Lewis GK (2002) Cholera toxin and heat-labile enterotoxin activate human monocyte-derived dendritic cells and dominantly inhibit cytokine production through a cyclic AMP-dependent pathway. Infect Immun 70: 5533–5539.
17. Ela Sala A, He J, Laricchia-Robbio L, Gorini S, Iwasaki A, et al. (2009) Cholera toxin inhibits IL-12 production and CD8α+ dendritic cell differentiation by cAMP-mediated inhibition of IRF8 function. J Exp Med 206: 1227–1235.
18. Negri DR, Pinto D, Vendetti S, Patrizio M, Sanchez M, et al. (2009) Cholera toxin and Escherichia coli heat-labile enterotoxin, but not their nontoxic counterparts, improve the antigen-presenting cell function of human B lymphocytes. Infect Immun 77: 1924–1935.
19. Wei M, Shinkura R, Doi Y, Maruya M, Fagarasan S, et al. (2011) Mice carrying a knock-in mutation of *Aicda* resulting in a defect in somatic hypermutation have impaired gut homeostasis and compromised mucosal defense. Nat Immunol 12: 264–270.
20. Singh A, Holvoet S, Mercenier A (2011) Dietary polyphenols in the prevention and treatment of allergic diseases. Clin Exp Allergy 41: 1346–1359.
21. Sharma S, Chopra K, Kulkarni SK, Agrewala JN (2007) Resveratrol and curcumin suppress immune response through CD28/CTLA-4 and CD80 co-stimulatory pathway. Clin Exp Immunol 147: 155–163.
22. Morinaga N, Yahiro K, Noda M (2010) Resveratrol, a natural polyphenolic compound, inhibits cholera toxin-induced cyclic AMP accumulation in Vero cells. Toxicon 56: 29–35.
23. Masilamani M, Wei J, Bhatt S, Paul M, Yakir S, et al. (2011) Soybean isoflavones regulate dendritic cell function and suppress allergic sensitization to peanut. J Allergy Clin Immunol 128: 1242–1250.e1.
24. Zuercher AW, Holvoet S, Weiss M, Mercenier A (2010) Polyphenol-enriched apple extract attenuates food allergy in mice. Clin Exp Allergy 40: 942–950.
25. Patel KR, Scott E, Brown VA, Gescher AJ, Steward WP, et al. (2011) Clinical trials of resveratrol. Ann N Y Acad Sci 1215: 161–169.
26. Nakamura Y, Harama D, Shimokawa N, Hara M, Suzuki R, et al. (2011) Circadian clock gene Period2 regulates a time-of-day-dependent variation in cutaneous anaphylactic reaction. J Allergy Clin Immunol 127: 1038–1045.
27. Kanada S, Nishiyama C, Nakano N, Suzuki R, Maeda K, et al. (2011) Critical role of transcription factor PU.1 in the expression of CD80 and CD86 on dendritic cells. Blood 117: 2211–2222.
28. Nakamura Y, Miyata M, Ohba T, Ando T, Hatsushika K, et al. (2008) Cigarette smoke extract induces thymic stromal lymphopoietin expression, leading to T(H)2-type immune responses and airway inflammation. J Allergy Clin Immunol 122: 1208–1214.

# 19

# Antigenic Proteins Involved in Occupational Rhinitis and Asthma Caused by Obeche Wood (*Triplochiton Scleroxylon*)

**Ana Aranda[1], Paloma Campo[2*], Arantxa Palacin[3], Inmaculada Doña[2], Cristina Gomez-Casado[3], Luisa Galindo[2], Araceli Díaz-Perales[3], Miguel Blanca[2]**

**1** Allergy Research Laboratory, Carlos Haya Hospital, Málaga, Spain, **2** Unidad de Gestión Clínica Allergy, Carlos Haya Hospital, Málaga, Spain, **3** Biotechnology Department, Center for Plant Biotechnology and Genomics, Pozuelo de Alarcon, Madrid, Spain

## Abstract

***Background:*** Obeche wood dust is a known cause of occupational asthma where an IgE-mediated mechanism has been demonstrated.

***Objective:*** To characterize the allergenic profile of obeche wood dust and evaluate the reactivity of the proteins by *in vitro*, *ex vivo* and *in vivo* assays in carpenters with confirmed rhinitis and/or asthma

***Materials and methods:*** An in-house obeche extract was obtained, and two IgE binding bands were purified (24 and 12 kDa) and sequenced by N-terminal identity. Specific IgE and IgG, basophil activation tests and skin prick tests (SPTs) were performed with whole extract and purified proteins. CCD binding was analyzed by ELISA inhibition studies.

***Results:*** Sixty-two subjects participated: 12 with confirmed occupational asthma/rhinitis (ORA+), 40 asymptomatic exposed (ORA−), and 10 controls. Of the confirmed subjects, 83% had a positive SPT to obeche. There was a 100% recognition by ELISA in symptomatic subjects vs. 30% and 10% in asymptomatic exposed subjects and controls respectively ($p<0.05$). Two new proteins were purified, a 24 kDa protein identified as a putative thaumatin-like protein and a 12 kDa gamma-expansin. Both showed allergenic activity *in vitro*, with the putative thaumatin being the most active, with 92% recognition by ELISA and 100% by basophil activation test in ORA+ subjects. Cross-reactivity due to CCD was ruled out in 82% of cases.

***Conclusions:*** Two proteins of obeche wood were identified and were recognized by a high percentage of symptomatic subjects and by a small proportion of asymptomatic exposed subjects. Further studies are required to evaluate cross reactivity with other plant allergens.

**Editor:** Vladimir N. Uversky, University of South Florida College of Medicine, United States of America

**Funding:** Financial Support: Ministry of Health grant FIS/PI071175; Andalusian Health Division grants PI-0182/2008; grant from the Spanish Society of Allergy, Ministry of Science and Innovation-DGI, Spain (grant BIO2009-07050); and Thematic Network FIS-RIRAAF (RD07/0064). The funders had no role in study design, data collection and analysis, decision to publish, or preparation of the manuscript.

**Competing Interests:** None of the authors has any conflict of interest, nor have they received any money from a biotechnology and/or pharmaceutical manufacturer for the present study.

* E-mail: campomozo@yahoo.com

## Introduction

Wood is a known sensitizer widely extended in the construction and furniture industries worldwide [1,2]. Exposure to wood dust has been associated with the risk of developing asthma, an increase in airway hyperresponsiveness and decreased $FEV_1$ [3,4], even in apprentices [5]. The obeche (*Triplochiton scleroxylon*) is a tree from West Africa belonging to the *Sterculiaceace* family [6]. Several cases of occupational asthma due to inhalation of obeche dust have been reported, with positive skin prick tests (SPTs), specific IgE to wood extracts and positive bronchial challenges suggesting an IgE-mediated mechanism [6–10]. However, there is no standardized extract for accurate diagnosis and the nature of the IgE-binding components in obeche is not fully known. Two reports [6–9] first described IgE binding bands by means of SDS-PAGE and immunodetection assays. In the study by Quirce *et al*, allergic subjects mostly recognized a 28 kDa band [6], while other bands of 64, 57.8, and 17 kDa were recognized with less intensity. In addition, IgE reactivity was reduced only by 8.6% when a deglycosylated extract was used, which indicates a non-carbohydrate nature of these IgE binding proteins. The same 28 and 17 kDa reactive components were also found in two other studies [9,11]. One of these, that of Vidal *et al*, described the presence of the 28 kDa protein in both obeche and in fruit extracts (*Cyphomandra betacea Sendth* or tamarillo), and this protein was recognized *in vitro* by a carpenter with occupational asthma due to obeche who suffered anaphylaxis after ingestion of tamarillo [11]. However, no further experiments were conducted to identify these components. Later on, a high molecular weight class I chitinase was described (Trip s1), and still remains the only allergen identified so far [10]. This 38 kDa protein shares a high molecular similarity with Prs a 1 (avocado allergen) and with Hev b 6, and cross reactivity has been demonstrated in a small group of sensitized subjects [10,12]. However, this allergen was not recognized by most subjects in the aforementioned studies [6,9,11], so its relevance in other populations remains unknown. Thus, the allergenic content of obeche wood needs to be analyzed in detail.

The aim of this study was to further characterize the allergenic profile of obeche wood dust. We also evaluated the reactivity of the potentially allergenic proteins by *in vitro*, *ex vivo* and *in vivo* assays in a well-characterized population of carpenters with confirmed rhinitis and/or asthma due to obeche wood exposure and two control populations.

## Materials and Methods

### Production of in-house obeche extract

Obeche wood dust was extracted with phosphate-buffered saline (PBS) buffer for 1 h at 4°C, centrifuged at 10000× g for 30 min at 4°C. The supernatant was dialysed (cut-off point, 3.5 kDa) against $H_2O$ and freeze-dried. The protein concentration was quantified according to the method of Bradford (Pierce Biotechnology, In. Rockford, USA).

### Study population

This study involved carpenters and carpentry apprentices with respiratory symptoms (nasal and/or bronchial) due to occupational exposure to obeche wood, and with a diagnosis of occupational rhinitis/asthma confirmed by specific inhalation challenge with the in-house obeche extract at 1 mg/ml. Nasal challenges were performed according to published methods [13], and responses were monitored by acoustic rhinometry, visual analogue scale and symptoms score. Bronchial challenges were performed using a DeVilbiss nebulizer and responses were monitored by serial spirometry [14]. Nasal and bronchial challenges were performed with the same extract in 5 controls showing negative responses. A group of asymptomatic exposed subjects, with negative SPT to obeche extract who worked in the same factories or school as the symptomatic subjects were invited to participate, and a number of them were randomly selected for the study. A group of non-exposed asymptomatic subjects was also recruited as a control group. All participants completed an occupational questionnaire, as described [15]. Spirometry was performed using a Spirobank spirometer (RDSM, Hasselt, Belgium) following the guidelines [16]. Skin prick tests (SPTs) (ALK-Abelló, Spain) were performed [17] with a battery of common aeroallergens that included grass pollen, trees, dust mites, molds, dog/cat dander and latex. Also, SPT with thaumatin-containing food extracts (banana, peach, hazelnut, chestnut, kiwi, apple and melon, ALK-Abelló, Spain) were performed. Written informed consent was obtained from all subjects and the ethical committee of our institution approved the study.

### Isolation of allergens

Obeche extract was fractionated by anion-exchange chromatography on a Bio-Scale™ Mini Macro-Prep® High Q column (BioRad, Hercules, CA, USA) equilibrated 20 mM ethalonamine, pH 9, and eluted with 1 M NaCl in the same buffer. Retained fractions were identified by SDS-PAGE and immunodetection with a serum pool from confirmed obeche-sensitised patients. The non-retained material was separated by RP-HPLC on Europa protein C4 column (25×0.7 mm; particle size 5 μm; Teknokroma, Barcelona, Spain). Elution was performed with a linear gradient of acetonitrile in 0.1% (v/v) trifluoroacetic acid (0–10% for 15 min and 10–100% for 150 min, at a flow rate of 0.5 ml/min). Peaks were processed along with the retained ion exchange fractions. The purified proteins were quantified by a commercial bicinchoninic acid test (Pierce, Cheshire, UK) and their purity was tested by SDS-PAGE, N-terminal amino acid sequencing with an Applied Biosystems 477A gas-phase sequencer (Applied Biosystems, CA, USA), and mass spectrophotometric analysis with a Biflex III Spectrometer (Bruker-Franzen Analytik, Bremen, Germany), using standard methods.

### SDS-PAGE and immunodetection

Obeche extract (30 μg) and purified proteins (5 μg) were separated on SDS-PAGE [18]. Proteins were electrotransferred to polyvinylidene difluoride membranes. Blocked membranes (Blocking solution, Sigma, St.Louis, USA) were incubated with a pool of sera from symptomatic exposed subjects with positive specific IgE to obeche (1:5 dilution). The IgE binding was revealed with anti-human IgE-peroxidase conjugate (Biosource, Camarillo, CA, USA; 1:3000 dilution) and chemiluminiscence (Amersham Supersignal West Pico Chemiluminutoescent Substrate, Rockford, USA). Further, blocked membranes were incubated with different polyclonal antibodies and then treated with goat anti-rabbit IgG-peroxidase conjugate (Dako, Carpinteria, CA, USA; 1:10000 dilution) and revealed by means of chemiluminiscence.

### Skin prick tests with obeche extract and purified allergens

SPTs with the in-house obeche dust extract (1 mg/ml protein in a 1:1 [v/v] PBS buffer/glycerol solution) or with purified proteins (20 μg/ml) were carried out [17]. Histamine dihydrochloride (10 mg/ml) and PBS buffer/glycerol solution served as positive and negative controls, respectively. Ten non-exposed asymptomatic subjects were tested with this obeche extract and purified proteins, and the responses were all negative.

### Specific immunoglobulin E and G determination

Specific IgE and IgG antibodies to obeche wood dust extract were determined in each individual serum in triplicate by direct ELISA method [19]. Obeche extract was tested at 20 μg/ml and purified proteins at 5 μg/ml as solid phase, and serum at 1:10 dilution for measurement of IgE and at 1:50 dilution for measurement of IgG. Blocking solution was used as a negative control. Specific IgE levels greater than 0.19 OD units and specific IgG levels greater than 0,25 OD units (mean [OD]+3× S.D. to blocking) were considered positive. Sera from subjects with confirmed occupational rhinitis and/or asthma were selected to analyze the IgE binding activity of the purified proteins as solid phase following the same protocol described above.

### ELISA inhibition studies with CCD determinants

Sera from subjects with confirmed occupational asthma/rhinitis were pre-incubated with different inhibitors (in-house obeche extract and bromelain, Sigma, St. Louis, USA) at final concentrations of 100, 10 and 1 μg/ml at room temperature for 3 h [19]. Later on, the inhibitor mixtures (including sera with no inhibitor as a positive control) were added to plates coated with obeche extract a 20 μg/ml and incubated at 37°C overnight. The assay was completed by incubating with rabbit anti-human IgE antibody (1:3000; DAKO A/S, Denmark). IgE binding was detected using o-phenylenediamine tablets (OPD, DAKO) and the reaction was stopped by adding 2 M chloric acid. The absorbance (OD) in each well was measured at 490 nm. The percentage inhibition of IgE binding was calculated using the following formula: % inhibition = (serum not inhibited-serum inhibited/serum not inhibited) ×100.

### Basophil activation test

The basophil activation test (BAT) was performed as described [20], using different concentrations of obeche extract (50, 25, 12.5 and 6.25 μg/ml) and of purified proteins (10, 5 and 2,5 μg/ml). The optimal concentrations of extract and purified proteins were chosen based on dose-response curves and cytotoxicity studies. Results were considered as positive when the stimulation index (SI), calculated as the ratio between the percentage of degranulated basophils with the allergens and the negative control, was >2 in at least one of the dilutions.

### Statistical analysis

Differences between groups were compared by the Student t test for continuous variables and by Chi square test for categorical variables using the SPSS software package (SPSS Corporation, Chicago, IL); p values<0.05 were considered statistically significant.

## Results

### Clinical characteristics of study population

Sixty-two subjects participated in the study:

1. Subjects with confirmed occupational rhinitis and/or asthma (n = 12). These subjects had a diagnosis of either occupational rhinitis (n = 7) or asthma (n = 5) as confirmed by specific nasal or bronchial challenges, all having immediate isolated nasal or bronchial responses. These subjects comprised the occupational rhinitis/asthma group (ORA+).
2. Subjects who were occupationally exposed to obeche wood without any respiratory symptoms and with a negative SPT to obeche extract (n = 40). These subjects comprised the non occupational rhinitis/asthma (ORA−) group.
3. Control group of non-exposed, asymptomatic subjects (CG, n = 10).

The characteristics of the ORA+ subjects were compared to the ORA- group and the control group (see **Table 1**). ORA+ subjects were older and had a significantly longer exposure time when compared with the asymptomatic group (p<0.05). ORA+ subjects had higher total IgE levels compared to ORA− and CG although this difference was not significant. The percentage of smokers and the $FEV_1$ were similar in all groups. Both ORA+ and ORA− subjects had a high percentage of positive SPT to pollen (ORA+:75%, 67% grass pollen; ORA−: 49%, 60% grass pollen).

### Measurement of specific IgE antibodies against obeche wood

Specific IgE antibodies to obeche wood were measured by ELISA in all ORA+, ORA− and CG subjects. As shown in **Figure 1a**, 100% of the ORA+ subjects had specific IgE antibodies against obeche extract, with the highest mean OD of the three groups (solid line shows the positivity cut-off point, dotted lines show mean OD for each group). On the other hand, only 30% of the ORA− subjects had specific IgE antibodies (p<0.05 ORA+ *vs.* ORA−). The control group of unexposed subjects showed the lowest mean value, below the cut-off point of positivity, with only one serum showing a positive value. Thus, detection of specific IgE antibodies was significantly higher (p<0.05) in symptomatic subjects as compared to asymptomatic subjects and controls. **Figure 1b** shows the measurement of specific IgG. We observed 100% positive results in ORA+ subjects and 80% in ORA− subjects. However, 40% of unexposed subjects also showed positive results, with the mean value of this group below the threshold of positivity (p<0.05).

### In-house obeche extract showed two principal IgE binding bands

To better characterize the molecular basis of obeche sensitization, the in-house extract was separated by SDS-PAGE and stained with Coomassie (**Figure 2A**). Replicas were electrotransferred and incubated with a pool of sera of sensitized subjects. Two principal bands seemed to be recognized with the highest intensity by serum pool: a 24 kDa and a band with an apparent molecular weight of 12 kDa. In order to identify the nature of these IgE-binding bands, their purification was investigated through different ionic exchange chromatographic techniques. The high molecular weight protein was the most difficult to purify since it was extremely unstable. For this reason, the amount of this purified protein was very small and therefore it was not possible to obtain enough protein to analyze its allergic activity *in vivo* by skin prick test in all subjects. However, the two proteins were purified in sufficient quantity to demonstrate their allergenic activity by *in vitro* (ELISA and BAT) assays. Their purity was checked sequencing their N-terminal amino acids and analyzing their real molecular weight by mass spectrometry.

### A gamma-expansin was identified as new allergen of obeche

The protein with the lowest molecular weight (12 kDa) presented 11642.5 Da by mass spectrometry, and its N-terminal amino acid was sequenced and rendered IQGTATFYTPPYVPS. This sequence matched in homology with gamma-expansins of alder (*Alnus glutinasa*; GU06293.1) and of lemon tree (*Citrus jambluri*; AF015782). Members of the same protein family have been associated with grass pollen allergy (group 1 of grass allergens) although their sequence identity with the new allergen is poor [21].

### The 24 kDa IgE binding protein could belong to the thaumatin-like family

The highest protein showed 23590.3 Da and its N-terminal corresponded to AQITVTYNGQNG. However, the number of residues was not enough to find identity with known sequences deposited in data banks. For this reason, SDS-PAGE bands were excised and in-gel trypsin digestion followed by offline LC-MALDI-TOF/TOF analysis was performed, but results did not add any relevant information about the identity of the proteins. Since attempts to characterize the purified proteins were not successful, an indirect strategy was attempted. Several protein-specific antibodies were used against the 24 kDa protein. These included rabbit polyclonal antibodies to chestnut TLP (1:30,000 dilution; 1 h; anti-TLP; kindly provided by Dr. L. Gómez, ETSIM, UPM, Madrid) or chestnut chitinases antibodies (dilution 1: 500; 1 h; anti-Chi), or with anti-complex asparagine-linked glycan serum (1:30,000 dilution; 1 h; anti-CCD). The 24 kDa band was recognized by a pool of sera (anti-IgE) (**Figure 2B**), by anti-thaumatin-like proteins (anti-TLP) (**Figure 2C**), antibodies and by anti-carbohydrate complex determinant (anti-CCD) (**Figure 2E**). In contrast, we detected no positive recognition with other antibodies, such as antibodies produced against chestnut-chitinases (anti-Chi) (**Figure 2D**). This result suggested that a TLP could be implicated in the obeche dust sensitization,

**Table 1.** Demographic and clinical characteristics of subjects with confirmed occupational rhinitis/asthma (ORA+) *vs.* asymptomatic exposed (ORA−) and controls (CG). SPT: skin prick test; SD: standard deviation; *: p<0.05.

| | ORA+ | ORA− | CG |
|---|---|---|---|
| | n = 12 | n = 40 | n = 10 |
| **Age, mean (SD)*** | 42,3 (13) | 20,05 (2,8) | 36,33 (7,2) |
| **Sex, M/F*** | 10/2 | 40/0 | 2/8 |
| **Smokers, (%)** | 41,7% | 29,3% | 30% |
| **Total IgE, mean (range)** | 250 (54–688) | 192 (3–1270) | 64 (3–270) |
| **Mean exposure to wood, months*** | 238 | 42 | 0 |
| **Mean $FEV_1$, %** | 93% | 94% | 95% |
| **Positive SPTs to pollen, %** | 75% (67% grass) | 49% (60% grass) | 30% (33% grass) |

and its recognition by anti-CCD could confirm this possibility. In order to clarify this aspect, two control proteins were used: Prs a1, class I chitinase and avocado allergen; and Act d2, TLP and kiwi allergen. Both were incubated with the corresponding antibodies and with the pool of obeche sensitized sera (**Figure 2B**). The avocado-protein was not recognized by IgE, nor could we detect any positive band when the extract was incubated with anti-chitinase antibodies. However, Act d 2 was recognized by the obeche-sensitized serum pool, and a reactive band was observed when the extract was incubated with anti-TLP antibodies. Thus, the 24 kDa band may be a TLP.

## Relevance of CCD determinants in the measurement of specific IgE to obeche wood

In order to determine the influence of cross-reactive carbohydrate determinants (CCDs) in the measurement of specific IgE to obeche wood in symptomatic subjects, ELISA inhibition studies were performed using obeche extract as solid phase and CCDs as inhibitors in all ORA+ patients (n = 12). Results were obtained in 11 cases, but in one case the correct interpretation of results was not possible, probably due to the low levels of IgE. A significant number of sera (9/11, 82% of cases) showed no inhibition of specific IgE binding when incubated with bromelain, but showed a specific IgE binding to obeche proteins in more than 80% of the

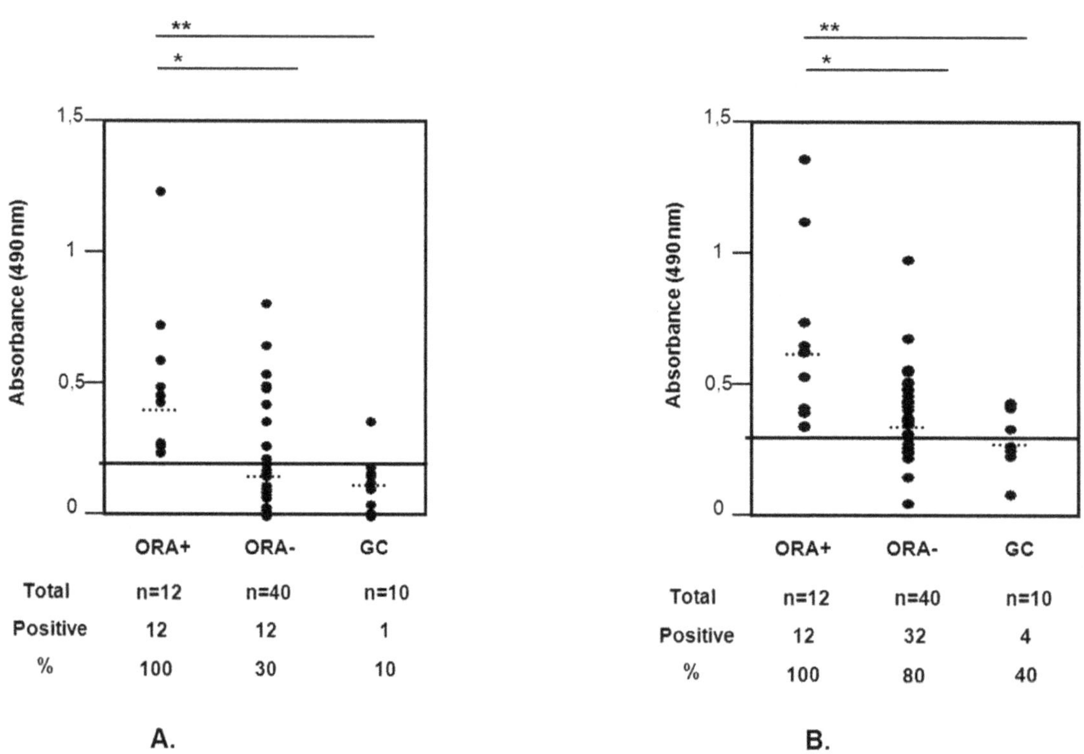


**Figure 1. Measurement of specific antibodies to obeche wood dust.** Means are represented by dotted lines and a horizontal line indicates cut-off value. *p<0.05 symptomatic vs asymptomatics; **p<0.05 symptomatic vs controls. **1A**. Levels of specific IgE in ORA+, ORA− and CG subjects; **1B**. Levels of specific IgG in ORA+, ORA− and CG subjects.

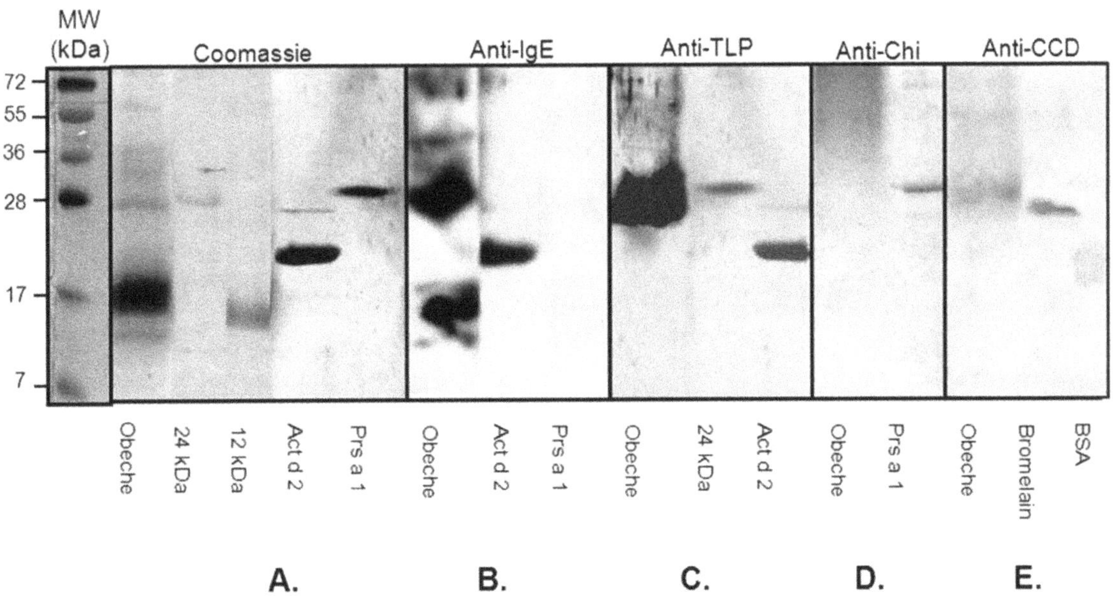


**Figure 2. Immunodetection of proteins in obeche wood dust. 2A**. *In-house* obeche wood dust extract (40 µg; Obeche), purified protein (5 µg; 24 kDa; 12 kDa) or purified allergens Act d 2 and Prs a 1 (5 µg) were separated by SDS-PAGE and stained with Coomassie blue (Coomassie). Replicas from the extract were electrotransferred and incubated with serum pool of selected exposure subjects (anti-IgE) (**2B**) or with antibodies produced against chestnut thaumatin-like protein (anti-TLP) (**2C**), against chestnut chitinases (anti-Ch) (**2D**) or anti N-glycan antibodies (anti-CCD) with bromelain and bovine serum albumin (BSA) as positive and negative controls (**2E**).

cases. Only two sera showed significant percentage of inhibition of specific IgE binding ≥50% when incubated with bromelain (subjects #4 and 10, see **Table 2**), showing that in these two cases the positive results may be attributed to cross–reactivity with CCDs (see **Figure 3**).

## Purified IgE binding proteins of obeche were recognized by exposed subjects

Allergenic activity of purified proteins was studied by ELISA using individual sera from the 12 symptomatic subjects (**Figure 4A**). The putative TLP was recognized by 92% of the subjects, and the gamma-expansin showed a positive response in 67%. This result was confirmed when the proteins were used in BAT (**Figure 4B**) in symptomatic subjects with total extract and with purified proteins (24 and 12 kDa). A positive activation of basophils was observed in 90% of ORA+ subjects in the presence of the obeche extract. The putative TLP protein was again the most active when it was incubated with basophils from exposed subjects, being recognized by 100% of the symptomatic subjects. The 12 kDa protein showed less activation capacity (70%). The optimal concentrations were chosen based on dose-response curves and cytotoxicity studies. Results of ELISA and BAT measurements for each subject are summarized in **Table 2**. Also, results were analyzed considering whether ORA+ subjects had rhinitis or rhinitis and asthma. As shown in Table 2, subjects with rhinitis recognized more the 12 kD band by ELISA compared to subjects with asthma (75% vs.50% respectively). However, rhinitis subjects recognized less the 12 kD band by BAT than asthmatic subjects (43% vs 100%). Also, the 24 kD band was recognized similarly by both groups regarding the technique used. Therefore, there are no significant differences between both groups.

## Skin prick testing with in-house extract and purified proteins

Skin prick testing with whole obeche extract at 1 mg/ml was positive in 83% of the ORA+ subjects, with no positive responses in the non-exposed asymptomatic controls. The allergenic capacity of the obeche-purified proteins was confirmed by SPT in 9 out of 12 ORA+ workers, obtaining 44% of positive responses to the purified putative TLP protein, while 11% recognized the gamma-expansin protein. Results of SPTs for each subject are summarized in **Table 2**.

## Reactivity of SE subjects to thaumatin-containing food extracts

Since the identified 24 kDa protein was a potential TLP, as demonstrated by specific antibodies, the presence of cross-reactivity with thaumatin-containing foods and food allergy was investigated. ORA+ workers were questioned about food allergy history, and SPTs were performed with commercial banana, peach, hazelnut, chestnut, kiwi, apple and melon extracts. Almost half of ORA+ patients reported a history of food allergy (see **Table 2**). SPTs to food extracts were positive in 40% of these subjects, mostly to peach, chestnut, hazelnut and kiwi extracts.

# Discussion

Occupational asthma is the most common occupational respiratory disease in developed countries [22]. Wood dust has been identified as a risk factor for the development of asthma [23], and in some cases it is caused by IgE-mediated sensitization to protein compounds of wood dust [6–10,24–26]. In the present study, an in-house obeche extract was produced that was recognized by SPT in 83% and by ELISA in 100% of subjects with confirmed occupational rhinitis and/or asthma, and by a small subset of asymptomatic exposed subjects (30% by ELISA).

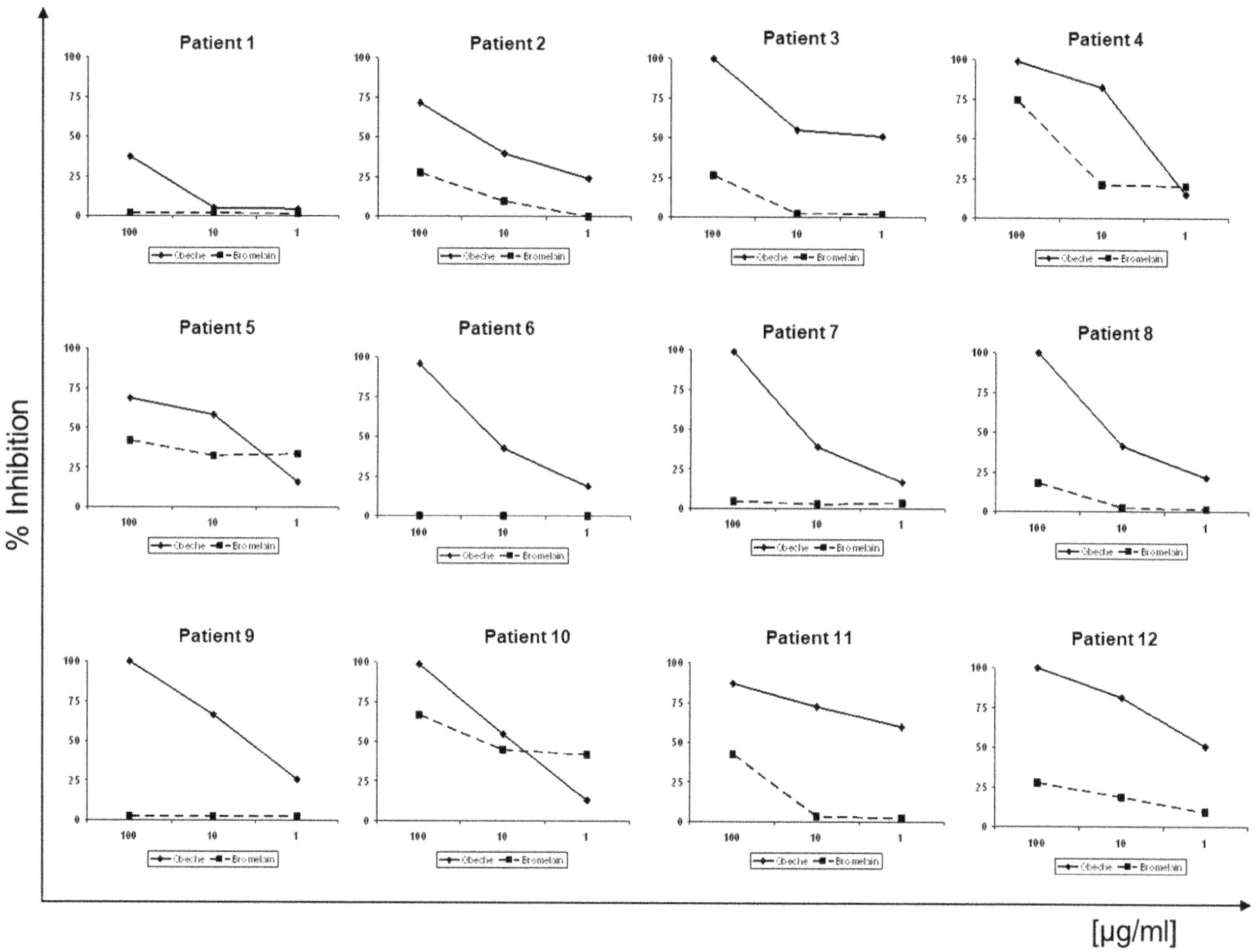


**Figure 3. ELISA inhibition studies in ORA+ subjects.** Bromelain (CCD, solid line) and obeche (dotted line) are inhibitors and obeche extract is the solid phase.

The detailed characterization of the allergenic activity of obeche wood dust revealed two principal bands of 24 and 12 kDa, which were recognized by ELISA in 92% and 67% of the ORA+ subjects, respectively. Unfortunately, there was not a sufficient amount of protein to test the asymptomatic subjects to obtain the reactivity to these proteins in that group. As reported, bands with apparent molecular weight of 28 and 17 kDa have been identified as principal IgE-binding proteins related to obeche sensitization [6,9], and these could correspond to our bands of 24 and 12 kDa. Surprisingly, no major IgE-binding band was observed that could be identified as Trip sl in the present study. In addition, no recognition was shown when the in-house extract of obeche was incubated with antibodies produced against chestnut chitinase. This difference in protein recognition may be explained by several hypotheses; the first possibility is that the allergen recognition profile may differ depending on geographic characteristics, as has been described in some food allergens such as LTPs [27]. Another possible explanation is that methodological differences in dust extraction and the fact that chitinases are highly thermolabile proteins may result in the absence of 38 kDa IgE-bands in the present study and others [6,9–11]. And finally, the geographical origin of the wood may influence the protein content of the extract, SDS-Page demonstrated that Trip s1 was mostly detected in wood samples coming from Ghana (*wawa*) but not in the samples coming from Cameroon (*ayous*) [28]. However, protein bands of 28 and 12 kDa were detected in dust samples from both wawa and ayous woods.

Identification of the 12 kDa protein revealed that it belonged to the gamma-expansin family [29], showing homology with tree-members of this family. Expansins refer to a family of non-enzymatic proteins found in the plant cell wall [30], and which includes small proteins grouped in two large (alpha and beta-expansins) and two small (gamma-, and epsilon- expansins) subfamilies [31]. A subset of beta-expansins has evolved a special role in grass pollen, where they are known as group 1 grass pollen allergens [21]. In contrast, the amino acid N-terminal and the trypsin-peptides obtained from the putative TLP had no correspondence with any known sequence deposited in the data bank. However, its recognition by anti-chestnut TLP antibodies suggests that it could belong to the thaumatin-like family, although more experimental analysis will be necessary to clarify its nature. Thaumatins are proteins described as plant defence proteins (PR5) against pathogen attacks and as panallergens responsible for cross-reactivity among foods and pollens [31], which may explain why some asymptomatic exposed subjects recognized the proteins mostly *in vitro* in our study [32–34]. For this reason, food allergy was also investigated in the ORA+ group, where 42% of the subjects reported a history of food allergy, and 40% had positive

**Table 2.** Results of *in vivo* and *in vitro* tests with obeche extract and purified proteins in subjects with confirmed occupational rhinitis and asthma (ORA+; R = rhinitis; R+A = rhinitis and asthma).

| Subjects # | Symptoms | SPT extract | SPT 12 kDa | SPT 24 kDa | ELISA extract | ELISA 12 kDa | ELISA 24 kDa | BAT extract | BAT 12 kDa | BAT 24 kDa | +SPT grass | Food allergy history | SPT TLP-related food | SPT+ food | CCD recognition |
|---|---|---|---|---|---|---|---|---|---|---|---|---|---|---|---|
| **1** | R+A | + | – | + | + | – | + | + | + | + | + | no | – | – | n/a |
| **2** | R | + | nd | nd | + | + | + | nd | nd | nd | + | no | nd | nd | no |
| **3** | R+A | + | nd | nd | + | + | – | nd | nd | nd | + | no | nd | nd | no |
| **4** | R+A | + | – | – | + | – | + | + | + | + | + | no | + | Peach,chestnut,hazelnut,kiwi, melon | yes |
| **5** | R+A | + | – | – | + | + | + | + | + | + | – | yes | + | Peach,chestnut,apple | no |
| **6** | R | + | + | + | + | + | + | + | + | + | + | no | – | – | no |
| **7** | R | + | – | + | + | + | + | + | – | + | – | yes | + | banana,kiwi | no |
| **8** | R | – | – | – | + | – | + | – | – | + | + | yes | + | hazelnut | no |
| **9** | R | + | – | + | + | + | + | + | + | + | – | yes | – | chestnut | no |
| **10** | R | – | – | – | + | + | + | + | – | + | – | yes | – | – | yes |
| **11** | R | + | – | – | + | – | + | + | + | + | – | no | – | – | no |
| **12** | R | + | nd | nd | + | + | + | + | + | + | – | no | – | – | no |

Results regarding food allergy assessment and CCD recognition are also included.

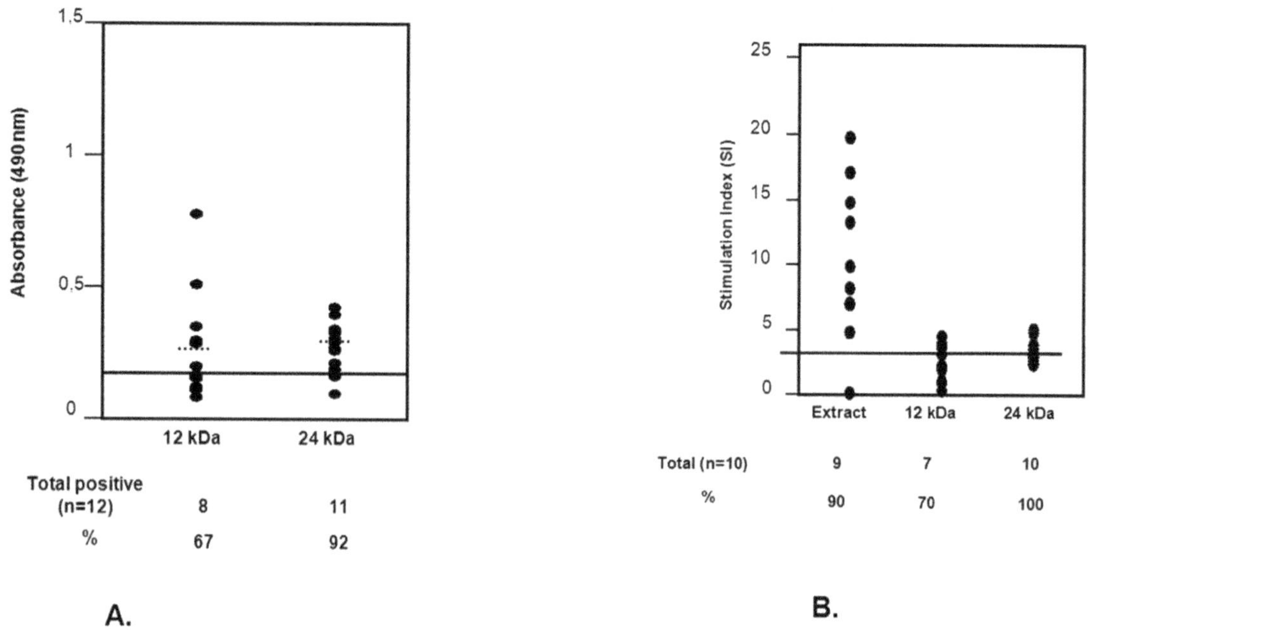


**Figure 4. Allergenic activity of purified proteins of obeche wood dust. 4A**. IgE-binding (ELISA) to purified obeche proteins (24 and 12 kDa). Solid line shows the positivity cut-off point, dotted lines show mean OD for each group. **4B**. Basophil activation tests using the *in-house* obeche wood dust extract and purified proteins (24 and 12 kDa). The solid line shows the threshold of positivity.

SPT's to several TLP-containing foods including peach, chestnut, hazelnut and kiwi, although the structural similarity among these TLPs and the 24 kDa protein in obeche is still unknown.

Regardless of their biochemical nature, the putative TLP and the obeche gamma-expansin were recognized by ELISA in 92% and 67% of workers with confirmed occupational rhinitis or asthma (ORA+), obtaining similar results in the BAT (100% for 24 kDa and 70% for 12 kDa protein, respectively). The results show that the protein with the highest molecular weight is the most active. However, the *in vivo* recognition was lower for both proteins, obtaining percentages of positive responses in the ORA+ group of 44% for the 24 kDa protein and only 11% for the 12 kDa protein.

The role of the cross-reactive carbohydrate determinants (CCDs) in sensitization allergy to wood proteins has been evaluated in other woods [35], showing a high rate of sensitization to CCDs in workers with *in vitro* sensitization to several woods but not among workers with a single sensitization or clinically relevant symptoms [36]. The putative thaumatin described in the present study may be glycosilated, based on the results of the incubation with anti-CCD antibodies. However, in our study, more than 80% of cases showed a specific IgE binding to obeche proteins that were not inhibited by bromelain, as demonstrated by ELISA-inhibition studies. A previous study that also described the 28 kDa as the most relevant protein in a very similar population showed that the use of a deglycosylated extract only reduced the IgE binding activity by 8.6%. Therefore, in the case of these obeche wood proteins, CCD sensitization does not seem relevant in most patients.

In conclusion, a 24 kDa putative TLP and a 12 kDa gamma-expansin were identified in obeche wood, showing a high percentage of recognition by *in vitro* studies and a modest *in vivo* recognition by subjects with confirmed rhinitis/asthma caused by obeche wood. This study will contribute to better characterize this wood, since there is a need of standardized, well-characterized extracts to correctly diagnose this disease, which is currently underestimated. Consequently, further studies are needed to establish the sensitivity and specificity parameters of these diagnostic techniques and further characterization of these and other wood allergens.

## Acknowledgments

The authors would like to thank Ian Johnson Johnstone for his help with the final English version of this manuscript. They also thank Mrs. Arias and Mr. García-Montes, and the staff and students from CEMER School (Cordoba, Spain) for their support and collaboration in this study.

## Author Contributions

Designed and coordinated the study and the protocol to collect sera: PC AD-P MB. Corrected the manuscript and suggested important contributions to define the final version: PC AD-P MB. Carried out the allergen purification: AA AP CG-C. Collected patients' sera and performed challenge tests: PC ID LG. Performed the experiments: AA AP CG-C. Analyzed the data: AA AP CG-C. Wrote the paper: AA PC AD-P.

## References

1. Chan-Yeung M, Malo JL (2006) Western Red cedar (*Thuja plicata*) and other wood dusts. IN: "Asthma in the workplace" 3rd edition Pages 505–524 Bernstein IL, Chan-Yeung M, Bernstein D, editors Taylor & Francis Group Publishers NY
2. Kauppinen T, Vincent R, Liukkonen T, Grzebyk M, Kauppinen A, et al. (2006) Occupational exposure to inhaled wood dust in the member status of the European Union. Ann Occup Hyg; 50: 549–61
3. Malmberg PO, Rask-Andersen A, Larsson KA, Stjernberg N, Sundblad BM, et al. (1996) Increased bronchial responsiveness in workers sawing Scots pine. Am J Respir Crit Care Med; 153(3): 948–52
4. Schlünssen V, Jacobsen G, Erlandsen M, Mikkelsen AB, Schaumburg I, et al. (2008) Determinants of wood dust exposure in the Danish furniture industry-Cross sectional studies 6 years apart. Ann Occup Hyg; 52(4): 227–238

5. Campo P, Aranda A, Rondon C, Doña I, Diaz-Perales A, et al. (2010) Work-related sensitization and respiratory symptoms in carpentry apprentices exposed to wood dust and diisocyanates. Ann Allergy Asthma Immunol, 105: 24–30
6. Quirce S, Hinojosa M, Marañón F, Ferrer A, Fernández-Caldas E, et al. (2000) Identification of obeche wood (Triplochiton scleroxylon) allergens associated with occupational asthma. J Allergy Clin Immunol; 106: 400–1
7. Hinojosa M, Losada E, Moneo I, Dominguez J, Carrillo T, et al. (1986) Occupational asthma caused by African maple (Obeche) and Ramin: evidence of cross reactivity between these two woods. Clin Allergy; 16:145–53
8. Reijula K, Kujala V, Latvala J (1994) Sauna builder's asthma caused by obeche (Triplochiton scleroxylon) dust. Thorax; 49:622–3
9. Ferrer A, Marañón F, Casanovas M, Fernández-Caldas E (2001) Asthma from inhalation of Triplochiton scleroxylon (Samba) wood dust. J Investig Allergol Clin Immunol.; 11: 199–203.
10. Kespohl S, Sander I, Merget R, Petersen A, Meyer HE, et al. (2005) Identification of an obeche (Triplochiton scleroxylon) wood allergen as a class I chitinase. Allergy; 60: 808–14
11. Vidal C, González-Quintela A, Rodriguez V, Armisén M, Liñares T, et al. (2006) Anaphylaxis to Cyphomandra betacea Sendth (tamarillo) in an obeche wood (*Triplochiton scleroxylon*) allergic patient. Ann Allergy Asthma Immunol.;96: 870–3.
12. Venturini M, Gastaminza G, Kespohl S, Bernedo N, Garmendia M, et al. (2004) Cross-reactivity between obeche wood (*Triplochiton scleroxylon*) and natural rubber latex. Allergy; 59: 225–8
13. Rondon C, Romero JJ, Lopez S, Antunez C, Martin-Casañez E, et al. (2007) Local IgE production and positive nasal provocation test in patients with persistent nonallergic rhinitis. J Allergy Clin Immunol.; 119(4): 899–905
14. Fernandez-Nieto M, Quirce S, Carnes J, Sastre J (2006) Occupational asthma due to chromium and nickel salts. Int Arch Occup Environ Health.; 79(6):483–6
15. Burney PG, Laitinen LA, Perdrizet S, Huckauf H, Tattersfield AE, et al. (1989) Validity and repeatability of the IUATLD (1984) bronchial symptoms questionnaire: an international comparison. Eur Resp J; 940–945
16. Miller MR, Hankinson J, Brusasco V, Burgos F, Casaburi R, et al. (2005) Series "ATS/ERS Task Force: standarization of lung function testing" Standardization of Spirometry. Eur Resp J; 26: 319–338.
17. Dreborg S, Frew A (1993) EAACI Position Paper: Allergen Standardization and skin tests; 48: 49–54.
18. Laemmli UK (1970) Cleavage of structural proteins during the assembly of the head of bacteriophage T4. Nature; 227:680–5
19. Díaz-Perales A, Lombardero M, Sánchez-Monge R, García-Selles FJ, Pernas M, et al. (2000) Lipid-transfer proteins as potential plant panallergens: cross-reactivity among proteins of Artemisia pollen, Castanea nut and Rosaceae fruits, with different IgE-binding capacities. Clin Exp Allergy; 30:1403–10
20. Torres MJ, Padial A, Mayorga C, Fernández T, Sanchez-Sabate E, et al. (2004) The diagnostic interpretation of basophil activation test in immediate allergic reactions to betalactams. Clin Exp Allergy; 34:1768–75.
21. Cosgrove DJ, Bedinger P, Durachko DM (1997) Group I allergens of grass pollen as cell wall-loosening agents. Proc. Natl. Acad. Sci. USA; 94: 6559–6564.
22. Kauppinen T, Vincent R, Liukkonen T, Grzebyk M, Kauppinen A, et al. (2006) Occupational exposure to inhalable wood dust in the member states of the European Union. Ann Occup Hyg.; 50: 549–61
23. Pérez-Ríos M, Ruano-Ravina A, Etminan M, Takkouche B (2010) A meta-analysis on wood dust exposure and risk of asthma. Allergy; 65: 467–73
24. Tse KS, Chan H, Chan Yeung M (1982) Specific IgE antibodies in workers with occupational asthma due to Western red cedar. Clin Allergy; 12: 249–258.
25. Quirce S, Parra A, Antón E, Fernández-Nieto M, Jerez J, et al. (2004) Occupational asthma caused by tali and jatoba wood dusts. J Allergy Clin Immunol; 113: 361–3.
26. Skovsted TA, Schlünssen V, Schaumburg I, Wang P, Staun-Olsen P, et al. (2003) Only few workers exposed to wood dust are detected with specific IgE against pine wood. Allergy;58: 772–9
27. Fernández-Rivas M, Bolhaar S, González-Mancebo E, Asero R, van Leeuwen A, et al. (2006) Apple allergy across Europe: how allergen sensitization profiles determine the clinical expression of allergies to plant foods. J Allergy Clin Immunol Aug; 118(2): 481–8
28. Kespohl S, Sander I, Schulze J, Poppe M, Brüning T, et al. (2008) Development of an obeche wood allergen quantification assay for the assessment of allergen exposure in workplaces. Scand J Work Environ Health; 34:387–95.
29. Ceccardi TL, Barthe GA, Derrick KS (1998) A novel protein associated with citrus blight has sequence similarities to expansin. Plant Mol Biol, 38:775–783
30. Sampedro J, Cosgrove D (2005) The expansin superfamily. Genome Biology; 6:242–253
31. Li Y, Darley C, Ongaro V, Fleming A, Schipper O, et al. (2002) Plant Expansins Are a Complex Multigene Family with an Ancient Evolutionary Origin. Plant Physiol; 128: 854–864.
32. Breiteneder H (2004) Thaumatin-like proteins: a new family of pollen and fruit allergens. Allergy; 59: 479–481
33. Gavrovic-Jankulovic M, Cirkovic T, Vuckovic O, Atanaskovic-Markovic M, Petersen A, et al. (2002) Isolation and biochemical characterization of a thaumatin-like kiwi allergen. J Allergy Clin Immunol; 110: 805–810
34. Palacín A, Tordesillas L, Gamboa P, Sanchez-Monge R, Cuesta-Herranz J, et al. (2010) Characterization of peach thaumatin-like proteins and their identification as major peach allergens. Clin Exp Allergy; 40:1422–30
35. Kespohl S, Kotschy-Lang N, Tomm JM, von Bergen M, Maryska S, et al. (2012) Occupational IgE-mediated softwood allergy: characterization of the causative allergen. Int Arch Allergy Immunol.;157: 202–8.
36. Kespohl S, Schlünssen V, Jacobsen G, Schaumburg I, Maryska S, et al. (2010) Impact of cross-reactive carbohydrate determinants on wood dust sensitization. Clin Exp Allergy; 40(7): 1099–106

# 20

# The Involvement of Thaumatin-Like Proteins in Plant Food Cross-Reactivity: A Multicenter Study Using a Specific Protein Microarray

**Arantxa Palacín[1], Luis A. Rivas[2], Cristina Gómez-Casado[1], Jacobo Aguirre[2], Leticia Tordesillas[1], Joan Bartra[3], Carlos Blanco[4], Teresa Carrillo[5], Javier Cuesta-Herranz[6], José A. Cumplido Bonny[5], Enrique Flores[7], Mar G. García-Alvarez-Eire[8], Ignacio García-Nuñez[9], Francisco J. Fernández[7], Pedro Gamboa[10], Rosa Muñoz[3], Rosa Sánchez-Monge[1], Maria Torres[11], Susana Varela Losada[8], Mayte Villalba[11], Francisco Vega[4], Victor Parro[2], Miguel Blanca[9], Gabriel Salcedo[12], Araceli Díaz-Perales[1]***

**1** Centro de Biotecnología y Genómica de Plantas, Campus de Montegancedo, Pozuelo de Alarcón, Madrid, Spain, **2** Departamento de Evolución Molecular, Centro de Astrobiología (INTA-CSIC), Torrejón de Ardoz, Madrid, Spain, **3** Unitat d'Allèrgia, Servei Pneumologia i Allèrgia Respiratòria, Hospital Clínic, Universitat de Barcelona, Institut d'Investigacions Biomèdiques August Pi i Sunyer (IDIBAPS), Centro de Investigaciones Biomédicas en Red de Enfermedades Respiratorias (CIBERES), Barcelona, Spain, **4** Servicio de Alergia, Hospital Universitario de la Princesa, Instituto de Investigación Sanitaria Princesa (IP), Madrid, Spain, **5** Servicio de Alergología, Hospital Universitario de Gran Canaria Dr. Negrín, Las Palmas de Gran Canaria, Spain, **6** Servicio de Alergia, Fundación Jiménez Díaz, Madrid, Spain, **7** Unidad de Alergia, Hospital General Universitario, Alicante, Spain, **8** Unidad de Alergología, Complexo Hospitalario, Ourense, Spain, **9** Laboratorio de Investigación, Fundación IMABIS-Carlos Haya Hospital, Hospital Civil, Málaga, Spain, **10** Servicio de Alergia, Hospital de Basurto, Bilbao, Spain, **11** Departamento de Bioquímica y Biología Molecular I, Facultad de Químicas, Universidad Complutense, Madrid, Spain, **12** Departamento de Biotecnología, ETSI Agrónomos, Universidad Politécnica, Madrid, Spain

## Abstract

Cross-reactivity of plant foods is an important phenomenon in allergy, with geographical variations with respect to the number and prevalence of the allergens involved in this process, whose complexity requires detailed studies. We have addressed the role of thaumatin-like proteins (TLPs) in cross-reactivity between fruit and pollen allergies. A representative panel of 16 purified TLPs was printed onto an allergen microarray. The proteins selected belonged to the sources most frequently associated with peach allergy in representative regions of Spain. Sera from two groups of well characterized patients, one with allergy to Rosaceae fruit (FAG) and another against pollens but tolerant to food-plant allergens (PAG), were obtained from seven geographical areas with different environmental pollen profiles. Cross-reactivity between members of this family was demonstrated by inhibition assays. Only 6 out of 16 purified TLPs showed noticeable allergenic activity in the studied populations. Pru p 2.0201, the peach TLP (41%), chestnut TLP (24%) and plane pollen TLP (22%) proved to be allergens of probable relevance to fruit allergy, being mainly associated with pollen sensitization, and strongly linked to specific geographical areas such as Barcelona, Bilbao, the Canary Islands and Madrid. The patients exhibited >50% positive response to Pru p 2.0201 and to chestnut TLP in these specific areas. Therefore, their recognition patterns were associated with the geographical area, suggesting a role for pollen in the sensitization of these allergens. Finally, the co-sensitizations of patients considering pairs of TLP allergens were analyzed by using the co-sensitization graph associated with an allergen microarray immunoassay. Our data indicate that TLPs are significant allergens in plant food allergy and should be considered when diagnosing and treating pollen-food allergy.

**Editor:** Bin Xue, University of South Florida, United States of America

**Funding:** Ministerio de Ciencia e Innovación (project BIO2009-07050) and FIS-Thematic Networks and Co-operative Research Centers: RIRAAF (RD07/0064). C. Gómez Casado and L. Tordesillas were supported by training grants from the Spanish Government (FPI and FPU programmes, MEC, respectively). J. Aguirre was supported by the Ministerio de Ciencia e Innovación (project FIS2011-27569) and Comunidad de Madrid, R&D Programme of Activities, grant MODELICO-CM S2009ESP-1691. The funders had no role in the study design, data collection or analysis, the decision to publish, or the preparation of the manuscript.

**Competing Interests:** The authors have declared that no competing interests exist.

* E-mail: araceli.diaz@upm.es

## Introduction

Cross-reactivity is an important problem for the diagnosis and treatment of allergy, and in the daily routine of patients, due to our lack of knowledge about the original sensitization source. Cross-reactivity in plant food allergy is mediated by panallergens belonging to widely distributed protein families. Identifying the patterns of association between different allergen sources from pollen and foods is a priority because of its importance for understanding how allergy is triggered.

*Rosaceae* fruit allergy, represented by peach, is the most prevalent plant ingested allergy in Spain and the south of Europe. It has become notably common in the last years [1]. Pru p 3, the lipid transfer protein (LTP) of peach, is considered to be the main allergen in this fruit, and is recognized by 60–70% of allergic patients [2,3]. This allergen exhibits cross-reactivity with a wide range of plant foods and some pollen sources, such as mugwort and plane, in a high proportion of patients [3,4,5]. However, despite the identification of the major allergen responsible for most peach-associated allergies, we still do not understand the coexistence of cross-reactivity between peach and some fruits or pollens such as grasses.

Recently, members of the thaumatin-like protein (TLP) family have been identified as important allergens in peach fruit [6]. TLPs have also been described as allergens in various fruits, such as apple, cherry, kiwi, olive and banana, and in pollens such as cypress and possibly others. This family is thought to be a panallergen family responsible for cross-reactivity between pollen and fruit, although this is not currently backed up by sufficient experimental evidence [7].

The proteins of the thaumatin-like family have molecular masses of 20–30 kDa, with a very stable three-dimensional structure that is maintained by six disulphide bridges. They have been described as plant defense proteins (PR-5) against pathogen-attacks, especially fungal. Some thaumatins are glycoproteins, and this could account for their allergenic capacity [8].

The involvement of this protein family in cross-reactivity has been determined by *in vitro* techniques, such as ELISA assays, that require large quantities of allergens and serum volume. The onset of microarray techniques with large panels of purified allergens, some of them from the same family, has been a major advance in the diagnosis of allergic diseases [9,10]. Thus, it is possible to measure simultaneously IgEs, specific to many molecules, using tiny amounts of allergen and sera, thereby enabling a large number of samples to be screened at the reasonable cost. The wealth of information generated by microarrays also demands more powerful analytical strategies to identify associations within the data [11,12]. For this reason, we have made use of the graph theory to study and visualize the co-sensitization of different sera for TLP allergens. A graph, or network, is composed of nodes and connecting links [13,14]. These links might be directed or undirected, and weighted or unweighted, depending on the nature of the system under study. In the graphs used in this work, nodes represent allergens, and links (which are undirected and weighted) represent the co-sensitization of sera for pairs of allergens. Recently, these graphs have been used to describe the cross-reactions in an antibody microarray immunoassay in a sandwich format [15], and, in fact, there is an extensive literature about their usefulness for analyzing biological systems [16,17,18,19,20]. In our particular case, we have focused on developing the potential of graph theory for analyzing TLP microarrays and for applying them in the field.

The principal objective of this study was to establish the role of TLPs in fruit allergy and their putative involvement in cross-reactivities with other foods and/or pollens. For this purpose, 16 members of this family were purified and printed on a protein microarray. The panel of proteins was chosen with respect to the specific features of the sensitization of the population under evaluation [2]. The TLP microarray was tested with the sera from 329 allergic patients from seven regions of Spain, and considering with respect to their different pollen profiles.

## Results

### Purification of TLP Members from Different Foods and Pollens

Peach allergy is usually associated to sensitization to other fruits such as apple, kiwi and banana, and to nuts such as hazelnut, chestnut and walnut [2]. Moreover, over 70% of peach-allergic patients in Spain also suffering from pollinosis, mainly from grasses, mugwort, olive and cypress [2]. Considering these associations, 16 TLPs were purified, from both foods and pollens, according to previously described methods (Table 1). Some of these food-related TLPs had been previously identified as allergens (www.allergen.org, IUIS; www.allergome.com): Act d 2 [8], Cup a 3 [21], Mal d 2 [22], Mus a 4 [23], Pru av 2 [24], Pru p 2.0101 [6], Pru p 2.0201 [6], a wheat TLP [25] and olive TLP [26]. The purified wheat TLP in this study proved to be different from the one associated with baker's asthma. In this paper, the allergenic activities of the other purified TLPs (such as the proteins from mugwort, birch and plane pollens, and from hazelnut, chestnut, cabbage, lettuce and olive) have been studied for the first time (Table 1). Unfortunately, no TLP from grass pollen could be purified, even though it is one of the most frequently associated with peach allergy.

Other allergens were included in the microarray: Pru p 3 (LTP, peach allergen), Art v 3 (LTP, mugwort allergen), Act d 1 (cysteine protease, kiwi allergen), Ana c 2 (pineapple allergen and marker of carbohydrate cross-reactive determinants (CCD)), Bet v 1 (PR10 from birch pollen), Cuc m 2 (melon fruit profilin), Pers a 1 (avocado latex-fruit allergen) and Pho d 2 (palm-pollen profilin).

### Frequency of Recognition of TLPs by Allergic Patients

Seven regions of Spain were chosen on the basis of their characteristic major pollens (Table 2, pollen count average for the previous 10 years), and two groups of patients were included in the study, prospectively among adult population (Table 2): fruit-allergic (FAG) patients and non-food pollen-allergic (PAG) patients. The first group was subdivided into two subgroups depending on whether patients were allergic to pollen (n = 169) or not (n = 43). An additional group of food-tolerant volunteers without pollinosis (n = 35; five per region) was recruited as a negative control.

A microarray approach was chosen as the best *in vitro* high-throughput immunological assay to test a large number of proteins and sera, based on the small quantities of protein and sera required. The microarray was constructed by printing TLP proteins onto activated glass slides, following previously published methods [27]. Each protein was recognized by at least one serum, but none of them gave a positive response with sera from the healthy control group (data not shown).

Generally, TLPs were not highly prevalent in the allergic populations examined in this study (Figure 1). Most of the TLPs (10/16) were recognized by fewer than 10% of the patients. Despite this, they were mainly associated with fruit allergy. The fruit-allergic patients recognized more TLPs than pollinic food-tolerant subjects (2 versus 0.5 on average, respectively). Curiously, patients from Barcelona were significantly different, showing higher polysensitization to these allergens (4 TLPs on average) than did subjects from the other regions (Mann-Whitney U test: $p = 0.001$).

Inhibition assays using the peach TLP, Pru p 2.0201, and chestnut and plane pollen TLPs as inhibitors confirmed the cross-reactivity between the members of this family (Figure 2). Pru p 2.0201 seemed to be the starting point for TLP sensitization since it was able to inhibit IgE binding to the other allergens tested (Figure 2).

Fruit allergic group was more likely to have a positive response to Pru p 2.0201(41% *vs.* 15%), chestnut (24% *vs.* 15%) and plane TLP (22% *vs.* 8%) than did patients from the pollen allergic group, who were pollinic subjects but plant-food tolerant attending to microarray results ($\chi^2 = 0.002$, 0.017 and 0.003, respectively). Individuals affected by fruit and pollen allergy more frequently recognized TLPs than did those without respiratory allergy. In the

**Table 1.** Purified proteins included in the TLP microarray.

| Protein | Family | Specific/common name | N-terminal or internal peptide sequence | Accession number | Reference |
|---|---|---|---|---|---|
| **Act d 2** | TLP | *Actinidia deliciosa*/Kiwi | ATFNI | P83958 | [35] |
| **Cup a 3** | TLP | *Cupressus arizonica*/cypress | VKFDIKNQXRYT | Q69CS2 | [21] |
| **Mal d 2** | TLP | *Malus domestica*/Apple | AKITFTNNXP | Q3BCT8 | [22] |
| **Mus a 4** | TLP | *Musa acuminata*/Banana | ATFEIVNRXSYTVWAAAVPGGGRQLNQ | 1Z3Q | [35] |
| **Pru av 2** | TLP | *Prunus avium*/Cherry | ATISFKNNCP | P50694 | This paper |
| **Pru p 2.0201** | TLP | *Prunus persica*/Peach | R.SVDAPSPWSGR.F AKITFTNKQS | gi190613905 | [6] |
| **Pru p 2.0101** | TLP | *Prunus persica*/Peach | K.ASTCPADINKVCPAPLQVKG AKITFTNK | gi190613911 | [7] |
| **Birch pollen TLP** | TLP | *Betula verrucosa*/Birch | K.NSTFTCSGGPDYVITFCP | Q9FSG7 | This paper |
| **Chestnut TLP** | TLP | *Castanea sativa*/Chestnut | STVIFYNKC | P50699 | [38] |
| **Cabbage TLP** | TLP | *Brassica oleraceae*/Cabbage | ATFEIVNRXS | P02884 | This paper |
| **Hazelnut TLP** | TLP | *Corylus avellana*/Hazelnut | K.NSGFTCSGAFIAAARS NTVWPGTLTGDQKPQLSLTAFELASKA | P83336 | This paper |
| **Lettuce TLP** | TLP | *Lactuca sativa*/Lettuce | ANFNIHNNXP | P83959 | This paper |
| **Mugwort pollen TLP** | TLP | *Artemisia vulgaris*/Mugwort | ATITVXNRXS | Q946Z0 | This paper |
| **Olive TLP** | TLP | *Olea europaea*/Olive | ATFDIVNQCTYTVWAAASPGG | ACZ57583 | [39] |
| **Plane pollen TLP** | TLP | *Platanus acerifolia*/Plane | RCSFTVWPAATPVGGGRQ | P31110 | This paper |
| **Wheat TLP** | TLP | *Triticum aestivum*/Wheat | KASQSVDAPSPWSGRF | P83336 | This paper |
| **Act d 1** | Cystein protease | *Actinidia deliciosa*/Kiwi | LPSYV | P00785 | [35] |
| **Ana c 2** | Cystein protease | *Ananas comosus*/Pineaple | MAEYGRVYKDNDE | BAA21929 | Commercial |
| **Art v 3** | LTP | *Artemisia vulgaris*/Mugwort | ALTXSDV | P0C088 | [4] |
| **Bet v 1** | PR10 | *Betula verrucosa*/Birch | ARLFKAFILDGDNL | P15494 | Commercial |
| **Cuc m 2** | Profilin | *Cucumis melon*/Melon | MSWGAYVDDHLMC | AJ565931 | [40] |
| **Pers a 1** | Class I chitinase | *Persea americana*/Avocado | EQHGR | P93680 | [41] |
| **Pho d 2** | Profilin | *Phoenix dactylifera*/Palm | MSWGAYVDEHLMC | AJ417566 | Commercial |
| **Pru p 3** | LTP | *Prunus persica*/Peach | ITCGQE | Q9LED1 | [42] |

case of Pru p 2.0201, 41% of patients allergic to pollen and fruit - had a positive response in contrast to 33% of individuals in the same group without pollen allergy. Pru p 2.0201 was the most prevalent allergen, being recognized by 32% of all the patients (FAG+PAG) studied. A close association between sensitization to Pru p 2.0201 and to Pru p 3 was observed ($\chi^2 = 0.005$).

## Response Pattern by Geographical Area

To study the differences in the TLPs recognition in patients with fruit allergy, we selected patients from 7 geographical areas with different pollen profiles (Table 3). The analysis of prevalence by geographical area revealed some specific features about recognition frequencies in fruit allergy group of patients (Figure 3).

Significant differences were observed in response to Pru p 2.0201 ($\chi^2 < 0.0001$), ranging from 18–23% in patients from Alicante/Ourense respectively, to 70% in those from the Canary Islands. These results contrasted with the prevalences of Pru p 2.0101, the other peach TLP, which was less than 10% in every region, except for the FAG patients from Bilbao (35%; $\chi^2 = 0.012$) and from Malaga (18%; $\chi^2 = 0.120$). In fact the frequencies of both peach TLPs (Pru p 2.0201 and Pru p 2.0101) were especially high in patients with pollen sensitization but with plant food tolerance (PAG) from Bilbao. The same pattern was observed for the lettuce TLP. This allergen was recognized by 40% of PAG subjects from Bilbao, although almost no recognition was detected in FAG patients (<5%). This raises the possibility that respiratory allergies affect the recognition of TLP allergens. However, this suggestion needs more evidences.

Chestnut TLP and plane TLP were found to be important in fruit sensitizations. The former proved to be a significant allergen in fruit-allergic patients from Barcelona and Bilbao, with recognition frequencies of more than 50%, and from the Canary Islands, with almost 40% recognition. In Barcelona, 48% of pollen-allergic patients with plant-food tolerance had a positive response. In all other study areas, limited recognition was observed. The case of the plane TLP was quite different. The most striking recognition level (around 30%) was exhibited by fruit-allergic patients from Alicante, Barcelona, Bilbao and the Canary Islands. This allergen was the only pollen TLP that appeared to be important in fruit allergy.

## Graph-based Analysis of the TLP Microarray Immunoassay

We made use of the graph theory for two main reasons. Firstly, it is a simple and useful way of representing TLP-microarray immunoassay data, and secondly, because we wanted to gain insight into the co-sensitization patterns of the TLP allergens in the selected population. The steps for building the co-sensitization graph associated with our TLP microarray immunoassay (Figure 4) are explained in detail in the Materials and Methods. In short, two

**Table 2.** Characteristics of the patient sample.

| | Total[1] | FAG[2] | | PAG[3] |
|---|---|---|---|---|
| | | Pollen | Non-pollen | |
| Number of patients | 329 | 169 | 43 | 117 |
| Sex[4] | 112M 217F | 57M 112F | 15M 28F | 40M 77F |
| Age range | 08–62 | 18–59 | 08–56 | 15–62 |
| **Food Allergy Symptoms (%)** | | | | |
| Rhinitis | 61 | 95 | 0 | 87 |
| Asthma | 27 | 34 | 4 | 43 |
| Oral allergy syndrome | 35 | 52 | 54 | 0 |
| Anaphylactic reaction | 14 | 18 | 25 | 0 |
| Urticaria | 31 | 63 | 28 | 2 |
| Angio-edema | 10 | 16 | 14 | 0 |
| Gastrointestinal | 5 | 9 | 6 | 0 |
| Others | 2 | 4 | 2 | 0 |
| **SPT (%)*** | | | | |
| Mugwort pollen | 42 | 50 | 31 | 45 |
| Cypress pollen | 24 | 28 | 13 | 31 |
| Grass pollen | 55 | 51 | 27 | 88 |
| Plane pollen | 36 | 54 | 23 | 31 |
| Olive pollen | 34 | 45 | 18 | 39 |
| Pellitory pollen | 7 | 5 | 4 | 13 |

[1]Total, all patients;
[2]FAG, Fruit-allergic patients;
[3]PAG, Pollen-allergic food-tolerant patients;
[4]M, male; F, female;
*SPTs with purified protein were performed in a selected group of patients of 50 FAG, 20 PAG and 20 non-pollen food-tolerant subjects.

allergens are connected by a link in the graph if at least one serum gave a positive reaction to both allergens, and the weight of such a link is a measure of the degree of similarity or correlation between the sera that reacted positively to each of the allergens -that is, such weight depends on whether these two sets have common elements or not-. Therefore, the maximum weight 1 was assigned when both allergens were recognized by exactly the same group of reacting sera (irrespective of the size of the group).

The co-sensitization graph showed to be totally connected (i.e., all allergens were connected with all other allergens), meaning at least one serum reacted positively to any pair of allergens, or in other words, that there were no incompatible pairs of co-sensitizations. Therefore, there are $(23\times22)/2=253$ links in the graph. However in order to clarify the interpretation of the results only the 25 links with weights greater than 0.50 were plotted in Figure 4.

The TLP allergens connected with the highest weights were cabbage-TLP/Lettuce TLP (0.69) and hazelnut-TLP/Mus a 4 (0.67). By contrast, the strongest link connected the non-TLP allergens Cuc m 2 and Pho d 2 (0.80), both belonging to the family of, profilins. The lowest co-sensitizations were found between Mal d 2/Pru p 2.0201 (0.12), wheat-TLP/Pru p 2.0101 (0.14), and wheat-TLP/Mal d 2 (0.16).

The average weights (Table 4) were a measure of the degree of co-sensitization that an allergen showed with the rest of the allergens in the graph. Pru av 2, cabbage TLP and Lettuce TLP had the highest average weights (all above 0.4), meaning that their co-sensitizations with the rest of the network are especially relevant. The case of the non-TLP allergens is remarkable, as they have relatively large average weights (especially Ana c 2 (CCD marker) with a value of 0.38), even when they were used as control proteins in the experiments. Finally, we should mention the case of olive TLP and Pru p 3, the allergens linked with the lowest average weight (both 0.29).

## Discussion

The study of cross-reactivity in allergy using protein-microarray strategies is a powerful method with advantages over other immunological approaches [9,11]. A large number of allergens and sera from many patients can be tested in the same assay, with the additional advantages of lower costs and the more rapid processing of samples [12,28,29,33].

In Spain, fruit allergy is clearly associated with LTP sensitization, especially to Pru p 3 [2,3], the peach allergen. However, LTPs are not the only proteins involved in fruit/food sensitization. Other families of allergens, such as profilins [30,31,32], have been described as being important in the development of food allergy in this area.

Members of the TLP family can have a role as allergens in a wide panel of plant food and several pollens, although there is little experimental evidence in plant foods and/or pollen cross-reactivities [6,7]. In this paper, we have tried to establish the role of this protein family in plant food allergy and in cross-reactivity between foods and pollens. A large number of patients were selected from different Spanish regions and a representative panel of TLPs based on the most frequent sensitizations associated with peach allergy [2] was printed in a protein microarray.

In order to study the association between the different allergens in a visual and intuitive manner, we have presented our results in a co-sensitization graph. In this, the nodes represent the different allergens, and the weight of the link that connects two allergens measures whether the sera that reacted positively to one allergen also gave a positive reaction to the other. Therefore, the weight of each link gives us a quantitative impression of the co-sensitization of sera for that pair of allergens.

The analysis of the recognition profile revealed that fruit-allergic (FAG, independent of their respiratory sensitization) subjects showed a strong positive response to several TLPs, although this response tended to be more frequent in patients with pollinosis. However, people with isolated pollen allergy (PAG) showed no predominant recognition pattern. They had a low level of positive responses to TLPs.

Only six of the 16 TLPs studied (the two peach, chestnut, lettuce, cabbage and plane TLPs) yielded recognition frequencies greater than 10%. Of particular interest is the significantly small number of responders we obtained with Mal d 2 and Pru av 2 (5%), which are both important allergens in central and northern Europe [7,34]. This low response may be related to the allergic profile of the patients included in this work, who were mainly sensitized to peach.

The peach TLP, Pru p 2.0201, gave more than 40% positive responses in fruit-allergic patients, with values of up to 50% in areas such as Barcelona, Bilbao, the Canary Islands and Madrid. This protein seems to act as the gateway for sensitizing members of this family. An unexpected pattern of association between the two LTP allergens (Pru p 3 and Art v 3) and the TLP Pru p 2.0201 was observed. The recognition of Pru p 3 and Pru p 2.0201 was closely associated ($\chi^2=0.005$), and the weight of its co-sensitization link was 0.61.

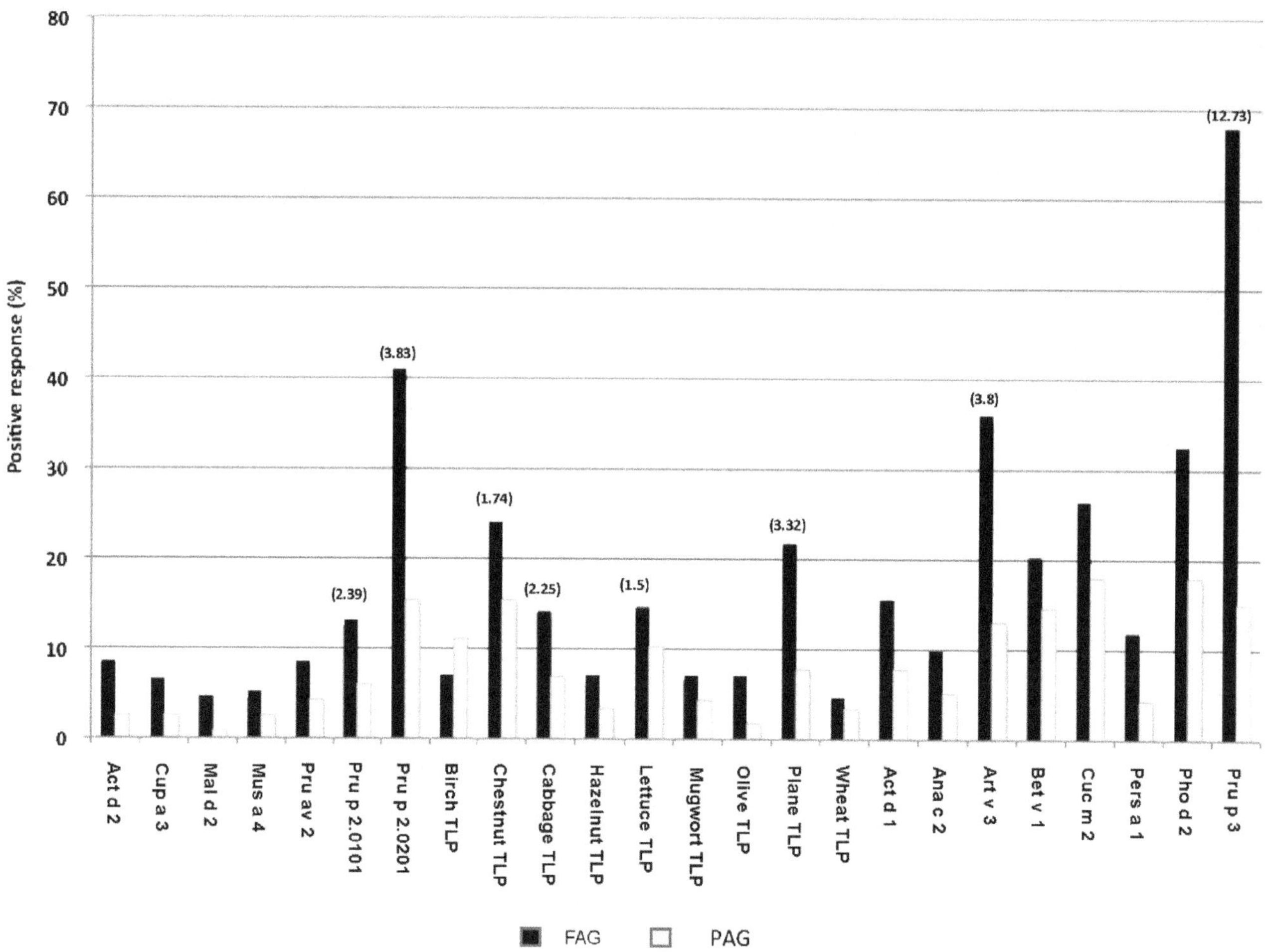


**Figure 1. Frequency of sensitization obtained by the TLP microarray using sera from both fruit-allergic (FAG) patients, and non-food pollen allergic (PAG) subjects.** Odds ratios are presented in parentheses (95% CI; $p<0.001$).

While most of the patients sensitized to this peach TLP (Pru p 2.0201) showed a positive response to Pru p 3, the opposite was observed for Pru p 3 to the other peach TLP, Pru p 2.0101, whose weight was very low (0.35). This allergen had a low frequency of positive responses (<15%), with the exception of FAG patients from Bilbao (35%). Both peach TLPs are linked with a low co-sensitization weight (0.40), although both of them share more than 94% of amino acid identity, with only eight different residues [7,30]. Thus, a different mode of sensitization may operate, which would be interesting to study in more detail.

The chestnut TLP yielded a higher positive response in patients from Barcelona and Bilbao, mainly in the FAG group, but also in the PAG group from Barcelona. The plane TLP was the only pollen included in this study that was associated with fruit allergy, especially in areas such as Alicante, Barcelona, Bilbao and Madrid. The other pollen TLPs, like mugwort and birch, had low responses in our population, although patients sensitized to these were included.

As mentioned above, TLPs were related to fruit allergy predominantly with pollen, but they also had sensitization profiles associated with the study geographical areas. Patients from Barcelona, Bilbao and the Canary Islands showed a higher positive response to these allergens than subjects from the other areas. Alicante and Ourense were situated at the other end of the peninsula. Patients from these areas had the lowest frequency of TLP recognition (around 20%, with the exception of plane TLP in Alicante). The patterns of TLP recognition, related to the different geographical areas, suggest a possible influence of local pollen in TLP sensitization.

Studies with large protein and serum panels are needed to clarify the role of cross-reactive allergens, and provide immunological evidence to clinical observations. In this way we can begin to detail the actors involved. In this work, we have shown that few members of the thaumatin family have an important role in fruit/pollen allergy in the studied areas, even if they can act as modifiers of sensitization profiles.

## Materials and Methods

### Selection and Purification of Allergens

Considering the allergies most frequently associated with peach sensitization in Spain, 16 TLPs were purified from foods and pollen relevant to the population under study, based on previously published methods [6,8,23,35] (Table 1).

Other allergens were included in the microarray: Pru p 3 (LTP, peach allergen), Art v 3 (LTP, mugwort allergen), Act d 1 (cysteine protease, kiwi allergen), Ana c 2 (pineapple allergen and marker of carbohydrate cross-reactive determinants (CCD)), Bet v 1 (PR10 from birch pollen), Cuc m 2 (melon fruit profilin), Pers a 1 (avocado latex-fruit allergen) and Pho d 2 (palm-pollen profilin).

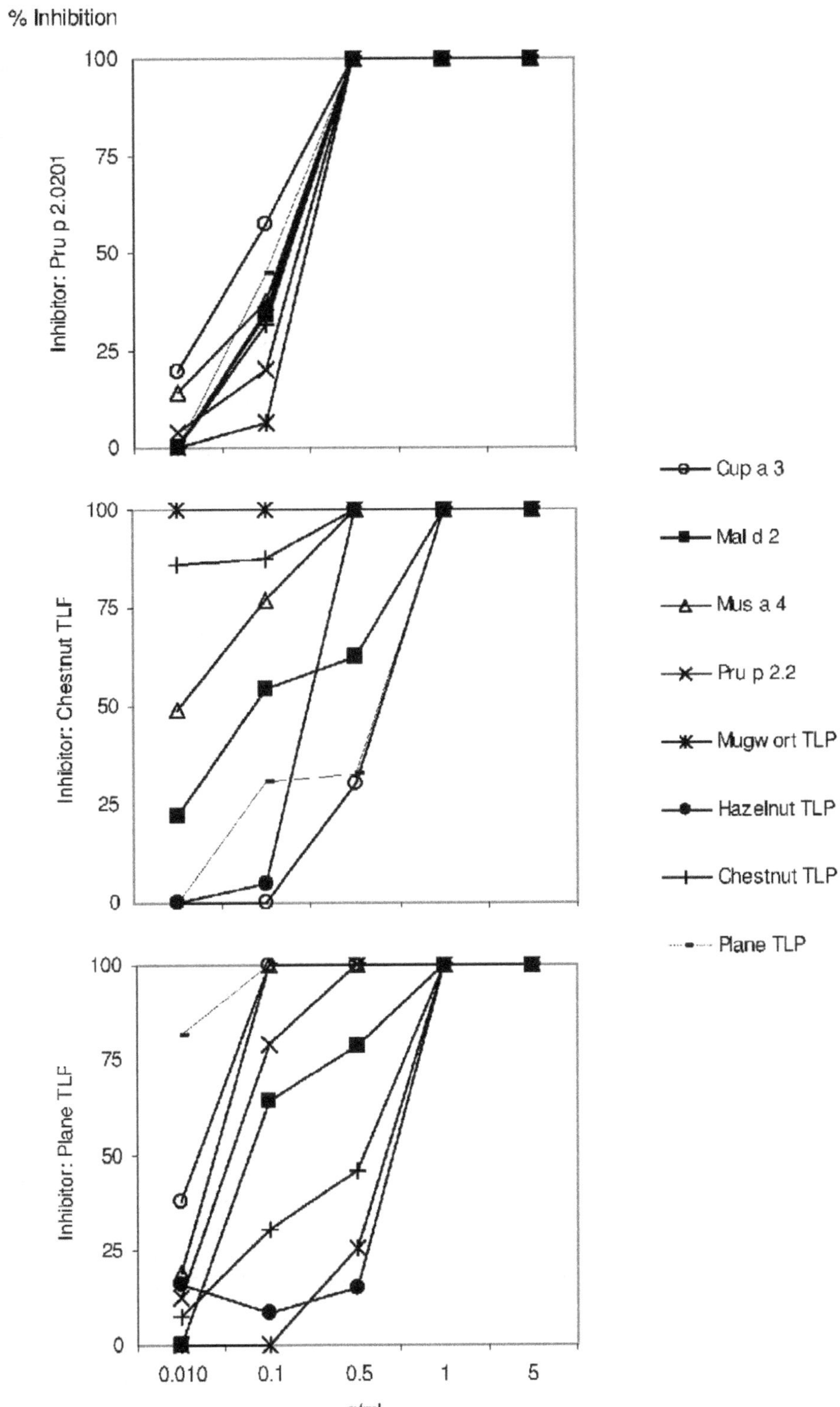


**Figure 2. IgE binding inhibition of the TLP microarray, when serum pool (n = 21; three per area) or individual sera were preincubated for 3 h at room temperature with increasing amounts of Pru p 2.0201, and chestnut and plane -pollen TLPs.**

All purified proteins were identified by trypsin peptide- and/or N-terminal amino acid-sequencing and mass spectrometry (MALDI-TOF).

## Characteristics of the Regions Under Study

Seven regions of Spain were chosen on the basis of their characteristic major pollens (Table 3, pollen count average for

**Table 3.** Pollen counts (grains/m$^3$ of air) of the regions included in the study.

| Region Pollen* | Alicante (2001–2011) | Barcelona (2001–2011) | Bilbao (2001–2011) | Canary I. (2008–2011) | Madrid (2001–2011) | Málaga (1995–1999) | Ourense (1996–1999) |
|---|---|---|---|---|---|---|---|
| Grass | – | – | – | – | 200 | – | – |
| Birch | – | – | 100 | – | – | – | 120 |
| Plane | – | 1800 | – | – | 1050 | 225 | – |
| Oak | – | 375 | 330 | – | 520 | – | 100 |
| Pine | 375 | 200 | 620 | 100 | 160 | – | 130 |
| Cypress | 175 | 525 | – | – | 200 | 250 | 470 |
| Mugwort | – | – | – | 150 | – | – | – |
| Pellitory | – | – | – | 110 | – | – | – |
| Olive | 355 | 125 | – | – | 473 | 1250 | – |
| Palm | 220 | – | – | – | – | – | – |

Data were obtained as the average of the previous n years, from the Comité de Aerobiología-SEAIC (http://www.polenes.com/concentraciones.html) and from PIA-Punto de información de Aerobiología-UAB (http://lap.uab.cat/aerobiologia/).
*Average of pollen counts (grains/m$^3$). The time period is indicated in brackets.

the previous 10 years). In Ourense and Bilbao, in the north of Spain, the most abundant pollens are from pine and oak, but the most distinctive feature is that birch pollen can be found in both regions; Barcelona, on the Mediterranean coast, is characterized by the presence of plane, oak and cypress pollen; Madrid, in the central region, has a high predominance of plane, oak and olive pollen; Málaga, in the south, has a high level of olive pollen; Alicante (Elche) is dominated by pine, olive and palm pollen; and finally, the Canary Islands, in the Atlantic Ocean, are characterized by mugwort and pellitory pollen.

## Characteristics of the Allergic Population Included

Two groups of patients were included in the study, prospectively among adult population (Table 2): fruit-allergic (FAG) patients and non-food pollen-allergic (PAG) patients. Criteria for inclusion in the FAG group (n = 212 patients) were: a consistent history of adverse reaction to fruit, indicative of IgE-mediated allergy, giving positive results to the skin-prick test and open food challenge, following the diagnostic algorithm recommended by official allergy academies [36,37]. Patients suffering severe systemic reactions to peach, and those with typical, recent and repeated reactions who had positive skin-prick tests did not undergo an oral challenge test to diagnose plant food. This group was divided into two subgroups depending on whether patients were allergic to pollen (n = 169; following the same criteria as for PAG, described below) or not (n = 43).

Criteria for inclusion in the PAG group (117 patients) were: a compatible clinical history of pollinosis confirmed by positive skin-prick tests to pollen allergens, but without any symptoms of plant food allergy and with a negative response to food extracts by SPTs. These patients showed mainly positive responses to mugwort, olive and grass pollen.

An additional group of food-tolerant volunteers without pollinosis (n = 35; five per region) was recruited as a negative control. Most of them (n = 27) were atopic, suffered from dust mite and animal dander allergies.

SPT responses were performed following EAACI recommendations [36]. The Ethics Committee of each hospital approved the study: the Ethic Committee of Hospital Clinic de Barcelona; the Ethic Committee of Hospital Universitario de la Princesa; the Ethic Committee of Hospital Universitario de Gran Canaria Dr. Negrín; the Ethic Committee of Fundación Jiménez Díaz; the Hospital General de Alicante; the Ethic Committee of Complexo Hospitalario de Ourense the Ethic Committee of Hospital Civil, Málaga; the Ethic Committee of Hospital de Basurto, Bilbao; the Ethic Committee of Universidad Politécnica de Madrid (Spain). Patients and control volunteers also gave their written informed consent to their participation.

## PrintingProduction of Allergen Microarray and Immunoassays

Purified proteins were printed (0.25 mg/ml and 0.125 mg/ml in 1X Protein Binding Buffer (Whatman, USA) containing 0.02% Tween 20) on epoxy-activated glass slides (TeleChem International, Sunnyvale, CA, USA) with 16 microarrays per slide, using a MicroGrid II TAS microarrayer (BioRobotics, Genomic Solutions, US). Several protein concentrations (1, 0.75, 0.5, 0.25 and 0.125 mg/ml) were tested and those that resolved the best were chosen (data not shown). Labeled pre-immune antibody was spotted as a guide dot to support automatic image analysis. Gaskets (TeleChem International, Sunnyvale, CA, USA) were attached to the slides to create a barrier between the 16 microarrays and sealed to prevent evaporation. Each microarray well was incubated for 1 hour at room temperature with blocking

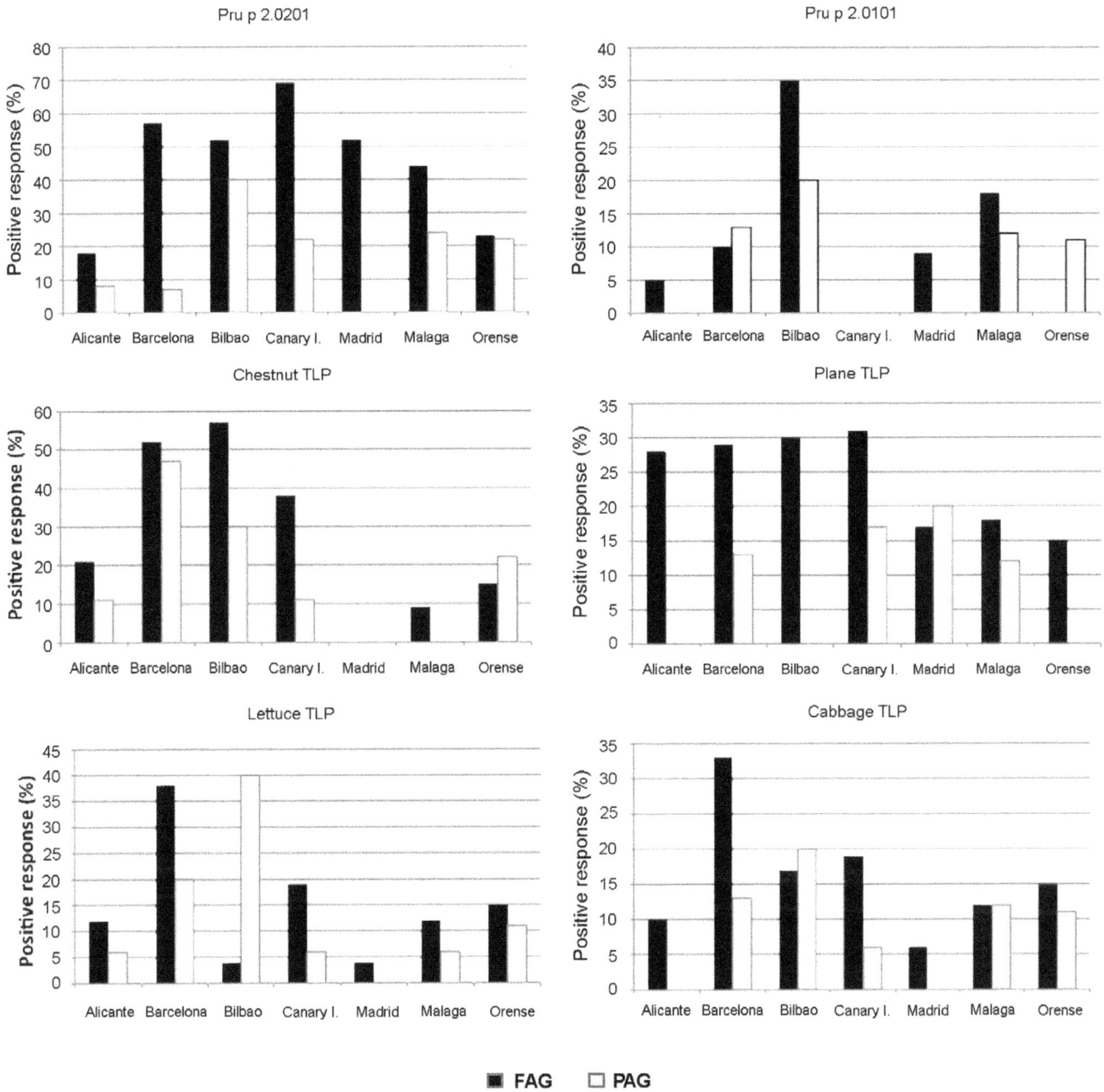


**Figure 3. Frequency of sensitization in the different geographical areas using the homemade microarray and sera from fruit-allergic (FAG) patients, and non-food pollen-allergic (PAG) subjects.** Only TLPs with more than 10% positive response were represented: Pru p 2.0201, Pru p 2.0101, chestnut, plane, lettuce and cabbage TLPs.

solution (Sigma, St. Louis, CO, USA), then incubated overnight with 80 µL of serum at 4°C. To detect bound IgE antibodies, the slides were incubated for 1 hour at room temperature with anti-human IgE labeled with PE-DY 647 (Thermo Scientific, Rockford, IL, USA) diluted 1:100. As a blank control, one microarray well per slide was always incubated solely with PBS (Sigma, St. Louis, CO, USA) instead of serum and, after washing, incubated with the fluorescence secondary antibody. PBS containing 0.1% Tween 20 was used as washing solution. Three points from the same sample were included in each microarray, and three replicates of each assay were performed (Pearson correlation = 0.83; $p<0.0001$).

The inhibition assays were performed in the same way but using sera preincubated with different quantities (5, 1, 0.5, 0.250, 0.125 mg/mL) of inhibitors (Pru p 2.0201, chestnut and plane-pollen TLPs).

Spots with obvious defects and those replicate spots having a signal-to-noise ratio less than 3, as measured by GenePix$^{TM}$ software (Genomics Solutions, US), were removed from the analysis. Only those allergen spots in which at least two of the three replicates fulfilled the analytical criteria were considered for quantification. The IgE binding of each allergen spot was calculated as the final fluorescence intensity, obtained by subtracting the local background $B$ from the observed value, measured by GenePix$^{TM}$ software and then the fluorescence

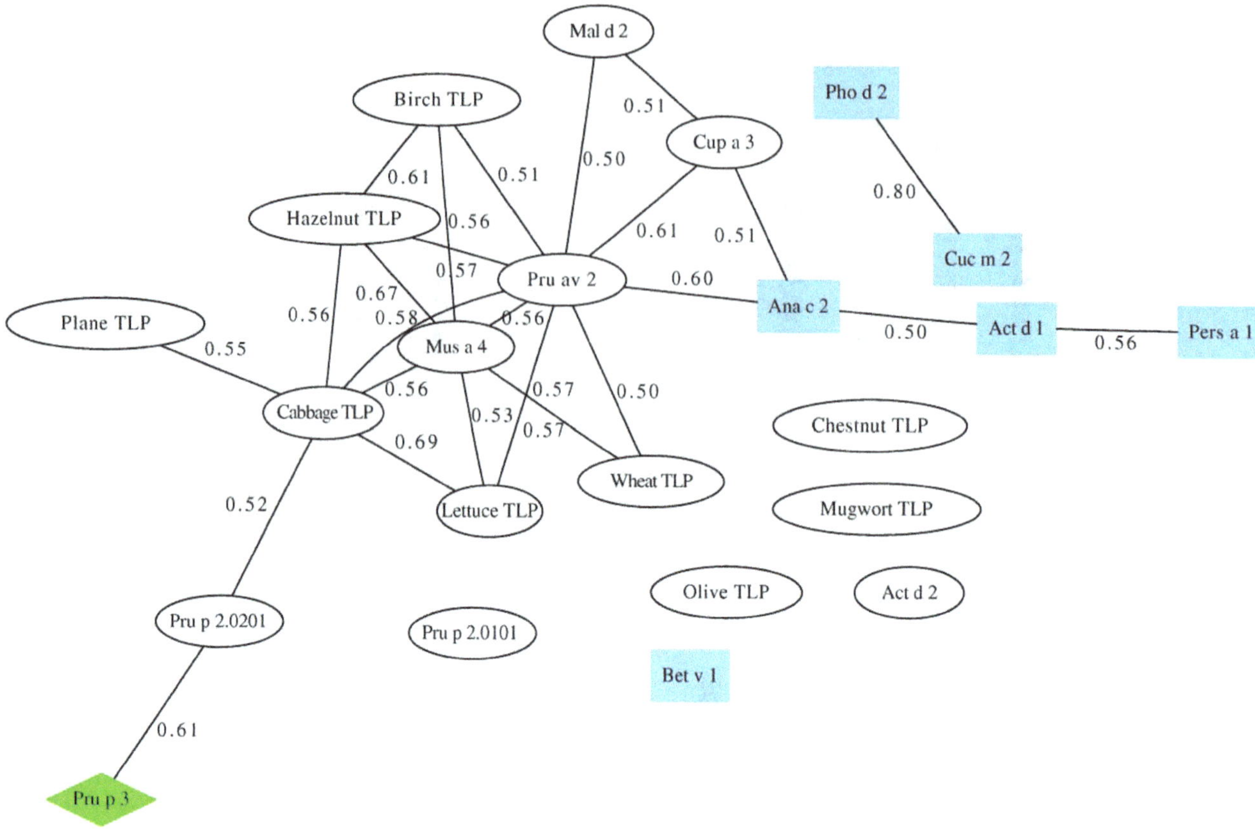


**Figure 4. Co-sensitization graph of TLP allergens.** Each node represents one allergen (TLP as white ellipses, non-TLP allergens as blue square nodes, and LTP-allergen Pru p 3 as a green diamond) and the links represent co-sensitization of one or more sera for the linked allergens. The weight of each link, ranging between 0 and 1, measures the degree of co-sensitization. For the sake of clarity, only the 25 links of weight greater than 0.50 out of the total 253 existing links were plotted.

intensity from the blank control by applying the next equation: $I = (F_{645}{-}B)_{\text{sample}} - (F_{645}{-}B)_{\text{blank}}$. Fluorescence intensity levels >200 units were considered to be positive (highest value of mean +3×SD of negative control spots, those containing only blocking solution).

## Graph-based Analytical Study of the Associations between TLPs. Building up the Co-sensitization Graph Associated with a TLP Microarray Immunoassay

A weighted and undirected co-sensitization graph $\mathcal{G}_{\mathcal{A}}$ is associated with a TLP microarray immunoassay for studying the co-sensitization between TLPs in the following manner. We define the elements of the matrix of fluorescence intensities $\boldsymbol{I}$ as the fluorescences $I_{ij}$ obtained when the serum IgE $i$ binds to the allergen $j$ as explained above. Therefore, each column of $\boldsymbol{I}$ represents the average of two different microarray immunoassays in which the same patient serum is incubated on the TLP microarray and revealed with fluorescently labeled anti-human IgE. We call $\boldsymbol{B}$ the matrix defined by $B_{ij} = 1$ when $A_{ij} > 0$ and $B_{ij} = 0$ otherwise.

Bipartite graphs are those with nodes of two or more different natures, where links only connect nodes of different type. The graph $\mathcal{B}$ associated with matrix $\boldsymbol{B}$ is of this kind. Nodes of type S represent the $N_S = 329$ sera and nodes of type A represent the $N_A = 23$ allergens (16 TLPs, 6 non-LTP allergens, and Pru p 3). Two nodes $i$ (serum) and $j$ (allergen) are connected in the bipartite graph $\mathcal{B}$ if $B_{ij} = 1$, which means that subject $i$ has shown a positive allergic reaction to the allergen $j$.

The bipartite graph $\mathcal{B}$ (not shown in this paper) can be projected into two smaller graphs $\mathcal{G}_S$ and $\mathcal{G}_{\mathcal{A}}$, each of them with nodes of only one type (sera and allergens, respectively). The present study focuses on the projected allergen graph $\mathcal{G}_{\mathcal{A}}$, and we have called it the co-sensitization graph (the construction of the projected serum graph $\mathcal{G}_S$ would be similar). The links in graph $\mathcal{G}_{\mathcal{A}}$ connect two allergens $m$ and $n$ if, in the original bipartite graph $\mathcal{B}$, these two allergens were connected to one or more common sera. The weight $w_{m,n}$ of such a link between $m$ and $n$ takes values from 0 to 1 and measures the *similarity* between the neighbours of allergens $m$ and $n$ in the bipartite graph. We have used the definition of the cosine distance between two vectors to calculate $w_{m,n}$:

$$w_{m,n} = \frac{B_m \cdot B_n}{|B_m| \cdot |B_n|} = \frac{\sum_{k=1}^{N_S} B_{k,m} \cdot B_{k,n}}{\sqrt{\sum_{k=1}^{N_S} B_{k,m}^2 \cdot \sum_{k=1}^{N_S} B_{k,n}^2}}$$

where $B_m$ and $B_n$ are the $m$- and $n$-columns of matrix $B$ respectively. Note that the weight $w_{m,n}$ is zero, and therefore there is no link between allergens $m$ and $n$, when $B_m$ and $B_n$ have no common elements (that is, when not even one serum has a positive reaction to both allergens $m$ and $n$), while $w_{m,n}$ reaches its maximum value of one when both vectors are identical (that is,

**Table 4.** Average weight of allergens included in the co-sensitization graph.

| Protein | Family | Average weight |
|---|---|---|
| Pru av 2 | TLP | 0.43 |
| Cabbage TLP | TLP | 0.42 |
| Lettuce TLP | TLP | 0.40 |
| Ana c 2 | Cysteine proteinase | 0.38 |
| Plane pollen TLP | TLP | 0.37 |
| Cup a 3 | TLP | 0.36 |
| Pers a 1 | Class I chitinase | 0.35 |
| Act d 1 | Cysteine protease | 0.35 |
| Mus a 4 | TLP | 0.34 |
| Hazelnut TLP | TLP | 0.34 |
| Pho d 2 | Profilin | 0.34 |
| Chestnut TLP | TLP | 0.33 |
| Birch pollen TLP | TLP | 0.33 |
| Cuc m 2 | Profilin | 0.33 |
| Mal d 2 | TLP | 0.33 |
| Pru p 2.0201 | TLP | 0.32 |
| Mugwort pollen TLP | TLP | 0.32 |
| Bet v 1 | PR10 | 0.31 |
| Wheat TLP | TLP | 0.30 |
| Act d 2 | TLP | 0.30 |
| Pru p 2.0101 | TLP | 0.30 |
| Pru p 3 | LTP | 0.29 |
| Olive TLP | TLP | 0.29 |

when allergens $m$ and $n$ are recognized by the same group of reacting sera).

Finally, an important quantity is the average weight of a node, which is calculated as.

$$\bar{w}_l = \frac{\sum_{k=1}^{N_A} w_{l,k}}{N_A}$$

The average weight of an allergen $l$ measures the average robustness of the co-sensitizations between $l$ and the rest of the allergens represented in the graph.

### Statistical Analysis

Fluorescence levels obtained from each patient's serum were analyzed by contingency tests. Pearson correlation coefficients were considered as a measure of reproducibility. Associations of frequencies were assessed with the Chi-square ($\chi 2$) test. Differences in the quantitative variables were analyzed by the Mann-Whitney U test. Significance was concluded for values of $p<0.05$.

## Author Contributions

Conceived and designed the experiments: GS JB JCH MB ADP. Performed the experiments: AP CGC LT RSM MT MV LAR VP JA. Analyzed the data: ADP AP LAR JA CGC. Contributed reagents/materials/analysis tools: JB RM CB FV JCH TC JACB FJF EF IGN MB SVL MGAE PG. Wrote the paper: ADP.

## References


1. Fernández Rivas M (2009) Food allergy in Alergologica-2005. J Investig Allergol Clin Immunol 19 Suppl 2: 37–44.
2. Cuesta-Herranz J, Barber D, Blanco C, Cistero-Bahima A, Crespo JF, et al. (2010) Differences among pollen-allergic patients with and without plant food allergy. Int Arch Allergy Immunol 153: 182–192.
3. Salcedo G, Sánchez-Monge R, Barber D, Díaz-Perales A (2007) Plant non-specific lipid transfer proteins: an interface between plant defence and human allergy. Biochim Biophys Acta 1771: 781–791.
4. Díaz-Perales A, Lombardero M, Sánchez-Monge R, García-Selles FJ, Pernas M, et al. (2000) Lipid-transfer proteins as potential plant panallergens: cross-reactivity among proteins of Artemisia pollen, Castanea nut and Rosaceae fruits, with different IgE-binding capacities. Clin Exp Allergy 30: 1403–1410.
5. Lauer I, Miguel-Moncin MS, Abel T, Foetisch K, Hartz C, et al. (2007) Identification of a plane pollen lipid transfer protein (Pla a 3) and its immunological relation to the peach lipid-transfer protein, Pru p 3. Clin Exp Allergy 37: 261–269.
6. Palacín A, Tordesillas L, Gamboa P, Sánchez-Monge R, Cuesta-Herranz J, et al. (2010) Characterization of peach thaumatin-like proteins and their identification as major peach allergens. Clin Exp Allergy 40: 1422–1430.
7. Breiteneder H (2004) Thaumatin-like proteins – a new family of pollen and fruit allergens. Allergy 59: 479–481.
8. Palacín A, Quirce S, Sánchez-Monge R, Fernández-Nieto M, Varela J, et al. (2008) Allergy to kiwi in patients with baker's asthma: identification of potential cross-reactive allergens. Ann Allergy Asthma Immunol 101: 200–205.
9. Hiller R, Laffer S, Harwanegg C, Huber M, Schmidt WM, et al. (2002) Microarrayed allergen molecules: diagnostic gatekeepers for allergy treatment. FASEB J 16: 414–416.
10. Skamstrup Hansen K, Poulsen LK (2011) Component resolved testing for allergic sensitization. Curr Allergy Asthma Rep 10: 340–348.
11. Salcedo G, Díaz-Perales A (2010) Component-resolved diagnosis of allergy: more is better? Clin Exp Allergy 40: 836–838.
12. Scala E, Alessandri C, Bernardi ML, Ferrara R, Palazzo P, et al. (2011) Cross-sectional survey on immunoglobulin E reactivity in 23,077 subjects using an allergenic molecule-based microarray detection system. Clin Exp Allergy 40: 911–921.
13. Boccaletti S, Latora V, Moreno Y, Chavez M, Hwang DU (2006) Complex networks: structure and dynamics. Phys Rep 424: 175–308.
14. Dorogovtsev SN, Goltsev AV, Mendes JFF (2008) Critical phenomena in complex networks. Rev Mod Phys 80: 1275–1335.
15. Jeong H, Mason SP, Barabasi AL, Oltvai ZN (2001) Lethality and centrality in protein networks. Nature 411: 41–42.
16. Rivas LA, Aguirre J, Blanco Y, Gonzalez-Toril E, Parro V (2011) Graph-based deconvolution analysis of multiplex sandwich microarray immunoassays: applications for environmental monitoring. Environ Microbiol 13: 1421–1432.
17. Albert R (2005) Scale-free networks in cell biology. J Cell Sci 118: 4947–4957.
18. Huber W, Carey VJ, Long L, Falcon S, Gentleman R (2007) Graphs in molecular biology. BMC Bioinformatics 8 Suppl 6: S8.
19. Arenas A, Díaz-Guilera A, Kurths J, Moreno Y, Zhou C (2008) Synchronization in complex networks. Phys Rep 469: 93–153.
20. Aguirre J, Buldú JM, Stich M, Manrubia SC (2011) Topological structure of the space of phenotypes: the case of RNA neutral networks. PLoS One 6: e26324.
21. Cortegano I, Civantos E, Aceituno E, del Moral A, López E, et al. (2004) Cloning and expression of a major allergen from Cupressus arizonica pollen, Cup a 3, a PR-5 protein expressed under polluted environment. Allergy 59: 485–490.
22. Menu-Bouaouiche L, Vriet C, Peumans WJ, Barre A, Van Damme EJ, et al. (2003) A molecular basis for the endo-beta 1,3-glucanase activity of the thaumatin-like proteins from edible fruits. Biochimie 85: 123–131.
23. Palacín A, Quirce S, Sánchez-Monge R, Bobolea I, Díaz-Perales A, et al. (2011) Sensitization profiles to purified plant food allergens among pediatric patients with allergy to banana. Pediatr Allergy Immunol 22: 186–195.

24. Fuchs HC, Bohle B, Dall'Antonia Y, Radauer C, Hoffmann-Sommergruber K, et al. (2006) Natural and recombinant molecules of the cherry allergen Pru av 2 show diverse structural and B cell characteristics but similar T cell reactivity. Clin Exp Allergy 36: 359–368.
25. Lehto M, Airaksinen L, Puustinen A, Tillander S, Hannula S, et al. (2010) Thaumatin-like protein and baker's respiratory allergy. Ann Allergy Asthma Immunol 104: 139–146.
26. Palomares O, Alcantara M, Quiralte J, Villalba M, Garzón F, et al. (2008) Airway disease and thaumatin-like protein in an olive-oil mill worker. N Engl J Med 358: 1306–1308.
27. Rivas LA, García-Villadangos M, Moreno-Paz M, Cruz-Gil P, Gómez-Elvira J, et al. (2008) A 200-antibody microarray biochip for environmental monitoring: searching for universal microbial biomarkers through immunoprofiling. Anal Chem 80: 7970–7979.
28. Sanz ML, Blazquez AB, García BE (2011) Microarray of allergenic component-based diagnosis in food allergy. Curr Opin Allergy Clin Immunol 11: 204–209.
29. Shreffler WG (2011) Microarrayed recombinant allergens for diagnostic testing. J Allergy Clin Immunol 127: 843–849; quiz 850–841.
30. Gadermaier G, Hauser M, Egger M, Ferrara R, Briza P, et al. (2011) Sensitization prevalence, antibody cross-reactivity and immunogenic peptide profile of api g 2, the non-specific lipid transfer protein 1 of celery. PLoS One 6: e24150.
31. Hauser M, Roulias A, Ferreira F, Egger M (2010) Panallergens and their impact on the allergic patient. Allergy Asthma Clin Immunol 6: 1.
32. Asero R, Monsalve R, Barber D (2008) Profilin sensitization detected in the office by skin prick test: a study of prevalence and clinical relevance of profilin as a plant food allergen. Clin Exp Allergy 38: 1033–1037.
33. Beyer K, Teuber SS (2005) Food allergy diagnostics: scientific and unproven procedures. Curr Opin Allergy Clin Immunol 5: 261–266.
34. Fernández-Rivas M, Bolhaar S, Gonzalez-Mancebo E, Asero R, van Leeuwen A, et al. (2006) Apple allergy across Europe: how allergen sensitization profiles determine the clinical expression of allergies to plant foods. J Allergy Clin Immunol 118: 481–488.
35. Palacin A, Rodriguez J, Blanco C, Lopez-Torrejon G, Sánchez-Monge R, et al.(2008) Immunoglobulin E recognition patterns to purified Kiwifruit (Actinidinia deliciosa) allergens in patients sensitized to Kiwi with different clinical symptoms. Clin Exp Allergy. 2008 Jul;38(7): 1220–8.
36. EAACI Sub-, Immunology CoSTotEAoAaC (1989) Skin tests used in type I allergy testing Position paper. Allergy 44: 1–59.
37. Committee AFR (1999) Food Adverse Reaction Committee of Sociedad Española de Alergia e Inmunología SEAIC 14: 50–62.
38. García-Casado G, Collada C, Allona I, Soto A, Casado R, et al. (2000) Characterization of an apoplastic basic thaumatin-like protein from recalcitrant chestnut seeds. Physiologia Plantarum 110: 172–180.
39. Tordesillas L, Sirvent S, Díaz-Perales A, Villalba M, Cuesta-Herranz J, et al. (2011) Plant lipid transfer protein allergens: no cross-reactivity between those from foods and olive and parietaria pollen. Int Arch Allergy Immunol 156: 291–296.
40. López-Torrejón G, Crespo JF, Sánchez-Monge R, Sánchez-Jimenez M, Alvarez J, et al. (2005) Allergenic reactivity of the melon profilin Cuc m 2 and its identification as major allergen. Clin Exp Allergy 35: 1065–1072.
41. Díaz-Perales A, Blanco C, Sánchez-Monge R, Varela J, Carrillo T, et al. (2003) Analysis of avocado allergen (Prs a 1) IgE-binding peptides generated by simulated gastric fluid digestion. J Allergy Clin Immunol 112: 1002–1007.
42. Díaz-Perales A, Sanz ML, García-Casado G, Sánchez-Monge R, García-Selles FJ, et al. (2003) Recombinant Pru p 3 and natural Pru p 3, a major peach allergen, show equivalent immunologic reactivity: a new tool for the diagnosis of fruit allergy. J Allergy Clin Immunol 111: 628–633.

# 21

# Peyer's Patches and Mesenteric Lymph Nodes Cooperatively Promote Enteropathy in a Mouse Model of Food Allergy

**Haruyo Nakajima-Adachi[1,2,13]*, Akira Kikuchi[1], Yoko Fujimura[1], Kyoko Shibahara[1,13], Tsuyoshi Makino[3], Masae Goseki-Sone[4], Miran Kihara-Fujioka[1], Tomonori Nochi[2], Yosuke Kurashima[2,5], Osamu Igarashi[2], Masafumi Yamamoto[6], Jun Kunisawa[2,5,7,8], Masako Toda[9], Shuichi Kaminogawa[10], Ryuichiro Sato[1], Hiroshi Kiyono[2,5,7,11,12], Satoshi Hachimura[1,13]**

**1** Department of Applied Biological Chemistry, Graduate School of Agricultural and Life Sciences, The University of Tokyo, Tokyo, Japan, **2** Department of Microbiology and Immunology, Institute of Medical Science, The University of Tokyo, Tokyo, Japan, **3** Biotechnical Center (BT Center), Japan SLC, Inc., Shizuoka, Japan, **4** Department of Food and Nutrition, Faculty of Human Sciences and Design, Japan Women's University, Tokyo, Japan, **5** Core Research for Evolutional Science and Technology (CREST), Japan Science and Technology Agency, Tokyo, Japan, **6** Department of Microbiology and Immunology, Nihon University School of Dentistry at Matsudo, Chiba, Japan, **7** International Research and Development Center for Mucosal Vaccines, Institute of Medical Science, The University of Tokyo, Tokyo, Japan, **8** Laboratory of Vaccine Materials, National Institute of Biomedical Innovation, Osaka, Japan, **9** Vice President's Research Group "Molecular Allergology", Paul-Ehrlich-Institut, Langen, Germany, **10** Department of Food Bioscience and Biotechnology, Nihon University, Kanagawa, Japan, **11** Department of Medical Genome Science, Graduate School of Frontier Science, The University of Tokyo, Tokyo, Japan, **12** Graduate School of Medicine, The University of Tokyo, Tokyo, Japan, **13** Research Center for Food Safety, Graduate School of Agricultural and Life Sciences, The University of Tokyo, Tokyo, Japan

## Abstract

***Background and Objective:*** To improve the efficacy and safety of tolerance induction for food allergies, identifying the tissues responsible for inducing intestinal inflammation and subsequent oral tolerance is important. We used OVA23-3 mice, which express an ovalbumin-specific T-cell receptor, to elucidate the roles of local and systemic immune tissues in intestinal inflammation.

***Methods and Results:*** OVA23-3 mice developed marked enteropathy after consuming a diet containing egg white (EW diet) for 10 days but overcame the enteropathy (despite continued moderate inflammation) after receiving EW diet for a total of 28 days. Injecting mice with anti-IL-4 antibody or cyclosporine A confirmed the involvement of Th2 cells in the development of the enteropathy. To assess the individual contributions of Peyer's patches (PPs), mesenteric lymph nodes (MLNs), and the spleen to the generation of effector $CD4^+$ T-cells, we analyzed the IL-4 production, proliferation in response to ovalbumin, and $CD4^+$ T-cell numbers of these tissues. EW feeding for 10 days induced significant IL-4 production in PPs, the infiltration of numerous $CD4^+$ T-cells into MLNs, and a decrease in $CD4^+$ T-cell numbers in spleen. On day 28, $CD4^+$ T-cells from all tissues had attenuated responses to ovalbumin, suggesting tolerance acquisition, although MLN $CD4^+$ T-cells still maintained IL-4 production with proliferation. In addition, removal of MLNs but not the spleen decreased the severity of enteropathy and PP-disrupted mice showed delayed onset of EW-induced inflammatory responses. Disruption of peripheral lymphoid tissues or of both PPs and MLNs almost completely prevented the enteropathy.

***Conclusions:*** PPs and MLNs coordinately promote enteropathy by generating effector T-cells during the initial and exacerbated phases, respectively; the spleen is dispensable for enteropathy and shows tolerogenic responses throughout EW-feeding. The regulation of PPs may suppress the initiation of intestinal inflammation, subsequently restricting MLNs and inhibiting the progression of food-allergic enteropathy.

**Editor:** Sergei Grivennikov, Fox Chase Cancer Center, United States of America

**Funding:** The authors received financial support from the Restart Postdoctoral Program of the Japan Society for the Promotion of Science and from The Food Science Institute Foundation and Food Safety Commission. The funders had no role in study design, data collection and analysis, decision to publish, or preparation of the manuscript.

**Competing Interests:** The author (Tsuyoshi Makino), who is employed by Biotechnical Center (BT Center), Japan SLC, Inc. contributed to developing the mesenteric lymphadenectomy procedure.

* Email: aryu@mail.ecc.u-tokyo.ac.jp

## Introduction

The prevalence of food allergies is increasing, particularly in westernized countries [1]. Among the prospective allergen-specific treatments for food allergies that have been investigated in current clinical practice, specific oral tolerance immunotherapy has attracted considerable interest [2]. However, several reports suggest that this immunotherapy can provoke severe adverse reactions (e.g. gastrointestinal inflammation and anaphylaxis) to the allergenic diet necessary to induce specific oral tolerance. For specific oral tolerance immunotherapy to be safe and effective, the mechanisms underlying the induction of food allergies and subsequent development of oral tolerance must be elucidated in detail, including identification of the tissue involved, so that targeted therapy with decreased risk to patients can be developed [3,4].

The intestinal immune tissue is a primary site of sensitization to food allergens. Gut-associated lymphoid tissues (GALT) may play an important role in causing food allergic intestinal inflammation and subsequent induction of oral tolerance [5,6]. GALT comprises both immune-inductive sites–Peyer's patches (PPs), isolated lymphoid follicles, and mesenteric lymph nodes (MLNs)–and effector sites, which include the lamina propria and intestinal epithelium. How GALT itself responds to food allergens, the relationship between the intestinal and systemic (e.g., splenic) responses to food allergens disseminated from GALT, and the role this association plays in determining tolerance versus inflammation remain unclear as yet. Previous studies revealed that effector cells from spleen, a key systemic immune tissue [7], or MLN [8] or PP cells [9] caused gastrointestinal inflammation. These results suggest both GALT and spleen act as effector tissues, but how these tissues function–both independently and cooperatively–has not been elucidated clearly [6].

Traditional food allergy mouse models involve primary sensitization with a food antigen and adjuvant, followed by oral administration of the antigen. However, this process fundamentally alters the immune responses of the mice [10], complicates direct analysis of the antigen-specific local or systemic immune responses that are triggered by orally administered antigen, and complicates efforts to elucidate the mechanisms of food allergy. Detailed analysis of the mechanisms underlying food-allergic intestinal inflammation and subsequent oral tolerance requires an improved mouse model.

In our previous study, we established a model of food allergy by using OVA23-3 mice, a transgenic line that expresses a T-cell receptor specific for ovalbumin (OVA; a leading egg allergen) [11,12]. Disproportionate Th2-skewed responses and food-allergic enteropathy with weight loss can be induced in OVA23-3 mice simply by feeding them an egg-white (EW)-based diet [12,13]. Furthermore, continued feeding of the EW diet is accompanied by reversal of extant inflammation. This enteropathy is similar to food protein-induced enteropathy of infancy [14]. Compared with traditional mice models, the OVA23-3 model is characteristic in manifesting the enteropathy by feeding diet alone, whereby we can follow the immune responses initiated from feeding diet in the absence of extraneous and potentially confounding effects due to adjuvant. To identify the key tissues in both food-allergic enteropathy and subsequent oral tolerance, we here examined the responses of $CD4^+$ T-cells purified from PPs, MLN, and spleen of intact EW-diet-fed OVA23-3 mice and of those from which we removed various lymphoid tissues. Our data revealed that both the MLNs and PPs of GALT are integral to the development of food-allergic intestinal inflammation through their cooperative roles in generating and maintaining IL-4-producing $CD4^+$ T-cells. In addition, we learned that the spleen contributes to the induction of systemic tolerance to EW diet in OVA23-3 mice, but is dispensable for the development of enteropathy. In particular, our chronologic analysis clearly showed that PPs are an important tissue as an accessible target in inducing oral tolerance to inhibit subsequent aggravation of the inflammatory responses in MLNs.

## Materials and Methods

### Ethics statements

We followed the ARRIVE Guidelines for preparing current experiments and submitting this manuscript. The all aspects of current experiments including anesthesia, euthanasia and the withholding of perioperative analgesia were approved by the Animal Use Committee of the Faculty of Agriculture at The University of Tokyo and we followed the guidelines of The University of Tokyo for the care and use of animals (approval no. P11-533). During surgery, mice were anesthetized by isoflurane, which was performed under aseptic condition. Perioperative analgesia was withheld, due to its pharmacological effects on inducing enteropathy and maintaining intestinal homeostasis, which was a primary parameter evaluated in the study [15~18]. When necessary for cellular and histological analysis, mice were euthanized by cervical dislocation by experts. Although the mice developed weight loss and enteropathy by day 10 of feeding the egg-white diet, they did not exhibit any other clinical signs (e.g., hunched body position, ruffled fur, decreased mobility/activity, severe weight loss) and recovered from the inflammation upon continued feeding of the diet for a total of 28 days. Therefore, our experiments without setting preemptive humane endpoints were approved.

### Mice

OVA23-3 mice were generously provided by S. Habu (Tokai University School of Medicine, Japan) [11]. Heterozygous OVA23-3 mice (obtained by backcrossing homozygous OVA23-3 mice with BALB/cA mice [CLEA Japan, Tokyo, Japan]) were maintained under specific pathogen-free and controlled conditions at The University of Tokyo (sterilized deionized drinking water; sterilized commercial chow; room temperature; 22°C, 12:12-h light:dark cycle). These conditions were monitored daily. Each cage (182×260×128 mm, [catalog no. CL-0103-2, CLEA Japan, Tokyo, Japan]) contained 5 or fewer mice.

### Generation of OVA23-3 mice devoid of PPs or peripheral lymphoid tissue (pLT)

To generate OVA23-3 mice devoid of PPs ($PP^-$ mice), female BALB/c mice were bred with homozygous OVA23-3 mice; on gestational day 14.5, the female mice were injected intravenously with 1 mg of anti-IL-7Ralpha monoclonal antibody (mAb; A7R34, generated and donated by S. Nishikawa [Kyoto University, Japan]) [19]. The frequencies of $CD4^+$ and $CD8^+$ T-cells in thymic, splenic, intestinal epithelial and mesenteric lymphocytes were comparable between PP-normal and PP-deficient of BALB/c or OVA23-3 mice (data not shown). To generate OVA23-3 mice devoid of pLT ($pLT^-$ mice), female BALB/c mice were bred with homozygous OVA23-3 mice; on gestational days 11, 14, and 17, female mice were injected intravenously with 200 microgram each of LTbetaR-Ig and TNFR55-Ig fusion proteins (these regents were gifts from P. D. Rennert [Biogen Idec, Inc., Cambridge, MA]) [20,21]. The disruption of PP or pLT organogenesis in the offspring was confirmed by observation under a stereomicroscope (Leica Microsystems Japan, Tokyo, Japan) or by intravenously injecting 200 microliter of 1% Evans blue in PBS into EW-fed OVA23-3 mice to visualize lymph nodes.

### Surgery

The organogenesis of MLNs or spleen cannot be disrupted by injection of mAb or fusion proteins into pregnant mice because specialized differentiation pathways of these tissues remain unclear. Therefore, we used surgery so that we might define the roles of the individual tissues. Mesenteric lymphadenectomy [22] and splenectomy of OVA23-3 mice (age, 6 to 7 weeks old) was performed in collaboration with Japan SLC (Hamamatsu, Japan). Mice were used in experiments once they had regained their postsurgical weight loss, 7 to 10 days after from the surgery. During surgery, mice were anesthetized by isoflurane, which was performed under aseptic condition, and abdominal tissues were bathed with sterile warm (37°C) PBS to prevent drying, and mice recovered from anesthesia and surgery in a warmed (40°C) clean cage. After surgery, mice were monitored (weight and activity) and the incision was cleaned daily. The completeness of lymphadenectomy was confirmed by observation under a stereomicroscope (Leica Microsystems Japan, Tokyo, Japan) or by intravenously injecting 200 microliter of 1% Evans blue in PBS into EW-fed OVA23-3 mice to visualize lymph nodes.

### EW diet and OVA uptake

For 28 d, male OVA23-3 mice (age, 6 to 8 weeks) were fed experimental solid diets in which the 20% protein fraction comprised EW (EW diet) or casein (CN; control diet) [12]. Mice were allocated to each group so that average weight did not differ significantly between groups and were weighted daily through day 10 and then every 4 to 7 days until the end of the 28-day experimental period. When necessary for cellular and histological analyses, mice were weighed, euthanized, and their tissues removed for further analysis. Sera were stored at −80°C. Serum OVA-specific IgE levels were analyzed by ELISA as described previously [12] and measurement of the serum concentration of OVA (OVA uptake) is described in File S1.

### Treatment with cyclosporine A and anti-IL-4 mAb

Cyclosporine A (Astellas Pharma, Tokyo, Japan) was dissolved (final concentration, 1 μg/μL) in elution buffer (0.05% Tween-80 and 10% ethanol in 0.9% NaCl) and administered intraperitoneally every other day throughout the 10-day experimental period. Anti-IL-4 mAb (1 mg; clone 11B11) [23] or control Ab (1 mg; rat IgG, Cappel, Cochranville, PA, USA) was administered intravenously on the day before and on day 7 of feeding the diet.

### Intestinal histology

Segments (3 cm each) of jejunum (just after or 8 cm distal to the duodenum) were harvested, opened longitudinally, fixed with 10% formalin, and stained with hematoxylin and eosin for morphologic evaluation [12].

### Measurement of alkaline phosphatase activity

The 1-cm section of jejunum that lay 7 cm distal to the duodenum was harvested, opened longitudinally, and washed with sterile cold PBS. Using 2 glass slides, we scraped the intestinal mucosa from these segments and stored it at -80°C prior to homogenization. The mucosa were homogenized in 10 mM Tris-buffered saline (pH 7.3) containing 1% Triton X-100 and 1 mM phenylmethylsulfonylfluoride and then centrifuged at 7,000 ×*g* for 15 min. Alkaline phosphatase activity in the supernatants of the intestinal tissue homogenates was analyzed by using an enzyme substrate (10 mM *p*-nitrophenyl phosphate in 100 mM 2-amino-2-methyl-1, 3-propanediole HCL buffer containing 5 mM $MgCl_2$; pH 10.0) at 37°C [24]. Enzyme activity was defined as the rate of hydrolysis of *p*-nitrophenyl phosphate and expressed in units (1 U = 1 μmol *p*-nitrophenol formed in 1 min). The protein concentration of each sample was standardized to 1 mg by using BCA protein assay reagent (Pierce, Rockford, IL, USA).

### Assessment of $CD4^+$ T-cell functions

$CD4^+$ T-cells were prepared from MLNs, PPs, and spleen, and their proliferation, cytokine production, and infiltration into various tissues were evaluated according to procedures provided in File S1 [12]. Protocols for isolating small intestinal lymphocytes and for measuring $CD4^+$ T-cell number and rate in small intestinal lymphocytes [25] are provided also in File S1.

### Statistical analysis

Results are presented as mean ± 1 SD. The Mann–Whitney *U* test, Steel, and Shirley–Williams tests were used for nonparametric analysis. Differences were considered significant when the *P* value was less than 0.05 or 0.01, depending on the test.

## Results

### IL-4-producing $CD4^+$ T-cells were indispensable for the clinical manifestation of food allergy in OVA23-3 mice

As described in our previous study [12], OVA23-3 mice demonstrated marked enteropathy, with weight loss (i.e., <10% of baseline body weight), from day 4 until day 7 to 10 after they began receiving the EW diet. Although particularly apparent in the jejunum, inflammation occurred throughout the small intestine and manifested as enteropathy involving goblet-cell hyperplasia, crypt elongation, villous atrophy and inflammatory cell infiltration (Figure 1). As the mice continued to receive the EW diet until day 28, they regained body weight and demonstrated repair of injured intestinal tissues, although moderate inflammation remained. As indicated previously [12], the cells that infiltrated into the small intestine were eosinophils, mast cells, neutrophils, macrophages, and $CD4^+$ T-cells (Figure S1 and Result S1). Excess $CD4^+$ T-cells function may contribute to the infiltration of other cells. Serum OVA-specific IgE responses were increased ($P<0.01$) on day 21 compared with the level before receiving EW diet. On day 28, the IgE responses were significantly ($P<0.05$) decreased compared with the level on day 21, but still elevated higher ($P<0.05$) than the level before receiving EW diet. (Figure S2 and Result S2).

We previously showed that EW-fed RAG-2 deficient OVA23-3 mice, in which nearly 100% of $CD4^+$ T-cells are OVA-specific, developed a similar enteropathy to that of the OVA23-3 mice in the current study [12]. Therefore, our results indicate that OVA-specific $CD4^+$ T-cells are involved in the induction and resolution of weight loss and intestinal inflammation in this model, because more than 90% of the peripheral $CD4^+$ T cells in OVA23-3 mice are OVA-specific [11].

In our previous study, the clinical manifestation of EW-fed OVA23-3 mice was associated with Th2 $CD4^+$ T-cell responses [12]. Other studies have used IL-4-deficient mice to illustrate the role of IL-4 in food allergic diarrhea [26,27] or aversion to oral administered OVA [28]. To verify the importance of Th2 cells in our model, we treated OVA23-3 mice with cyclosporine A, an inhibitor of T-cell activation, or anti-IL-4 mAb. Both treatments markedly decreased the expected weight loss and intestinal inflammation in EW-fed OVA23-3 mice (Figure 2A and 2B). These results suggest that IL-4-producing $CD4^+$ T-cells are indispensable effector cells in the induction of disease symptoms of EW-fed OVA23-3 mice.

### MLN $CD4^+$ T-cells, but not PP or splenic $CD4^+$ T-cells, maintained IL-4 production during feeding of the EW diet

To analyze the contribution of the primary inductive sites of GALT and a tissue central to systemic immunity to the generation

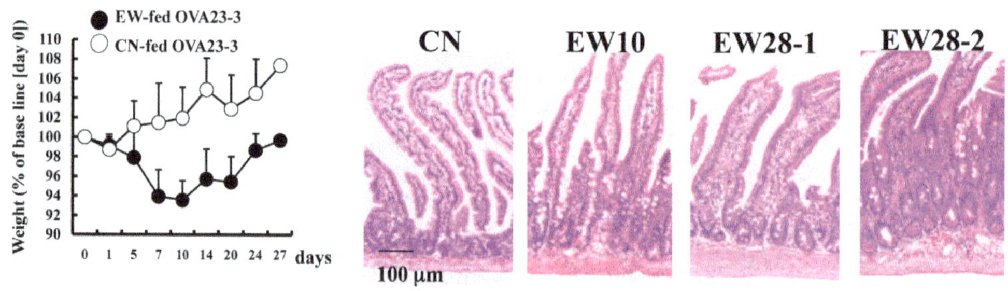


**Figure 1. An OVA-specific mouse model of food allergy demonstrates enteropathy followed by oral tolerance.** Weight changes and jejunal sections (hematoxylin and eosin stain) throughout EW-diet feeding of OVA23-3 mice (open circles: CN-fed, n = 5; solid circles: EW-fed, n = 7). The data shown are representative of four independent experiments.

of effector T cells, we examined CD4+ T-cell function–specifically, cell number, proliferation and IL-4 production–in the MLNs, PPs, and spleen of OVA23-3 mice after stimulation with OVA. These functions were assessed before the induction of inflammation (that is, during feeding of the CN diet) and during the marked (days 7 through 10 of feeding the EW diet) and moderate (day 28 of the EW diet) phases of inflammation.

The number of splenic CD4+ T-cells was decreased on day 10 ($P<0.1$) and 28 ($P<0.05$) in EW-diet-fed mice compared with the CN-diet group. In contrast, the number of CD4+ T-cells in PPs remained consistently low throughout EW-diet feeding, whereas

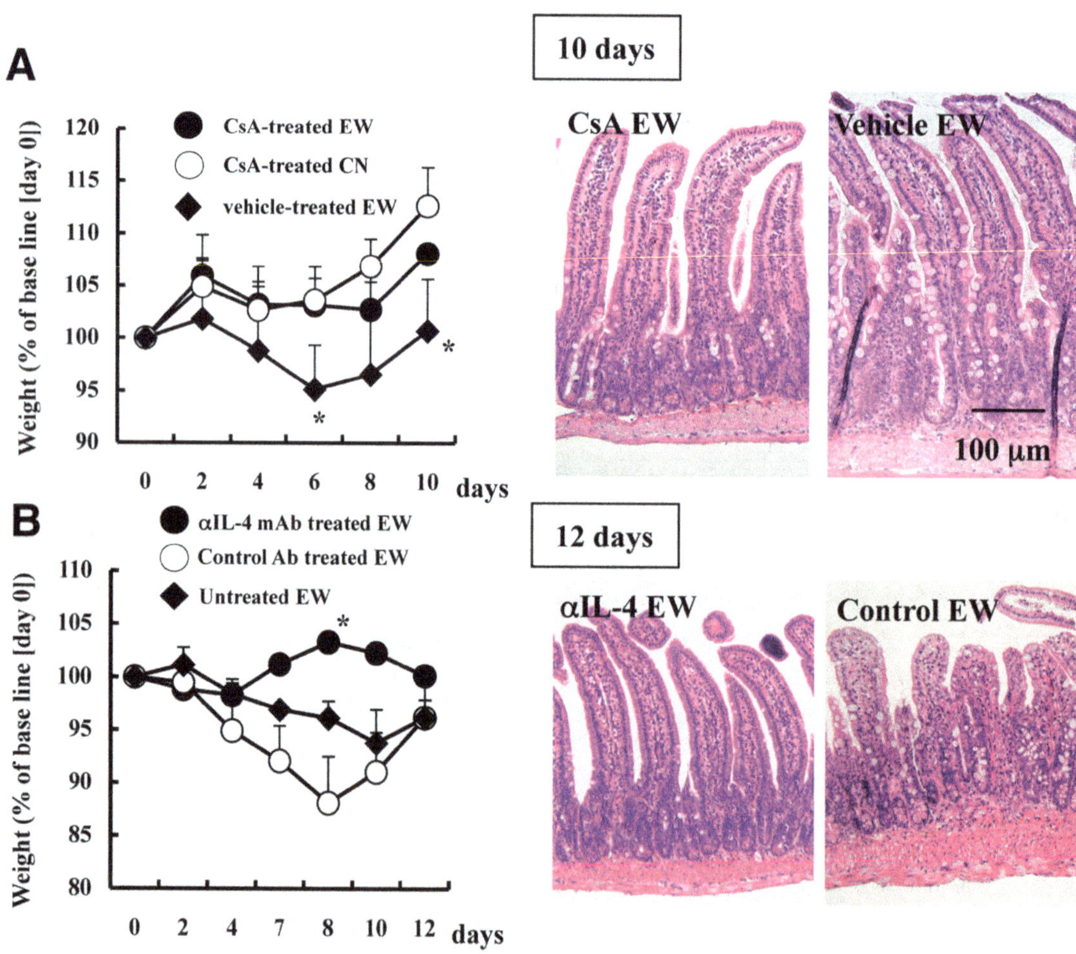


**Figure 2. Roles of T-cells and IL-4 in food-allergic intestinal inflammation.** Weight changes and jejunal sections (hematoxylin and eosin stain) of EW- or CN-fed OVA23-3 mice treated with (A) cyclosporine A (CsA) or (B) anti-IL-4 mAb. Morphologic changes were analyzed between days 10 and 12. (A) Open circles: CsA-treated, CN-fed (CN, n = 3); solid circles: CsA-treated, EW-fed (EW, n = 5); solid diamonds: vehicle (control)-treated EW-fed (n = 4). (B) Open circles: Control Ab-treated (EW, n = 3); solid circles: anti IL-4-treated (EW, n = 3); solid diamonds, untreated (EW, n = 2). *, Value is significantly ($P<0.05$) different from that for vehicle-treated EW or control Ab-treated EW mice. All data are representative of three independent experiments.

that in MLNs increased significantly ($P<0.05$) on day 10 compared with cell counts in CN-fed mice and decreased ($P<0.05$) on day 28 from that on day 10 of EW diet. The number of $CD4^+$ T-cells in MLNs increased significantly ($P<0.01$) compared with those in spleen and PPs on day 10 and remained elevated ($P<0.01$) on day 28 of the diet (Figure 3A, left panel).

The proliferation of $CD4^+$ T-cells from the PPs, MLNs, and spleen on day 10 was similar between CN-fed and EW-fed OVA23-3 mice. However, on day 28, $CD4^+$ T-cell proliferation was significantly ($P<0.05$) lower in EW-fed compared with CN-fed mice. However, $CD4^+$ T-cells from MLNs maintained the highest ($P<0.01$) level of proliferation among the 3 lymphoid tissues evaluated (Figure 3A, right panel). These results suggest a central role for MLNs, but not spleen or PPs in the intestinal inflammation.

IL-4 production by $CD4^+$ T-cells from EW-fed OVA23-3 mice on day 10 was increased ($P<0.05$) compared with that in CN-diet groups in all 3 tissues; the difference was particularly apparent in PP $CD4^+$ T-cells ($P<0.01$ compared with MLNs and spleen on day 10, Figure 3B). This finding suggests that, compared with those from MLNs or spleen, $CD4^+$ T-cells from PPs play an important role in early inflammatory responses. On day 28, IL-4 production in $CD4^+$ T-cells from spleen and PPs was dramatically lower ($P<0.01$) than that in $CD4^+$ T-cells from MLNs, suggesting persistent role for MLNs in the inflammatory responses.

These results suggest that 1) the establishment of the enteropathy was dependent on the generation of IL-4-producing $CD4^+$ T-cells in GALT; 2) long-term feeding of EW diet induced $CD4^+$ T-cell tolerance through inhibition of IL-4 production in an OVA-specific manner; and 3) the induction of T-cell tolerance was followed by attenuation of intestinal inflammation and weight loss in EW-fed OVA23-3 mice.

## MLNs are required for the induction of intestinal inflammation in a mouse model of food allergy

The inflammatory $CD4^+$ T-cell functions in GALT and the maintenance of persistent $CD4^+$ T-cell responses to dietary OVA in MLNs suggest that MLNs promote the development of enteropathy in OVA23-3 mice during EW-diet feeding. To examine this potential role, we surgically removed the MLNs from OVA23-3 mice and then fed the EW diet to the lymphadenectomized mice. Notably, MLN-ectomized EW-fed OVA23-3 mice showed significantly ($P<0.05$) less weight loss than did sham-operated EW-fed mice (Figure 4A). Moreover, compared with sham-operated mice, MLN-ectomized EW-fed OVA23-3 mice had milder intestinal inflammation, that is, only crypt hyperplasia on day 7 (Figure 4B, upper) and less cell infiltration on day 28 (Figure 4B, lower). The EW diet remarkably increased the size of the MLNs in sham-operated OVA23-3 mice (Figure 4C, center panel). In contrast, MLNs were not visible in MLN-ectomized EW-fed OVA23-3 mice, indicating that the

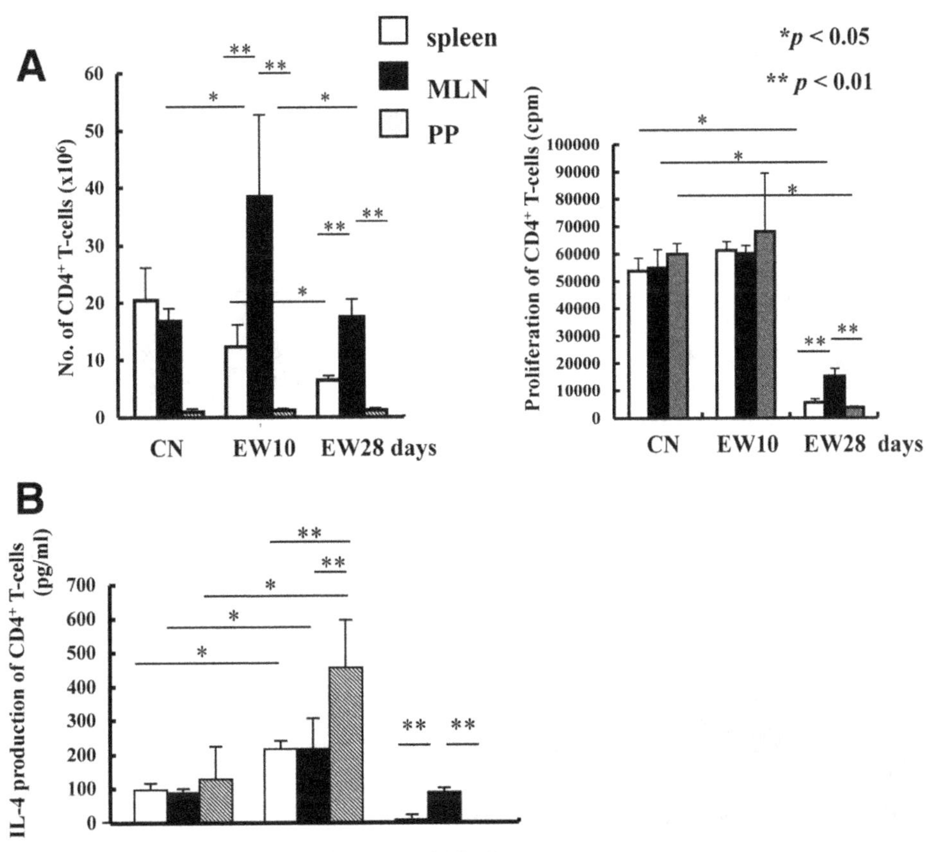


**Figure 3. Roles of $CD4^+$ T-cells from PPs, MLNs, and spleen differ in EW-fed OVA23-3 mice.** (A) Number of $CD4^+$ T-cells (mean$\pm$1 SD) that infiltrated into (left, $n=3$) and the proliferation of $CD4^+$ T-cells (mean$\pm$1 SD) purified from (right, $n=4$) the PPs, MLNs, and spleens of OVA23-3 mice on the EW or the CN diet over time. (B) IL-4 production (mean$\pm$1 SD) by $CD4^+$ T cells from each tissue of OVA23-3 mice ($n=4$) on the EW or the CN diet over time. All data are representative of two independent experiments.

tissues had been removed successfully through lymphadenectomy (Figure 4C, right panel). The swelling of the MLNs during severe inflammation in the EW-fed OVA23-3 mice may relate to the significant ($P<0.01$) increase in the number of $CD4^+$ T-cells in MLNs on day 10 compared with those of spleen and PPs (Figure 3A). These results indicate that MLNs are indispensable for the induction of marked weight loss and intestinal inflammation in this mouse model of food allergy.

## PPs initiate the induction of intestinal inflammation in food-allergic mice

The high levels of IL-4 production of PP $CD4^+$ T-cells on day 10 of the EW diet and the moderate intestinal inflammation found in the MLN-ectomized mice suggest that PPs play a role in establishing intestinal inflammation in EW-fed OVA23-3 mice. To this end, we generated $PP^-$ OVA23-3 mice by disrupting PP organogenesis, and fed them the EW diet. $PP^-$ EW-fed OVA23-3 mice began to demonstrate weight loss on day 5 or 6, markedly later than did $PP^+$ (normal) EW-fed OVA23-3 mice, which showed onset of weight loss on day 3 or 4. The normal growth of both CN-fed $PP^-$ and $PP^+$ OVA23-3 mice showed that weight loss was specific to the EW diet and was dependent on the presence of PPs. $PP^-$ OVA23-3 mice began to recover from their weight loss on day 8 of the EW diet, which was earlier than did $PP^+$ OVA23-3 mice (day 10; Figure 5A). This result suggests that PPs, through their role in the initial induction of inflammatory responses after orally administered OVA, delayed the recovery from weight loss in $PP^+$ OVA23-3 mice.

To verify that the initial induction of the enteropathy occurred in PPs, inflammatory responses in the jejunum on day 3 or 4 of the EW diet were examined. $PP^+$ but not $PP^-$ OVA23-3 mice showed morphologic changes, including cell infiltration, villous atrophy, and an increased number of goblet cells (Figure 5B). In addition, alkaline phosphatase activity, an indication of inflammation [29], was significantly ($P<0.05$) lower in $PP^-$ EW-fed than $PP^+$ EW-fed OVA23-3 mice (Figure 5C). We then assessed the influence of PP disruption on $CD4^+$ T-cell function in MLNs. On day 3 of the EW diet, MLN $CD4^+$ T-cells from $PP^-$ EW-fed OVA23-3 mice showed greater proliferation ($P<0.1$) (Figure 5D, left panel) and significantly ($P<0.05$) enhanced IL-4 production compared with those from $PP^+$ EW-fed mice (Figure 5D, right panel). PP disruption did not alter OVA uptake by epithelial cells or its transport into sera (Figure S3 and Result S3). These results suggest that the delayed onset of inflammation in $PP^-$ OVA23-3 mice reflects the lack of an immediate response of PP $CD4^+$ T-cells against OVA; aggravation of the enteropathy likely developed only after antigen and antigen-presenting cells reached the MLNs to initiate the activation of and IL-4 production by MLN $CD4^+$ T-cells and their migration into the lamina propria. In addition, these findings show that PPs are involved early in induction of enteropathy in this mouse model of food allergy.

## Coordinated contribution from PPs and MLNs is crucial to the development of enteropathy in a mouse model of food allergy

Neither disruption of PP organogenesis nor mesenteric lymphadenectomy alone completely abolished the EW-diet induced intestinal inflammation in OVA23-3 mice. To determine whether PPs and MLNs cooperate to induce enteropathy, we generated OVA23-3 mice devoid of both PPs and MLNs ($PP^-$ MLN-ectomized mice). When fed the EW diet, $PP^-$ MLN-ectomized OVA23-3 mice showed no associated weight loss or morphologic changes in the small intestine. In particular, the small intestinal villi of the EW-fed $PP^-$ MLN-ectomized OVA23-3 mice were well-

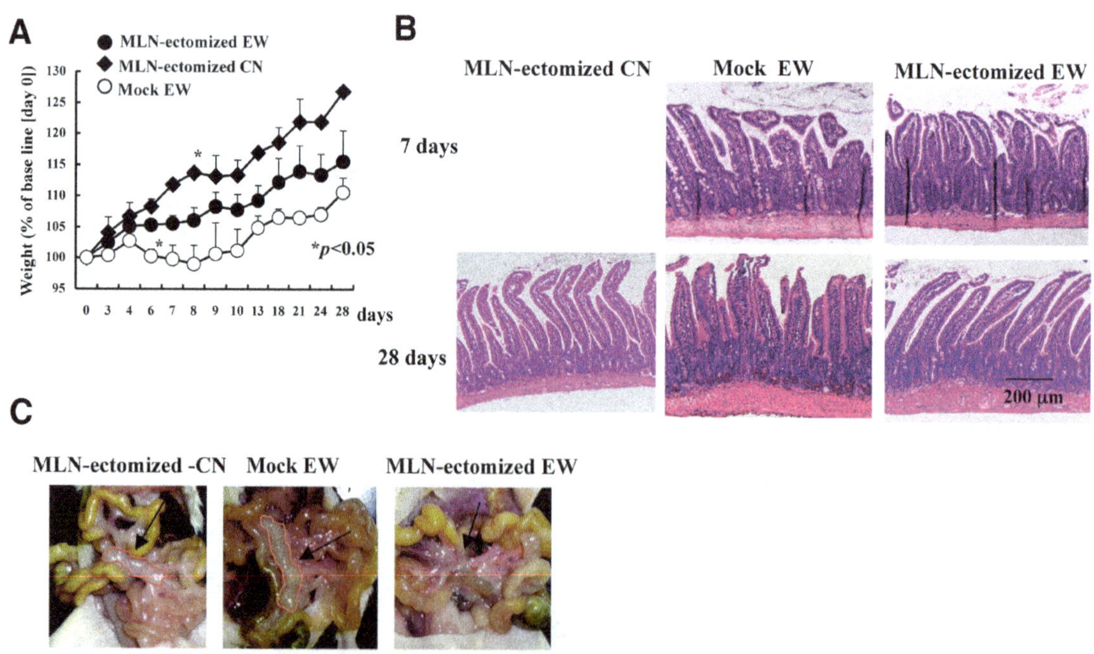


**Figure 4. Potential contribution of MLNs to the intestinal inflammatory immune response.** (A) Weight changes of MLN-ectomized EW-fed (EW, n = 7); sham-operated EW-fed (Mock, n = 4); and MLN-ectomized CN-fed (CN, n = 3) mice. *, Value is significantly ($P<0.05$) different between those for MLN-ectomized EW and sham-operated EW groups or those for MLN-ectomized EW and MLN-ectomized CN groups. (B) Jejunal sections obtained on day 7 (during inflammation, upper panels) or on day 28 (during tolerance, lower panels). (C) Arrows indicate MLNs or site of mesenteric lymphadenectomy in OVA23-3 mice on day 7 of the EW (Mock EW or MLN-ectomized EW) or CN (MLN-ectomized CN) diet. All data are representative of two independent experiments.

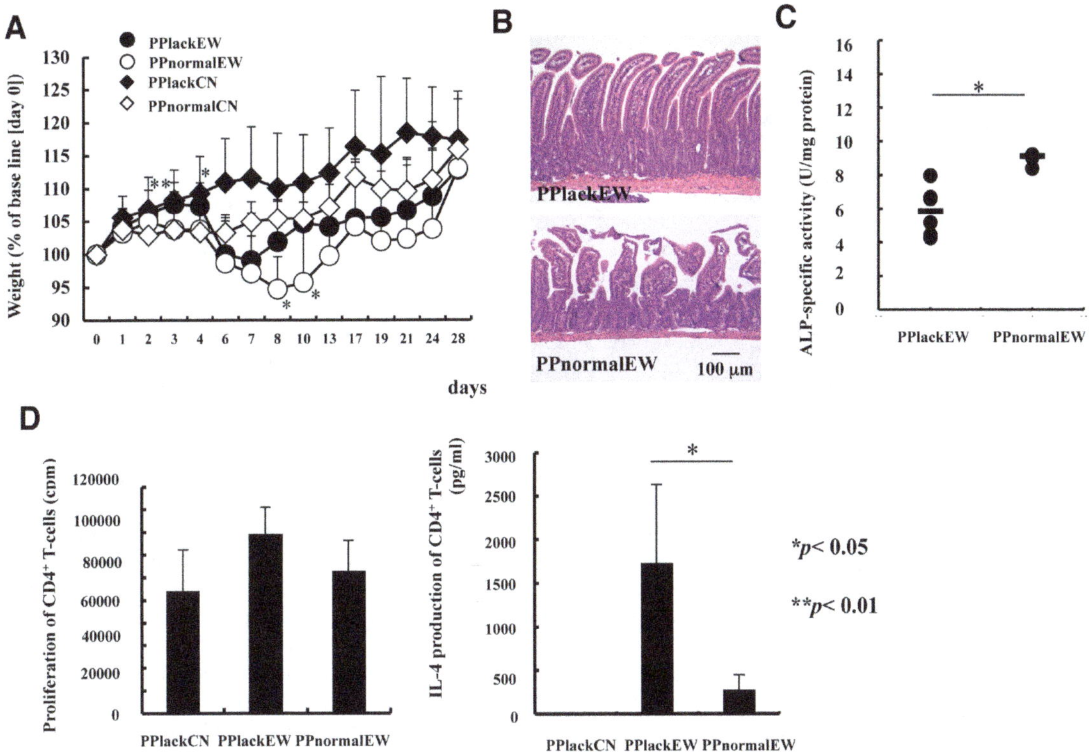


**Figure 5. Manifestation of food allergy in EW-fed PP⁻ OVA23-3 mice.** (A) Weight change in EW-fed $PP^-$ (PPlackEW, n = 18); EW-fed $PP^+$, (PPnormalEW, n = 17; CN-fed $PP^-$ (PPlackCN, n = 8); and CN-fed $PP^+$ (PPnormalCN, n = 8) mice. Value significantly (*, $P<0.05$; **, $P<0.01$) different between those for $PP^-$ and $PP^+$ EW-fed OVA23-3 mice. (B) Jejunal sections. (C) alkaline phosphatase activity in the jejunum (PPlackEW, n = 6; PPnormalEW, n = 3). (D) Proliferation of (left panel) and IL-4 production by (right panel) MLN $CD4^+$ T-cells from $PP^-$ or $PP^+$ EW-fed OVA23-3 mice on day 3. Data are representative of two or three experiments.

organized compared with those of $PP^+$ MLN-ectomized OVA23-3 mice (Figure S4, Result S4, and Figure 4). Mice devoid of pLT by treatment with LTβR-Ig and TNFR55-Ig fusion proteins were generated as described previously to examine the functions of MLNs and PPs [21]; these mice retain their spleens and isolated lymphoid follicles [20,21]. When fed the EW diet, $pLT^-$ OVA23-3 mice did not develop weight loss or intestinal inflammation (Figure S5 and Result S4). These results indicate that both PPs and MLNs cooperatively promote EW-associated enteropathy in OVA23-3 mice. In addition, splenectomized EW-fed mice showed marked enteropathy similar to that in EW-fed sham-operated mice (Figure 6). In addition, the prevention of inflammation in the EW-fed $pLT^-$ OVA23-3 mice, which have spleens and isolated lymphoid follicles only (in the absence of PP and MLNs), supported the dispensable role of the spleen in inflammation. These results confirm that the concurrent absence of both PPs and MLNs led to the lack of clinically apparent food allergy and that the spleen is dispensable in regard to the enteropathy of EW-fed OVA23-3 mice.

## Discussion

Our current study is the first to show the relation between GALT and spleen in the establishment of food-allergic enteropathy in response to orally administered OVA, clarifying the integral roles of MLNs and PPs, but not the spleen. Although the sensitivity of the immune response in each intestinal lymph node population (e.g. pancreatico-duodenal) other than MLNs may influence the ultimate degree of inflammation [30], preparation of MLN-ectomized, $PP^-$, $PP^-$ MLN-ectomized, and $pLT^-$ OVA23-3 mice revealed the necessary coordination between PPs and MLNs in the development of intestinal inflammation. Because the prevention of inflammation was more complete in the absence of both PPs and MLNs than in the absence of either tissue alone, we surmise that PPs contributed to the development of the inflammation by cooperating with MLNs.

Whereas both PP and MLN seem to contribute in generating effector T-cells to establish intestinal inflammation, we posit that their roles are sequential. Specifically, we consider that the responses of PPs are immediate because from results of current study, they are the early and direct inductive sites for orally administered OVA, whereas those of MLNs augment and maintain the PP-induced inflammation thereafter. However the severity of the enteropathy was attenuated in EW-fed $PP^+$ MLN-ectomized mice compared with $PP^+$ $MLN^+$ that is, untreated) EW-fed OVA23-3 mice. In light of the results from CN-fed MLN-ectomized mice, we believe that the surgery itself had no effect on the development of inflammation induced by EW diet feeding in MLN-ectomized OVA23-3 mice. Therefore, although later in the cascade than are PPs, MLNs nonetheless appear to be pivotal in exacerbating the enteropathy and maintaining the associated symptoms.

PPs may not be absolutely required for the development of the enteropathy, as indicated by the blunted response in $PP^-$ OVA23-3 mice. However, weight loss and inflammatory responses were exacerbated in control or MLN-ectomized OVA23-3 mice compared with $PP^-$ or $PP^-$ MLN-ectomized mice, suggesting that PPs provide an important contribution to enteropathy. The morphology of PPs, particularly the interfollicular region, enables

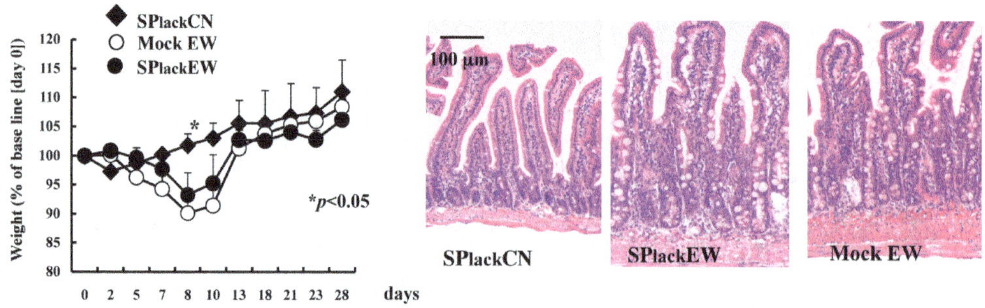


**Figure 6. The spleen is dispensable for the establishment of enteropathy in EW-fed OVA23-3 mice.** Weight change (left panel) and jejunal sections (right panel, day 7) of splenectomized EW-fed (SPlackEW, n = 5), splenectomized CN-fed (SPlackCN, n = 3), and sham-operated EW-fed (Mock EW, n = 4) OVA23-3 mice. *, Significant ($P<0.05$) difference between values for splenectomized CN-fed and EW-fed mice.

the direct activation of CD4$^+$ T-cells at this site of OVA uptake by M cells, which overlie PPs and which are involved in food intake [31]. Inflammatory dendritic cells in PPs [9,32] may facilitate the induction of PP CD4$^+$ T-cells to produce the high levels of IL-4 noted on day 10 in EW-fed OVA23-3 mice. The tissues removed from OVA23-3 mice and effects of that removal on the establishment of enteropathy are summarized in Table S1.

The current results also revealed significant differences in the properties of PPs, MLNs, and spleen during the tolerance acquisition phase that followed the enteropathy. Spleen, which is dispensable in regard to intestinal inflammation, appears to contribute to the induction of systemic oral tolerance. On day 28, the induction of systemic tolerance was confirmed by the attenuation of both splenic CD4$^+$ T-cell responses (Figure 3A) and serum OVA-specific IgE levels in EW-fed OVA23-3 mice (Figure S2). Concurrent decrease in serum IgE levels with the acquisition of tolerance also occurred in another food allergy model generated through immunization of OVA and alum [33] and in clinical studies of allergen-specific immunotherapy [34]. Even in MLN-ectomized EW-fed OVA23-3 mice, tolerance was induced in splenic CD4$^+$ T-cells (Figure S6 and Result S5). On day 10 of the EW diet, although splenic CD4$^+$ T-cells were activated and produced IL-4 in response to OVA, the number of CD4$^+$ T-cells that infiltrated into the spleen was decreased compared with that in CN-fed OVA23-3 mice. These suggested either T-cell depletion or the induction of apoptosis is a key feature of tolerance induction [35].

In contrast, the induction of tolerance in GALT seemed blunted compared with that in spleen but had a greater effect on PPs than on MLNs in our system. MLNs may be susceptible to excess IL-4 production and thus maintain inflammation in the context of continuous administration of food allergens, even though strong systemic tolerance was induced. In the induction of oral tolerance, the suppression of persistent MLN inflammatory IL-4 responses of effector CD4$^+$ T-cells, even after the establishment of systemic tolerance, may have clinical significance in regard to preventing adverse reactions [36,37]. Distinct from other studies, our current study revealed concurrent differences in the behavior of CD4$^+$ T cells between systemic (tolerance) and local (maintenance of priming) tissues in EW-fed OVA23-3 mice. By further improvement, the OVA23-3 mouse model may facilitate delineation of the decisional factors in the blunted T-cell immune responses against oral administered antigens that subsequently cause inflammation versus tolerance. In addition, because antigen-specific T-cells may play an important role in triggering and driving IgE-mediated diarrhea [38], clarifying the mechanism underlying the T-cell mediated intestinal inflammation and developing ways to regulate T-cell responses in food allergy would promote the advancement of specific oral tolerance immunotherapy. Our study further suggests that systemic sensitization by routes other than the intestinal route (e.g., through skin) is needed to induce severe IgE-mediated systemic food-allergy like anaphylaxis [39].

In conclusion, for the effective acquisition of tolerance in food allergy and to improve the induction of tolerance through rational strategies built on clarification of the mechanism, the persistent MLN-associated inflammatory responses must be controlled. However, our study clearly indicates that regulating immune responses in MLNs alone was insufficient, because both PPs and MLNs contribute to the development of the T-cell mediated intestinal inflammation of food allergy. In this regard, PPs are the early and direct inductive sites of immune responses on the intestinal epithelium for uptake of OVA. In addition, PPs reportedly uptake aggregated milk proteins and induce Th2 response [31]. Therefore, regulation of the T-cells in PPs may, through the subsequent attenuation of persistent MLN-driven inflammatory responses, be an easily accessible tool for treating or preventing the exacerbation of intestinal inflammation. An M-cell-targeting delivery system or tolerogenic dendritic cell induction techniques may be valuable in cases involving soluble antigens, such as OVA [40~42].

## Supporting Information

**Figure S1 The number of or rate of CD4$^+$ T-cells in the small intestinal lymphocytes infiltrating into the small intestinal lamina propria of EW-fed OVA23-3 mice during 28 days.**
(TIF)

**Figure S2 Serum concentrations of OVA-specific IgE Abs of EW-fed normal OVA23-3 mice.**
(TIF)

**Figure S3 OVA uptake in PP$^-$ OVA23-3 mice.**
(TIF)

**Figure S4 PPs and MLNs cooperatively induce enteropathy in EW-fed OVA23-3 mice.**
(TIF)

**Figure S5 Inhibition of organogenesis in both PPs and MLNs obstructs enteropathy in EW-fed OVA23-3 mice.**
(TIF)

**Figure S6 Proliferation of splenic CD4$^+$ T-cells in EW-fed MLN-ectomized OVA23-3 mice.**
(TIF)

**Table S1 Roles of lymphoid tissues in the establishment of enteropathy in EW-fed OVA23-3 mice.**
(TIF)

**File S1 Materials and Methods; Measurement of OVA uptake; Preparation and culture of CD4+ T-cells; Preparation of lamina propria lymphocytes and staining of CD4+ T cells.**
(PDF)

**Result S1 Result of Figure S1; Infiltration of $CD4^+$ T cells into the lamina propria of the small intestine of EW-fed OVA23-3 mice.**
(PDF)

**Result S2 Result of Figure S2; Serum concentrations of OVA-specific IgE Abs of EW-fed normal OVA23-3 mice.**
(PDF)

**Result S3 Result of Figure S3; Deficiency of PPs did not influence on ability of OVA uptake in intestinal epithelial cells.**
(PDF)

**Result S4 Result of Figures S4 and S5; Coordinated contribution from PPs and MLNs is crucial to the development of enteropathy in a mouse model of food allergy.**
(PDF)

**Result S5 Result of Figure S6; Proliferation of splenic $CD4^+$ T-cells in EW-fed MLN-ectomized OVA23-3 mice.**
(PDF)

## Acknowledgments

We thank S. Habu for providing OVA23-3 mice, H. Ishikawa for providing valuable reagents and helping in producing $PP^-$ mice, and S. Nishikawa for providing anti-IL-7R mAb. We also thank T. Nagatake and G. Pontes (The University of Tokyo) for technical advice.

## Author Contributions

Conceived and designed the experiments: HNA. Performed the experiments: HNA AK YF KS TM MKF YK. Analyzed the data: HNA AK YF KS MKF. Contributed reagents/materials/analysis tools: YK TM TN MGS MY OI SK RS HK SH. Wrote the paper: HNA. Discussed the data and reviewed the manuscript: HNA AK YF MGS HK SH. Reviewed the manuscript: MT RS SK YK TN OI JK.

## References

1. Wang J, Sampson HA (2011) Food allergy. J Clin Inv 121: 827–835.
2. Nowak-Wegrzyn A, Sampson HA (2011) Future therapies for food allergies. J Allergy Clin Immunol 127: 558–573.
3. Scurlock AM, Vickery BP, Hourihane JO, Burks AW (2010) Pediatric food allergy and mucosal tolerance. Mucosal Immunol 3: 345–354.
4. Bedoret D, Singh AK, Shaw V, Hoyte EG, Hamilton R, et al. (2012) Changes in antigen-specific T-cell number and function during oral desensitization in cow's milk allergy enabled with omalizumab. Mucosal Immunol 5: 267–276.
5. Pabst O, Mowat AM (2012) Oral tolerance to food protein. Mucosal immunol 5: 232–239.
6. Steele L, Mayer L, Cecilia Berin M (2012) Mucosal immunology of tolerance and allergy in the gastrointestinal tract. Immunol Res 54: 75–82.
7. Kweon MN, Yamamoto M, Kajiki M, Takahashi I, Kiyono H (2000) Systemically derived large intestinal CD4(+) Th2 cells play a central role in STAT6-mediated allergic diarrhea. J Clin Invest 106: 199–206.
8. Knight AK, Blázquez AB, Zhang S, Mayer L, Sampson HA, et al. (2007) CD4 T cells activated in the mesenteric lymph node mediate gastrointestinal food allergy in mice. Am J Physiol Gastrointest Liver Physiol 293: G1234–43.
9. Temblay JN, Bertelli E, Arques JL, Regoli M, Nicoletti C (2007) Production of IL-12 by Peyer patch-dendritic cells is critical for the resistance to food allergy. J Allergy Clin Immunol 120: 659–665.
10. Kool M, Soullié T, van Nimwegen M, Willart MAM, Muskens F, et al. (2008) Alum adjuvant boosts adaptive immunity by inducing uric acid and activating inflammatory dendritic cells. J Exp Med 205: 869–882.
11. Sato T, Sasahara T, Nakamura Y, Osaki T, Hasegawa T, et al. (1994) Naive T-cells can mediate delayed-type hypersensitivity response in T cell receptor transgenic mice. Eur J Immunol 24: 1512–1516.
12. Nakajima-Adachi H, Ebihara A, Kikuchi A, Ishida T, Sasaki K, et al. (2006) Food antigen causes TH2-dependent enteropathy followed by tissue repair in T-cell receptor transgenic mice. J Allergy Clin Immunol 117: 1125–1132.
13. Nakajima-Adachi H, Koike E, Totsuka M, Hiraide E, Wakatsuki Y, et al. (2012) Two distinct epitopes on the ovalbumin 323–339 peptide differentiating CD4+T cells into the Th2 or Th1 phenotype. Biosci Biotechnol Biochem 76: 1979–1981.
14. Morita H, Nomura I, Matsuda A, Saito H, Matsumoto K (2013) Gastrointestinal food allergy in infants. Allergol Int 62: 297–307.
15. Newberry RD, Stenson WF, Lorenz RG (1999) Cyclooxygenase-2-dependent arachidonic acid metabolites are essential modulators of the intestinal immune response to dietary antigen. Nat Med 5: 900–6.
16. Goldstein JL, Eisen GM, Lewis B, Gralnek IM, Zlotnick S, et al. (2005) Video capsule endoscopy to prospectively assess small bowel injury with celecoxib, naproxen plus omeprazole, and placebo. Clin Gastroenterol Hepatol 3: 133–141.
17. Maiden L, Thjodleifsson B, Theodors A, Gonzalez J, Bjarnason I (2005) A quantitative analysis of NSAID-induced small bowel pathology by capsule enteroscopy. Gastroenterology 128: 1172–1178.
18. Costes LM, Boeckxstaens GE, de Jonge WJ, Cailotto C (2013) Neural networks in intestinal immunoregulation. Organogenesis 9: 216–223.
19. Yoshida H, Honda K, Shinkura R, Adachi S, Nishikawa S (1999) IL-7 receptor alpha+ CD3(–) cells in the embryonic intestine induces the organizing center of Peyer's patches. Int Immunol 11: 643–655.
20. Rennert PD, Browning JL, Mebius R, Mackay F, Hochman PS (1996) Surface lymphotoxin alpha/beta complex is required for the development of peripheral lymphoid organs. J Exp Med 184: 1999–2006.
21. Yamamoto M, Kweon MN, Rennert PD, Hiroi T, Fujihashi K, et al. (2004) Role of gut-associated lymphoreticular tissues in antigen-specific intestinal IgA immunity. J Immunol 173: 762–769.
22. Worbs T, Bode U, Yan S, Hoffmann MW, Hintzen G, et al (2006) Oral tolerance originates in the intestinal immune system and relies on antigen carriage by dendritic cells. J Exp Med 203: 519–527.
23. Ohara J, Paul WE (1985) Production of a monoclonal antibody to and molecular characterization of B-cell stimulatory factor-1. Nature 315: 333–336.
24. Haraikawa M, Sogabe N, Tanabe R, Hosoi T, Goseki-Sone M (2011) Vitamin K1 (phylloquinone) or vitamin K2 (menaquinone-4) induces intestinal alkaline phosphatase gene expression. J Nutr Sci Vitaminol 57: 274–279.
25. Gohda M, Kunisawa J, Miura F, Kagiyama Y, Kurashima Y, et al. (2008) Sphingosine 1-phosphate regulates the egress of IgA plasmablasts from Peyer's patches for intestinal IgA responses. J Immunol 180: 5335–43.
26. Cardoso CR, Provinciatto PR, Godoi DF, Ferreira BR, Teixeira G, et al. (2009) IL-4 regulates susceptibility to intestinal inflammation in murine food allergy. Am J Physiol Gastrointest Liver Physiol 296: G593–600.
27. Brandt EB, Munitz A, Orekov T, Mingler MK, McBride M, et al. (2009) Targeting IL-4/IL-13 signaling to alleviate oral allergen-induced diarrhea. J Allergy Clin Immunol 123: 53–58.
28. Dourado LPA, Saldanha JCS, Gargiulo DL, Noviello M de LM, Brant CC, et al. (2010) Role of IL-4 in aversion induced by food allergy in mice. Cell Immunol 262: 62–68.
29. Matsunaga T, Harada T, Hokari S, Komoda T (2002) Alkaline phosphatases reduce toxicity of lipopolysaccharides in vivo and in vitro through dephosphorylation. Clin Biochem 35: 455–461.
30. Morton AM, Sefik E, Upadhyay R, Weissleder R, Benoist C, et al. (2014) Endoscopic photoconversion reveals unexpectedly broad leukocyte trafficking to and from the gut. Proc Natl Acad Sci U S A 111: 6696–701.
31. Roth-Walter F, Berin MC, Arnaboldi P, Escalante CR, Dahan S, et al. (2008) Pasteurization of milk proteins promotes allergic sensitization by enhancing uptake through Peyer's patches. Allergy 63: 882–890.
32. Chambers SJ, Bertelli E, Winterbone MS, Regoli M, Man AL, et al. (2004) Adoptive transfer of dendritic cells from allergic mice induces specific immunoglobulin E antibody in naïve recipients in absence of antigen challenge without altering the T helper 1/T helper 2 balance. Immunology 112: 72–79.
33. Burggraf M, Nakajima-Adachi H, Hachimura S, Ilchmann A, Pemberton AD, et al (2011) Oral tolerance induction does not resolve gastrointestinal inflammation in a mouse model of food allergy. Mol Nutr Food Res 55: 1475–83.
34. Akdis M, Akdis CA (2014) Mechanisms of allergen-specific immunotherapy: multiple suppressor factors at work in immune tolerance to allergens. J Allergy Clin Immunol 133: 621–31.
35. Dubois B, Goubier A, Joubert G, Kaiserlian D (2005) Oral tolerance and regulation of mucosal immunity. Cell Mol Life Sci 62: 1322–1332.
36. Möhrenschlager M, Ring J (2011) Food allergy: an increasing problem for the elderly. Gerontology 57: 33–36.

37. Hu W, Katelaris CH, Kemp AS (2007) Recurrent egg allergy in adulthood. Allergy 62: 709–715.
38. Blázquez AB, Knight AK, Getachew H, Bromberg JS, Lira SA, et al. (2010) A functional role for CCR6 on proallergic T cells in the gastrointestinal tract. Gastroenterology 138: 275–278.
39. Beck LA, Leung DY (2000) Allergen sensitization through the skin induces systemic allergic responses. J Allergy Clin Immunol 106: S258–63.
40. Suzuki H, Sekine S, Kataoka K, Pascual DW, Maddaloni M, et al. (2008) Ovalbumin-protein sigma 1 M-cell targeting facilitates oral tolerance with reduction of antigen-specific CD4+ T cells. Gastroenterology 135: 917–925.
41. Fecek RJ, Marcondes Rezende M, Busch R, Hassing I, Pieters R, et al. (2010) Enteric reovirus infection stimulates peanut-specific IgG2a responses in a mouse food allergy model. Immunobiology 215: 941–948.
42. Ruiter B. Shreffler WG (2012) The role of dendritic cells in food allergy. J Allergy Clin Immunol 129: 921–928.

22

# *In silico* Identification of IgE-Binding Epitopes of Osmotin Protein

**Prerna Sharma[1], Shailendra Nath Gaur[2], Naveen Arora[1]***

1 Allergy and Immunology Section, CSIR-Institute of Genomics and Integrative Biology, Delhi, India, 2 Department of Respiratory Medicine, Vallabhbhai Patel Chest Institute, University of Delhi, Delhi, India

**Abstract**

The identification of B-cell epitopes is an important step to study the antigen- antibody interactions for diagnosis and therapy. The present study aimed to identify B- cell epitopes of osmotin using bioinformatic tools and further modify these regions to study the allergenic property. B-cell epitopes were predicted based on amino acid physicochemical properties. Three single point mutations M1, M2, and M3 and a multiple point mutant (M123) were selected to disrupt the IgE binding. These mutants were cloned, expressed and proteins purified to homogeneity. The IgE binding of the purified proteins was evaluated by ELISA and ELISA inhibition with patients' sera. Three regions of osmotin M1 (57–70 aa), M2 (72–85 aa) and M3 (147–165 aa) were identified as potential antibody recognition sites using *in silico* tools. The sequence similarity search of the predicted epitopes of osmotin using Structural Database of Allergenic proteins (SDAP) showed similarity with known allergens from tomato, kiwifruit, bell pepper, apple, mountain cedar and cypress. Mutants M1, M2 and M3 showed up to 72%, 60% and 76% reduction, respectively in IgE binding whereas M123 showed up to 90% reduction with patients' sera. The immunoblot of M123 mutant showed 40% reduction in spot density as compared to osmotin. All mutants showed decreased inhibition potency with M123 exhibiting lowest potency of 32% with osmotin positive pooled patients' sera. The three B- cell epitopes of osmotin predicted by *in silico* method correlated with the experimental approach. The mutant M123 showed a reduction of 90% in IgE binding. The present method may be employed for prediction of B- cell epitopes of allergenic proteins.

**Editor:** Christian Schönbach, Kyushu Institute of Technology, Japan

**Funding:** The work covered in this manuscript was funded by the Council for Scientific and Industrial Reasearch (CSIR). The URL for the funder's website is "http://rdpp.csir.res.in/csir_acsir/Home. aspx". The funders had no role in study design, data collection and analysis, decision to publish, or preparation of the manuscript.

**Competing Interests:** The authors have declared that no competing interests exist.

* E-mail: naveen@igib.res.in

## Introduction

The prevalence of food allergy is increasing worldwide and as many as 8% of children and 2% of adults are affected in western countries [1]. Primary treatment of food allergy is strict avoidance of the diets containing food allergens. Recently new strategies have been designed to reduce allergic reactions [2]. Specific immunotherapy is not used to treat food allergies because of the risk of severe side effects, including anaphylactic shock [3]. Several studies have shown the development of hypoallergenic molecules with reduced or no allergenic potential, which may be useful for specific immunotherapy [4], [5].

The knowledge of the B-cell epitopes can be applied in diagnosis, therapy or development of effective vaccines for immunotherapy [6]. In case of food allergens, digestion/heating may lead to loss of the structure of the protein thereby rendering the conformational epitopes inactive. Thus sequential epitopes play an important role for diagnosis of food allergy. Moreover, it is difficult to study the conformational epitopes of allergens as considerable efforts are required for validation [7]. Epitopes can be identified by many methods but computational tools provide a promising and rapid alternative [8]. These epitopes may be modified to reduce allergenicity of an allergen. These variants can be produced by disruption of IgE binding epitopes either by chemical modification [5] or genetic engineering [9]. The key requirement is to identify IgE-binding epitopes on food allergens. The recombinant allergens have similar structure and immunologic properties as that of native counterparts, hence these can be modified to reduce the allergenicity while maintaining important immunologic properties [10]. Earlier studies on recombinant food allergens have demonstrated reduced allergenicity of shrimp [4], peanut allergen [11], apple [12], olive [13], etc.

Osmotin is a stress-responsive multifunctional protein from tobacco (*Nicotiana tabacum*). It accumulates in cells on osmotic stress adaptation and provides osmotolerance to plants [14]. It belongs to pathogenesis related-5 (PR-5) protein family and exhibits antifungal activity as it permeabilizes the plasma membrane and dissipates the membrane pH gradient of the fungal species [15]. These two properties of osmotin have been exploited for developing transgenic crops such as tobacco [16], strawberry [17], wheat [18], cotton [19], tomato [20], and mulberry [21]. In our previous study we had identified osmotin as a potential allergen using bioinformatic and immunobiochemical methods [22]. In the present study we identified sequential epitopes of osmotin by *in silico* approach. The potential IgE binding residues in these epitopes were mutated to reduce allergenicity of osmotin.

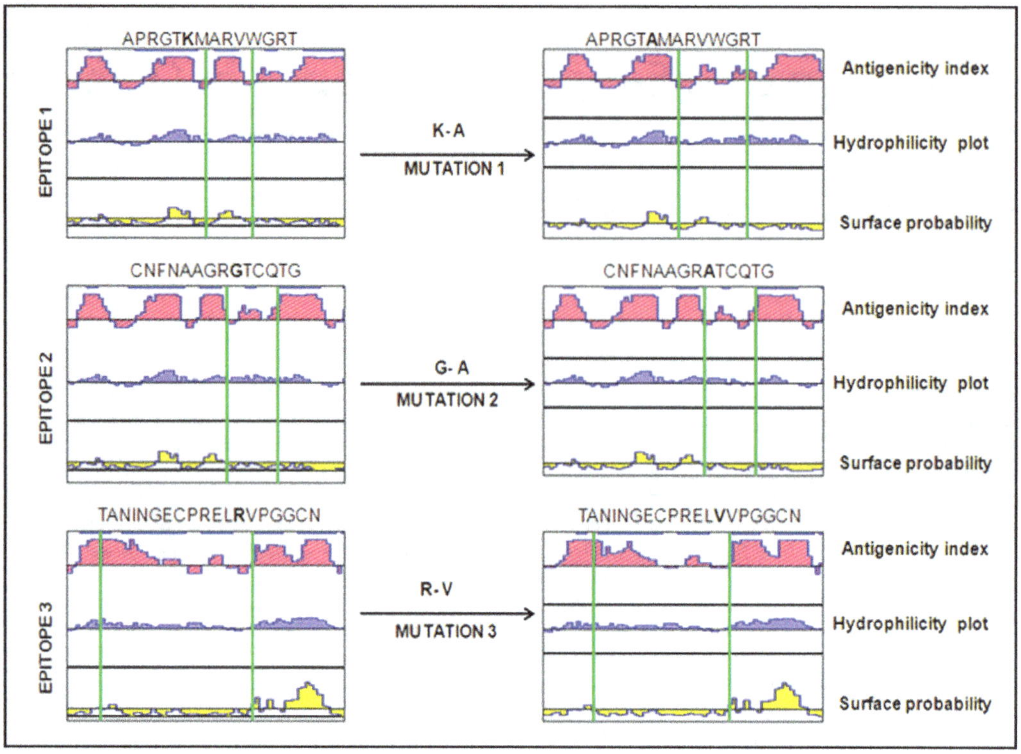


**Figure 1. Comparative analysis of antigenic index of osmotin epitopes and its mutants by DNAstar protean system.** The region between vertical lines show the three regions mutated by site directed mutagenesis. Mutation in epitope regions shows reduction in antigenic index in DNAstar program.

## Materials and Methods

### Ethics statement

The study protocol was approved by human ethics committee of the Institute of Genomics and Integrative Biology, Delhi. Informed written consent was obtained from the patients and healthy subjects that participated in the study. The study did not involve any minors/children.

### B-cell epitope prediction

B-cell epitopes are classified as either continuous or discontinuous. A number of algorithms have been developed for predicting the continuous B-cell epitopes based on physico-chemical properties like hydrophilicity (Parker method), flexibility (Karplus and Schulz method), accessibility (Emini method) and turns (Pellequer method) [23]. The prediction methods of the linear or continuous epitopes have improved over the years. The linear B- cell epitopes were predicted by different servers namely, BcePred (based on a combination of physico-chemical properties), BepiPred 1.0b (based on hydorophilicity scale with a Hidden Markov Model), ABCpred (uses artificial neural networks), and BCPred (uses support vector machine) [23]. DNASTAR Lasergene version 7.2. (DNASTAR Inc., Madison, WI, USA) was also used which uses amino acid propensity scales of Hopp -Woods (hydrophilicity), Emini (Surface probability), Jameson-Wolf (antigenic index) and Karplus-Schulz (flexibility). The epitopes identified frequently by most of the tools were selected.

### Site directed mutagenesis of osmotin

Osmotin was mutated at three residues to generate three single point mutants M1, M2 and M3. A fourth mutant M123 with all three point mutations was also generated. Mutagenesis was performed using oligonucleotide primers and mutation-specific oligonucleotide primers accommodating each mutation. Internal amino acid substitution in osmotin was performed by a three step PCR reaction. The first two steps of PCR reaction was carried out with an internal mutant primer and one of the flanking primers. Final products of these two steps were purified from agarose gel, mixed and amplified using flanking primers. The fourth mutant with all three point mutations was generated step wise using mutant M2 as template. The mutation 1 was generated using forward primer 5′ATCAATGCGCCACGATTTACTAAAAAG3′ and reverse primer 5′CATTTTAGTAAATCGTGGCGCATTG3′, mutant 2 was generated using forward primer 5′ATGCTGCTGGTAGGTTTACGTGCCAA3′ and reverse primer 5′TTTGGCACGTAAA CCTACCAGCAGCA3′, mutant 3 using forward primer 5′ACGGCTAATATATTCGGCGAATGTCC3′ and reverse primer 5′GGACATTCGCCGAATATATTAGCCGTAC3′ and the flanking primers 5′GAATTGAATTCGATGGGCAACTTGAGATCTTCTTTTG3′with *EcoR I* site and 5′GCTCGAG CTCCTTAGCCACTTCATCACTTCCAG 3′ with *Xho I* site. The PCR products were digested with *EcoRI* and *XhoI* enzymes, subcloned in pET22b+ vector and sequenced to confirm the mutations. Constructs containing the mutations in the epitopes were used for the expression of fully modified recombinant osmotin protein mutants.

### Expression and purification of mutants

The constructs of M1, M2, M3 and M123 mutant sequences in pET22b+ vector were transformed into BL-21 *Escherichia coli* cells. The cells were grown till 0.6 O.D., induced with 1 mM isopropyl-beta-D-thiogalactopyranoside for 3 h, harvested and the pellet was suspended in binding buffer containing 50 mM $NaH_2PO_4$, 300 mM NaCl, 10 mM imidazole (pH 8.0), sonicated and centrifuged. The supernatant was incubated for 2 h with 2 ml Ni-NTA equilibrated with binding buffer. The column was washed with buffer containing 20 mM imidazole, 300 mM NaCl and 50 Mm $NaH_2PO_4$ (pH 8.0) and bound proteins were eluted using buffer containing 250 mM imidazole, 300 mM NaCl and 50 mM $NaH_2PO_4$. The purified mutant proteins were resolved on 12% SDS-PAGE, transferred to nitrocellulose membrane and probed with osmotin positive patients' pooled sera. Densitometry of the immunoblot was performed by Gene Tools software from SynGene (Synoptics Ltd, Cambridge, UK).

## Circular dichroism (CD) spectroscopy

Osmotin protein and its mutant M123 were dialyzed against 10 mM $KH_2PO_4/K_2HPO_4$ buffer (pH 7.4). Circular dichroism spectroscopy was performed on a J-815 S spectropolarimeter (Jasco) with constant nitrogen flushing at 25°C. Wavelength was analysed with a step width of 0.2 nm and a band width of 1 nm. The spectral range was 200–240 nm at a scan speed of 50 nm/min. The final spectra were corrected by subtracting the corresponding baseline spectrum obtained under identical conditions. Average of three scans was taken and the mean residue molar ellipticity was calculated.

## Sera collection

The patients of allergic rhinitis and asthma aged 15–50 years were skin prick tested with various aeroallergens and food extracts to detect sensitization. The guidelines of the American Thoracic Society were followed for diagnosis of asthma [24]. The patients having any two of the symptoms, viz. sneezing, rhinorrhea, nasal blockage, postnasal drip, etc. for most of the time since the last two years were diagnosed as rhinitis. Blood samples were collected from patients showing marked positive skin reactions to different food extracts and healthy subjects at the outpatient department, V.P. Chest Institute, Delhi, a referral chest hospital.

## Specific IgE estimation

Specific IgE binding for the mutants and osmotin protein was determined by ELISA. Briefly the proteins were incubated in carbonate buffer overnight at 4°C in a microtitre plate (Nunc, Roskilde, Denmark). After washing with PBS– Tween 20 (0.05%), the nonspecific sites were blocked with 3% defatted milk for 3 h at 37°C. The plate was washed again and incubated with 100 µl diluted (1:10 v/v) sera of food allergic patients which were positive to osmotin, overnight at 4°C. Normal human sera (n = 4) were used as negative control. The plate was washed and incubated with antihuman IgE-horse radish peroxidase (1:1000 v/v, Sigma) for 3 h at 37°C. The plate was washed with PBS- Tween 20 and followed by PBS and colour was developed with orthophenylene diamine in citrate – phosphate buffer, pH 5.0. The reaction was stopped after 30 min by adding 5 N $H_2SO_4$ and the absorbance was read at 492 nm.

## ELISA inhibition

ELISA inhibition with the mutants was performed to determine the allergenic potency and relative ability of the mutants for IgE binding. The microtitre plate was coated with purified osmotin protein and blocked with 3% defatted milk. Further it was incubated with pre- incubated mixture of 1:10 v/v osmotin positive pooled patients' sera (n = 5) and graded amounts of

**Table 1.** Peptide similarity search of the three predicted epitopes of osmotin with known allergens in SDAP database.

| S. No. | Predicted osmotin Epitopes | Allergen | *PD* Sequence Similarity Index | Matching region |
|---|---|---|---|---|
| 1 | APRGTKMARVWGRT | Lyc e NP24 | 0.39 | **APRGTKMAR**i**WGRT** |
| | | Cap a 1 | 2.01 | **AP**p**GTKMAR**i**WGRT** |
| | | Cap a 1w | 3.47 | **AP**p**GT**a**MAR**i**WGRT** |
| | | Act c 2 | 7.31 | pgag**TK**g**ARVW**p**RT** |
| 2 | CNFNAAGRGTCQTG | Lyc e NP24 | 0.00 | **CNFNAAGRGTCQTG** |
| | | Act c 2 | 2.92 | **CNF**dg**AGRG**k**CQTG** |
| | | Jun a 3 | 3.26 | **C**t**F**d**A**s**G**k**G**s**CQTG** |
| | | Cap a 1 | 3.39 | **CNF**dg**AGRG**w**CQTG** |
| | | Cup s 3.0101 | 4.34 | **C**t**F**d**A**s**G**g**G**s**C**rs**G** |
| | | Cup a 3 | 4.34 | **C**t**F**d**A**s**G**k**G**s**C**rs**G** |
| | | Mus a 4.0101 | 4.49 | CSFDGSGRGRCQTG |
| | | Mal d 2 | 7.08 | **C**std**AAG**kft**C**e**T**a |
| 3 | TANINGECPRELRVPGGCN | Lyc e NP24 | 1.21 | **TANINGECPR**a**L**k**VPGGCN** |
| | | Cap a 1w | 2.42 | **TANINGECP**gs**LRVPGGCN** |
| | | Act c 2 | 2.46 | **TA**d**ING**q**CP**n**ELR**a**PGGCN** |
| | | Cap a 1 | 3.24 | v**ANINGECP**gs**LRVPGGCN** |
| | | Mus a 4.0101 | 5.07 | aad**ING**q**CP**ga**L**ka**PGGCN** |
| | | Cup a 3 | 5.73 | kad**IN**av**CP**s**EL**k**V**d**GGCN** |
| | | Jun a 3 | 5.79 | kad**IN**av**CP**s**EL**k**V**d**GGCN** |

The table shows similarity of the predicted B- cell epitopes of osmotin with peptides of known allergens with a PD value less than 8.5 in SDAP database. Matching amino acids are depicted in bold and upper case. Unmatched amino acids in lower case.

osmotin and each of the purified mutants i.e. 0.1, 1, 10, 100 and 1000 ng as inhibitor. Sera of non-allergic subjects were used as control. The remaining steps were the same as followed for ELISA. Inhibition was presented as percentage decrease in absorbance of sample with inhibitor to that of sample without inhibitor and allergenic potency was defined by establishing the concentration of protein required for 50% inhibition.

### Statistical analysis

Statistical analysis of results was done by using GraphPad Prism and GraphPad Instat software (GraphPad Software, San Diego, CA, USA). The statistically significant difference was determined using one way ANOVA followed by Bonferroni comparison test between osmotin and the mutant M123 challenged mice groups. The p value $<0.05$ was considered as significant.

## Results

### Mapping of IgE-binding epitopes

IgE binding regions were identified by sequence based tools which fall in common regions of the sequence map. Three stretches of amino acids 57–70, 72–85 and 147–165 recognized by at least four tools were predicted as B- cell epitopes. Residues 60 (Gly → Phe), 80 (Gly → Phe) and 151(Asn → Phe) in each epitope were selected for substitution mutation. These epitopes on mutation using *in silico* approach showed reduction in the antigenic index in DNAstar program (Fig. 1). In Structural Database of Allergenic Proteins (SDAP; 737 sequences; http://fermi.utmb.edu/SDAP/), these epitopes showed similarity with tomato allergen Lyc (NP24), kiwi fruit allergen (Act c 2), cypress allergen (Cup s 3.0102), bell pepper allergen (Cap a 1), apple allergen (Mal d 2) and mountain cedar allergen (Jun a 3) with a *PD* (property distance) value of less than 8.5 (Table 1).

### Expression and purification of the mutants

Four osmotin mutants M1, M2, M3 and M123 proteins were expressed in *E. coli* and purified as His-tag proteins. The yield obtained of these proteins were 2.5 mg/L, 2 mg/L, 2 mg/L, 3 mg/L of the culture. The protein expression in the culture after induction at 1h, 2 h and 3 h with IPTG was visualized by SDS-PAGE (Fig. 2). The purified recombinant proteins were resolved on SDS-PAGE (Fig. 3a) and reacted with osmotin positive pooled patients' sera on immunoblot (Fig. 3b). The intensity of spots on the blot was measured by densitometric scan and osmotin was set as a reference point. The mutant M123 showed 40% reduction in the spot density followed by M1, M3 and M2 as compared to osmotin (Figure 3c).

### Circular dichroism analysis of purified recombinant osmotin and mutant M123

Figure 4 shows the comparison of the osmotin protein and M123 mutant by circular dichroism analysis. The far-UV spectra showed similar characteristics. Minima were obtained at 208 nm, 218 nm and 222 nm. It shows the presence of both α- helices and β- sheets in the secondary structure of the osmotin protein. The CD spectrum of the M123 mutant was similar to osmotin indicating that the mutant has probably adopted the same folded state.

### IgE binding of the mutants with osmotin positive patients' sera

IgE-binding of the four mutants was compared with that of osmotin by ELISA. The mutants showed a reduction in specific

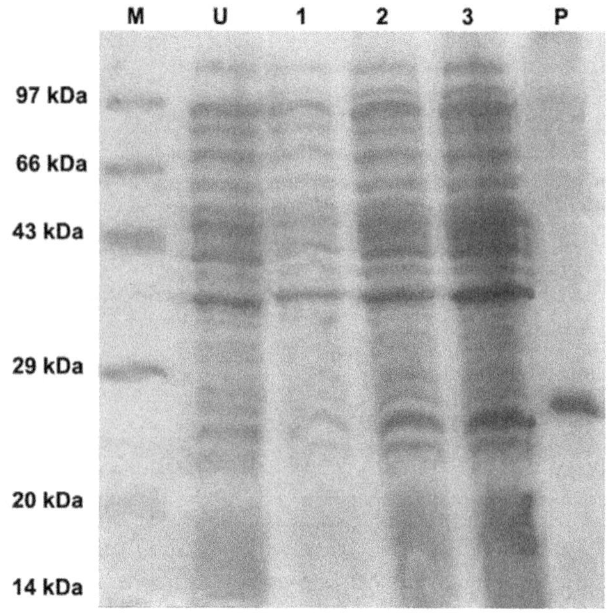


**Figure 2. SDS-PAGE analysis of protein expression in culture.** The uninduced and induced stages of expression of osmotin protein was resolved on 12% gel and stained with Coomassie brilliant blue. Lane M was loaded with Molecular weight marker. Lane U uninduced protein expression. Lane 1, 2, 3 shows expression after induction for 1 h, 2 h, 3 h respectively and lane P represents purified protein.

IgE binding between 25%–72% (M1), 22%–60% (M2), 43%–76% (M3) and 50%–90% (M123) as compared to osmotin (Fig. 5). All the mutants showed significant reduction in IgE binding as compared to osmotin ($p<0.001$) with mutant M123 having maximum reduction.

### Potency of osmotin mutants

IgE-binding and immunoblot of the mutants were further substantiated by ELISA inhibition assay. Pooled osmotin positive patients' sera preincubated with different amounts of the four mutants were added to ELISA plate coated with osmotin. Here, wild-type osmotin gave 66% inhibition at 1000 ng of protein. In contrast, all mutants showed decreased ability to inhibit IgE binding. M1, M2, M3 and M123 reached a maximum inhibition of 39%, 53%, 43% and 32% respectively at 1000 ng/ml inhibitor concentrations. Osmotin required 4 ng of protein to reach the $EC_{50}$. Only M2 showed the inhibition with an $EC_{50}$ of 500 ng whereas the other mutants did not reach the $EC_{50}$ value (Fig. 6).

## Discussion

The knowledge of epitopes is a prerequisite for understanding mechanism of antigen antibody interactions. Various methods like X-ray crystallography, enzymatic fragmentation, synthetic overlapping peptides, site-directed mutagenesis and phage display may be used to determine B- cell epitopes. However, these approaches are time consuming, exhaustive and require many experiments. Hence, we used computational methods to predict the location of B- cell epitopes. Earlier studies have shown the use of bioinformatic approach to predict eptiopes which correlated well with the experimental approach [8], [25]. In the present study, three IgE binding regions of osmotin were identified and validated by *in vitro* experiments. Further, residues in these regions were mutated to study the allergenic properties.

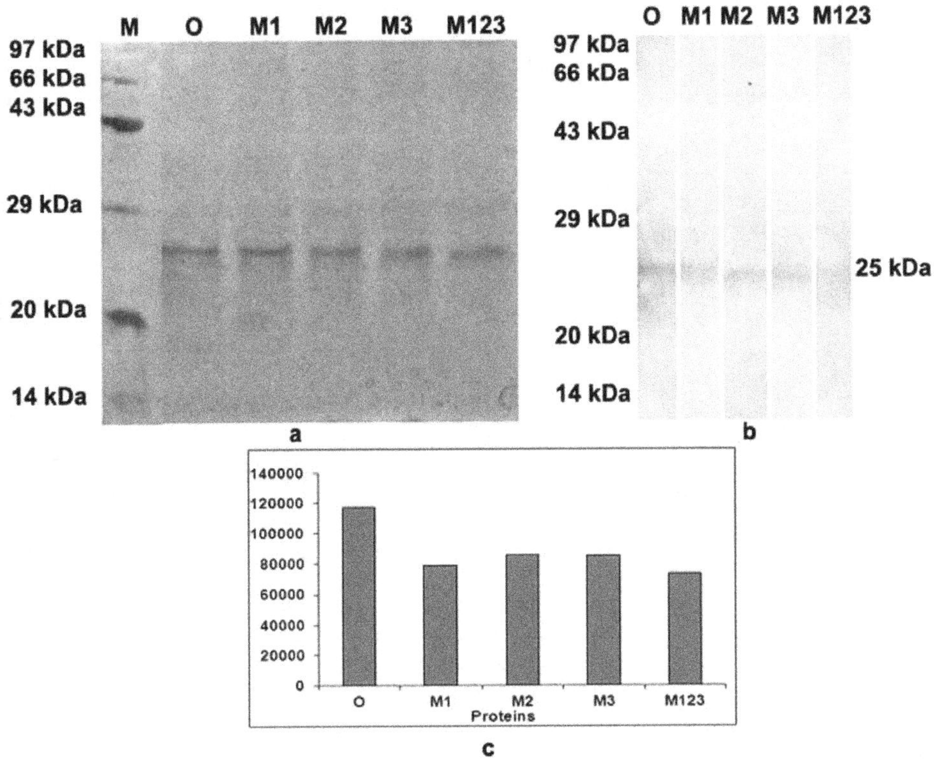


**Figure 3. SDS-PAGE profile of purified osmotin and the three mutants.** (a) The proteins were resolved on 12% gel and stained with Coomassie brilliant blue. (b) SDS-PAGE resolved protein was transferred on to nitrocellulose membrane and probed with osmotin positive patients' pooled sera. Lane M was loaded with Molecular weight marker. Lanes O, M1, M2, M3, M123 were loaded with osmotin and the mutants respectively. (c) Graph showing densitometric scan of spots of the blot.

Linear epitopes are more relevant as compared to conformational epitopes for food allergens as these allergens are encountered by the immune system only after they are subjected to digestion/heating [26]. Further it is difficult to validate computationally predicted epitopes except by cocrystallographic approach [7]. Conformational epitopes are preferred in case of globular allergens such as aeroallergens or food allergens involved in oral allergy syndrome [27]. It has been demonstrated that many food allergens like Ara h 1, Ara h 2, Ara h 3 [28], shrimp allergen Pen a 1 [29], hen's egg ovomucoid [30] and milk allergen [31] have linear epitopes that binds to IgE. Many algorithms have been developed to predict linear epitopes on a protein sequence based on propensity values of amino acid properties of hydrophilicity, antigenicity, segmental mobility, flexibility and accessibility [27]. In our study, we selected three linear epitopes commonly recognized by most of the sequence based tools. The three epitopes predicted comprise approximately 50% hydrophobic residues and 25% charged residues. The SDAP sequence similarity search of the predicted epitopes of osmotin showed similarity with known allergens which are members of the PR-5

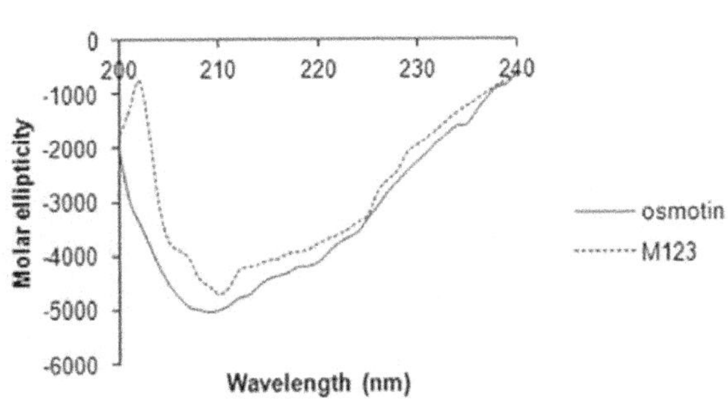


**Figure 4. Circular dichroism analysis.** Far-UV CD analysis of purified osmotin protein and M123 mutant. Results are expressed as mean residue ellipticity (y-axis) at a given wavelength (x-axis).

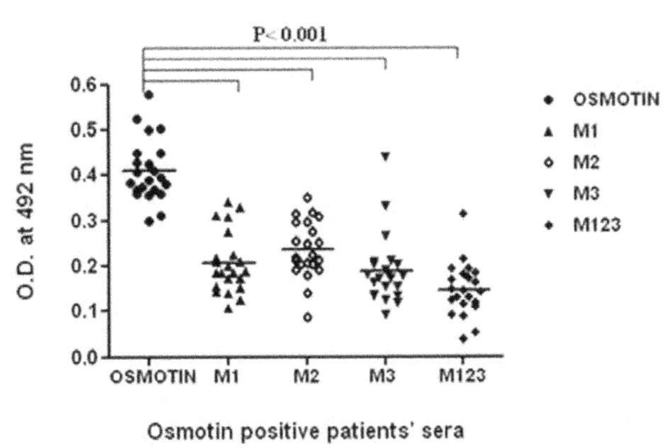


**Figure 5. IgE affinity of osmotin, M1, M2, M3, M123 with food allergic patients' sera (n = 22).** Specific IgE values against the respective proteins in patients' sera by ELISA. Specific IgE values ≥3 times of control were taken as cutoff for the positive results. (—) median value. Statistical difference in IgE binding among osmotin and the mutants is p<0.001 was considered statistically significant.

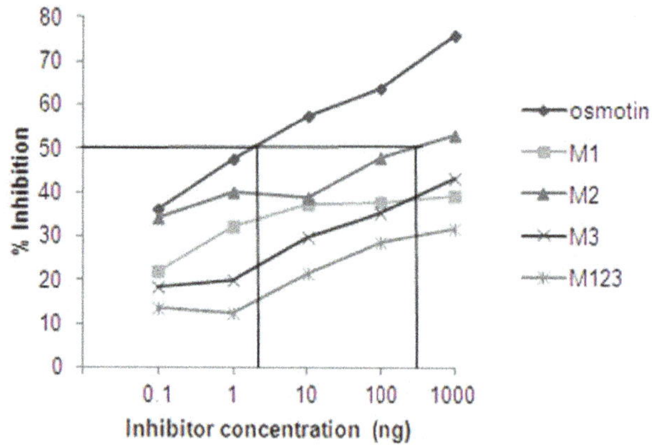


**Figure 6. IgE reactivity of osmotin, M1, M2, M3 and M123.** For IgE inhibition, osmotin positive patients' pooled sera were incubated with 0.1–1000 ng of osmotin protein and mutants as inhibitor. The assay was carried out with purified osmotin protein coated on microtitre plate. Competition of IgE binding to osmotin on the solid phase was quantified by ELISA. The ($EC_{50}$) value for Osmotin is 4 ng and for M2 is 500 ng.

protein family. Maleki et al., 2011 reported that peptides with a *PD* value similarity (<8.5) to known IgE epitopes could contribute to IgE binding and cross-reactivity [32]. This indicates that osmotin may share cross reactive epitopes with other similar proteins. In our earlier study osmotin showed IgE binding with sera of tomato and apple allergic patients confirming the predicted epitopes [22].

In the present study, three single point mutants (M1, M2 and M3) and a triple point mutant, M123 was subcloned and protein purified to homogeneity. These were developed by mutating a single residue in each of the three IgE binding predicted areas. Previous study has shown that single point allergen mutants do not lead to significant changes in protein structure but reduces allergenicity [33]. Mutational analysis of Pen a 1 showed that at least three substitutions per epitope were necessary to abolish the IgE Ab reactivity in >99% of the mutated epitopes [4]. In our study, all the mutants of osmotin showed reduction in IgE binding with patients' sera. The pattern of IgE binding of the mutants was not similar among all the patients suggesting the contribution was not same for all the mutations. However, the triple mutant of osmotin showed maximum reduction of up to 90% in the IgE binding as compared to osmotin. The reduction in IgE binding may be attributed to the phenylalanine substitution that is non reactive and tend to bury in hydrophobic cores of the protein molecule [34].

The *Brassica* pollen allergen Bra r 1 showed 74% and 94% inhibition of IgE binding with two patients' sera respectively at the highest inhibitor concentration. The double mutant of Bra r 1 showed 13% and 19% inhibition indicating reduced affinity of the IgE antibodies [35]. Peach allergen, Pru p 3 mutated at single position showed no change in IgE binding pattern whereas the triple mutant showed a 5 times reduction in IgE binding and inhibition potency [36]. Allergic response is elicited due to the multiple epitopes on an allergen, therefore multiple mutations are required to inhibit IgE binding completely. In the present study, triple mutant M123 of osmotin showed up to 90% reduction as compared to osmotin whereas single point mutants showed reduction of up to 76% in IgE binding. The circular dichroism spectra of the recombinant osmotin and M123 mutant showed that the secondary structure was not affected by three substitutions.

The potential of introduced foreign or engineered proteins in genetically modified crops to cause allergy has been of concern worldwide [37]. Many food allergens have been modified to generate the hypoallergenic mutants that showed reduced IgE binding. Osmotin has been shown as a potential allergen using *in silico* and *in vitro* studies [22]. It is still being used for developing transgenic crops owing to its properties of osmotic stress tolerance and antifungal activity. Therefore, genetically modified foods containing osmotin may not get clearance from regulatory bodies. Osmotin with no IgE binding having biological activity may be employed in developing genetically modified crops.

Specific immunotherapy against allergic disorders requires frequent injections of allergen extract to slowly build up the maintenance dose [38]. Allergen specific immunotherapy with purified protein has shown potential but may cause anaphylactic reactions. This can be prevented by modifying the IgE binding epitopes of the protein. In the present study IgE binding linear epitopes of osmotin were modified to have a hypoallergenic. These mutant proteins will have potential for immunotherapy.

In conclusion, three B- cell epitopes of osmotin were predicted by *in silico* method that correlated well with the experimental approach. Osmotin mutant M123 showed a reduction of 90% in IgE binding. The present method may be employed for prediction of B- cell epitopes of allergenic proteins.

## Acknowledgments

The authors thank Prof. K.C. Bansal, Indian Agricultural Research Institute, New Delhi, for providing the osmotin gene.

## Author Contributions

Conceived and designed the experiments: NA PS. Performed the experiments: PS SNG NA. Analyzed the data: PS NA. Contributed reagents/materials/analysis tools: PS SNG NA. Wrote the paper: PS SNG NA.

## References

1. Cianferoni A, Spergel JM (2009) Food allergy: review, classification and diagnosis. Allergol Int 58: 457–466.
2. Vrtala S (2008) From allergen genes to new forms of allergy diagnosis and treatment. Allergy 63: 299–309.
3. Nelson HS, Lahr J, Rule R, Bock A, Leung D (1997) Treatment of anaphylactic sensitivity to peanuts by immunotherapy with injections of aqueous peanut extract. J Allergy Clin Immunol 99: 744–751.
4. Reese G, Viebranz J, Leong-Kee SM, Plante M, Lauer I, et al. (2005) Reduced Allergenic Potency of VR9-1, a Mutant of the Major Shrimp Allergen Pen a 1 (Tropomyosin). J Immunol 175: 8354–8364.
5. Toda M, Reese G, Gadermaier G, Schulten V, Lauer I, et al. (2011) Protein unfolding strongly modulates the allergenicity and immunogenicity of Pru p 3, the major peach allergen. J Allergy Clin Immunol 128: 1022–1030.
6. Xiao Y, Lu Y, Chen YH (2001) Epitope-vaccine as a new strategy against HIV-1 mutation. Immunol Lett 77: 3–6.
7. Wang HW, Lin YC, Pai TW, Chang HT (2011) Prediction of B-cell linear epitopes with a combination of support vector machine classification and amino acid propensity identification. J Biomed Biotechnol 2011: 432830.
8. Nair S, Kukreja N, Singh BP, Arora N (2011) Identification of B cell epitopes of alcohol dehydrogenase allergen of *Curvularia lunata*. PLoS One 6: e20020.
9. Thalhamer T, Dobias H, Stepanoska T, Pröll M, Stutz H, et al. (2010) Designing hypoallergenic derivatives for allergy treatment by means of in silico mutation and screening. J Allergy Clin Immunol 125: 926–934.
10. Valenta R, Niederberger V (2007) Recombinant allergens for immunotherapy. J Allergy Clin Immunol 119: 826–830.
11. King N, Helm R, Stanley JS, Vieths S, Luttkopf D, et al. (2005) Allergenic characteristics of a modified peanut allergen. Mol Nutr Food Res 49: 963–971.

12. Bolhaar ST, Zuidmeer L, Ma Y, Ferreira F, Bruijnzeel-Koomen CA, et al. (2005) A mutant of the major apple allergen, Mal d 1 demonstrating hypo-allergenicity in the target organ by double-blind placebo-controlled food challenge. Clin Exp Allergy 35: 1638–1644.
13. Marazuela EG, Rodríguez R, Barber D, Villalba M, Batanero E (2007) Hypoallergenic mutants of Ole e 1, the major olive pollen allergen, as candidates for allergy vaccines. Clin Exp Allergy 37: 251–260.
14. Cornelissen BJC, Hooft van Huijsduijnen RA, Bol JFA (1986) Tobacco mosaic virus-induced tobacco protein is homologous to the sweet-tasting protein thaumatin. Nature 321: 531–532.
15. Abad LR, D'Urzo MP, Liu D, Narasimhan ML, Reuveni M, et al. (1996) Antifungal activity of tobacco osmotin has specificity and involves plasma membrane permeabilization. Plant Sci 118: 11–23.
16. Barthakur S, Babu V, Bansal KC (2001) Overexpression of osmotin induces proline accumulation and confers tolerance to osmotic stress in transgenic tobacco. J Plant Biochem Biotechnol 10: 31–37.
17. Hussaini AM, Abdin MZ (2008) Overexpression of tobacco osmotin geneleads to salt stress tolerance in strawberry (*Fragaria* X *ananassa* Duch.) plants. Indian J Biotechnol 7: 465–471.
18. Noori SAS, Sokhansanj A (2008) Wheat plants containing an osmotin gene show enhanced ability to produce roots at high NaCl concentration. Russ J Plant Physiol 55: 256–258.
19. Parkhi V, Kumar V, Sunilkumar G, Campbell LM, Singh NK, et al. (2009) Expression of apoplastically secreted tobacco osmotin in cotton confers drought tolerance. Mol Breed 23: 625–639.
20. Goel D, Singh AK, Yadav V, Babbar SB, Bansal KC (2010) Overexpression of osmotin gene confers tolerance to salt and drought stresses in transgenic tomato (*Solanum lycopersicum* L.). Protoplasma 245: 133–141.
21. Das M, Chauhan H, Chhibbar A, Rizwanul Haq QM, Khurana P (2011) High-efficiency transformation and selective tolerance against biotic and abiotic stress in mulberry, *Morus indica* cv. K2, by constitutive and inducible expression of tobacco osmotin. Transgenic Res 20: 231–246.
22. Sharma P, Singh AK, Singh BP, Gaur SN, Arora N (2011) Allergenicity assessment of osmotin, a pathogenesis-related protein, used for transgenic crops. J Agric Food Chem 59: 9990–9995.
23. El-Manzalawy Y, Honavar V (2010) Recent advances in B-cell epitope prediction methods. Immunome Res 6 Suppl 2: S2.
24. American Thoracic Society (1991) Lung function testing: selection of reference values and interpretative strategies. Am Rev Respir Dis 144: 1202–1218.
25. Sharma V, Singh BP, Gaur SN, Pasha S, Arora N (2009) Bioinformatics and immunologic investigation on B and T cell epitopes of Cur l 3, a major allergen of *Curvularia lunata*. J Proteome Res 8: 2650–2655.
26. Bannon GA (2004) What makes a food protein an allergen? Curr Allergy Asthma Rep 4: 43–46.
27. Pomes A (2010) Relevant B cell epitopes in allergic disease. Int Arch Allergy Immunol 152: 1–11.
28. Sicherer SH, Sampson HA (2007) Peanut allergy: emerging concepts and approaches for an apparent epidemic. J Allergy Clin Immunol 120: 491–503.
29. Ayuso R, Lehrer SB, Reese G (2002) Identification of continuous, allergenic regions of the major shrimp allergen Pen a 1 (tropomyosin). Int Arch Allergy Immunol 127: 27–37.
30. Jarvinen KM, Beyer K, Vila L, Bardina L, Mishoe M, et al. (2007) Specificity of IgE antibodies to sequential epitopes of hen's egg ovomucoid as a marker for persistence of egg allergy. Allergy 62: 758–765.
31. Busse PJ, Järvinen KM, Vila L Beyer K, Sampson HA (2002) Identification of sequential IgE-binding epitopes on bovine alpha (s2)-casein in cow's milk allergic patients. Int Arch Allergy Immunol 129: 93–96.
32. Maleki SJ, Teuber SS, Cheng H, Chen D, Comstock SS, et al. (2011) Computationally predicted IgE epitopes of walnut allergens contribute to cross-reactivity with peanuts. Allergy 66: 1522–1529.
33. Chan SL, Ong TC, Gao YF, Tiong YS, Wang de Y, et al. (2008) Nuclear magnetic resonance structure and IgE epitopes of Blo t 5, a major dust mite allergen. J Immunol 181: 2586–2596.
34. Betts MJ, Russell RB (2003) Amino acid properties and consequences of subsitutions. In: Barnes MR, Gray IC, Editors. Bioinformatics for Geneticists. Wiley Chichester UK. pp. 289–316.
35. Okada T, Swoboda I, Bhalla PL, Toriyama K, Singh MB (1998) Engineering of hypoallergenic mutants of the *Brassica* pollen allergen, Bra r 1, for immunotherapy. FEBS Lett 434: 255–260.
36. García-Casado G, Pacios LF, Díaz-Perales A, Sánchez-Monge R, Lombardero M, et al. (2003) Identification of IgE-binding epitopes of the major peach allergen Pru p 3. J Allergy Clin Immunol 112: 599–605.
37. Herman EM (2003) Genetically modified soybeans and food allergies. J Exp Bot 54: 1317–1319.
38. Srivastava D, Arora N, Singh BP (2009) Current immunological approaches for management of allergic rhinitis and bronchial asthma. Inflamm Res 58: 523–36.

# 23

# Beyond Labelling: What Strategies Do Nut Allergic Individuals Employ to Make Food Choices? A Qualitative Study

**Julie Barnett[1]*, Konstantina Vasileiou[1], M. Hazel Gowland[2], Monique M. Raats[3], Jane S. Lucas[4]**

**1** Department of Information Systems and Computing, Brunel University, Middlesex, United Kingdom, **2** Allergy Action, Farnborough, United Kingdom, **3** School of Psychology, Faculty of Arts and Human Sciences, University of Surrey, Guildford, Surrey, United Kingdom, **4** Clinical and Experimental Sciences, Faculty of Medicine, University of Southampton, University Hospital Southampton NHS Foundation Trust, Southampton, United Kingdom

## Abstract

***Objective:*** Food labelling is an important tool that assists people with peanut and tree nut allergies to avoid allergens. Nonetheless, other strategies are also developed and used in food choice decision making. In this paper, we examined the strategies that nut allergic individuals deploy to make safe food choices in addition to a reliance on food labelling.

***Methods:*** Three qualitative methods: an accompanied shop, in-depth semi-structured interviews, and the product choice reasoning task – were used with 32 patients that had a clinical history of reactions to peanuts and/or tree nuts consistent with IgE-mediated food allergy. Thematic analysis was applied to the transcribed data.

***Results:*** Three main strategies were identified that informed the risk assessments and food choice practices of nut allergic individuals. These pertained to: (1) qualities of product such as the product category or the country of origin, (2) past experience of consuming a food product, and (3) sensory appreciation of risk. Risk reasoning and risk management behaviours were often contingent on the context and other physiological and socio-psychological needs which often competed with risk considerations.

***Conclusions:*** Understanding and taking into account the complexity of strategies and the influences of contextual factors will allow healthcare practitioners, allergy nutritionists, and caregivers to advise and educate patients more effectively in choosing foods safely. Governmental bodies and policy makers could also benefit from an understanding of these food choice strategies when risk management policies are designed and developed.

**Editor:** José César Perales, Universidad de Granada, Spain

**Funding:** This study was funded by the United Kingdom Food Standards Agency under project code T07058 (http://www.food.gov.uk/). The funder had no role in study design, data collection and analysis, decision to publish, or preparation of the manuscript. They provided comment on a full draft of this paper.

**Competing Interests:** The authors have declared that no competing interests exist.

* E-mail: Julie.Barnett@brunel.ac.uk

## Introduction

Food allergy is an important public health problem [1]. Although there are difficulties in estimating prevalence, and there is some variation between countries [2], in Europe and the United States food allergies are estimated to affect up to approximately 8% of children and 2% of adults [3,4]. Peanut and tree nuts are the most common cause of severe and life-threatening food allergic reactions [5]. The prevalence of peanut allergy, tree nut allergy or both (henceforth 'nut allergies') is around 1% in North American and UK populations [6,7,8,9] and seems to be increasing [7,8,10,11]. Between 1999 and 2006, 18 out of 48 deaths which were caused by allergic reactions to foods in the UK [12], and more than 90% of fatal reactions in the US between 1994 and 1999, were provoked by peanuts or tree nuts [13]. For ease – and despite the fact that peanuts are actually legumes – the word 'nuts' is henceforth used as a convenient generic.

The quality of life of children and adolescents with a nut allergy including their families can be severely compromised [14,15] since constant vigilance about diet needs to be exercised, whilst the risk of accidental exposure and the fear of a fatal reaction cannot completely be eliminated and controlled [16]. Parents of children with a nut allergy report higher levels of impairment in their quality of life and more disruptions of familial and social relations than do parents of children with a rheumatologic disease [17]. Similarly, higher levels of disease-related anxiety were found in children with a nut allergy compared with children with diabetes [18]. Recent research in adults has revealed the difficulties and challenges that nut allergic individuals face when eating out [19] and when travelling abroad [20] where a series of often competing considerations need to be balanced.

The clinical manifestation of allergic reactions includes symptoms affecting the skin (e.g. urticarial), respiratory tract (e.g. dyspnoea, throat tightness), gastrointestinal tract (e.g. vomiting, diarrhoea), and/or the cardiovascular system (e.g. hypotensive shock) [3]. Anaphylactic reactions are life-threatening episodes involving the cardiovascular or respiratory systems, which should be treated immediately by injection of intramuscular adrenaline

[3,4]. Nut allergies are not currently curable and consequently management primarily involves effective allergen avoidance and the provision of self-injectable adrenaline for severe reactions [1,21]. However, patients do not always carry their adrenaline devices or use them appropriately [22,23], and even when correctly administered, reactions can be fatal. Therefore, recognizing and avoiding foods containing nuts remains the key self-management strategy.

Labelling on the packaging of food products is an important tool that helps nut allergic individuals to make safe purchases. Although consumers do not normally pay much regard to labels, specific dietary requirements, such as food allergies, increase their attention to food labels [24]. Nonetheless, nut allergic people often encounter a series of difficulties in identifying correctly the allergens on the labels [25,26], and in interpreting advisory labelling such as 'may contain' [27]. Moreover, an examination of 20,241 products in US revealed the ambiguities and the variety of terminologies used in advisory labelling [28] confirming the challenges that nut allergic individuals face when buying foods. Recently, qualitative research in the UK [29,30] examined the ways in which nut allergic adults used information on the packaging to inform their food choices, corroborating many of the difficulties mentioned previously in the literature. It is evident, however, that labelling was used in conjunction with a series of other decision making strategies. But, whilst food choice strategies and 'rules of thumb' have been studied extensively among consumers in general [31,32,33,34], little is known in relation to nut allergic individuals. A recent focus-group study compared the food choice behaviours and eating experiences of adults diagnosed with food allergies to those of non-allergic consumers. The results demonstrated that food allergic people usually encounter difficulties in finding safe foods; their experiences around eating are less satisfactory and spontaneous since a high level of organisation and preparation is constantly required [35].

This paper has sought to characterise the nature of strategies employed by nut allergic individuals when choosing foods that extend beyond labelling. By using a variety of qualitative methods, we aimed to examine in depth how nut allergic individuals reason about food risk and how they choose and purchase foods.

## Methods

### Ethics Statement

The research received ethical approval from the National Research Ethics Service (09/H1109/64) and the University of Surrey Ethics Committee.

### Study Population

The study population included individuals, aged 16 or over, with a clinical history of reactions to peanuts and/or tree nuts which was compatible with IgE-mediated allergy. The participants were recruited from three sources in South England: (a) the paediatric and adult allergy clinics at University Hospital Southampton NHS Foundation Trust, (b) three General Practitioners (GP) Surgeries, and (c) the staff and students at the University of Surrey. Letters were sent to 411 individuals explaining the aim of the research and inviting them to complete a screening questionnaire. For the interested reader, the screening questionnaire is provided as File S1. Seventy-seven respondents returned this (response rate 18.73%) of which 54 were eligible to take part following examination of the information by an allergy specialist (JSL). Of the 54 eligible individuals, 32 consented to participate in the study. Participants' consent was obtained in written form.

Participants' eligibility, based on the information provided in the postal screening questionnaire, was assessed by the allergy specialist as follows: respondents were required to be aged 16 years or older with a clinical history compatible with IgE-mediated reactions to peanuts or tree nuts. Participants recruited from the specialist allergy clinic had positive skin prick tests and/or specific IgE measurements. Recruits from the University of Surrey and from primary care settings were required to have been diagnosed with peanut or tree nut allergy by a medical practitioner, and prescribed rescue medication. Individuals with allergies or intolerance to foods in addition to peanut or tree nuts were excluded because this would affect their consumer choices. The exception was inclusion of participants with oral allergy syndrome (OAS) to fruits and/or vegetables. Unlike egg or milk for example, avoidance of fruit and vegetables was unlikely to create significant dilemmas during the shopping tasks.

Of the 32 participants who took part in the study, 9 were males and 23 females, aged between 16 and 70 years old. Five participants had only peanut allergy, 9 had only tree nut allergy, and 18 had both. The severity of their worst-ever reaction was rated as mild, moderate or severe using a classification previously employed for peanut allergy [36]. Eighteen participants described severe reactions, 12 moderate and 2 mild.

### Methods of Data Collection

Three different qualitative methods were used to collect data:

**A. The accompanied shop (AS).** Participants were followed, observed and audio-recorded in their routine weekly shop by an experienced qualitative researcher. Accompanying consumers while shopping is an established technique in consumer studies that enables direct observation of actual behaviour [37]. Participants in this research were additionally asked to think aloud about their purchase decisions, having being familiarised with and trained in the 'think aloud' method. File S2 provides the details of how participants were trained to the 'think aloud' protocol and how they were instructed to conduct the accompanied shop. To ensure that the accompanied shop was as naturalistic as possible, the researcher's input at this stage was minimal, consisting mainly of prompts such as 'what are you thinking?' when participants stopped thinking aloud.

The 'think aloud' technique allows the elicitation of a concurrent with-the-behaviour-observed verbal report. Ericsson & Simon's [38] classical work advocated the value of verbal data deriving from introspection for the examination of the cognitive processes involved in problem-solving scenarios. Since then, the 'think aloud' technique has been used extensively in several fields, including food choice research [39] usually after being adapted to serve particular research questions and in combination with other techniques [40].

**B. A semi-structured interview (SSI).** Issues arising during the accompanied shop were followed up in a face-to-face interview. This allowed us to examine interesting behaviours noted by the researcher during the accompanied shop that was relevant to our research questions (e.g. avoiding certain products or even parts of the supermarket). The SSI also explored the ways the participants were managing their food choices and consumption across various eating-related situations (e.g. eating-out, holidays), as well as the history of their allergies and their views on labelling.

**C. The Product Choice Reasoning Task (PCRT).** Participants were presented with 13 products, each of which embodied a recognized dilemma for people avoiding nuts/peanuts. These are described in detail in Barnett et al [29].

Participants were asked whether and why they would or would not consume each one of the products.

Fuller detail of the methods can be found in Barnett et al [41].

Employing this configuration of methods allowed the in-depth examination of both reported and actual food choices and the reasoning behind them. All research phases were audio recorded and fully transcribed. The accompanied shop was directly followed by the interview and the Product Choice Reasoning Task which were conducted in participants' homes.

## Analytic Procedure

Thematic analysis [42,43] was used to explore the data. Given that the aim was to examine what strategies the nut allergic individuals are employing to make sense of, and manage the risk of allergic reactions when choosing food, a realist epistemological stance to participants' speeches was adopted. This means that people's accounts were considered as being reflective of their thoughts, cognitions, and reported behaviours and that language provided the means through which the researchers were able to access these.

Initially, the researchers (JB and KV) familiarised themselves with the data through repeated reading of the transcripts, and noted interesting and relevant-to-the-research-question points. Further analysis was conducted during a series of regular meetings. Codes were formed and assigned, assisted by computer software [44], to the relevant textual segments. Finally, themes and subthemes were developed by aggregating semantically identical codes; further revision and refinement of the themes took place in order to be internally homogenous, distinct from each other [45] and reflective of the data.

# Results

Risk reasoning and food choice practices were located in relation to three main themes: (a) *product qualities*, (b) *past experience*, and (c) *sensory appreciation*. Food choices, however, were not exclusively defined by safety considerations; participants reported other considerations, which often competed with those pertaining to risk forming a fourth theme, named *beyond safety*.

Respondents' quotes below are identified by a. their coding number (e.g. 4015), b. their sex (M for males, F for females), c. the severity of allergy (S for severe, M for moderate and MI for mild), d. their age, and e. the corpus of data from which the quote is drawn (Accompanied shop – AS, Semi-Structured Interview – SSI, and Product Choice Reasoning Task - PCRT).

## Product Qualities

Several product-related indicators were employed, sometimes in combination, to inform participants' risk assessments. These concerned the *product category*, the *brand*, the *producer and/or the provider* of the food, and the *country of origin*, and operated to provide guidance as to the desirability of purchase and consumption.

The broader *product category* was among the most salient categorisations that informed risk judgments. Certain product categories, such as bakery, chocolate, cereals, desserts, processed or ready-made meals, were considered as particularly problematic, as they were strongly associated with nuts, signalling the necessity for closer examination usually by looking the labels. Hesitation and worry around consumption of these products was often reported, while total rejection was not uncommon:

> *If it's like a savoury type thing, particularly bready stuff, for some reason, that's what freaks me out a little bit, and I'll just say…bready things, biscuits, cakes, I'll just say, "No thanks". (4015, MS34, PCRT)*

Fresh vegetables, fruits, and dairy, on the other hand, were product categories that rarely posed any safety concerns and were generally trusted immediately as safe.

The *brand* also informed risk reasoning. Well-known and reputable brand names clearly functioned to indicate safety. Notably, in some instances a trusted brand acted as such a strong indicator of safety that it could override precautionary labelling or the influence of a problematic product category:

> *Yeah, I'd eat these. Normally – oh, it says "Not suitable for peanut allergy sufferers"… I'd probably still eat them though because if they're – like [brand name] is a trusted name, and I highly doubt they actually would. I'd probably still eat them, yeah. (1011, FS18, PCRT)*

Conversely, products associated with a lesser known brand, even when they were not problematic *per se*, raised suspicions which were resolved either through avoidance or further checks of labels:

> *For a first look, I'd probably be like, "Oh yeah, I can eat them," and then I'd just be like, "Oh, hang on, it's not a main brand – I probably should have a look at it." (1008, FM16, PCRT)*

The trust accorded to well-known brands was associated with the assumed safety standards of the manufacturing processes and the perceived thoroughness and adequacy of labelling practices, although participants did not claim any knowledge of manufacturing or labelling processes:

> *That's a brand that I would be comfortable that their food labelling and their standards are adequate. (1029, FS26, PCRT)*

The *provider* of the products – which in some cases coincided with the producer – was an additional resource for risk judgments. Big companies such as supermarkets were often trusted due to the belief that they have strong interests to protect their reputation and enough resources to check the products:

> *…so if I'm buying any sort of products where it relates to nuts, I would definitely only buy them in the supermarket, because I'm pretty much trusting that someone is checking and that the risk of me finding them in the food is less. (3008, FM45, SSI)*

A smaller number of participants, however, perceived small, and usually local, producers or providers as more trustworthy than big companies.

The last product quality repeatedly articulated in risk reasoning was the *country of origin*. Foreign products were almost always treated with hesitation and were avoided compared to native products:

> *Em, anything that's foreign is a no – I just won't buy it. (4015, MS34, SSI)*

Even if the particular allergen was apparently not an ingredient the overarching designation as foreign led to rejection. Foreign products activated beliefs that in other countries there is a lower level of awareness or recognition of the problem of nut allergies and a higher tendency to use nuts in products:

> *They look like they're probably made somewhere else because the initial language here is not English. I have no idea how they...if they have any concept of allergies. (5009, FS38, PCRT)*

Reluctance to consume foreign products was also explained in terms of unfamiliarity with the standards of production and regulation applied in other countries:

> *To be honest, if it was a foreign product, which had equally good labelling, I might be more reluctant because I'm not familiar with the standards that they would be obliged to comply with (1029, FS26, PCRT).*

## Past Experience

Past experience was a second, and particularly powerful, resource for nut allergic individuals that dictated safe food choices in an efficient and confident manner. Experiential knowledge accumulated over the course of years invited absolute trust in foods, often without reference to labels:

> *I could almost say yes without looking at the ingredients for these ones because I've eaten them lots of times before. (1068, FM34, PCRT)*

Several participants were alert to the possibility that manufacturers may change product ingredients. Some reported that they still checked the labels for potential changes, even though past experience warranted safe consumption, but others ignored this possibility, especially when they had recently consumed the product:

> *If I know that it's something I've had quite recently, then I'm not bothered about it. I'll just have it straightaway, pick it up without reading it. (1016, FS18, SSI)*

Importantly, uneventful past experience of consuming a product was such a powerful indicator of future safe consumption that precautionary labelling was ignored or discounted:

> *Yeah, I can see here it says that it's not suitable for peanut allergy sufferers and it may have traces of peanut or other nuts, but I've never ever had an allergy to [product name], and so my automatic reaction is yeah, I'd try it. (3008, FM45, PCRT)*

Conversely, novel products led, at least some participants, to attend to 'contains' or 'may contain' labelling.

Positive experiences of consumption led to the routinisation of food choices and the establishment of habitual food purchase patterns. Although participants recognized that this strategy limited the trial of new foods, they were generally content since time and effort were saved:

> *So yes, I do tend to stick with things I know, and probably not adventurous with trying many new things [laughing]! (1042, FS26, SSI)*

Negative past experiences were particularly instructive in creating an often intense aversion and rejection of the associated foods. This was often not simply restricted to the particular product that had caused the allergic reaction but was rather generalised to include other exemplars of the broader category in which the problematic food was classified, for example unrelated products within the same brand or product category, with similar ingredients, or even similar labelling:

> *It was a type of chocolate bar from [supermarket name] and I had a reaction to it, even though it just said "may contain", and then I never ate anything that said "may contain" again. (1112, FS21, SSI)*

## Sensory Appreciation

Reliance on senses such as taste, sight and smell was an additional and trusted strategy the participants employed to assess the riskiness of foods. This strategy was often used when the food was novel and there was thus some uncertainty around its safety. A sensory check provided a rapid initial assessment, yet the resulting evidence was in many cases regarded as unequivocal.

The PCRT was particularly revealing in showing that some products were directly associated with nuts simply from the way they looked. This created strong feelings of aversion to a degree that the product was ultimately rejected without further examination or seeking further validation through labelling:

> *It looks too much like nuts, so no. Actually, seeing – just on what it looks like, I wouldn't even, in the real world, read any ingredients. (4015, MS34, PCRT)*

The texture of the product was an additional cue signifying risk. The more plain and smooth the product looked the less risky it was perceived to be. By contrast, a granular texture in the product caused concern and activated avoidance:

> *Well, I think it looks risky because there's lots of bits in [laughing]! That sounds simplistic, but over the years, I've learnt that means trouble. (1031, FM30, PCRT)*

Olfactory evaluation was also used for risk judgments and was very much trusted as a signal of danger. Participants smelt the products and some even claimed that they had developed an acute sensitivity to detect nuts or products containing nuts with their odour even 'from a mile off'. This then provoked again avoidance and rejection of the product:

> *I'm just more aware, and I would trust my senses more with regards to my sense of smell, very much so...Those smells immediately send warning bells off in my head. (4015, MS34, SSI)*

Finally, a sort of 'taste test' was recurrently reported. Here participants tried a little bit of the product, waited to see whether there were any adverse reactions and depending on the outcome of the trial, they then either consumed or rejected the food. The taste test was deployed when participants felt uncertain about the safety of the food or lacked previous experience. For some, this strategy was still used, even when they knew that the product was safe, thus providing further reassurance:

*Even when I come to eat it, even if I know there's not actually any nuts in it, I'll taste a little bit and then wait a few minutes to see if anything happens…just to be really sure. (4001, FS24, SSI)*

## Beyond Safety

Arguably safety was the primary consideration in food choices. However, other factors influenced decision making. These pertained firstly to other product attributes that were taken into account in food purchases, secondly to contextual factors within which the nut allergic individuals assessed the risk of food consumption, and thirdly to their internal – physiological or psychological – states and the broader life stage. Taking into account these parameters led on occasions to a more risk adverse stance, whilst in other instances greater risk was embraced.

Much of the time participants were considering and valuing additional product attributes such as taste, cost, quality, health, convenience and ethics as well as the needs of other people for whom they were shopping. Although on many occasions these considerations were not related to problematic foods, in some instances there was evidence of how participants sought to incorporate these values alongside their risk assessments. Importantly, in the effort to balancing competing values some admitted that they were taking the risk, mainly when they liked the taste of a product:

*Generally I would do, apart from in the case of the soya nuts [laughing], because I like them so I take the risk! (1042, FS26, SSI)*

Assignations of risk were closely enmeshed with the context within which participants were operating. Two dimensions of the context were evaluated; firstly, respondents were more willing and relaxed to assume greater risk when they were close to medical facilities:

*I mean, if I was in the centre of town in a country where I know the medical facilities are good, then I'm much more relaxed, and I'll risk certain things. If I'm up a mountain in the middle of nowhere, even if it seems safe, I would be more reluctant to eat. (1029, FS26, SSI)*

Secondly, the presence of other people by whom participants and their allergy were known, and who were therefore trusted, was a further reassuring parameter that allowed people to take on greater risks:

*Usually, it's with my parents, and I'm happier eating out at a restaurant with my parents because they know me, they know…like no one knows you as well as your parents do – no one ever would. So I'm happier…like when we've been on holidays and stuff, I'd be happier to risk it when they're there because they know everything. They know my medical history. (1112, FS21, SSI)*

Interestingly, while the presence of others sometimes functioned as reassurance, in many instances it was a source of stress, and more particularly embarrassment, due to participants' belief that interrogating others about the content of food violated important social norms. The feelings of embarrassment and the unwillingness of people to attract attention or to offend others often obstructed the approach to managing risk:

*So I did actually have a bit, even though, really, by my rules I set myself, I wouldn't have eaten that normally, but because it was my birthday cake, I felt a bit guilty! (1161, FM22, SSI)*

It was evident that risk judgments made by participants were contingent upon attending to aspects of their internal state, personal characteristics or life situation. For instance, people mentioned that factors, such as hunger or tiredness, could impede a thorough risk assessment:

*If you're tired, you go round the supermarket, you're really wanting to get home, you do occasionally pick things up and you haven't read it clearly. (4013, FS37, SSI)*

Others related the way they managed their allergy to broader life contexts and significant transitions. A woman (1031, FM30, SSI) mentioned that she used to be much more adventurous with food choices before her baby was born as she had more time to check labels and try new foods. Another participant (1198, FM48, SSI) explained the difficulties of allergy being diagnosed as an adult as well as how a busy life with children militated against giving much attention to her own food choices. Finally, a young woman with severe allergy linked the way she managed her allergy to the general rise and fall of her stress levels:

*If I'm very stressed at work or stressed for whatever reason, I'll become more paranoid about it. It's like something that I focus my energy on or relax away from, depending on everything else that's going on in my life! (1029, FS26, SSI)*

## Discussion

Our results indicate the complexity of risk reasoning and the variety of strategies the nut allergic individuals use to inform their decision making. Participants relied heavily on their previous experience of consuming foods and the relevant knowledge they had developed, their senses as well as their evaluations of different product characteristics, namely the product category, the brand, the provider and the country of origin. These results chime with previous research, conducted with non-allergic consumers, which demonstrates that both past experience and sensory assessments of foods constitute particularly useful rules of thumb in food choices [34]. Applying a system of categorisations and evaluating foods accordingly has also been observed with lay people when they attempt to make sense of various food risks [46,47]. Additionally, the strategies that people use to make food choices are characterised by trust, dictate confident food consumption, and provide efficiency in decision making [34]; findings which are corroborated by our results. At the same time, this study indicates the complexity of the dilemmas that nut allergic people often face when choosing food, also alluded to in recent research with food allergic consumers [35]. The current study has shed further light on the food choice practices of people with nut allergies and adds to previous research that examines the strategies of non-allergic consumers in this area [31,32,33,34].

One of the strengths of the present research is the variety of qualitative methods used that enabled a detailed insight into the complexity of risk reasoning and food management practices [48]. The accompanied shop allowed us to observe the participants while shopping. This access to their shopping practices seeks to address the challenge of obtaining relevant behavioural data and avoids a sole reliance on self-reported attitudes or behaviour.

Additionally, since participants at this stage were simply informed that the focus was on their food management strategies rather than framing this in terms of risk, the accompanied shop proved to be an ideal setting within which other product-based considerations (e.g. taste, cost) were revealed thus further reducing the likelihood of socially desirable behaviours. The interview enabled an in-depth examination of issues emerging during the accompanied shop and provided participants with the opportunity to reflect on their reasoning around their food choices and risk managing behaviour. Finally, the Product Choice Reasoning Task was particularly useful in documenting the exact risk thinking as this was being shaped as well as the, often combined, deployment of the various strategies in decision making.

### Implications of the study

This study has clear implications for healthcare professionals (clinicians, allergists, allergy dieticians) that develop management plans and advise patients as to how to avoid problematic foods, while also maintaining a balanced and healthy diet. On the one hand, it is important to recognize that the strategies provide efficiency and confidence in food decision making, reducing the anxiety and thus they are likely to lead to established behaviour patterns. On the other hand, it is also crucial to acknowledge that the strategies are contingent on contextual factors and are additionally influenced by physiological and socio-psychological needs that sometimes impede thorough and extensive risk assessments and consequently lead to accidental ingestion of the allergens. Understanding and taking into account the day to day strategies that shape nut allergic individuals' food choice practices will enable healthcare professionals to advise their patients more effectively by drawing attention to potential pitfalls and by fostering the use of successful and functional strategies.

Food manufacturers, importers, distributors and retailers also have a responsibility to ensure that the foods they sell are safe for all consumers, including those with food allergies. Policy makers and governmental bodies would also benefit from an understanding of these food choice strategies when risk management policies are developed. It is notable for example that people with nut allergies are most likely to turn to labelling in the context of uncertainty when more habitual strategies do not lead to a confident decision. Under these circumstances it is vital that labelling is available, clear and trustworthy.

## Supporting Information

**File S1** Screening questionnaire. (DOCX)

**File S2** Think aloud training & accompanied shop instructions. (DOCX)

## Acknowledgments

We acknowledge the support of the Anaphylaxis Campaign and also the contribution of Jo Leftwich and Kate Muncer who collected the data on which the analysis is based.

## Author Contributions

Provided advice as an allergic consumer to the project throughout: MHG. Provided clinical expertise as an allergist for the study design and analysis: JSL. Provided expertise regarding consumers' food choice strategies: MMR. Contributed to reviewing and commenting on early drafts of the paper: MHG MMR JSL. Conceived and designed the experiments: JB MHG MMR JSL. Analyzed the data: JB KV. Wrote the paper: JB KV.

## References

1. Boyce JA, Assa'ad A, Burks AW, Jones SM, Sampson HA (2010) Guidelines for the diagnosis and management of food allergy in the United States: Report of the NIAID-sponsored expert panel. J Allergy Clin Immunol 126(6): S1–S58.
2. Rona RJ, Keil T, Summers C, Gislason D, Zuidmeer L, et al. (2007) The prevalence of food allergy: A meta-analysis. J Allergy Clin Immunol 120: 638–46.
3. Al-Muhsen S, Clarke AE, Kagan RS (2003) Peanut allergy: An overview. CMAJ 168(10): 1279–1285.
4. Sampson HA (2002) Clinical Practice. Peanut allergy. N Engl J Med 346(17): 1294–1299.
5. Sicherer SH, Furlong TJ, Munoz-Furlong A, Burks AW, Sampson HA (2001) A voluntary registry for peanut and tree nut allergy: Characteristics of the first 5149 registrants. J Allergy Clin Immunol 108(1): 128–132.
6. Sicherer SH, Muñoz-Furlong A, Burks AW, Sampson HA (1999) Prevalence of peanut and tree nut allergy in the US determined by a random digit dial telephone survey. J Allergy Clin Immunol 103(4): 559–562.
7. Sicherer SH, Munoz-Furlong A, Sampson HA (2003) Prevalence of peanut and tree nut allergy in the United States determined by means of a random digit dial telephone survey: A 5-year follow-up study. J Allergy Clin Immunol 112(6): 1203–1207.
8. Grundy J, Matthews S, Bateman B, Dean T, Arshad SH (2002) Rising prevalence of allergy to peanut in children: Data from 2 sequential cohorts. J Allergy Clin Immunol 110(5): 784–789.
9. Ben Shoshan M, Kagan RS, Alizadehfar R, Joseph L, Turnbull E, et al. (2009) Is the prevalence of peanut allergy increasing? A 5-year follow-up study in children in Montreal. J Allergy Clin Immunol 123(4): 783–788.
10. Sicherer SH, Munoz-Furlong A, Godbold JH, Sampson HA (2010) US prevalence of self-reported peanut, tree nut, and sesame allergy: 11-year follow-up. J Allergy Clin Immunol 125(6): 1322–1326.
11. Venter C, Arshad SH, Grundy J, Pereira B, Clayton CB, et al. (2010) Time trends in the prevalence of peanut allergy: Three cohorts of children from the same geographical location in the UK. Allergy 65: 103–108.
12. Pumphrey RS, Gowland MH (2007) Further fatal allergic reactions to food in the United Kingdom, 1999–2006 [letter to the editor]. J Allergy Clin Immunol 119(4): 1018–1019.
13. Bock SA, Muñoz-Furlong A, Sampson HA (2001) Fatalities due to anaphylactic reactions to foods. J Allergy Clin Immunol 107(1): 191–193.
14. Cummings AJ, Knibb RC, King RM, Lucas JS (2010) The psychosocial impact of food allergy and food hypersensitivity in children, adolescents and their families: A review. Allergy 65: 933–945.
15. Cummings AJ, Knibb RC, Erlewyn- Lajeunesse M, King RM, Roberts G, et al. (2010) Management of nut allergy influences quality of life and anxiety in children and their mothers. Pediatr Allergy Immunol 21: 586–594.
16. Teufel M, Biedermann T, Rapps N, Hausteiner C, Henningsen P, et al. (2007) Psychological burden of food allergy. World J Gastroenterol 13(25): 3456–3465.
17. Primeau MN, Kagan R, Joseph L, Lim H, Dufresne C, et al. (2000) The psychological burden of peanut allergy as perceived by adults with peanut allergy and the parents of peanut-allergic children. Clin Exp Allergy 30: 1135–1143.
18. Avery NJ, King RM, Knight S, Hourihane JO (2003) Assessment of quality of life in children with peanut allergy. Pediatr Allergy Immunol 14: 378–382.
19. Leftwich J, Barnett J, Muncer K, Shepherd R, Raats MM, et al. (2011) The challenges for nut-allergic consumers of eating out. Allergy 41: 243–249.
20. Barnett J, Botting N, Gowland MH, Lucas JS (2012) The strategies that peanut and nut-allergic consumers employ to remain safe when travelling abroad. Clin Transl Allergy 2: 12.
21. Sampson HA (1996) Managing peanut allergy demands aggressive intervention in prevention and treatment. BMJ 312: 1050–1051.
22. Gallagher M, Worth A, Cunningham-Burley S, Sheikh A (2011) Epinephrine auto-injector use in adolescents at risk of anaphylaxis: a qualitative study in Scotland, UK. Clin Exp Allergy 4: 869–877.
23. Macadam C, Barnett J, Roberts G, Stiefel G, King R, et al. (2012) What factors affect the carriage of epinephrine auto-injectors by teenagers? Clin Transl Allergy 2(1): 3.
24. Enright G, Good H, Williams N (2010) Qualitative research to explore people's use of food labelling information: Final report. Social Science Research Unit, Food Standards Agency.
25. Joshi P, Mofidi S, Sicherer SH (2002) Interpretation of commercial food ingredient labels by parents of food-allergic children. J Allergy Clin Immunol 109(6): 1019–1021.
26. Cornelisse-Vermaat JR, Voordouw J, Yiakoumaki V, Theodoridis G, Frewer LJ (2007) Food-allergic consumers' labelling preferences: A cross-cultural comparison. Eur J Public Health 18(2): 115–120.
27. Noimark L, Gardner J, Warner JO (2009) Parents attitudes when purchasing products for children with nut allergy: A UK perspective. Pediatr Allergy Immunol 20: 500–504.

28. Pieretti MM, Chung D, Pacenza R, Slotkin T, Sicherer SH (2009) Audit of manufactured products: Use of allergen advisory labels and identification of labeling ambiguities. J Allergy Clin Immunol 124(2): 337–341.
29. Barnett J, Leftwich J, Muncer K, Grimshaw K, Shepherd R, et al. (2011) How do peanut and nut allergic consumers use information on the packaging to avoid allergens? Allergy 66(7): 969–978.
30. Barnett J, Muncer K, Leftwich J, Shepherd R, Raats MM, et al. (2011) Using 'may contain' labelling to inform food choice: A qualitative study of nut allergic consumers. BMC Public Health 11: 734.
31. Connors M, Bisogni CA, Sobal J, Devine CM (2001) Managing values in personal food systems. Appetite 36(3): 189–200.
32. Falk LW, Bisogni CA, Sobal J (1996) Food choice processes of older adults: A qualitative investigation. J Nutr Educ 28: 257–265.
33. Furst T, Connors M, Bisogni CA, Sobal J, Falk LW (1996) Food choice: A conceptual model of the process. Appetite 26: 247–266.
34. Green J, Draper A, Dowler E (2003) Short cuts to safety: Risk and 'rules of thumb' in accounts of food choice. Health, Risk Soc 5(1): 33–52.
35. Sommer I, MacKenzie H, Venter C, Dean T (2012) Factors influencing food choices of food allergic consumers: Findings from focus groups. Allergy doi:10.1111/j.1398-9995.2012.02883.x.
36. Hourihane JO, Kilburn SA, Dean P, Warner JO (1997) Clinical characteristics of peanut allergy. Clin Exp Allergy 27: 634–639.
37. Otnes C, McGrath MA, Lowery TM (1995) Shopping with consumers: Usage as past, present, and future research technique. J Retailing Consumer Services 2(2): 97–110.
38. Ericsson KA, Simon HA (1984) Protocol analysis: Verbal reports as data. Cambridge: Massachusetts.
39. Higginson CS, Rayner MJ, Draper S, Kirk TR (2002) The nutrition label – which information is looked at? Nutr Food Sci 32(3): 92–99.
40. Nielsen J, Clemmensen T, Yssing C (2002) Getting access to what goes on in people's heads? Reflections on the think-aloud technique. Nordic Conference of Computer-Human Interaction October 19–23.
41. Barnett J, Leftwich J, Muncer K, Raats M, Shepherd R et al (2010) Understanding the food choice reasoning of nut allergic consumers. Final Technical Report T07058. Food Standards Agency. Available: http://www.food.gov.uk/science/research/allergy-research/allergy-labelling/t07058/.
42. Boyatzis RE (1998) Transforming qualitative information: Thematic analysis and code development. Thousand Oaks, CA: Sage.
43. Braun V, Clarke V (2006) Using thematic analysis in psychology. Qual Res Psychol 3: 77–101.
44. NVivo qualitative data analysis software [computer program]: Version 9 QSR International Pty Ltd.: 2008.
45. Patton MQ (1990) Qualitative evaluation and research methods. 2nd ed. Newbury Park, CA: Sage.
46. Lupton DA (2005) Lay discourses and beliefs related to food risks: an Australian perspective. Sociol Health Illn 27(4): 448–467.
47. Horlick-Jones T, Walls J, Kitzinger J (2007) Bricolage in action: learning about, making sense of, and discussing, issues about genetically modified crops and food. Health Risk Soc 9(1): 83–103.
48. Gallagher M, Worth A, Sheikh A (2009) Clinical allergy has much to gain from engagement with qualitative research. Allergy 64: 1117–1120.

# PERMISSIONS

All chapters in this book were first published in PLOS ONE, by The Public Library of Science; hereby published with permission under the Creative Commons Attribution License or equivalent. Every chapter published in this book has been scrutinized by our experts. Their significance has been extensively debated. The topics covered herein carry significant findings which will fuel the growth of the discipline. They may even be implemented as practical applications or may be referred to as a beginning point for another development.

The contributors of this book come from diverse backgrounds, making this book a truly international effort. This book will bring forth new frontiers with its revolutionizing research information and detailed analysis of the nascent developments around the world.

We would like to thank all the contributing authors for lending their expertise to make the book truly unique. They have played a crucial role in the development of this book. Without their invaluable contributions this book wouldn't have been possible. They have made vital efforts to compile up to date information on the varied aspects of this subject to make this book a valuable addition to the collection of many professionals and students.

This book was conceptualized with the vision of imparting up-to-date information and advanced data in this field. To ensure the same, a matchless editorial board was set up. Every individual on the board went through rigorous rounds of assessment to prove their worth. After which they invested a large part of their time researching and compiling the most relevant data for our readers.

The editorial board has been involved in producing this book since its inception. They have spent rigorous hours researching and exploring the diverse topics which have resulted in the successful publishing of this book. They have passed on their knowledge of decades through this book. To expedite this challenging task, the publisher supported the team at every step. A small team of assistant editors was also appointed to further simplify the editing procedure and attain best results for the readers.

Apart from the editorial board, the designing team has also invested a significant amount of their time in understanding the subject and creating the most relevant covers. They scrutinized every image to scout for the most suitable representation of the subject and create an appropriate cover for the book.

The publishing team has been an ardent support to the editorial, designing and production team. Their endless efforts to recruit the best for this project, has resulted in the accomplishment of this book. They are a veteran in the field of academics and their pool of knowledge is as vast as their experience in printing. Their expertise and guidance has proved useful at every step. Their uncompromising quality standards have made this book an exceptional effort. Their encouragement from time to time has been an inspiration for everyone.

The publisher and the editorial board hope that this book will prove to be a valuable piece of knowledge for researchers, students, practitioners and scholars across the globe.

# LIST OF CONTRIBUTORS

**Heidi Kaulfürst-Soboll and Antje von Schaewen**
Institute of Plant Biology and Biotechnology, University of Münster, Münster, Germany

**Melanie Mertens and Randolf Brehler**
Department of Dermatology, University of Münster, Münster, Germany

**Claudia Alessandri, Paola Palazzo, Danila Zennaro, Chiara Rafaiani, Rosetta Ferrara, Maria Livia Bernardi, Mario Santoro, Sara Zuzzi, Ivana Giangrieco and Adriano Mari**
Center for Molecular Allergology, IDI-IRCCS, Rome, Italy

**Stefano Sforza, Francesca Lambertini, Sara Paolella and Arnaldo Dossena**
Department of Organic and Industrial Chemistry, University of Parma, Parma, Italy

**Arantxa Palacín, Cristina Gómez-Casado, Leticia Tordesillas, Rosa Sánchez-Monge and Araceli Díaz-Perales**
Centro de Biotecnología y Genómica de Plantas (UPM-INIA), Campus de Montegancedo, Pozuelo de Alarcón, Madrid, Spain

**Luis A. Rivas, Jacobo Aguirre and Victor Parro**
Departamento de Evolución Molecular, Centro de Astrobiología (INTA-CSIC), Torrejón de Ardoz, Madrid, Spain

**Joan Bartra and Rosa Muñoz**
Unitat d'Alèrgia Servei Pneumologia i Alèrgia Respiratòria Universitat de Barcelona, Institut d'Investigacions Biomèdiques August Pi i Sunyer (IDIBAPS), Centro de Investigaciones Biome´dicas en Red de Enfermedades Respiratorias (CIBERES), Barcelona, Spain

**Carlos Blanco and Consolación de Frutos**
Servicio de Alergia, Hospital Universitario de la Princesa, Instituto de Investigación Sanitaria Princesa (IP), Madrid, Spain

**Teresa Carrillo**
Servicio de Alergología, Hospital Universitario de Gran Canaria Dr. Negrín, Las Palmas de Gran Canaria, Spain

**Javier Cuesta-Herranz**
Unidad Servicio de Alergia, Fundación Jiménez Díaz, Madrid, Spain

**Francisco J. Fernández**
Allergy Section, General University Hospital, Miguel Hernández University, Elche, Spain

**Genoveva García Álvarez-Eire and Susana Varela-Losada**
Unidad de Alergología, Complexo Hospitalario, Ourense, Spain

**Miguel Blanca and María J. Torres**
Research Laboratory, Fundación IMABIS-Carlos Haya Hospital; Hospital Civil, Málaga, Spain

**Pedro Gamboa**
Servicio de Alergia, Hospital de Basurto, Bilbao, Spain

**Sofía Sirvent and Rosalía Rodríguez**
Departamento de Bioquímica y Biología Molecular I, Facultad de Químicas, Universidad Complutense, Madrid, Spain

**Gabriel Salcedo**
Departamento de Biotecnología, ETSI Agrónomos, Universidad Politécnica, Madrid, Spain

**Swantje C. Duncker, David Philippe, Christine Martin-Paschoud, Mireille Moser, Annick Mercenier and Sophie Nutten**
Nestlé Research Center, Nestec Ltd., Vers-chez-les-Blancs, Lausanne, Switzerland

**Stine Kroghsbo, Nanna B. Andersen, Tina F. Rasmussen and Charlotte B. Madsen**
National Food Institute, Technical University of Denmark, Søborg, Denmark

**Susanne Jacobsen**
Enzyme and Protein Chemistry, Department of Systems Biology, Technical University of Denmark, Lyngby, Denmark

**Jodie B. Abramovitch, Nirupama Varese, Robyn E. O'Hehir and Jennifer M. Rolland**
Department of Immunology, Monash University, Melbourne, Victoria, Australia

Department of Allergy, Immunology and Respiratory Medicine, The Alfred Hospital and Monash University, Melbourne, Victoria, Australia

**Sandip Kamath, Celia Zubrinich and Andreas L. Lopata**
School of Pharmacy and Molecular Science, James Cook University, Townsville, Queensland, Australia

**Qiang Zeng and Sheng-Yong Dong**
International Medical Center, Chinese PLA General Hospital, Beijing, China

**Liu-Xin Wu**
The Second Laboratory, PLA Air Force Institute of Aviation Medicine, Beijing, China

**Hong Li**
Health Management Center, Fujian Provincial Hospital, Fuzhou, Fujian, China

**Zhi-Jian Sun**
Health Management Center, Shandong Provincial Hospital, Jinan, Shandong, China

**Jing-Bo Li**
Health Management Center, Southwest Hospital, The Third Military Medical University, Chongqing, China

**Hong-Xia Jiang**
Health Management Center, Xiangya Hospital, Central South University, Changsha, Hunan, China

**Zhi-Heng Chen**
Health Management Center, The Third Xiangya Hospital of Central South University, Changsha, Hunan, China

**Qi-Bin Wang**
Health Management Center, Shandong Electric Power Center Hospital, Jinan, Shandong, China

**Wei-Wei Chen**
Treatment and Research Center for Infectious Diseases, 302 Hospital of PLA, Beijing, China

**Jenna L. Van Gramberg, Michael J. de Veer, Els N. T. Meeusen and Robert J. Bischof**
Biotechnology Research Laboratories, Department of Physiology, Monash University, Clayton, Australia

**Robyn E. O'Hehir**
Department of Allergy, Immunology and Respiratory Medicine, Alfred Hospital and Monash University, Melbourne, Australia

**Francisca Gomez, Paloma Campo, Miguel Blanca and Maria José Torres**
Allergy Service, IBIMA, Regional University Hospital of Malaga, UMA, Malaga, Spain

**Ana Aranda and James Perkins**
Research Laboratory, IBIMA, Regional University Hospital of Malaga, UMA, Malaga, Spain

**Cristobalina Mayorga**
Allergy Service, IBIMA, Regional University Hospital of Malaga, UMA, Malaga, Spain
Research Laboratory, IBIMA, Regional University Hospital of Malaga, UMA, Malaga, Spain

**Araceli Diaz-Perales and Maria Garrido**
Biotechnology Department, Center for Plant Biotechnology and Genomics, Pozuelo de Alarcon, Madrid, Spain

**Natalia Blanca-Lopez**
Allergy Service, Infanta Leonor Hospital, Madrid, Spain

**Franziska Roth-Walter and Gerlinde Hofstetter**
Comparative Medicine, Messerli Research Institute of the University of Veterinary Medicine Vienna, Medical University Vienna and University Vienna, Vienna, Austria

**Luis F. Pacios, Cristina Gomez-Casado and Araceli Diaz-Perales**
Biotechnology Department, Center for Plant Biotechnology and Genomics, Technical University of Madrid, Madrid, Spain

**Georg A. Roth**
Department of Anesthesiology, General Intensive Care and Pain Medicine, Medical University of Vienna, Austria

**Josef Singer**
Comparative Immunology and Oncology, Department of Pathophysiology and Allergy Research,
Center of Pathophysiology, Infectiology and Immunology, Medical University of Vienna, Vienna, Austria

**Erika Jensen-Jarolim**
Comparative Medicine, Messerli Research Institute of the University of Veterinary Medicine Vienna, Medical University Vienna and University Vienna, Vienna, Austria
Comparative Immunology and Oncology, Department of Pathophysiology and Allergy Research,
Center of Pathophysiology, Infectiology and Immunology, Medical University of Vienna, Vienna, Austria

**Jungang Xie, Larisa C. Lotoski, Ruey-Chyi Su and Jude Uzonna**
Department of Immunology, University of Manitoba, Winnipeg, Canada

**Rishma Chooniedass**
Department of Pediatrics and Child Health, University of Manitoba, Winnipeg, Canada

**F. Estelle R. Simons, Allan B. Becker and Kent T. HayGlass**
Department of Immunology, University of Manitoba, Winnipeg, Canada
Department of Pediatrics and Child Health, University of Manitoba, Winnipeg, Canada

**Joel Liem**
Windsor Allergy Asthma Education Centre, Ontario, Canada

**Chenwen Cai, Jun Shen, Di Zhao, Yuqi Qiao, Antao Xu, Shuang Jin, Zhihua Ran and Qing Zheng**
Key Laboratory of Gastroenterology & Hepatology, Ministry of Health, Division of Gastroenterology and Hepatology, Ren Ji Hospital, School of Medicine, Shanghai Jiao Tong University, Shanghai Institute of Digestive Diseases, 145 Middle Shandong Road, Shanghai 200001, China

**Christine Y. Y. Wai, Nicki Y. H. Leung and Ka Hou Chu**
School of Life Sciences, The Chinese University of Hong Kong, Shatin, Hong Kong SAR, China

**Marco H. K. Ho**
Department of Pediatrics and Adolescent Medicine, The University of Hong Kong, Hong Kong SAR, China

**Laurel J. Gershwin**
Department of Pathology, Microbiology and Immunology, School of Veterinary Medicine, University of California Davis, Davis, California, United States of America

**Shang An Shu and Patrick S. C. Leung**
Division of Rheumatology/Allergy, School of Medicine, University of California Davis, Davis, California, United States of America

**Milena Weber, Margarete Focke-Tejkl and Rudolf Valenta**
Division of Immunopathology, Department of Pathophysiology and Allergy Research, Center of Pathophysiology, Infectiology and Immunology, Medical University of Vienna, Vienna, Austria

**Sandra Pahr and Susanne Vrtala**
Division of Immunopathology, Department of Pathophysiology and Allergy Research, Center of Pathophysiology, Infectiology and Immunology, Medical University of Vienna, Vienna, Austria
Christian Doppler Laboratory for the Development of Allergen Chips, Medical University of Vienna, Vienna, Austria

**Regina Selb and Verena Niederberger**
Department of ENT, Medical University of Vienna, Vienna, Austria

**Gerhard Hofer, Andela Dordić and Walter Keller**
Institute of Molecular Biosciences, Karl-Franzens University Graz, Graz, Austria

**Nikolaos G. Papadopoulos and Stavroula Giavi**
Allergy Department, 2nd Pediatric Clinic, University of Athens, Athens, Greece

**Mika Mäkelä and Anna Pelkonen**
Skin and Allergy Hospital, Helsinki University Central Hospital, Helsinki, Finland

**Hanna Berkner, Christian Seutter von Loetzen, Maximilian Hartl and Paul Rösch**
Department of Biopolymers, University of Bayreuth, Bayreuth, Bavaria, Germany

**Stefanie Randow, Michaela Gubesch, Lothar Vogel, Felix Husslik, Andreas Reuter, Stefan Vieths and Dirk Schiller**
Division of Allergology, Paul-Ehrlich-Institut, Langen, Hesse, Germany

**Jonas Lidholm**
Immuno Diagnostics Division, Thermo Fisher Scientific Inc., Uppsala, Uppsala län, Sweden

**Barbara Ballmer-Weber**
Department of Dermatology, Allergy Unit, University Hospital Zürich, Zürich, Zürich, Switzerland

**Enrico Scala, Claudia Alessandri, Paola Palazzo, Debora Pomponi, Marina Liso, Maria Livia Bernardi, Rosetta Ferrara, Danila Zennaro, Mario Santoro, Chiara Rasi and Adriano Mari**
Center for Molecular Allergology, IDI-IRCCS, Rome, Italy

**Elisabeth Hoflehner, Marina Binder, Ursula Wiedermann and Michael Duchêne**
Institute of Specific Prophylaxis and Tropical Medicine, Center for Pathophysiology, Infectiology and Immunology, Medical University of Vienna, Vienna, Austria

**Wolfgang Hemmer and Reinhart Jarisch**
Floridsdorfer Allergiezentrum, Vienna, Austria

**Vera Mahler**
Department of Dermatology, University of Erlangen-Nuremberg, Erlangen, Germany

**Raphael C. Panzani**
Centre de recherche en allergologie, Marseille, France

**Yui Okada**
Department of Immunology, University of Yamanashi Faculty of Medicine Chuo, Yamanashi, Japan
The Institute of Enology and Viticulture, University of Yamanashi, Koufu, Yamanashi, Japan

**Kyoko Oh-oka, Yuki Nakamura and Kayoko Ishimaru**
Department of Immunology, University of Yamanashi Faculty of Medicine Chuo, Yamanashi, Japan

**Masashi Hisamoto and Tohru Okuda**
The Institute of Enology and Viticulture, University of Yamanashi, Koufu, Yamanashi, Japan

**Shuji Matsuoka**
Deparment of Pathology, Juntendo University School of Medicine, Bunkyo-ku, Tokyo, Japan

**Ko Okumura, Hideoki Ogawa and Atsuhito Nakao**
Atopy Research Center, Juntendo University School of Medicine, Bunkyo-ku, Tokyo, Japan

**Ana Aranda**
Allergy Research Laboratory, Carlos Haya Hospital, Málaga, Spain

**Paloma Campo, Inmaculada Doña, Luisa Galindo and Miguel Blanca**
Unidad de Gestión Clínica Allergy, Carlos Haya Hospital, Málaga, Spain

**Arantxa Palacin, Cristina Gomez-Casado and Araceli Díaz-Perales**
Biotechnology Department, Center for Plant Biotechnology and Genomics, Pozuelo de Alarcon, Madrid, Spain

**Arantxa Palacín, Cristina Gómez-Casado, Leticia Tordesillas, Rosa Sánchez-Monge and Araceli Díaz-Perales**
Centro de Biotecnología y Genó mica de Plantas, Campus de Montegancedo, Pozuelo de Alarcón, Madrid, Spain

**Luis A. Rivas, Jacobo Aguirre and Victor Parro**
Departamento de Evolución Molecular, Centro de Astrobiología (INTA-CSIC), Torrejón de Ardoz, Madrid, Spain

**Joan Bartra and Rosa Muñoz**
Unitat d'Allérgia, Servei Pneumologia i Allèrgia Respiratòria, Hospital Clínic, Universitat de Barcelona, Institut d'Investigacions Biomèdiques August Pi i Sunyer (IDIBAPS), Centro de Investigaciones Biomédicas en Red de Enfermedades Respiratorias (CIBERES), Barcelona, Spain

**Carlos Blanco and Francisco Vega**
Servicio de Alergia, Hospital Universitario de la Princesa, Instituto de Investigación Sanitaria Princesa (IP), Madrid, Spain

**Teresa Carrillo and José A. Cumplido Bonny**
Servicio de Alergología, Hospital Universitario de Gran Canaria Dr. Negrín, Las Palmas de Gran Canaria, Spain

**Javier Cuesta-Herranz**
Servicio de Alergia, Fundación Jiménez Díaz, Madrid, Spain

**Enrique Flores and Francisco J. Fernández**
Unidad de Alergia, Hospital General Universitario, Alicante, Spain

**Mar G. García-Alvarez-Eire and Susana Varela Losada**
Unidad de Alergología, Complexo Hospitalario, Ourense, Spain

**Ignacio García-Nuñez and Miguel Blanca**
Laboratorio de Investigación, Fundación IMABIS-Carlos Haya Hospital, Hospital Civil, Málaga, Spain

**Pedro Gamboa**
Servicio de Alergia, Hospital de Basurto, Bilbao, Spain

**Maria Torres and Mayte Villalba**
Departamento de Bioquímica y Biología Molecular I, Facultad de Químicas, Universidad Complutense, Madrid, Spain

**Gabriel Salcedo**
Departamento de Biotecnología, ETSI Agrónomos, Universidad Politécnica, Madrid, Spain

**Akira Kikuchi, Yoko Fujimura, Miran Kihara-Fujioka and Ryuichiro Sato**
Department of Applied Biological Chemistry, Graduate School of Agricultural and Life Sciences, The University of Tokyo, Tokyo, Japan

**Tomonori Nochi and Osamu Igarashi**
Department of Microbiology and Immunology, Institute of Medical Science, The University of Tokyo, Tokyo, Japan

**Tsuyoshi Makino**
Biotechnical Center (BT Center), Japan SLC, Inc., Shizuoka, Japan

**Masae Goseki-Sone**
Department of Food and Nutrition, Faculty of Human Sciences and Design, Japan Women's University, Tokyo, Japan

**Yosuke Kurashima**
Department of Microbiology and Immunology, Institute of Medical Science, The University of Tokyo, Tokyo, Japan
Core Research for Evolutional Science and Technology (CREST), Japan Science and Technology Agency, Tokyo, Japan

**Masafumi Yamamoto**
Department of Microbiology and Immunology, Nihon University School of Dentistry at Matsudo, Chiba, Japan

**Jun Kunisawa**
Department of Microbiology and Immunology, Institute of Medical Science, The University of Tokyo, Tokyo, Japan
Core Research for Evolutional Science and Technology (CREST), Japan Science and Technology Agency, Tokyo, Japan
International Research and Development Center for Mucosal Vaccines, Institute of Medical Science, The University of Tokyo, Tokyo, Japan
Laboratory of Vaccine Materials, National Institute of Biomedical Innovation, Osaka, Japan

**Masako Toda**
Vice President's Research Group "Molecular Allergology", Paul-Ehrlich-Institut, Langen, Germany

**Shuichi Kaminogawa**
Department of Food Bioscience and Biotechnology, Nihon University, Kanagawa, Japan

**Hiroshi Kiyono**
Department of Microbiology and Immunology, Institute of Medical Science, The University of Tokyo, Tokyo, Japan
Core Research for Evolutional Science and Technology (CREST), Japan Science and Technology Agency, Tokyo, Japan
International Research and Development Center for Mucosal Vaccines, Institute of Medical Science, The University of Tokyo, Tokyo, Japan
Department of Medical Genome Science, Graduate School of Frontier Science, The University of Tokyo, Tokyo, Japan
Graduate School of Medicine, The University of Tokyo, Tokyo, Japan

**Satoshi Hachimura and Kyoko Shibahara**
Department of Applied Biological Chemistry, Graduate School of Agricultural and Life Sciences, The University of Tokyo, Tokyo, Japan
Research Center for Food Safety, Graduate School of Agricultural and Life Sciences, The University of Tokyo, Tokyo, Japan

**Haruyo Nakajima-Adachi**
Department of Applied Biological Chemistry, Graduate School of Agricultural and Life Sciences, The University of Tokyo, Tokyo, Japan
Department of Microbiology and Immunology, Institute of Medical Science, The University of Tokyo, Tokyo, Japan
Research Center for Food Safety, Graduate School of Agricultural and Life Sciences, The University of Tokyo, Tokyo, Japan

**Prerna Sharma and Naveen Arora**
Allergy and Immunology Section, CSIR-Institute of Genomics and Integrative Biology, Delhi, India

**Shailendra Nath Gaur**
Department of Respiratory Medicine, Vallabhbhai Patel Chest Institute, University of Delhi, Delhi, India

**Julie Barnett and Konstantina Vasileiou**
Department of Information Systems and Computing, Brunel University, Middlesex, United Kingdom

**M. Hazel Gowland**
Allergy Action, Farnborough, United Kingdom

**Monique M. Raats**
School of Psychology, Faculty of Arts and Human Sciences, University of Surrey, Guildford, Surrey, United Kingdom

**Jane S. Lucas**
Clinical and Experimental Sciences, Faculty of Medicine, University of Southampton, University Hospital Southampton NHS Foundation Trust, Southampton, United Kingdom

# Index

CPSIA information can be obtained
at www.ICGtesting.com
Printed in the USA
BVHW012342141019
561126BV00001B/1/P

9 781682 864517